1,001 Health-Care Questions Women Ask

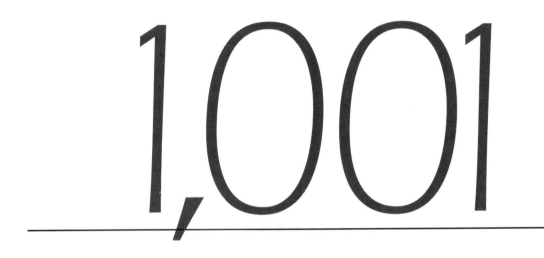

Health-Care Questions Women Ask

Third Edition

Joe S. McIlhaney Jr., M.D.
with Susan Nethery

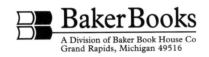

Baker Books

A Division of Baker Book House Co
Grand Rapids, Michigan 49516

Published by Baker Books
a division of Baker Book House Company
P.O. Box 6287, Grand Rapids, MI 49516-6287

Previously published in 1985 and 1992 under the title *1250 Health-Care Questions Women Ask.*

Printed in the United States of America

Library of Congress Cataloging-in-Publication Data

McIlhaney, Joe S.
    1,001 health-care questions women ask / Joe S. McIlhaney, Jr., with Susan Nethery. — 3rd ed.
      p.   cm.
    Includes index.
    ISBN 0-8010-5810-4 (paper)
    1. Gynecology—Miscellanea. 2. Pregnancy—Miscellanea. 3. Childbirth—Miscellanea. 4. Women—Health and hygiene—Miscellanea.
I. Nethery, Susan. II. Title.
RG121.M396   1998
618—dc21   98-3257

The medical, health, and supportive procedures in this book are based on the training, personal experiences, and research of the author and on recommendations of responsible medical and nursing sources. But because each person and situation is unique, author and publisher urge the reader to check with a qualified health professional before using a procedure where there is any question as to its appropriateness. In regard to treatment or medication, always check with a physician.
The author and publisher assume no responsibility for adverse effects or consequences resulting from the use of any of the suggestions, preparations, procedures, or legal data in this book.

For current information about all releases from Baker Book House, visit our web site:
           http://www.bakerbooks.com

To Marion, uncommonly gifted by God.

Marion's keen mind,
her wisdom,
her strength of character,
and her love for the Lord
have helped make
our years
as man and wife
a wonderful experience
of growth together.

Contents

Part Two:
Bearing a Child

Part Three:
Special Concerns

Illustrations

Preface

Change! This is the one word everyone uses about medical care today. Most of the time doctors and patients are talking about change in the way medical care is provided—HMOs, PPOs, PHOs—the alphabet soup is endless.

Almost lost in the talk about the packaging of medical care by these various organizations is the medical care itself. Is the medical care you receive actually improving? Is medical science making new discoveries that make your life safer, healthier? The answer is a strong yes! Great strides are being made in medical science for your benefit. The change is shown by comparing the first edition of this book published in 1985 to this 1998 edition. Striking contrast is seen in the discussions of laparoscopic surgery, the environment for the birth of a baby, and the provision of care for infertile couples. These and numerous other changes in medicine for women have allowed you to have better medical care provided with less discomfort, less time in the hospital, and a greater chance of success than ever before in the history of humankind.

It is for these reasons that this book is so important to you. Since medical care is changing so quickly, you need some way to keep up, to understand it. This is especially true if you have a medical problem and need medical care. As I said in the introduction to the first edition, "This book is my sincere effort to provide you with information that will keep you from making wrong choices about your medical care and personal health. Bad decisions in this area can adversely affect you physically, mentally, and emotionally the rest of your life." My desire to help you in this way still burns deep within me. I have attempted to bring every significant change in women's health care to your attention in this book so you can look forward to the healthiest, brightest future possible.

You will notice that we have put this book on a diet! It is smaller. We have eliminated some topics that you can find answers to in other resources. We have distilled the book to provide the most important information you need about medical issues in the very best way.

My desire for you is that the knowledge and understanding you get from this book will make your interaction with your physicians and hospital more comfortable. Susan Nethery was my invaluable editor, assistant, and encourager in writing the original edition of this book. Debbie Bible and the editorial staff at Baker Book House were key in taking hundreds of pages of changed text and making it into a comprehensive volume. Dr. Tim Harstad, a maternal-fetal medicine specialist and a dear friend, made invaluable suggestions for the chapters dealing with pregnancy. Once again, my executive secretary of over twenty years, Charlotte Matthews, played an essential role in putting my ideas on paper. The "other women" in my life, my daughters Lynne, Anne, and Caren, have competently and maturely guided me over the years to a deeper understanding of women's issues. Finally, all my love and thanks go to Marion, my wife of thirty-eight years. She continues to be my biggest source of encouragement and strength.

Joe S. McIlhaney Jr., M.D.
July 1998

Part One

The Female Body in Change

1

Basic Anatomical Facts

Although most women today have reasonably good knowledge of the structure of their bodies, there remains a great deal of interesting and helpful information that the average woman usually does not know about her own anatomy (structure) and physiology (function). Because most people are unsure about these aspects of their bodies, it is important to include some background information.

Lack of this knowledge can cause many problems for women. A woman cannot properly care for herself if she doesn't understand her body. A woman may be embarrassed by her sexuality if she is unaware of the beauty, purpose, and importance of her body's form and function. A lack of such understanding may also breed fears that only knowledge can dispel.

The goal of this chapter is not pure anatomical knowledge, but rather anatomical knowledge as it contributes to self-understanding and then to self-acceptance. As we explain how the reproductive and sexual parts of a woman's body are put together, we will provide a general account of the physical makeup of the female body. This will be followed with a description of the different parts of a woman's anatomy, how they developed, and how they change through life.

1 What are my sexual and reproductive organs?

The sexual and reproductive parts of your body include the following: the vulva, the vagina, the uterus, the fallopian tubes, the ovaries, and the breasts. Our discussion of those major body parts will be broken up into several subtopics:

vulva	vagina
mons pubis	hymen
labia	uterus
clitoris	cervix
vestibular bulbs	corpus of the uterus
urethral opening	fallopian tubes
Bartholin's glands	ovaries
anus	breasts
perineum	

External Female Sexual and Reproductive Organs

2 What is the vulva?

The vulva is the area of your body between your legs that can be seen when your legs are spread apart. This area serves as the entrance to the vagina. The vulvar tissues cover that entrance and the opening to the bladder (the urethra). The vulva is comprised of several parts, which are discussed in the following questions.

3 What is the mons pubis?

The hair-covered area at the top of the vulva (mons veneris or mons pubis) is often called the pubic mound. This area is the most obvious part of a woman's genital area when she is standing or lying with her legs together; technically it is not part of the vulva but is its border on the front side of the body.

Mons is Latin for "mountain," and the protuberance of this area is obviously the reason for its name. This prominence is due to the fact that the pubic bone underlying this area is covered by a mound of fatty tissue. This fat serves as a cushion during intercourse, keeping pressure from the man's body from being applied directly against the woman's pubic bone.

It is normal for a woman's hair growth to be confined to the mons, but it is just as normal for it to extend up to her umbilicus (navel). Although abnormal hormones can cause heavier hair growth extending up to the umbilicus, this kind of hair growth is most commonly genetic. A gynecologist should be consulted if the hair growth is unusually heavy or if it bothers a woman. If this hair growth does extend to the umbilicus and is a problem to a woman, she can shave it off or use a depilatory cream to dissolve the hair, using caution to avoid getting the cream on sensitive vulvar skin. A more permanent method of removing this is electrolysis. This technique is safe and usually very effective.

4 What are the labia?

The word *labia* comes from the Latin for "lips." A woman has labia majora (major lips) and labia minora (minor lips). The labia majora are the thicker lips on the outside of the vulva, and the outside margins of the labia majora mark the outer limits of what is considered the vulva. The labia majora have hair growth on the outside surfaces but not on their inner surfaces. The bulk of the labia majora consists of fat.

Between the labia majora are the labia minora. These two thin and sensitive folds of skin surround the entrance to the vagina. They have no hair growth. The labia minora of women who have not borne children are usually hidden by the labia majora; women who have had babies usually have labia minora that project beyond the labia majora. Even in virginal women, or in women who have not delivered babies, however, the labia minora may become enlarged by normal growth, or from manipulation or masturbation, and then project beyond the labia majora.

Did you ever wonder what purpose the labia have other than guarding the entrance of the vagina? They serve two other interesting functions. First, they guide the flow of urine as it leaves the body. Women who have had their labia surgically removed "splatter" urine—a messy and bothersome situation.

The other function of the labia is to provide pleasure. Because of their sensitivity to touch, most women find pleasure when their husbands touch their labia gently. When a woman is sexually aroused, the labia become engorged, adding to sexual pleasure.

The labia are therefore important and dynamic parts of a woman's body.

5 What is the clitoris?

The clitoris (klit´-o-ris) is a small pencil-shaped body of tissue that is about an inch long. If you spread your labia minora apart and look at the top (front) where they come together, just below the hair of the mons pubis, you will see the small hood that overlies the clitoris. The tip of the clitoris can normally be seen peeking out from under this hood. The urethra opening, or outlet of the bladder, is below the clitoris and between it and the vagina.

Since the tip of the clitoris is sensitive, gentle stimulation normally produces sexual arousal. The clitoris contains erectile tissue (tissue that can become engorged with blood), which causes the clitoris to become enlarged during sexual excitement.

Sexual stimulation of the clitoris does not always have to be directly applied to be effective. Because the labia minora form a hood over the clitoris, and because this hood is actually attached to the clitoris, movement of the labia minora will usually cause clitoral stimulation. During intercourse, as the pressure of the man's penis causes movement of the labia minora, stimulation of the clitoris is produced, whether or not the clitoris is touched. The same results occur during foreplay when the man gently pulls and stimulates the labia minora. In this way he is stimulating both the labia minora and the clitoris.

It is interesting to note that once a woman has experienced orgasm and has established orgasm as her response to sexual activity, the presence of the clitoris is not absolutely necessary for achieving orgasm or sexual fulfillment. Consequently, if a woman develops a growth that requires surgical removal of the clitoris, she can continue to have satisfactory sexual responsiveness.

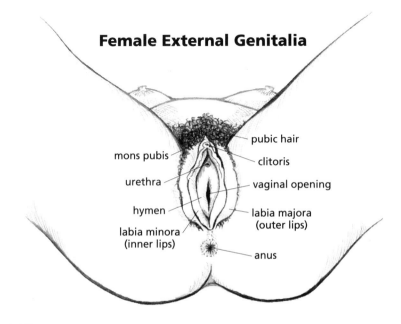

Female External Genitalia

pubic hair

mons pubis

clitoris

urethra

vaginal opening

hymen

labia majora
(outer lips)

labia minora
(inner lips)

anus

6 What are the vestibular bulbs?

These two accumulations of tissue are located under the skin just inside the labia minora (but outside the hymen) on either side of the entrance to the vagina. These areas are important for sexual responsiveness and sensitivity. Like the clitoris, they contain erectile tissue that becomes engorged with blood with sexual arousal. This increases sensitivity of the vulvar area. They also cause protrusion of the vulva, making the vaginal tract longer during intercourse. In addition, they produce tightening of the outer third of the vagina. This action not only causes the vagina to "grip" the penis during intercourse, but also helps hold semen in the vagina, increasing the chance of pregnancy.

7 What is the urethra and where is the urethral opening?

The urethra is the tube through which urine flows out of the bladder. While lying on your back and using a mirror, the urethral opening or "meatus" can be seen just above the vaginal opening and just below the clitoris. If you spread your labia minora and look above the vagina, you can see the slightly puckered, vertical slit that marks the urethral opening.

Because the urethral opening is located so close to the vaginal entrance and is therefore in the path of sexual stimulation, bladder infections associated with intercourse are fairly common. The urethra is short (about 1½ inches long). As the penis is moving back and forth near the opening to the urethra, germs can be massaged into the bladder through the urethra. Also, friction against the urethra and the urethral opening during intercourse can cause irritation of the urethra and burning during urination, even when there are no germs and infection involved.

When a woman cleans herself after urination or a bowel movement, she should wipe from front to back. This decreases the chance of bacteria from the anal area contaminating the urethra and causing a bladder infection.

8 What are Bartholin's glands?

There are two Bartholin's glands (vulvo-vaginal glands), one located on either side of the vaginal opening, just outside the hymen and inside the labia minora. The glands produce mucus, a slippery secretion. Although they secrete a small amount of mucus all the time, during sexual excitement they produce a significant amount of mucoid material for lubrication. Abscess of the Bartholin's glands and Bartholin's gland cysts are fairly common among women. (See Q. 592–593.)

9 What is the anus?

The anus is located at the rearmost portion of the vulva. It is not actually part of the vulva but marks its rearward border. The anus is the opening at the lowest portion of the intestinal tract; it is from the anus that stool leaves the body. External hemorrhoids (dilated blood veins) often occur around the anal opening. Anal or rectal sex refers to the man's penis entering the rectum through the anus instead of being inserted into the vagina.

10 What is the perineum?

The perineum is the name of the thick layer of muscle that underlies the skin of the vulvar area and is the floor of the abdominal cavity. These muscles keep the intestines from falling out of the body. It is also these muscles that are in part responsible for keeping the vagina from turning inside out. Finally, it is these muscles that a woman exercises when she does "Kegel's exercises" to tighten up the vagina and give better support to the rectum and bladder. (See Q. 615–616.)

When doctors speak of the perineum being cut or lacerated, they are generally talking about the perineal body—the area under the skin between the anus and the vagina. An incision into this perineal body is called an episiotomy. Such an incision is done to prevent tears that may occur during delivery. When these tissues are cut or torn, they often must be sewn back together. This repair prevents the vaginal opening from gaping open after healing and also helps keep the vaginal tissues from prolapsing (falling) outside the vagina.

11 What is the vagina?

The vagina is an absolutely amazing part of a woman's body. As part of my obstetrical practice, for years I have watched beautiful little baby boys and girls pass down their mothers' "birth canals." I still don't understand how it can happen. How can the vagina stretch large enough to allow a baby's body through, then only six weeks later be tight enough for pleasurable sexual intercourse? As I describe the physical structure of the vagina, remember how marvelously it functions.

The vaginal opening is below (behind) the urethra and above (in front of) the place where the labia majora and minora come together in front of the anus. The vagina is basically a tube about three and one-half inches long, and its walls are made up of three different layers. The first is a delicate lining called a mucous membrane. Next is a thin layer of muscle, and the third layer is strong connective tissue that provides most of the strength of the vaginal walls.

The vagina is normally closed and does not contain air, but if a woman has had several children her vagina may tend to gape open, allowing air inside. This is normal and is in no way harmful.

When a woman is standing, the vagina points back and up toward the upper part of the buttocks. This is why it does not normally turn inside out; pressure from the abdomen tends to push the vagina back into the cradle of the curve of the sacral bones and not down toward the outside of the body.

The vagina has three primary functions. First, it serves as an outlet for the menstrual flow. It also provides a convenient place for tampons to absorb that menstrual flow, allowing most women to avoid the inconvenience of external protection. Second, it accommodates the penis during intercourse and, in so doing, receives the semen, providing it access to the cervix for sperm penetration. Finally, the vagina serves as an important part of the birth canal through which a baby is delivered.

Sometimes a woman wonders whether her vagina is large enough for intercourse with a man who has a relatively large penis. (Actually, there is very little variation in the size of men's erect penises). The vagina is quite capable of stretching enough to allow intercourse, no matter what size the penis is. If a baby's head can get out through the vagina, then a man's penis can get in!

The front wall of the vagina is in contact with the urethra and the bladder, separated from them by only thin layers of tissue. The back wall of the vagina is in contact with the rectum, and, again, only thin layers of tissue separate them. The upper vaginal lining is continuous with the lining of the cervix (the mouth of the uterus). The cervix projects about an inch down into the upper vagina.

Normally, a woman cannot see her vaginal walls without a speculum. However, if she has had children and her tissues are fairly relaxed, she may be able to observe these walls. To accomplish this she must use a mirror. Sitting with her legs spread apart, she must push as though she were going to have a bowel movement. In so doing, it might be possible to see the front and back walls of her vagina bulging down toward the opening as the labia spread apart.

Occasionally, with marked relaxation of the vaginal tissues, a woman will feel a bulge of tissue, about the size of a golf ball or a tennis ball or even larger, from her vagina. A woman with this problem needs to be checked by her physician. The problem of vaginal relaxation is not just relaxation of the vaginal tube itself. It is as much a problem of the organs surrounding the vagina (bladder, rectum, and uterus) collapsing in on the walls of the vagina as it is of the stretching of the vaginal tissues. (If you have a problem with vaginal looseness, see Q. 612–618.)

12 What is the hymen?

A great deal of folklore surrounds the subject of the hymen. If a woman has a tight hymen, the first time she has intercourse the hymen will tear and she will often bleed. This has led to the custom in some communities in the East of demanding that the bed coverings have blood on them the morning after newlyweds' first night together. I have never understood this. Many women do not have tight hymens and will not bleed with their first act of intercourse. A woman is a virgin if she has not had intercourse, even if the hymen is not tight and she does not bleed with first intercourse.

The hymen is a ring of soft tissue (mucous membrane) just inside the labia minora. If you are a virgin, you cannot see your hymen without spreading the labia minora apart. Even then, your vagina will look almost totally closed because of the hymen.

Occasionally the hymen may be so thick that it requires surgical incision to allow intercourse. This is normal but uncommon. Normally at first intercourse the hymen dilates by being both stretched and torn along its edges at several different points. After the first act of intercourse and for the rest of a woman's life, the small pieces of tissue that are the residual hymeneal tags remain around the vaginal opening.

The normal opening that a woman has in her hymen before she starts having intercourse or using tampons can be of many different types. Most common is one central opening, but there can also be several smaller openings. Occasionally there is no opening at all. This, of course, prevents the flow of menstrual blood from the vagina. If a girl at the appropriate age has symptoms of menstruation (cramping, bloating) but does not have any menstrual flow, she should see a physician immediately. This can be a dangerous situation. It can, if not corrected, eventually cause infertility.

Tampons do not tear a girl's hymen since they are made small enough in diameter to go through the hymeneal opening of a virgin. When a young woman uses tampons for many months or years, the hymen does tend to stretch open a little. This is actually an advantage, since it allows the first pelvic examination or the first act of intercourse to be more comfortable. A vaginal exam does not "break" the hymen either. It may stretch the opening a bit or even cause some minute tearing of the edges. The instruments used are made small enough to allow a pelvic examination without damaging the hymen.

Internal Female Sexual and Reproductive Organs

13 What is the uterus?

If the vagina is an amazing organ, then the uterus is an astounding one. It has a special lining that bleeds monthly, yet this lining is not damaged during pregnancy when no bleeding occurs for nine months.

During pregnancy, cervical mucus prevents germs from entering the uterus, keeping the baby's sanctuary infection-free.

The uterus grows in pregnancy from about half the size of an adult woman's fist to the size of a small watermelon. Through it there is an enormous blood flow carrying the baby's oxygen and nutrition. At delivery, however, the muscle fibers of the uterus clamp down on the blood vessels, preventing the mother from bleeding to death instantaneously.

The uterus is truly an amazing wonder of God's creation!

The uterus is made up of the cervix and the body (corpus). The cervix is the mouth of the uterus, and the corpus is the portion of the uterus that produces the menstrual flow and holds a baby during pregnancy. The uterus is normally about three and a half inches long. About one-third of this length is the cervix, and the remaining two-thirds is the body of the uterus.

The bulk of the uterus is muscle called the myometrium. The cavity of the uterus is lined by a delicate tissue called the endometrium. The outside of the body of the uterus is covered with the peritoneum, a lining that covers all the organs that lie inside the abdomen.

The uterus is located at the top of the vagina, between the bladder and the rectum. The bladder is attached to the lower part of the front of the uterus. When the uterus is removed at hysterectomy, or when a cesarean section is done, the bladder normally must be detached from the uterus and pushed away. On the back side, the uterus is not normally attached to the rectum, but merely lies in front of it.

14 What is the cervix?

The cervix is the doorway of the uterus. It is through the cervical canal that sperm swim into the uterus for fertilization and menstrual flow enters the vagina.

When you have intercourse with your husband and you feel a pleasant sensation of him hitting something that doesn't hurt, that is probably your cervix. Since the mouth of the cervix is very small, it is impossible for a man's penis to go through it during intercourse, just as it is impossible for tampons to go through it. The cervix has the amazing capability, however, of expanding during delivery to allow a baby to leave the uterus. Even after delivering babies for many years, I continue to marvel at the tremendous elasticity of the cervix.

You can feel your cervix with your fingers by reaching inside your vagina. The cervix feels very much like your nose, with a small dimple in the middle! If you have had a baby, the size of your cervix may be more like that of your chin. The

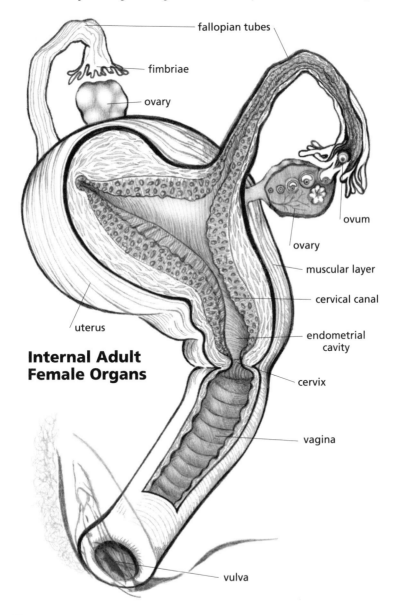

fallopian tubes

fimbriae

ovary

ovum

ovary

muscular layer

cervical canal

endometrial cavity

uterus

cervix

Internal Adult Female Organs

vagina

vulva

cervix feels firm, and the dimple in the middle is the opening into the uterus.

Although most of the uterus is muscle, the cervix is different—85 percent of it is made up of fibrous connective tissue. The lining of the cervix does not shed tissue and blood during menstruation as the lining of the uterus does, but it serves another important function: It produces mucus through which sperm can swim.

When semen from a male's ejaculation comes in contact with a woman's cervix, the sperm swim out of the semen and into the cervical mucus. From there they go up into the uterus. If the cervix did not produce this important mucus, it would

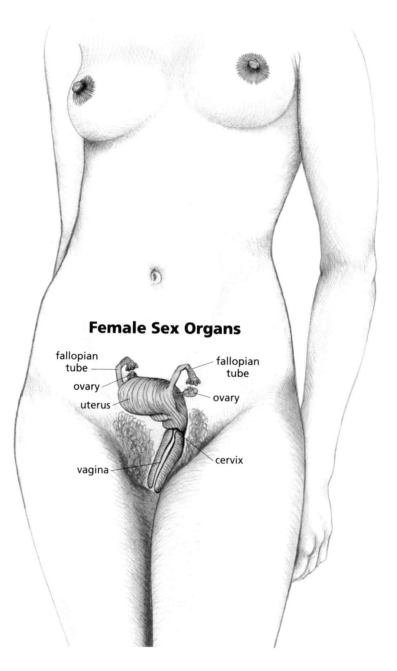

Female Sex Organs

fallopian tube

fallopian tube

ovary

ovary

uterus

vagina

cervix

be impossible for a woman to become pregnant in a normal fashion.

To obtain a Pap smear, the doctor inserts a vaginal speculum to hold the vaginal walls open, scrapes a spatula across the surface of the cervix, and collects cells for a pathologist to examine (see illustration, p. 88). The cervix is the second most common site of malignancy (cancer) of the genital organs in females, the first being the breast.

15 What is the corpus of the uterus?

The corpus of the uterus is its main body. There are three openings into the uterus: one from the cervix (at the lower end) and two from the fallopian tubes (at the upper corner on each side). The fallopian tube openings are quite small, but—with an instrument called a hysteroscope—a doctor can look through the cervix into the uterus and actually see them.

The uterus stays in position inside the body because ligaments are attached to various parts of the corpus. These ligaments, made of strong connective tissue that does not stretch easily, are much like the guy wires that hold television transmission towers in place.

Round ligaments come off the upper front part of the uterus on either side; uterosacral ligaments come from the lower back part of the uterus near the junction between the cervix and the corpus; cardinal ligaments come off the lower part of the uterus on either side, helping to support the upper vagina as well as the uterus; and utero-ovarian ligaments come off the uterus on either side, near attachment to the round ligaments. It is from these utero-ovarian ligaments that the fallopian tubes and ovaries hang.

Despite these attached ligaments, the uterus is fairly mobile. It can rise up out of the pelvis during pregnancy, but after its enlargement and displacement during pregnancy, the uterus goes back down into the pelvis to resume its former position and size when the pregnancy is over.

In past years, doctors have told patients that when their uterus was tilted back toward their backbone, they could experience problems with infertility, pain during intercourse, or some other "female" problem (see Q. 671). This is untrue. One-third of all women have a uterus that is tilted back; two-thirds have a uterus tilting forward. It does not make any difference in which direction the uterus is tilting, and it is not unusual for a woman to have a forward-tilting uterus one year and have it tilting back the next.

16 What are the fallopian tubes?

The fallopian tubes serve one purpose—transporting eggs. Without the fallopian tubes, there is no natural way for fertilized eggs to reach the uterus. (See Q. 236.)

The fallopian tubes are two wormlike tubes attached to either side of the uterus at the upper corners. Each tube is about four and a half to five inches long.

Fallopian tubes have walls made of delicate muscle fibers and an inner lining of thin mucous membrane. The outer lining of the tubes is peritoneum, the same delicate lining that covers all organs inside the abdominal cavity.

The inner lining is specialized. The cells that line the fallopian tubes have little hairlike projections called cilia. The wavelike synchronized beating of these cilia produce a current of fluid that moves down the fallopian tube, providing the propulsion for eggs to travel through the tube.

The outer diameter of a fallopian tube is much like a medium-sized earthworm. It is soft and flaccid, like a relaxed worm. The inner diameter of the tube is very small, and the portion attached to the uterus is so small that only a thin thread can pass through. The outer half of the tube is somewhat larger.

At the tip end of the fallopian tube is a flower blossomlike structure called the fimbria. This acts as a "vacuum cleaner," sucking the egg (ovum) from the ovary into the tube. The fimbria's "tentacles" sense from which part of the ovarian surface the egg is going to come; they move over that area of the surface of the ovary to pick up the egg as soon as it is exuded.

17 What are the ovaries?

Ovaries are the organs that are the source of a woman's eggs (ova) and most of her female hormones. They are located deep in the pelvis, behind the pubic bone. Incidentally, the ovaries are not straight back in your abdomen above your pubic bone; they are deeper and lower in your body than that. I emphasize this because many women complain to their gynecologists about "pain in the ovaries" when, in fact, the pain they are having is much higher in the abdomen than the ovaries could possibly be located. This type of higher abdominal pain usually originates from the intestines.

The ovaries, which are almond-shaped organs, are about one and a half inches by one inch by one-half inch prior to menopause. Your ovaries, which are firm, can usually be felt by the doctor when he or she has two fingers in your vagina and the other hand feeling your abdomen externally. When the ovaries are compressed, you will usually experience pain similar to the pain a man feels when his testicles are squeezed.

Each ovary has two parts—the cortex and the medulla. The outer layer of the ovary is the cortex. In this layer are located all the eggs that a woman will ever have, since she is born with her entire lifetime supply. Each month an egg ripens in a small cyst. When the egg is mature, ovulation occurs. Ovulation is the rupture of the cyst with consequent release of an egg.

The inner part of the ovary, the medulla, is responsible for producing some of the female hormones. Others are produced by the cortex and some by the follicle from which an egg has developed.

The blood supply to the ovaries comes directly from the aorta, the major artery of the body. The ovaries' blood supply does not come from the uterus. Because of this, ovarian function is not affected by hysterectomy (removal of the uterus), and after the uterus is removed the ovaries still continue producing normal amounts of hormones. The hormones produced by the ovaries are poured into a woman's blood supply through blood vessels flowing toward the sides of the body and then go into larger blood vessels through which they spread to the rest of the body.

The Breasts

18 What can you tell me about female breasts?

A woman's breasts are the focus of much attention, both cosmetically and sexually. Primarily, however, God made the female breasts to nurture babies, and even in a society of meticulously prepared, nutritionally calculated infant formulas, mother's milk is still the best source of nutrition for a newborn infant.

Externally, the female breast is made up of a mound of tissue. In the center of this mound is the areola (areola mammae), a circular, darker colored area, approximately one inch in diameter. In the center of the areola is the nipple. Around the nipple in the areola are ten or fifteen oil glands called the glands of Montgomery. These glands, which are in the skin, appear as small bumps in the areola. Secretions from these glands lubricate the nipple, helping to decrease dryness during nursing. There are also some small muscles in the areolar tissue that tend to make the nipple stiffen during nursing so that the baby can handle the nursing process more easily.

Sometimes a woman's nipples are elevated and sometimes they are depressed, or inverted. Either position is "normal," and nursing a baby is possible whether or not the nipple protrudes. Each of the fifteen or twenty milk-producing lobes of a breast empties via its own special duct through the end of the nipple. Before the duct reaches the nipple surface, however, there is an expansion called a *lactiferous sinus*. This widening serves as a reservoir for milk for the nursing process.

Beneath the areola and nipple is an area that is much softer than other areas of breast tissue. This softened area actually represents a decrease in the amount of supporting tissue because of the convergence in one place of all the ducts from the different portions of the breast. If you feel this area of your breast, you will find that it seems to "cave in" under the nipple area. This is normal, but it is also normal not to have this distinct depression.

A breast is mostly gland tissue; it is not just an accumulation of fat under a covering of skin. The

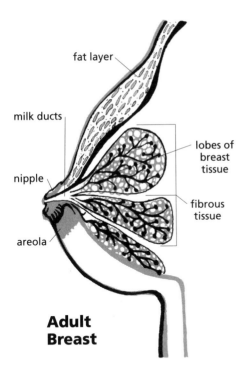

fat layer

milk ducts

nipple

areola

lobes of breast tissue

fibrous tissue

Adult Breast

gland portion of breast tissue is firm, just as a man's testicles (which are gland tissue) are firm. This firm, normal breast tissue is covered by fat. The fat is soft, but when one feels through the fat in palpating the breast, the nodularity of the lobules of breast tissue can be felt. When a woman is palpating her breasts and checking them for lumps, she need not be concerned about this firm, nodular tissue. It is normal; it is supposed to feel that way. She is looking for a more precise and well-defined marble of tissue that could be a growth or a cancer. Such a knot of tissue usually feels very different from normal lumpy breast tissue. If a woman feels something like a marble, she should let her doctor check it.

The breast is supported by fascia, sheets of fibrous tissue that hold muscles and various body organs in place. The breast itself is contained in a fascial envelope that is attached to the chest wall to give the breast support. It extends down into the breast itself and separates the fifteen or twenty lobules of the breast from each other.

It is common for breasts to be asymmetrical (unequal in size or shape). Such asymmetry is quite normal and healthy. If a woman is quite up-

set about the problem, the solution is to have augmentation mammoplasty (an operation in which an implant is used) to enlarge one breast or a reduction mammoplasty to make one breast smaller. These procedures are done by a plastic surgeon.

How Female Organs Develop and Change

19 How does the vulva look at birth?

At birth an infant girl's labia are swollen and prominent. The hymen is succulent (soft and swollen) and, because of its thickened condition, tends to protrude outward from the vagina. The swelling of the labia and the thickness of the hymen are a result of the hormones received from the mother, since these are female genital tissues and are sensitive to female hormones. Most of this thickness and prominence is gone after two weeks, and at six weeks all visible signs of stimulation from the mother's hormones have disappeared. Although the newborn girl's clitoris is still a little large in proportion to the rest of the vulva, it assumes a more proportionate size as the baby matures.

20 How does the vulva develop from birth to puberty?

The infant and child's external genital tissues stay essentially in a "resting phase" until about the seventh year of life. If the labia are spread, the tissues will look thin, shiny, and somewhat red. This redness is due to the high visibility of blood vessels in the thin tissues; it is not normally due to infection.

Between seven and nine years of age the vulvar tissues begin to mature. The mons pubis (fatty pad over the pubic bone) begins thickening. Genital hair will eventually develop over this thickening; by the time a girl starts her menstrual periods she will usually have a well-developed growth of pubic hair.

During this same time fat is deposited in the labia majora and, by the time monthly periods start, the labia majora are usually large enough to cover the opening to the vagina. Although the labia minora never become as thick as the labia majora, they lose their sharp edges during this time and become somewhat rounded and full. In addition, the clitoris loses its baby size and begins thickening and elongating.

During puberty, the vulvar tissues lose their redness and become pink in color. There is a great deal more moisture present, partly a result of the growth of the Bartholin's glands, which provide lubrication for the vaginal opening.

21 How do the vulvar tissues change at menopause?

The cause of change in the vulvar tissues—from those of the young child to those of the mature

Development of Pelvic Organs from Birth to Menopause

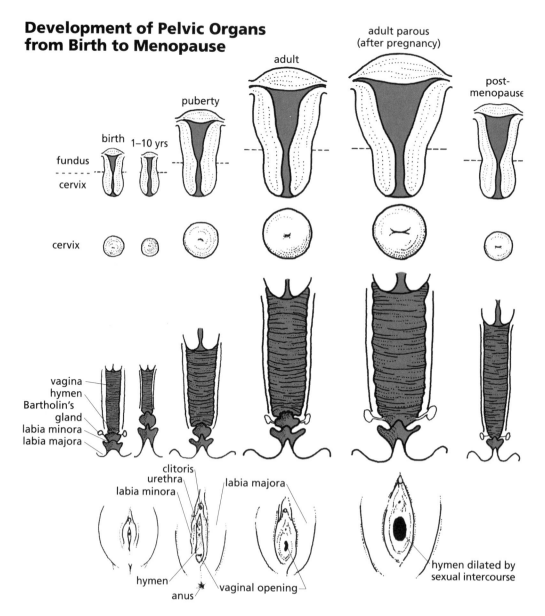

woman—is the presence of estrogen from the ovaries. When menopause occurs, or when the ovaries are removed by surgery, estrogen is no longer produced by the body in adequate amounts. When this estrogen deprivation occurs, the changes to a woman's vulva simulate in reverse those changes that occurred from childhood to maturity.

After the menopause, if a woman does not take estrogen replacement, the vulvar tissues gradually become thinner; the labia majora and the mons pubis both lose a good deal of their fatty tissue; and the labia minora become thinner, sharper, and less prominent. As a result of this atrophy, the entrance to the vagina may become smaller and tighter and cause pain with intercourse.

The urethral opening can "turn out" and become very red. This change is called a urethral caruncle. Doctors who are unaware of this may think it is a growth of some type, when it merely indicates a lack of estrogen. Application of estrogen cream will usually cause the urethral opening to build up, turn back in, and lose its redness.

The changes mentioned above can be reversed, or even prevented, if a woman takes estrogen regularly from menopause on. Occasionally, however, estrogen taken by mouth is not adequate to prevent discomfort with intercourse from mild persistent dryness; in this situation, vaginal estrogen cream can be used. It can be applied in the vagina and also on the vulva to prevent or ease any discomfort that might have resulted from menopause. (See chapter 5 on menopause for more information, especially Q. 223.) Of course, a vaginal lubricant with intercourse can also alleviate pain.

22 How does the vagina appear at birth?

When the infant girl is born, the hymen and vaginal tissues are thick, moist, and luxuriant. This is a result of estrogen from the mother's body that stimulated the baby's tissues during pregnancy. Six weeks after birth this effect on the baby's female organs is gone. From that point until puberty the tissues stay thin, slightly reddish, and dry-looking.

23 How does the vagina develop from childhood to menopause?

Between the ages of seven and nine the girl's ovaries begin producing estrogen, causing her hymen and vagina to thicken again and the tissues to become softer and more moist. The tissues maintain that change as the female goes through her reproductive years.

When the ovaries cease functioning at menopause, the female again has only small amounts of estrogen in her body. This lack of estrogen allows the process to reverse, and the hymen and vaginal tissues become very thin (atrophic). Because of this thinness, they are a little more susceptible to certain infections. The thinness can also result in relaxation of the tissues, which may cause a woman to develop relaxation of her bladder so that she loses urine when she coughs or sneezes. Additionally, thin vaginal tissue can cause pain with intercourse.

Many of these changes can be prevented or cured by the use of estrogen. This estrogen treatment is usually given as a pill. If the tissues do not respond well to oral medication, vaginal estrogen cream can be put directly into the vagina three times a week (see Q. 21, 223), or a vaginal lubricant can be used with intercourse.

24 How does the uterus develop from birth through menopause?

The uterus of a newborn is quite large in proportion to the rest of the baby girl's body. This is due to the presence of the mother's hormones in the infant's body at birth. The uterus becomes smaller during the next five or six weeks as the mother's hormones leave the baby's body. Then no active change takes place in the young girl's uterus until she is seven to nine years of age. When she begins to secrete female hormones from her ovaries, the uterus starts enlarging again.

During the reproductive period, a woman's uterus is about half the size of her fist. Prior to seven to nine years of age, the uterus is about one-third that size and, after a woman goes through menopause, the uterus becomes much smaller again. To a doctor, the uterus of a post-menopausal woman feels about half the size of that of a reproductive-age female. This uterine atrophy does not seem to affect the way a woman feels or her sexual responsiveness.

25 How do the fallopian tubes develop from birth through menopause?

The fallopian tubes of a newborn girl are string-like, very thin, and about an inch long. During childhood they grow proportionately to the rest of the body but maintain their thin, stringlike appearance. It is the estrogen produced at puberty that stimulates the tubes to assume their adult size. This stimulation causes the inner lining of the tubes to grow, thicken, and form hair cells (cilia) that are responsible for the current of fluid that flows through the tubes.

The fallopian tubes attain a length of about four and a half inches at maturity. Following menopause the fallopian tubes lose much of their bulk and seem to shorten a little. Just as the vaginal lining and the other genital organs become thinner and smaller, so do the fallopian tubes. This change does not seem to affect the way a woman feels or functions at all.

26 How do the breasts appear at birth?

As with other estrogen-sensitive tissues in the female body, the newborn's breasts may show signs of stimulation by the mother's estrogen. One or both of the baby's breasts may be slightly enlarged, and there may be some thickened breast tissue under the nipples. The baby's breasts may even secrete a little milk (a further result of the hormone stimulation from the mother), and there may be slight nipple pigmentation (a result of that same stimulation). All these hormone changes will normally be completely gone after a few weeks of life.

27 What changes in the breasts occur from childhood to menopause?

After the mother's hormones have been excreted from the baby's body and any breast stimulation that was present at birth has disappeared, no tissue is palpable under the small, infantile nipples. When a girl is between the ages of nine and eleven, estrogen from her ovaries stimulates the primitive breast tissue that was laid down before birth. This estrogen does the same thing to her breasts that it does to other parts of her body—it causes growth and change.

In this phase of maturation, the small breast glands experience further growth of their ducts. This will often appear as a small, round mound of flesh that is a flat, buttonlike nubbin of tissue located just under the nipple. This firm mound of tissue soon softens, and the girl will then experience further breast development. Because women have been warned to worry about breast lumps, a mother may panic at discovering this little knot of tissue that *is* her daughter's breast. It is indeed a lump, but such a knot is normal breast development.

Often one breast will begin developing before the other so that there is a nodule on only one side. This is normal, but the presence of a lump on only one side can cause parents and even physicians to think the lump is abnormal.

The amount of breast development by the time a female starts her periods varies a great deal. Some girls develop only small breasts by that time, while others have almost adult-sized breasts.

As the breasts reach their adult form, they undergo further development of the duct system. The ducts become longer and branch out to be prepared for pregnancy.

The estrogen causes not only breast tissue enlargement but also change in color of the areola and the nipples. The first change visible will be enlargement of the nipples. They become elevated above the areola, the darker area that surrounds the nipple. Soon after nipple enlargement, the second-stage branching of the ducts under the nipple causes thickening of that tissue, with further elevation of the nipple. The areola becomes a little darker and larger.

The areola thickens next. In 25 to 50 percent of girls entering puberty it almost seems to be swollen, with the appearance of a cap sitting on top of the developing breast. From this point on the breasts develop to their mature size. As previously mentioned, some girls' breasts have attained almost a mature size by the time they start their periods; others' breasts do not attain their adult size until long after the start of their periods.

Breasts in mammals develop along a milk line on either side of the body from the underarm (axilla) to the mons pubis. "Extra" nipples—and even extra breast tissue with nipples—can develop anywhere along this line. These accessory nipples exist in about 1 percent of all females.

Further changes in the breasts occur during pregnancy. The gland structure matures, enabling milk production. Also, the amount of milk a mother is able to produce is not dependent on the size her breasts were before pregnancy.

After menopause the breasts become thin and atrophic and lose much of their size and shape. As the years go by breast tissue is often replaced with fat. Most older women still have visible breasts, though they may contain more fat than breast tissue.

An Afterword

After considering the intricate development of a human being in the womb, we are reminded of Eve's words following the birth of Cain: "With the help of the LORD, I have brought forth a man" (Gen 4:1 NIV). Eve obviously understood that the development of a child in the womb was the result of God's creative genius.

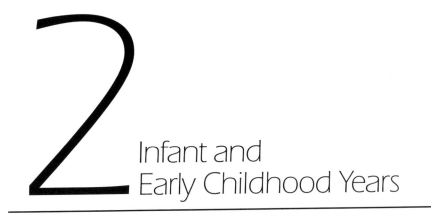

2 Infant and Early Childhood Years

Healthy baby girls glow! They are beautiful—and almost always normal. When they are not, they tug at our hearts even more.

When something is wrong with a newborn baby, parents are shocked and worried; they may see no way for a normal life for their child or themselves.

Sometimes we forget that we and our children can learn and grow a great deal through problems and pain. If you have a little girl who was born with, or has developed, a health problem and if you become bitter and succumb to angry despair, you increase your own stress and the stress on your child. Your anger can make the burden of your child's problems harder to bear. Bitterness on your part can also neutralize any lessons she and you might learn from the situation and stunts any emotional and spiritual growth you might otherwise attain.

Fortunately, most little girls are completely normal. If you look around a hospital nursery, you will see that almost all the babies are perfectly fine, in spite of all the things that *could* have gone wrong.

Early Genital Health Care

28 How do I know that my baby's female organs are normal?

There are several ways to ease your mind about this.

One way is to listen to the people who know. The obstetrician checks her at birth; the pediatrician examines her thoroughly; and during her hospital stay her diaper is changed by professionals in the nursery who know how baby girls' bottoms are supposed to look. If all these people do not see anything wrong with your baby on the outside, she is probably normal on the inside too.

The second way to assure yourself concerning her normality is to examine her yourself. It will not hurt your baby one bit to roll her around and look her over. You can examine her closely. It is perfectly okay for you to put a thumb on either side of her perineum (the area between the vagina and the anus) and press downward and outward, spreading her labia apart slightly. Remember that for the first few weeks after delivery the hymen is thickened and enlarged and will protrude a bit from the vagina. If you see anything that you think is not quite right, check with your pediatrician.

29 What will happen if something does seem to be wrong?

If you or the doctor feels that something about your baby's body is abnormal, testing should be done. Your physician may want to consult with other doctors regarding diagnosis and care. It is important that proper studies be done promptly, since some problems can affect your daughter's health and fertility if not corrected when she is young.

It is important that you and your doctor remember that even perfectly normal girls have variations in the way they are made. In a study by J. McCann, R. Wells, and J. Voris, published in the major journal *Pediatrics* (1990, 86:4228–439), many slight irregularities were noted in normal little girls. For instance, 56 percent had redness of the entrance into the vagina (the vestibule); 50 percent had little bands of tissue attached to the urethra (the urinary opening); 38 percent had some degree of sticking together of the labia

(labial agglutination); more than half of the girls had some irregularity of the hymen; 34 percent had mounds (normal thickenings); 33 percent had projections (extra tissue); and 18 percent had tags of extra tissue.

Out of the group of ninety-three girls, only one had a truly significant developmental abnormality (no opening in the hymen).

30 What kind of examination would a doctor do if either of us suspects a female organ problem?

A doctor would want to do a complete exam of your child, including careful examination of the genitalia. If a child has an abnormality in one area, she may also have an abnormality in another part of her body.

If your daughter is an infant or small child, she will feel most secure and the doctor can best examine her if you sit on the edge of the examining table with her in your lap. In this way, you can hold your daughter's legs apart while the doctor gently examines her vulvar area. The doctor usually cannot do a vaginal exam in the office but could, if necessary, pass a small catheter into the vagina to make sure that the hymen and vagina are properly developed. A rectal exam can be done to be sure there are no growths in the child's pelvis.

A child between the ages of three and eight can lie on the examining table with her bent legs pulled back to her abdomen. The doctor may ask her to hold her own labia apart and then put his or her fingers on the child's to facilitate seeing the area.

An eight- or nine-year-old child is usually big enough to lie on an examination table with her feet in the stirrups like an adult. Also, her vagina is large enough to allow a pediatric vaginal speculum to be inserted into it. This little instrument allows the doctor to view the entire vagina and cervix in the office, with little pain to the child.

If a girl has begun having menstrual periods, she can be examined with a small speculum similar to the instrument used for an adult.

Occasionally a girl must have a vaginal and pelvic exam and, because she is too young or too afraid, an office exam is impossible. A brief general anesthetic at the hospital or outpatient surgical facility can make such an exam possible and much less traumatic for everyone. Such an anesthetic in competent hands is quite safe. If your doctor recommends this, I encourage you to allow it.

31 Will a vaginal exam cause my daughter to "lose her virginity"?

No. Exams of this type done by gentle, caring doctors do no more than stretch the hymen a little. There may be a minute tearing of the edges of the hymen, which could result in a slight amount of bright red bleeding.

In any event, "loss of virginity" results from intercourse, not from a vaginal exam.

32 How likely is it that problems of the female organs will develop in an infant or child before the age of fertility?

Infants and children rarely have problems of the genital tract. When problems do occur, they are minor about 90 percent of the time. Most of the disorders that occur in young girls have to do with vulvar or vaginal irritations or infections. Many problems that a child can have will be discussed in the following questions.

Vulvar/Vaginal Problems in Young Girls

33 What vulvar or vaginal irritations or vaginal infections can occur in young girls?

The four most common are:

infections from lack of good hygiene
genital warts
herpes
impetigo

34 What is "good hygiene"? Why is it so important?

"Hygiene" refers to practices and conditions conducive to sound health. "Good hygiene" means taking steps to maintain good health and to prevent disease.

Good hygiene, particularly of the genital area, is important for everyone, but it is especially important for females. Daily washing of the vulva with warm water and a mild soap (which contains no perfumes or other chemicals) is important. If a girl or woman has a large amount of nonirritating, nonodorous vaginal secretions—a condition that can be totally normal—washing twice a day may be even more important. Careful drying is also wise.

Careful washing between the folds of skin in the vulvar area is especially important to avoid the development of irritation. Gently spreading the labia and washing between them is also helpful.

35 What causes diaper rash?

Newborns have sensitive skin that requires extra care. Diaper rash, for instance, is usually alleviated by changing diapers more frequently, temporarily avoiding rubber or plastic pants that hold moisture against the baby's bottom, and cleansing the area thoroughly. (Diaper rash is often caused by the ammonia released from urine-soaked diapers.) Disposable diapers, because of high absorbency, seem to have helped alleviate much of this problem.

If the baby's bottom seems particularly inflamed and does not respond to careful hygiene, fungus medication or antibiotic ointments may be helpful. It may be necessary to change from detergent to soap for washing diapers or underwear, to stop using medicated or perfumed soaps, and to eliminate any other medication that might be touching the baby's or young child's bottom. The baby may be sensitive or allergic to any of these things. Disposable diapers have made these problems much less common and when they do occur, they are easier to deal with.

36 Is it normal for a girl to have some discharge from her vagina?

As a girl's ovaries begin producing hormones, vaginal tissues begin to grow and produce moist secretions. These secretions can collect on the vulva, and they are normal as long as they do not cause itching or odor. Of course, if a girl does not keep herself clean and dry, any type of moisture (normal secretions, swimming pool water, and so on) can cause her vulva to become irritated.

37 What infections might cause "abnormal" discharge? What will the doctor do if my little girl develops a vaginal discharge or infection?

A normal discharge is moisture or secretions. When a discharge is abnormal it usually itches, burns, smells, or looks like pus (with a yellow or green color). Abnormal vaginal discharge can be caused by infection or by a girl having an object in her vagina such as a bean or a small marble. The same infections that can cause an adult woman to have a discharge can also cause a child to have a discharge. These infections include fungus (monilia or yeast), trichomonas, gonorrhea, chlamydia, vaginosis, pinworms, and other infections.

When you take your daughter to the doctor for a discharge problem, he or she will ask what the discharge is like and how long it has been present. The doctor will want to know if it itches, burns, or smells. Next, the doctor will want to examine the child to get an idea of the type of discharge present. In older children it is sometimes possible for the doctor to look into the girl's vagina. This is often not possible in younger girls. The doctor may be able to get a Q-tip into the girl's vagina to get some secretions to look at and to culture, but sometimes even that is not possible. If an adequate exam in the office is not possible and various treatments are not successful, the doctor may recommend an exam under general anesthesia. (See Q. 30.)

Fungus infections (yeast or monilia or candida) are fairly common in children. They will often start because a child has been on antibiotics. They can also develop when a child's bottom has been left wet too long. These infections cause irritation of the area, producing a red rash, with isolated spots of red infection around the edges. A fungal infection can usually be stopped with one of the common preparations used for adult fungus infections: Monistat, Gyne-Lotrimin, Vagistat, etc., which can be purchased without a prescription. If a child is older, it is possible to put medication into her vagina. If a child is receiving antibiotics frequently, it may be necessary to treat her with fungus medication every time she takes the antibiotics. If the fungus seems to be persistent, the girl should be checked for diabetes. Diabetes can cause a person to be more susceptible to vaginal fungus infections.

Trichomoniasis and vaginosis are infections that a doctor would diagnose by obtaining some secretions and looking at them under the microscope. Once he or she has determined which type of infection exists, it can be treated. Actually, both of these infections can be treated with Flagyl. It is possible that either one of these infections can spread to a child from the hands of an adult. Unfortunately, these infections can be spread to a child by sexual abuse from an infected male or female. This does not have to be penetration—it can be a result of the abuser's hands or genitals touching the external parts of a girl's bottom.

Gonorrhea and/or chlamydia can infect a child who has been sexually abused. If a girl has an abnormal discharge, and there is any possibility that she has been a victim of sexual abuse, tell the doctor so he or she can be alert to the possibility of these infections. The doctor then can culture the secretions for these germs and provide treatment if necessary.

Other germs can infect a girl's vagina. The germs that cause an upper respiratory tract infection may also cause a vaginal infection. Pediatricians frequently see vaginal infections develop a week to ten days after a girl has developed a sore throat and cough.

Young girls often have pinworm infections. These can not only infect the intestines and anus, but they can also get into the child's vagina and infect it. This infection can cause vaginal discharge and vulvar irritation. If you or the doctor suspect a pinworm infection, the doctor will want you to press a piece of sticky, transparent tape against your daughter's anus with a tongue depressor at night (which is when pinworms come out). By looking at this tape under a microscope, the doctor can see pinworm eggs if such an infection is present. The entire family will usually need treatment with Vermox if pinworms are found. Vermox should not be used by pregnant women.

38 What are venereal (genital) warts? Can a little girl get them? How are they treated?

Genital warts or condyloma acuminata look like ordinary warts (somewhat firm protuberances). They are called "venereal or genital" because they occur in the venereal (genital) area. Genital warts are becoming quite common in our population.

These warts are caused by a virus called HPV (human papillomavirus). (See the chapter on sexually transmitted diseases to learn more about this virus.)

Formerly physicians thought that condyloma acuminata in children was almost always a result of sexual abuse or sexual contact. Further studies, however, have shown that these growths in children can be acquired from the child's contact with the common warts a parent might have on his or her hands or feet. In fact, sexual transmission, though it does occur, may be much less common than was previously suspected. A frequent form of transmission seems to be from sharing beds, towels, and bathwater. One reliable study that demonstrated the nonsexual transmission of warts was reported by Shavonir Obalek in the *Journal of the American Academy of Dermatology* (1990, 23:205–13). If these warts occur and there is any suspicion of sexual abuse, prompt investigation is mandatory in order to stop the abuse.

It is important to have the warts treated because they can grow larger and spread if left alone; they can also cause irritation and discomfort. Surprisingly, though, warts can occasionally clear up spontaneously.

39 Can a baby or child get herpes?

Genital herpes (herpes virus type II) can occur in a baby or child. It may be passed from the mother's or father's hands to their child, though this is unusual. It can also result from sexual abuse.

If you have had herpes of your own vulvar tissues, you do not need to be terribly concerned about passing it on to your little girl. Using normal hygienic measures, such as washing your hands after touching your own vulvar area, should prevent passing the virus. It is probably best that you not bathe with your daughter if you have a herpes sore. Although unlikely, it may be possible to spread the virus in this way. Herpes virus has been cultured from hot tubs, and if it can remain alive there, it could remain active in a bathtub.

Although herpes infections may cause burning and discomfort, they will not permanently damage a little girl's body. Like an adult, however, she may have secondary herpes episodes or recurrent outbreaks for many months or even years.

40 What other disorders might affect the vulvar skin of my baby or child?

Several conditions can affect the skin of the vulva. Unfortunately, some are difficult to diagnose. If your child has a condition of the vulva that your family practitioner or gynecologist is unable to definitely diagnose, it might be good to get an opinion from a dermatologist.

Conditions of this sort include impetigo; psoriasis (rarely occurring before five years of age); seborrheic dermatitis (the same problem that causes dandruff); vitiligo (normal skin but without its pigmentation; skin appears almost pure white); lichen sclerosis; and molluscum contagiosum. (For the latter two problems, see Q. 576, 581.)

Although these problems sound serious, none of them are dangerous. Perhaps the greatest hazard would be for a doctor to overtreat the problems. In earlier days, for instance, lichen sclerosis was thought to predispose a person to cancer. We know now that it does not. It would be tragic if a well-meaning but uninformed doctor erroneously operated to remove your daughter's vulvar skin because of this problem!

41 Is it normal for a baby girl to have vaginal bleeding?

During the first week or ten days after birth, as her mother's hormones leave her body, a baby girl can have some "withdrawal" bleeding. This is normal and needs no evaluation unless bleeding begins again after the baby is two or more weeks old. If bleeding from the vagina occurs at any other time before puberty, she needs to see a doctor for an evaluation. She may have put a foreign object into her vagina or she could have a vaginal tumor, though such tumors are exceedingly rare. If she has other signs of sexual development plus vaginal bleeding, she may be having premature puberty.

42 My baby's labia seem stuck together. Is this dangerous?

No. This condition is called "labial agglutination" (labial adhesions); in this condition the edges of the labia minora stick to each other because they have become inflamed. This situation is not dangerous, nor does anything need to be done unless the urethral opening is obstructed and urine flow is partially blocked. (This could cause a bladder infection.)

Treatment, if necessary, is usually very simple. The doctor will probably give you a prescription for Premarin vaginal cream or a similar estrogen preparation, to be applied to the vulva each night for a couple of weeks. This results in a healthy thickening of the labia minora, allowing them to separate. Generally after separation the labia will not stick together again. If they do, the cream can be used again as needed. (In the past doctors thought they had to physically peel the labia apart. Doing this, however, did not solve the problem, as the labia would stick together again.)

Vulvar or Vaginal Injury in Children

43 What can cause damage to my daughter's vulva or vagina? What should be done about such damage?

One of the things that can cause the vulva of a newborn baby to appear damaged is a breech de-livery. When a little girl is born bottom first, her labia may be swollen and bruised. Although this looks bad, it is not dangerous. It should be left alone, as it will heal on its own.

Other causes of vaginal or vulvar injury are falls onto sharp objects, a beating or kicking or other physical abuse, and intercourse or rape.

44 What should be done if a young girl's vulva is injured by a beating or kicking or by an accidental fall?

Sadly, babies and young girls do get hurt. Physical injury that involves a girl's vulva will not normally cause any significant lasting damage; a large bruise is usually all that occurs.

When a doctor examines a girl who has been hurt, he or she may want to admit the child to a hospital and give her anesthesia so she can be examined and have any torn areas repaired. Often this is not required. The doctor may merely advise the child's mother to put ice on the area for the first twenty-four hours and, after that, have the child sit in a tub of warm water for twenty or thirty minutes, two times a day. Additionally, if a great deal of tissue has been damaged, the doctor may want her to receive antibiotics. (For more information on vulvar or vaginal injury, see Q. 595, 632.)

45 Can a young girl be badly damaged by intercourse or rape?

A girl cannot ordinarily have "normal" intercourse until she is at least eight years of age. From about this age on, a girl's vulva and vagina have been prepared to some extent for intercourse by her own natural hormones. When a child in this older age group has intercourse, the hymen is usually the only vulvar part that is torn.

Even if an older girl is raped, she usually does not have significant tears of her vagina. Tears can occur, however, especially if intercourse takes place when a girl is younger than about eight years of age. If rape, incest, or other sexual abuse is suspected, the girl should be examined by a physician who can evaluate her in a caring and sensitive way. If forcible intercourse has torn the external area of a girl younger than eight or nine, the doctor may want the girl admitted to the hospital for an internal examination, fearing that she might have internal tears. Antibiotics may be prescribed to prevent her acquiring syphilis, gonorrhea, or chlamydia from her attacker. A blood test for syphilis and HIV in three months would also be wise.

Adequate initial and follow-up counseling are needed to help the child overcome the emotional trauma of rape or other sexual abuse. Emotional support and help from her parents are vital. Such parents should read extensively on the subject and obtain counseling for themselves and their daughter. Everything possible must be done to help the child overcome the trauma of the event and enable her to grow up with a healthy attitude toward her own sexuality. (See Q. 184–195 for a complete discussion of rape and sexual assault.)

Female-Organ Abnormalities in Children

46 Can my daughter be born with her hymen closed?

Yes. This abnormality is called an "imperforate hymen." It is usually detected immediately after birth when the doctor examines the baby girl's vulvar area. A bulging hymen just inside the labia minora is an indication that the hymen is closed. Secretions in her vagina are filling it, causing the bulging.

If the imperforate hymen is not detected at birth, it may not be discovered until the girl starts her menstrual periods, at which time she may develop abdominal pain for a few days each month. This pain is caused by the accumulation of blood in the vagina and uterus at period time each month, a condition that can affect her future fertility. It is best, obviously, that this problem be discovered early, when a girl is still a baby. A simple surgical procedure is all that is required to open the hymen and fix the problem.

47 What other abnormalities of the female organs can be present at birth?

The abnormalities of the female organs that a baby girl can have at birth are multiple and varied, and virtually no two persons are born with the same abnormality. Because of these two facts, an in-depth discussion of congenital birth abnormalities is not possible here. Examples, however, are given below.

Labia that are larger or smaller than normal. This is a minor problem and is significant only if the labia are so oversized that they cause discomfort or embarrassment. In this case, a simple operation can be done to trim excessive tissue.

Failure of the vaginal, urethral, and anal openings to form properly. Occasionally openings for these important body parts may not develop properly. There may be no opening at all or they may open in an abnormal way. For example, the rectum may open into the vagina, or not at all; the urethra may open into the vagina; the bladder may open directly to the outside of the body. Many of these abnormalities are major and require specialized care.

Other abnormalities. Some of the other abnormalities gynecologists see in patients are discussed in Q. 48–54.

48 What should generally be done if my daughter is born with an abnormality of her female organs?

Don't delay proper treatment! A doctor should be able to lay out a plan of treatment that seems logical and well-thought-out to you. If there is any question, see a specialist such as a gynecologic endocrinologist or a pediatric surgeon. These are doctors who have special training in this area and can help avoid mistakes.

49 Can a girl be born with two vaginas?

It is not extremely rare for a girl to be born with two vaginas (septate vagina). I have seen several patients with this abnormality.

The problem is not usually found until a female is examined as an adult. The two vaginas generally cause no trouble, because one side or the other is usually large enough for normal intercourse and vaginal delivery. Surgery is usually not necessary for this particular problem.

50 Can a girl be born with other vaginal problems or *no* vagina?

Occasionally a female infant is born with no vagina. Although a girl with this problem usually has normal labia, clitoris, and urethral opening, most of the time she has no uterus, and perhaps no fallopian tubes.

It is important to discover this problem early, so that the girl can be prepared for the fact that she will need to have medical treatment to form a vagina. Finding this problem early allows for testing of chromosomes to determine if all of the cells in her body are female. In addition, sonogram and/or radiologic studies can be done to see if there is a uterus.

The vagina can develop with narrow places along its length. Such constrictions of the vagina can cause pain during intercourse. This problem is almost never found during childhood. A gynecologist may discover the problem on a woman's first visit for a routine checkup or because she comes to the office complaining of pain during intercourse. The vagina is reasonably elastic. Therefore a virginal woman with a constriction may want to have intercourse for a few months to see if her vagina will stretch and thus eliminate pain. If this doesn't work, repair can usually be accomplished with simple vaginal surgery.

51 What abnormalities of the uterus can be present at birth?

The embryonic formation of the uterus and vagina are very similar. The müllerian ducts come together in the midline, fusing and forming one organ. If the ducts do not meet and fuse normally, variations occur in the organs they form. If they do not come together in the midline to form a normal uterus, two half uteri can develop. If one mül-

lerian duct forms properly, but the other one does not, a woman may have a normal half-uterus on one side (which will usually function normally even in pregnancy), with a small, poorly developed half-uterus on the other.

Occasionally when there is incomplete fusion of the müllerian duct in the middle, a uterus may look normal but have a septum inside. This is a partition down the middle of the uterus, dividing it into two compartments. Treatment of these problems is unnecessary unless a woman cannot become pregnant or has repeated miscarriages.

52 Can a baby be born part girl and part boy?

A baby may be born with external genitalia that are not completely one sex or the other. This condition is called ambiguous genitalia. Unfortunately, these babies are often incorrectly called hermaphrodites.

When a baby is born with ambiguous genitalia, three abnormalities usually exist: first, an enlarged phallus (too small to be a normal penis but larger than a normal clitoris); second, folds of skin that are too large to be normal labia but too small to be a scrotum (there is usually a cleft down the middle that keeps the skin from looking like a scrotum); and finally, a urethra that empties neither at the end of the phallus like a male nor at the base of the phallus like a normal female.

The most common cause of ambiguous genitalia in a child that is truly a girl (female pseudohermaphrodite) is congenital adrenal hyperplasia. This is a condition in which the female fetus (while still inside her mother's uterus) produces an excess of a male hormone from her own abnormal adrenal glands. This hormone causes her external genitalia to become malelike, but leaves her uterus, tubes, and ovaries normal.

When I was in residency training, I reviewed all the charts on babies who had been admitted to Texas Children's Hospital in the Texas Medical Center in Houston for problems of their female organs. Most of the babies with ambiguous genitalia had been there because of congenital adrenal hyperplasia.

Certain drugs given during pregnancy can cause

a baby girl to have ambiguous external genitalia. These drugs do not interfere with the development of a girl's vagina, uterus, tubes, or ovaries. The drug most likely to cause this change is Provera. In addition, if a woman received testosterone (the primary male hormone) during her pregnancy, a baby girl would very likely be similarly affected.

Surgery can usually correct the genital abnormalities caused by this problem and allow the girl to look normal, have normal sex as an adult, and be able to bear children. Medical care can correct the problem of the abnormal adrenal glands.

53 What abnormalities of her ovaries can a baby girl have?

It is rare for a girl who has an otherwise normal female body to be born without ovaries, but the ovaries can be underdeveloped. When a female child has ovarian development abnormalities (gonadal dysgenesis), her ovaries cannot produce eggs or estrogen. At the time that puberty should occur, such girls must be given estrogen by mouth.

There are three types of gonadal dysgenesis, and none of them would normally be detected before the time of puberty.

Normal female chromosomes but poorly developed ovaries (pure gonadal dysgenesis). In this situation, the girl would appear normal at birth and would grow normally until the onset of puberty. Then, because her ovaries cannot produce hormones or eggs, she would not start menstrual periods and not develop sexual hair or breasts. A laparoscopy (see Q. 810), would show only streaks of white tissue where the ovaries should be. Estrogen would be given to help her develop breasts and normal adult sexual characteristics. The girl would function sexually in a normal way as an adult, but she would not be able to conceive. Her chromosomes are normal female chromosomes (46XX); the problem is poor development of the ovaries.

Abnormal chromosomes and undeveloped ovaries (Turner's syndrome). This is the most common form of gonadal dysgenesis. This girl is missing an X chromosome (see Q. 241). She has only forty-five chromosomes instead of the usual forty-six and her ovaries do not develop. Her chromosome makeup is written as 45XO (normal girls are 46XX). This adolescent's development would be like that described above for pure gonadal dysgenesis but, because of the chromosomal abnormality, there would be abnormalities in various parts of her body. The most characteristic abnormality is shortness—these girls would almost never grow to more than five feet. The second most common abnormality is webbing of the neck (skin and tissue extend from the sides of the neck out to the shoulders). Other signs that may occur include a high-arched palate, low-set prominent ears, or low hairline on the back of the head.

With proper care, these girls can function sexually in a normal way, but because their ovaries do not produce eggs or female hormones, they are unable to conceive. They will need to be given estrogen at the time puberty would normally start. A child born with Turner's syndrome is a very special child. While this problem is the most common human chromosome abnormality, occurring in 0.8 percent of all embryos, only about 3 percent of these fetuses survive the growth process in their mother's womb. The others miscarry. The three in a hundred are tough little survivors. However, many of them will die in infancy because they have a higher rate of other abnormalities.

Mixed abnormalities of the chromosomes with ovaries almost totally undeveloped. In this situation, "mixed gonadal dysgenesis," various combinations of chromosomes may be present in a girl's body. Occasionally there will be a Y chromosome present.

If a child has mixed gonadal dysgenesis with a Y chromosome, the ovaries, which *are* present but almost totally undeveloped, have a 30 percent chance of developing a malignancy. Such ovaries should be removed early in the child's life. Mixed gonadal dysgenesis (also called gonadal dysgenesis variants) are rare and occur in many forms. They are complicated situations that require truly expert care by a gynecologic endocrinologist.

54 Do inguinal hernias occur in girls?

Although more common in boys, these hernias do occasionally occur in girls.

An inguinal hernia is a weakness in the wall of the lower abdomen, allowing a protrusion of the internal lining of the abdominal cavity (the peritoneum). A saclike bulge develops into which the intestines and uterus can fall. This sac can be noticed when a child cries or is pushing down with a bowel movement. Such a hernia is seen as a bulge on either side of the body just above the pubic bone.

Occasionally a girl's ovary will drop down into the hernia sac. On examination of the hernia sac, a doctor would find this as a small, solid lump. About 3 percent of the time when such a mass is felt, it is present because the child is actually a male with pseudo-hermaphroditism, even though the external genitalia look totally female. Because of this possibility, chromosome studies may be indicated. Except for this problem, such protrusion of the ovary is not in any way dangerous.

A child of either sex who has an inguinal hernia needs to have it surgically repaired.

The "Facts of Life"

55 When should I tell my daughter "the facts of life"?

Sex education for your daughter begins the day she is born and continues for the rest of her life—whether or not you say a word to her about sex. Your attitudes, opinions, and reactions to sexual matters will be noted by your child, and your views will become a part of her attitudes, opinions, and reactions concerning sex.

Without doubt, your words on this subject are the most vitally important your child will ever hear. Recent studies clearly show that you have more influence on her future decisions about sex than any other factors in her life. So she will have a greater chance for a happy and healthy life, it is best that your transmission of sexual information to your daughter be done well (see chapter 13 on STD).

56 What guidelines do you suggest for the sexual and moral development of my daughter?

There are fourteen points that I advocate.

1. Beginning in infancy, treat your daughter's vulvar area as you would any other part of her body. Do not give the impression it is a "forbidden zone."

2. Don't make a big deal of your daughter touching or manipulating her vulva or clitoris. Children are curious and smart. They soon discover that touching their genitals brings pleasure, and it is natural that they will want to do it again. If your attitude is right and your explanations frank and open, it is unlikely that this will develop into something that will be an embarrassment in public or a problem of habitual masturbation. It is certainly appropriate to teach your child that scratching her bottom in public is not "appropriate manners."

3. Don't entertain false and obsessive modesty around the house. If your child sees you or your spouse nude, accept it as normal. I don't see any advantage, though, in family members running around the house without their clothes on just so they can be seen by others.

4. Use correct terms for sexual organs, but do not use rigid terminology. (When was the last time you referred to the hole in your abdomen as your "umbilicus"?) This will show your child that her sexual organs are a normal part of her body—not something about which she needs to be ashamed.

5. Don't be embarrassed by her questions. Since sexual organs and sexual functions are a normal part of life, learn to be comfortable when asked questions about them. However, don't make your answers too complicated. If a five-year-old asks what a vagina is, she does not want to hear about the whole process of intercourse and childbirth. Gear your explanation to her level of understanding. Merely answer all questions in a straightforward, simple way. If you don't know the answer to a particular question, tell your child you will find out and tell her later.

6. Explain to your daughter the body changes that will occur and the normal functions she can expect. Your eight-year-old girl should know that she will start breast development,

pubic hair growth, and menstruation so that she will not be frightened when these things occur. As she grows older, you should explain to her how intercourse is achieved, how pregnancy takes place, and how deliveries are accomplished.

7. Take advantage of events occurring around you. Many years ago the five-year-old daughter of a neighbor of ours asked her mother if there was any connection between the fact that her stomach had been large before the new baby came and now was smaller. This mother blew a great chance to explain some basic facts to the girl when she told her that there was *no* relationship between those two things! Actually, she blew a great chance much earlier. The little girl could have been encouraged to participate in the excitement of expecting a new baby by being allowed to feel the baby kicking and moving in her mother's tummy before it was born.

8. Show your love for your spouse. When children see their parents exhibiting love toward each other and having physical contact (kissing, caressing, hugging), they will learn to associate the two in a positive way. This helps develop the attitude that physical contact between a man and a woman is associated with love.

9. Take your daughter with you for your annual physical exam or for obstetric visits while you are pregnant. This can be a very positive aid in helping a young girl learn more about her own body. In doing this, she finds that the experience is not threatening, but is something that responsible adult women do. She can meet the physician who "takes care of Mommy" and learn that a doctor is a friend. When my patients have brought their daughters with them for their pelvic exams, the daughters almost always accept the visit and the examining room without undue bewilderment and without any significant fright.

10. Speak of having a baby as a miracle shared by a husband and wife. This will emphasize the fact that conception and the growth of a baby in a mother's uterus is a special thing, and that the mother and father have an important role in its development. It is good to speak of "a husband and wife" and not just of "a man and woman." This will help a child understand that the proper place for a baby's conception and birth is in marriage.

11. Continue with the pattern of discussing normal bodily events in a natural way as the girl grows older. For instance, when your daughter has learned that babies come from sexual intercourse, it is perfectly natural for you to explain to her that intercourse does not always result in pregnancy. A natural outgrowth of that conversation would be another conversation about marriage and then another about contraception. Your message to your children is important. If they don't hear about contraceptives from you, they will get their information from their friends or the media.

12. Teach modesty concerning the body and its functions. Most girls become modest about the time they begin developing sexual hair and breasts. They begin closing the door when they dress or use the bathroom. Consideration of this sense of privacy will help your daughter understand that she has a right to privacy. The right attitude in the home can help the girl develop proper modesty not only in her attitude to nudity but also in her approach to acceptable dress and behavior in society at large. It can also help her learn that no one else has a right to her body without her permission—good protection from sexual abuse.

13. Use appropriate aids. There are a number of excellent books, and at least one good series of tapes that can help you with the sex education program for your child. In addition, urge your church or any other organization with moral values similar to yours, to teach those values from early childhood and then to conduct sex-education classes for the children from at least fifth grade through high school. This allows someone else to support your message about sex. Also, it is good for the entire group to re-

ceive similar sex information and therefore have a common level of knowledge and to develop common values.

14. Have good rules about television viewing and using the Internet! One study of 450 sixth graders showed that 66 percent of them viewed sexually explicit shows at least once a month. Roughly 70 percent of these children said that their parents did not monitor the shows they watched. It is also very common today for children to view sexually explicit material on the Internet, much of which is pornographic. Common sense says that parental monitoring of television shows and Internet access is absolutely necessary if we want to keep our children's perspective on sex appropriate. It is a good idea for parents to watch TV and videos with their children. Parents can then discuss and explain sexual innuendos. These can be valuable learning times for the child. Parents can also discuss the dangers of the Internet and give guidelines for using personal computers at home, at school, in the library, or at a friend's house.

57 What books and tapes would be helpful to me in preparing my child for the changes of puberty?

Dr. James Dobson has an excellent series of tapes titled, "Preparing for Adolescence." He recommends that parents listen to these tapes with their children before those offspring enter puberty. Families that have used the tapes have found them helpful. These tapes may be obtained from most Christian bookstores.

Another good tape from Focus on the Family is "Understanding Physical and Sexual Development."

Excellent books on this subject are:

1. *Preparing for Adolescence*, James Dobson. It follows the same outline as the tape series.
2. The Concordia Sex Education series:

How to Talk Competently with Your Child About Sex
Why Boys and Girls Are Different (for 3–5-year-olds)
Where Do Babies Come From? (for 6–8-year-olds)
How You Are Changing (for 8–11-year-olds)
Sex and the New You (for 11–14-year-olds)
Love—Sex and God (for 14 and up)

3. *Decent Exposure—How to Teach Your Children About Sex*, Connie Marshner (Wolgemuth & Hyatt)
4. *How to Teach Your Child About Sex*, Grace Ketterman (Power Books)
5. *Sexuality and the Young Christian*, Joanne De Jonge (Baker Book House)
6. *Facts of Life: Teaching Your Children About Sex*, Focus on the Family
7. *A Gift for All Ages: A Family Handbook on Sexuality*, Clifford and Joyce Penner (Word)

An Afterword

In concluding the discussion on the female as a baby and child, I wish to stress again that most children are born completely normal. My purpose in mentioning some of the abnormalities that can occur is not to frighten parents but to enlighten them. Parents need to know that there is much that can be done for a child with birth defects.

Even as parents should not be fear-stricken over the possibility of having a child with abnormalities, neither should they be terrified of failing to provide "perfect" sex education for their child. As with any other aspect of childrearing, all parents can do is their best. If they do that they cannot be "failures" as parents.

Enjoy your little daughter! Her infancy and childhood will soon be a memory, and the innocence and charm of those special early years should be treasured. True, there is great responsibility in parenting a child. But the rewards are equally great, and there is nothing more precious than the trust and love of a little girl and the joy of seeing her grow into adulthood.

3
The Adolescent Years

An adolescent is a person in the process of growing from childhood to maturity. Obviously this involves many changes, and change is almost always a mixed blessing, bringing pleasure and pain, elation and depression, joy and sorrow. The metamorphosis of a child into an adult is not accomplished in isolation, however, since the process dramatically involves those closest to the adolescent.

Many parents live in fear of both the adolescent years and of adolescents themselves. All of us know parents of preteens who are dreading the approaching teenage years, and we know parents of teenagers who are wringing their hands in despair. Will our child be killed in a car wreck because a teenager is driving too fast? Will our daughter be a victim of date rape? Will she give in to the lure of drugs or alcohol? Will she believe the lies about the beauty of sex outside marriage or about the fulfillment of materialism?

A primary cause of parents' disabling fear may be their failure to teach their children that there is a moral foundation on which they can base their lives. Children need a strong foundation of morality and faith to survive the storms of life; without it, they are subject to every prevailing wind of doctrine and philosophy. They face destruction if they have no firm ground on which to stand. Common sense tells us faith can provide a solid foundation for life's choices, and scientific studies show this too.

I encourage you to pass on to your children the inner resource of a relationship with God.

The physical changes and social and ethical dilemmas of adolescence that often perplex and dismay both parent and child can be handled more smoothly with factual knowledge, proper guidance, and sound medical care. This chapter will provide some of the information and guidance needed by adolescent females and their parents.

The Changes and Timing of Puberty

58 What exactly *is* adolescence?

One dictionary defines adolescence as "growing from childhood to maturity." This growth involves every aspect of the child making that passage. For a young girl it includes:

Emotional growth. A child changes from a dependent person to an independent and mature adult.

Physical growth. A child's physical structure becomes an adult body, the most obvious sign being the changes in contour and size.

Sexual growth. The changing of a girl's body into that of an adult woman includes and involves the vital change from being incapable of pregnancy to, in most cases, being fertile and able to bear children.

Spiritual growth. A person may for the first time become aware of the hand of God in the creation and history of the world and in their own personal lives.

59 What is puberty?

Puberty refers to the period during which a girl's body changes from being unable to bear children to the state of being fertile. The physical changes in her body during this transition involve two things—the growth of the sexual organs of the body (vagina, uterus, and breasts) and the start-up of the sexual hormonal cycle that precipitates the release of eggs (ova) and prepares the uterus to receive fertilized eggs for the pregnancy process.

Physicians divide puberty into different growth stages. These processes, with their medical names, are shown in the accompanying table.

Puberty is considered complete when a girl has developed regular menstrual cycles with regular ovulation—and is, therefore, normally fertile.

60 When does puberty usually begin?

Studies indicate that when a girl's body composition shifts to a higher proportion of fat, she is more likely to start her menstrual periods. This shift occurs earlier in well-nourished children than in children whose overall nutrition has been poor. It has been noted by researchers that children on the whole have grown significantly larger during the past eighty years. This is one reason the age at which girls start their menstrual cycles has been decreasing. The increased size of children is not due merely to the overall better nutrition of children, however. It is also due to the better nutrition of expectant mothers.

Additionally, girls living closer to the equator, at lower altitudes, in urban areas, and who are mildly obese start puberty earlier than those in

Puberty Stages

Pubertal Change	Medical Name	Median Developmental Age
Breast budding	Adrenarche	9.8 years
Pubic hair	Adrenarche or Pubarche	10.5 years
Growth spurt	Somatic growth	11.8 years
Axillary hair growth	Thelarche or Pubarche	12.5 years
Uterine bleeding	Menarche	12.8 years

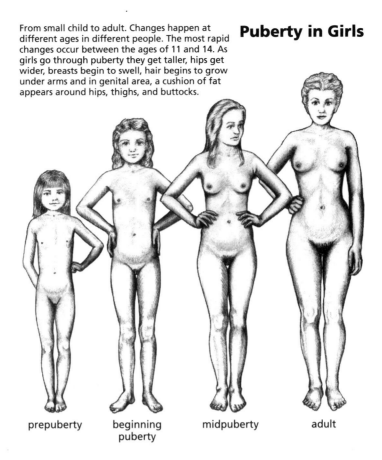

From small child to adult. Changes happen at different ages in different people. The most rapid changes occur between the ages of 11 and 14. As girls go through puberty they get taller, hips get wider, breasts begin to swell, hair begins to grow under arms and in genital area, a cushion of fat appears around hips, thighs, and buttocks.

Puberty in Girls

| prepuberty | beginning puberty | midpuberty | adult |

Northern latitudes, at higher elevations above sea level, in rural areas, and at normal weight. There is fairly good correlation between the time of onset of periods of mothers and daughters and between sisters. And, intriguingly, blind girls experience earlier menarche.

If puberty in a female begins before the age of eight, it is considered to be early, or precocious. On the other hand, if a girl has not begun breast budding by age thirteen, she may be experiencing abnormal sexual development. Also, if she has not begun menstruating by the age of fifteen, she may have some abnormality of sexual growth. Although these ages are not absolute, and a girl who is outside them may be totally normal, chances are that there is a problem.

It normally takes about four and one-half years for a girl to develop from the earliest signs of puberty (usually budding of breasts) to having regular menstrual periods. This time span may range from one and one-half to six years, so a mother or her child should not get upset if the development is progressing slowly. It is important that the mother and child realize that not only the age at which these things occur, but also the pattern may be different from the stated "norm." For example, it is not uncommon for a girl to develop pubic hair before breast budding, and axillary hair may not develop until after a girl has started her menstrual periods. If an adolescent understands that these variations are normal, she may not worry so much if she does not develop at the same rate and in the same way that her friends do.

61 What causes all the changes of puberty in a girl's body?

Research shows that the glands (hypothalamus, pituitary, and ovaries) in the body of a baby girl even before she is born, and certainly after birth, are able to produce the same concentrations of hormones into her body they will later produce when she becomes an adult. Why don't a baby's glands produce adult levels of hormones and cause her to grow breasts and have periods?

There are two reasons for the delay. First, the secretions of hormones by the hypothalamus and pituitary of a female infant and child are extremely sensitive to inhibition by estrogen. This means that even the small amounts of estrogen in an infant girl's body tell the hypothalamus and pituitary that the estrogen level is excessive. This is called inhibition and it shuts down the secretion of hormones from the pituitary and hypothalamus that might otherwise cause a baby's body to develop prematurely.

The second reason for the delay is that there is some type of secondary inhibitory influence on the hypothalamus (as yet undiscovered). This inhibitory influence keeps the hypothalamus from causing the pituitary to put out its hormones that make the ovaries produce eggs and estrogen. This inhibitory influence is referred to as a "central intrinsic inhibitor." Scientists do not know what this "factor" is or where it originates, nor do they know what makes it go away so adolescence can begin.

As Drs. Speroff, Glass, and Kase say in their *Clinical Gynecologic Endocrinology and Infertility* (4th ed., Baltimore: Williams & Wilkins, 1989), "The fascinating search for the factor(s) involved in the depression of the 'gonadostat' so crucial to the timing of puberty continues." This means that we really don't know what makes puberty start when it does. All the glands are mature enough even before a baby is born to produce puberty, but they are repressed until the child's body is mature enough to handle it.

When the hypothalamus (the gland located at the base of the brain that is the master control gland of both the female and male hormones) is allowed to "wake up," the first event of puberty begins. The hypothalamus releases a hormone GnRH (gonadotrophin-releasing hormone), which goes to the pituitary gland (a small grape-shaped gland that hangs off the underside of the hypothalamus) and stimulates it to release the two gonadotrophin hormones FSH (follicle-stimulating hormone) and LH (luteinizing hor-

mone). These hormones are released into the bloodstream, and then go to the ovaries and stimulate them to begin producing estrogen, which initiates the changes of puberty. At first, estrogen causes a growth spurt, then breast budding. Then, increased hormone secretion from both the adrenal glands and the ovaries cause pubic and axillary hair growth. Finally, menstrual periods come. The first few menstrual periods often occur without the young woman producing any eggs (without ovulation). She may then only ovulate about half the time during the first two years of her periods. Regular ovulation comes last in the series of events of puberty.

Drs. Speroff, Glass, and Kase state, "These hormonal changes are correlated with orthologic [physical] changes in the ovary, making coordination of this system one of the most remarkable events in biology." I agree!

---

62   What is the menstrual cycle?

The female menstrual cycle is an astounding integration of hormonal-physical events that occur in all normal women of reproductive age. The primary purpose of this cycle is to enable a woman to become pregnant so the human race can continue. The years of the monthly menstrual cycle are considered to be a woman's "reproductive" years. Normal pregnancy cannot occur except during these years as a result of this cycle.

The interaction of the hormones of a woman's body with her ovaries and the eggs they contain is amazing. But then to see how these function in concert with the breasts, fallopian tubes, uterus, and cervical mucus is even more amazing. Then to understand that this requires a biologic molecular environment to function almost relegates the entire process to the unbelievable—yet it works. I marvel at the creative intelligence of the God who created it.

The menstrual cycle can best be described as a "circle" of events that occurs every month. There are four elements in this "circle." (See diagram below and more complete explanations of each element in following questions.)

                                                                         The Female Body in Change

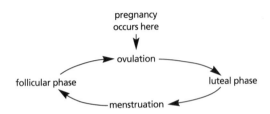

pregnancy occurs here

ovulation

follicular phase

luteal phase

menstruation

1. Follicular phase—the time of the cycle, about fourteen days long, during which the egg is developing in the follicle (small cyst containing an egg) of the ovary. This phase includes most of the days during which the menstrual bleeding occurs, because it is during the menstrual bleeding that development of the next egg begins.

2. Ovulation—the moment at which the egg is released from the follicle of the ovary.

3. Luteal phase—the time following ovulation, about fourteen days long, until the next period arrives or until a period is missed because of pregnancy. During this time the lining of the uterus is becoming better supplied with blood vessels and is getting thicker to support a pregnancy if pregnancy has occurred.

4. Menstruation—uterine bleeding (the period).

The entire process of a woman's reproductive cycle is fascinating. Each ovary contains thousands of eggs. When a female fetus is only twenty weeks along in her mother's uterus, she has more eggs (immature egg cells called oogonia) than she will ever have again in her life—about 6 to 7 million. At birth she has only about 2 million, and at the onset of puberty there are approximately 300,000 eggs left in the ovaries.

Even though a girl has lost 95 percent of her eggs by the time she reaches reproductive age, she still has more eggs than she will ever need in her lifetime. Assuming she will ovulate twelve times a year for, at most, forty-five years, her ovaries will release less than six hundred eggs.

Each egg in a woman's ovaries is contained in a primordial follicle, a unit consisting of one egg surrounded by a single layer of granulosa cells. A portion of the primordial follicles are developing toward maturity constantly, every day, from birth through the end of a woman's reproductive life, even during infancy, while on oral contraceptives, and while pregnant. While some of the follicles and their eggs complete development, most do not. About 8,000 eggs deteriorate each year throughout a woman's life until all the eggs contained in the ovaries die. Menopause starts when all eggs are gone.

The very earliest development of primordial follicles and their eggs is going on all the time and is not related to any type of cycle. Most of these primordial follicles develop only slightly and then die. When FSH is coming from the pituitary, however, it will catch a few of these eggs and their immature follicles at just the right stage of development to make them grow that month. Out of this group of maturing follicles one becomes dominant. While the others die, this one reaches maturity. There are exceptions to this orderly process. Occasionally no good follicles develop and a woman will not ovulate. Sometimes more than one follicle develops to maturity, and this can cause pregnancy with fraternal twins, triplets, etc.

Research has uncovered some interesting facts about a woman's eggs. During the last few weeks before she is born, the egg cells of a female fetus begin a maturing process called meiosis. All eggs (and sperm, in a male fetus) must go through this meiosis.

The first part of meiosis happens to each egg in the girl's body before she is born and then the process stops. No one knows why. All the eggs stay unchanged until just before ovulation. Even when an egg is in a follicle that is developing (later I will explain how a follicle develops), the egg does not reach maturity immediately. It is just along for the ride until about thirty-eight hours before ovulation when the pituitary produces a substance called luteinizing hormone (LH). Now, suddenly, after no change for twelve to as many as fifty years, the egg in the one follicle that is going to mature this particular month starts changing. In the thirty-eight hours before ovulation it begins maturing again and completes the meiotic process so that it will contain only one-half the number of chromosomes of a normal cell.

Menstruation Cycle

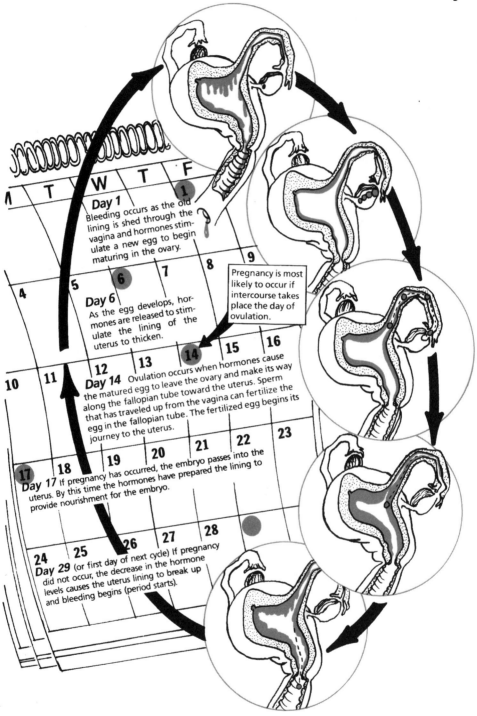

Day 1
Bleeding occurs as the old lining is shed through the vagina and hormones stimulate a new egg to begin maturing in the ovary.

Day 6
As the egg develops, hormones are released to stimulate the lining of the uterus to thicken.

Pregnancy is most likely to occur if intercourse takes place the day of ovulation.

Day 14 Ovulation occurs when hormones cause the matured egg to leave the ovary and make its way along the fallopian tube toward the uterus. Sperm that has traveled up from the vagina can fertilize the egg in the fallopian tube. The fertilized egg begins its journey to the uterus.

Day 17 If pregnancy has occurred, the embryo passes into the uterus. By this time the hormones have prepared the lining to provide nourishment for the embryo.

Day 29 (or first day of next cycle) If pregnancy did not occur, the decrease in the hormone levels causes the uterus lining to break up and bleeding begins (period starts).

All mature human sperm and all mature human eggs have half the number (twenty-three) of chromosomes of all other normal cells in a human body. This happens (as a result of meiosis) so that when a sperm and egg unite (at fertilization), the chromosome combination results in the "right number" (forty-six) of chromosomes in the first complete cell of the new baby's body.

63 What occurs during the follicular phase?

The purpose of the follicular phase is to develop one follicle and one egg (ovum) to maturity and have them ready for ovulation. It takes about fourteen days for this process to be completed.

The process of preparing an egg for ovulation actually starts on the day before the menstrual bleeding begins. At this point the body realizes that a pregnancy did not take place and a new egg must be made ready for release in the next ovulation period.

It is the drop in the female hormones, estrogen and progesterone, that signals the hypothalamus gland to begin another cycle. The hypothalamus then starts production of GnRH (gonadotrophin-releasing hormone). This hormone travels only a short distance in the bloodstream to the pituitary gland, causing it to release the follicle-stimulating hormone (FSH). This FSH travels in the bloodstream to the ovaries where it stimulates the development of an egg. (FSH is the hormone contained in Pergonal, Metrodin, and similar drugs used in many infertility protocols to make a woman's ovaries produce extra eggs.)

During the two weeks of its development, the dominant follicle produces increasing amounts of estrogen and releases it into the woman's body. This estrogen circulates in her bloodstream, flowing into her uterus, stimulating the uterine lining to develop in anticipation of a pregnancy. At the same time the dominant follicle is producing estrogen, it is growing as it fills with more and more fluid.

The dominant follicle (with its egg) that forms on an ovary is normally about three-quarters of an inch in diameter and can get even larger. A doctor can often feel these ovarian enlargements when doing a pelvic exam and may use the term *cyst* in referring to them. Such cysts are not to be confused with the growths and tumors that most women associate with the word. Occasionally an unscrupulous or incompetent doctor will tell a woman that she has an ovarian cyst and will insist that she have immediate surgery to have it removed (implying that it might be cancer), when it may be nothing more than a normal development of the ovary. If you have any reason to question your doctor's intent or ability, you should get a second opinion before you have surgery for an ovarian cyst. Furthermore, most ovarian cysts are normal fluid-filled sacs that will go away on their own and do not require surgery. If they are two to three inches in diameter, are causing pain, have been present for several months, and the ultrasound study looks suspicious, they could be a growth and might require surgery.

64 What occurs during ovulation?

The body's goal with ovulation is to get the mature egg out of the follicle (cyst) so that it can be picked up by the fallopian tube. At the end of the follicular phase, just before ovulation, there is a great deal of estrogen being secreted by the follicle. This high level of estrogen stimulates the pituitary to release a large amount of luteinizing hormone (LH) over a period of a few hours. Ovulation (release of the egg) occurs thirty-eight hours after this surge of LH reaches its peak.

At ovulation the dominant follicle ruptures, releases the egg, and then collapses. It does not die, however. This follicle now becomes a temporary gland called a corpus luteum, which serves a vital part in the reproductive process. It produces progesterone, the hormone that completes the process of preparing the lining of the uterus for pregnancy. Just as was the estrogen, the progesterone also is secreted by the ovary into the bloodstream and is circulated to the uterus to do its preparatory work. The corpus luteum gland is unusual in that it makes not only progesterone but estrogen and androgens (male-type hormones), which are produced in small amounts by ovaries of all normal women.

The process of ovulation begins as the amount of fluid in the follicle increases and the outer wall becomes thin and stretched. Hormones called prostaglandins increase in quantity in the follicle fluid and in some way seem to cause the follicle to rupture; additionally, contractions of muscle cells in the ovary apparently cause the fluid in the follicle and the egg to be squeezed out of the ovary. The rupture of the follicle and release of the egg from the ovary take only a few minutes. (Prostaglandin hormones are such a significant part of ovulation that a woman who is trying to get pregnant should not use drugs at midmonth that would inhibit prostaglandins. These drugs include aspirin, Tylenol, ibuprofen, Advil, Naprosyn, etc.)

When the follicle ruptures, the cystic fluid and the mature egg ooze out of the ovary and are picked up by the fallopian tube. Women frequently have slight bleeding from the ovary upon ovulation. This may cause abdominal pain for a day or two *(Mittelschmerz)*. It is this slight pain that signals to some women the occurrence of ovulation. Rarely does a woman have enough internal bleeding to be a problem, but it can happen. If a woman is having significant pain and seems to be bleeding inside her abdomen, the problem could be a bleeding corpus luteum, a tubal (ectopic) pregnancy, or some other dangerous problem. Because of this, severe pain with signs of internal bleeding often requires an operation. A laparoscopy can usually take care of the problem, but occasionally a large incision is required.

Interestingly, medical scientists have discovered that ovulation occurs most often during the morning hours in the spring and primarily during the evening hours in autumn and winter. From July to February, about 90 percent of women ovulate between 4 and 7 P.M.; in spring, half of women ovulate between midnight and 11 A.M.

65 What happens in the luteal phase?

The goal of the luteal phase is to prepare the lining of the uterus for reception of an impending pregnancy. To accomplish this, the ovary secretes large amounts of progesterone as well as estrogen. Not only does progesterone participate in preparing the uterine lining for implantation of the embryo, but it also does other things—such as suppressing the ovaries to prevent other follicles from developing until after the next period, and decreasing the irritability of the uterus so that it will hold a pregnancy and not squeeze it out.

As the luteal phase begins, the cells that line the inside of the follicle remain after the egg passes out of the follicle. These cells are called granulosa cells. Other cells, called theca-lutein cells, participate in the formation of the corpus luteum. All of these cells are responsible for production of both progesterone and estrogen.

After ovulation the granulosa cells change their appearance, developing a yellowish color. The theca-lutein cells become part of the corpus luteum and begin producing estrogen and progesterone. This production peaks eight days after ovulation and begins declining during the next two or three days if pregnancy does not occur.

If pregnancy occurs, HCG hormone (human chorionic gonadotrophin hormone) is released from the pregnancy tissues into the mother's bloodstream. HCG supports the corpus luteum to prevent its degeneration. The corpus luteum will then go on serving the pregnancy by producing vital hormones until the ninth or tenth week of pregnancy, when the placenta takes over all the production of hormones for maintaining the pregnancy. Then the corpus luteum degenerates.

If pregnancy does not occur, there is no HCG for the corpus luteum to "feed on" and it begins to degenerate, with a subsequent marked decrease in the production of progesterone and estrogen. The corpus luteum will continue to degenerate, and when the degeneration is complete, a menstrual period will start. The luteal phase normally lasts fourteen days from the day of ovulation.

66 What is menstruation and its function?

The goal of menstruation is to rid the uterus of the lining that has been built up during the previous month. This allows the development of a new lining that will be receptive to pregnancy the following month. Usually a menstrual period occurs from every twenty-seven to thirty days during a woman's reproductive life. Since 95 percent of all women menstruate from every twenty-one to every forty-five days, women who are within this range can consider their cycles normal. Menstrual periods occurring outside these boundary ranges may be abnormal and need evaluation.

When the corpus luteum degenerates, it no longer produces estrogen and progesterone; this is what initiates menstruation. When the amounts of these hormones in the bloodstream drop below a certain level, the blood vessels of the inside lining of the uterus go into spasm, stopping the flow of blood to the lining. The lining dies and begins sloughing out. This material is the menstrual "blood." Menstrual flow is made up of both dead tissue, formerly the lining of the inside of the uterus, and blood. Some of the menstrual flow is also fluid that has oozed through the raw surface of the uterine wall when its overlying surface broke down.

When menstrual flow ends, the endometrial lining grows once more, in response to the increasing levels of estrogen that are a result of the next follicular phase of the menstrual cycle. It is at this point, therefore, that the cycle begins all over again, developing another egg, a new lining to the uterus, and the hormonal changes necessary for pregnancy.

Menstruation usually continues for three to six days, but it is also normal for a woman's menstrual bleeding to last only one day or as long as seven or eight days. There is a great deal of individual variation in the amount of blood that is lost during a menstrual period. It is usually from one ounce to three ounces, but it can be more or less than that. If a woman is otherwise normal and is not becoming anemic because of blood lost during menstruation, having a heavy menstrual flow is just an inconvenience, not a danger.

Precocious Puberty

67 What if puberty occurs earlier than is considered normal?

If your daughter develops breasts or pubic hair before the age of eight, or if she begins menstrual bleeding before she is nine, she is starting puberty prematurely. If this happens, you should take her to a physician who specializes in problems of female adolescence. This would normally be a gynecologist, but some pediatricians are both interested and capable in this area of medicine. If a family practitioner or endocrinologist has taken a special interest in this area, he or she too might be appropriate for your daughter to see. A gynecologic endocrinologist would be one expert in this area.

Testing is necessary to make sure there is no life-threatening disease present, and to see if the process going on in your daughter's body is progressing or whether it was only a brief surge of hormone production that has already stopped and does not need to be treated.

In some families, puberty tends to start early, even before the age of eight. The reason for this is not known, but if this tendency toward early puberty has been a "family trait," you might expect your daughter to experience it. Do not worry about it as much as a family who has a child who starts this early when no one else in the family ever has.

68 What is the usual cause of precocious puberty?

In 75 percent of the cases of precocious puberty, the girl's internal time clock simply started the maturing process early. The process is begun in the hypothalamus (the tissue at the base of the brain responsible for starting puberty).

For some unknown reason, the hypothalamus will occasionally begin too-early production of the hormones that lead to full-blown sexual development. This process can start as early as birth and can occur at any age up to the time that normal puberty would start. There have even been rare cases of babies born with breasts who, during their first year of life, began developing pubic hair and menstruation.

69 What treatment should be instituted for precocious puberty when it is caused by the normal maturing process having begun too early?

The primary physical problem with this type of precocious puberty is that the girl will be short when fully grown. The problem does not interfere with reproductive ability and is not associated with premature menopause.

In the past, a drug called medroxyprogesterone acetate (Provera) was used to treat girls with precocious puberty not caused by disease process. This drug worked to slow breast and genital development and to prevent menstrual periods. It was not usually successful in slowing bone growth.

A newer treatment is the use of a drug called GnRH agonist (Lupron, Syneral, and similar drugs). This drug is safe, has almost no side effects, and causes no permanent change to a girl's hormones. It can be given in either injection or nasal spray form.

GnRH agonist suppresses the pituitary and keeps it from secreting gonadotrophins (FSH and LH), the hormones responsible for causing puberty. When it is time for puberty to occur, the drug is stopped and the pituitary is free to start producing FSH and LH again.

Treatment is aimed at delaying the girl's maturity so that she can grow normally and attain the height she would otherwise have reached.

70 What do I need to know about the emotional and social development of a girl with precocious puberty?

Girls who have precocious puberty or early normal puberty not only require adequate medical care, but they and their families need emotional support. They are children of only eight or nine who have developed breasts, pubic hair, and menstrual periods. They must use deodorants and protection for menstrual bleeding and wear bras. Such young girls can develop some of the emotional characteristics of teenagers, such as irritability, strained relations with parents, and poor self-image. Proper counsel can help parents and children cope with all this.

These children are not "little adults" just because they have sexual development. They do not want or need early sexual activity; they do not have abnormal sexual libido. It is important that parents, teachers, and friends interact with them as the young children that they are.

71 What might cause partial sexual maturation prior to the age of eight?

It is fairly common for a girl to experience sudden growth in one or both breasts, to develop some pubic hair, or to have a few episodes of bleeding from the uterus. When this occurs, and it is not followed by continued maturation of the sexual organs, the girl does not have true precocious puberty. She has experienced only a brief, temporary outpouring of sexual hormones, and such a situation happens frequently enough that it can almost be considered normal. Girls who have this temporary sexual development (partial sexual maturation) usually do start their true puberty earlier than other girls their age.

Why this brief surge of hormones occurs is a mystery. It could be that the girls who experience this do not have mature enough hormone systems at the time to progress to normal function. It is also possible that the girl has gotten into some estrogen tablets or birth-control pills and this estrogen has caused her symptoms. Such drug intake can be suspected if the girl's nipples and areolae have developed dark pigmentation. If this is what has happened, the girl would not need medical evaluation or treatment, since taking hormones for a short time would not hurt her or make her body start true puberty early.

Delayed Puberty

72 What should be done if my daughter's puberty seems to be abnormally delayed?

If your daughter has had absolutely no breast development, even breast budding, by the age of thirteen, or if she has not started her menstrual periods by the time she is fifteen, she may have a developmental problem. She probably needs to be examined by a physician. Since the variation in the onset of puberty is so great, however, your daughter's apparently delayed puberty may be totally normal.

Only 1 percent of all girls will not have started their periods by age eighteen or will not have had at least some breast budding by the age of thirteen. Any adolescent who lacks these signs of puberty probably has a medical problem and definitely needs to be evaluated by a physician.

If your daughter has this kind of delayed puberty and your doctor continues to tell you that she is normal and does not need an examination, he or she is obviously not familiar with this type of problem. You should find another physician who can be more helpful—an endocrinologist or a gynecologist who is interested in adolescent gynecology.

73 What causes delayed puberty?

The basic problem in this situation is that the girl's ovaries are not producing the estrogen necessary for the development of breasts and the initiation of menstrual periods. The lack of estrogen may be due to defective ovaries or to some other abnormal body function.

Hormone "time clock" set late. In this case the girl is normal in every way except that her hormonal functioning has not started as early as that of most of her friends. If all her tests are normal, including a pelvic examination, she can be assured that she is normal. She will begin puberty

and periods later on, and she will be as capable of having children as any other normal woman.

Abnormal ovaries. If a girl's ovaries are so abnormal that they cannot produce estrogen, she will not develop puberty. The most common cause of this is a condition called Turner's syndrome (see Q. 53), in which the girl has abnormal chromosomes. There are other, less common reasons for abnormal ovarian function. She may have no ovaries, for example. Most of these problems would not only keep a girl from experiencing puberty but would also prevent her from being able to become pregnant.

An ovarian problem that is not so severe but can prevent the onset of menstruation is polycystic ovarian syndrome (see Q. 830–833).

Finally, ovarian failure (premature menopause) can prevent the onset of periods. Patients with premature ovarian failure will usually, but not always, have a few periods before they cease all menstruation. (I have had one patient whose ovaries failed before she was twenty years old.)

Disease or health problems not located in the sex organs. Nutrition problems and disease in the rest of the body can affect the physiology so traumatically that the female organs are affected and will not begin functioning properly. An example of this is the poor nutrition produced by anorexia nervosa (see Q. 117) or by some intestinal diseases that prevent absorption of nutrients from the intestinal tract. In this situation a girl will probably not develop the onset of menses until these problems have been eliminated.

Diseases of the brain and of the base of the brain (hypothalamus) or of the pituitary gland can prevent the production of hormones necessary for initiating puberty, as can thyroid and adrenal disease.

Congenital abnormalities. Female babies can be born normal in every way except without a vagina or uterus, or with a uterus that has no opening, or with some other similar problem. These girls will develop normal secondary sexual characteristics (breast development, pubic hair, hair under the arms) but will not start menstrual bleeding.

74 What is involved in a medical evaluation for delayed puberty?

An evaluation for a girl who has delayed puberty (no breast development by thirteen, no menstrual periods by fifteen) includes the following steps.

The physician will want to know when menstrual periods began among other female family members, since mothers and daughters tend to start their periods around the same age. He or she will also ask about how much stress the girl is under, what kind of diet she has, whether she might be abusing drugs, whether or not she is having sexual intercourse (pregnancy can occur before the first period).

Next will probably be a complete examination, including the breasts and pelvic area. For an adequate exam of her pelvis, a laparoscopy may be necessary. (See Q. 810 for a description of this procedure.) The doctor will want to examine your daughter neurologically, which includes checking her reflexes and visual fields, and may also want to order an EEG and skull X-ray or a CT scan or MRI of the brain.

75 What treatment is advised for delayed puberty?

First, it is important that a girl have an adequate evaluation so that the cause of the delayed puberty can be diagnosed. The treatment depends on the problem. If she does not have a normally developed vagina and uterus, surgery may be necessary. (Q. 46–51 discuss this problem.)

If a girl has a medical problem, such as thyroid or adrenal gland disease, this would need to be treated.

If the problem is ovarian failure or ovaries that will not produce enough estrogen to initiate periods, she will need to be given estrogen. This should be discussed with a doctor who is competent in such treatment.

Finally, if a girl merely has a "time clock" that is set late, which means that all her other tests are normal, she can await the onset of her menstrual period for another two or three years.

The best course during this time is for the girl to continue seeing her physician each year to make sure some abnormality is not developing that was not detected in the initial evaluation.

It may also be wise for the girl to begin taking estrogen so that her development and her periods will start and she does not feel "abnormal."

Breast Development in the Adolescent

76 My daughter's breasts are developing, but one is much larger than the other. Is this normal?

No woman's breasts are totally symmetrical. In fact, you may have noticed that your own breasts are somewhat different in size and shape. This normal asymmetry between breasts is much exaggerated during the time that breasts are growing. (See Q. 26–27.)

If a girl has grown to maturity and her breasts are different enough in size to bother her, she can have augmentation of the smaller breast done to bring it up to the size of the larger breast, or reduction done on the larger breast. More simply, though, she can wear a bra with padding on one side.

77 Is it necessary that my daughter wear a bra?

There are two considerations about wearing bras.

As a girl's breasts are developing, she may or may not want to wear a bra. If her friends are wearing them, it is probably best to let her wear one even before she really needs it. Some girls are embarrassed if their developing nipples show through their T-shirts, and they want to wear a bra to cover them. If your daughter's nipples are quite noticeable, and you feel it is appropriate, mention this to your daughter even if she has not said anything. She may be too embarrassed to mention it herself.

Second, when a woman's breasts develop to

Stages of Breast Development

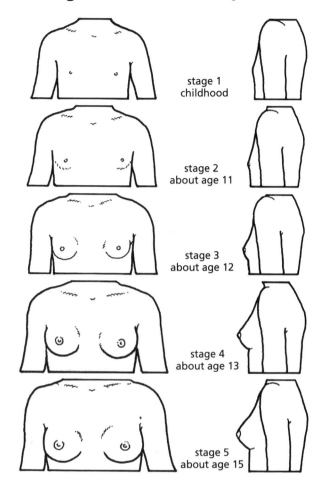

stage 1
childhood

stage 2
about age 11

stage 3
about age 12

stage 4
about age 13

stage 5
about age 15

Breast Changes of Puberty

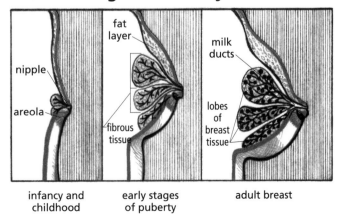

fat
layer

milk
ducts

nipple

areola

fibrous
tissue

lobes
of
breast
tissue

infancy and
childhood

early stages
of puberty

adult breast

their mature size, gravity starts pulling them down. Through the years this pull stretches the supporting ligaments and causes breasts to sag. Because of this physicians often encourage women to wear a bra for support. Women who have breast tenderness and women with heavy breasts often feel more comfortable wearing a bra. There is no real medical reason otherwise, however, for a girl or woman to wear a bra.

Menstrual Irregularities in Adolescence

78 My daughter has begun her periods, but they are irregular. Should anything be done?

One of the most common problems with girls going through puberty is irregular bleeding. About half of all girls will have irregular periods during the first twelve months after starting their menses because they do not ovulate every month. In fact, it may take eight or ten years before a girl's menstrual regularity is fully established.

If a girl's menstrual periods are heavy, overly long, infrequent, or irregular the first few years, there is probably nothing to worry about. If, however, you or your daughter feel that her menstruation is too abnormal or is too inconvenient, you should call your doctor and ask if an office visit is warranted.

79 Which patterns of menstrual bleeding are in the normal range? Which are not?

Patterns of menstrual bleeding that are considered normal, and about which you do not need to worry, are the following:

Periods that come as often as twenty-one days, or periods that come as infrequently as six weeks.

Periods that last only one or two days, or periods that last up to six or eight days.

Bleeding that is very light, or bleeding that is fairly heavy (six or eight soaked pads a day).

Bleeding patterns about which you would probably need consultation include the following:

Bleeding or spotting that occurs on a daily or almost-daily basis, or periods that come only every three or four months after the girl has been menstruating a year or more.

Bleeding that lasts more than six or eight days with every period.

Heavy bleeding (more than six or eight well-soaked pads a day), especially if the child seems to be getting unusually weak or tired.

80 What can cause irregular periods?

The usual cause of adolescent menstrual irregularities during the first few years is irregular ovulation. The probable reason for this is the immaturity of the hormone system. Just as the rest of the body takes a while to mature, so does the hormone system. When it matures and if the girl begins ovulation regularly, her periods will almost always become regular.

There are other conditions of the teenage body that can increase the chance of a girl's having irregular periods. Some of these are:

Dieting. A young girl can delay the establishment of regular ovulation by starting and maintaining a rigid reducing diet. Anorexia or bulimia can cause irregular menses or no menses.

Obesity. It is fairly common for a teenager to gain a good deal of weight around the time of puberty. This extra fat generates extra estrogen in her body, which can cause excessive buildup of the uterine lining, producing irregular spotting and bleeding.

Exercise. Vigorous exercise can affect a young woman's ovulation. If she has not yet developed regular ovulatory patterns and she begins exercising vigorously, she may have irregular bleeding and spotting.

Stress. It is fairly common for young women to skip periods in times of stress. I have had several patients, students at the University of Texas, who would have three normal periods during the summer and no periods during the nine months they were in school. The only explanation found was that the stress of school was preventing them from having periods.

Medical Problems. Some medical disorders can cause a girl to have abnormal or irregular vaginal bleeding. These include problems of the hormonal system, which can cause abnormal production of hormones from the pituitary, the thyroid, or the adrenal gland; blood-clotting abnormalities, which would be suspected if the girl's first period is frighteningly heavy; bleeding from an unsuspected pregnancy; growths in the uterus or vagina; and other, more unusual medical problems, such as TB or nephritis.

---

81 What can be done about irregular or abnormal bleeding?

After the doctor has discussed the girl's bleeding pattern, he or she will examine her. This exam can discover or rule out some things that can cause abnormal bleeding, such as tumors and growths.

The doctor will probably want a blood count to make certain the girl is not anemic, especially if she has a pattern of excessive bleeding. Other blood tests may be required if the doctor suspects hormonal abnormalities or other medical problems. If they are ordered at the same time, blood for all required tests can often be drawn at once.

The problem that will usually be found is that ovulation is not taking place regularly. In spite of irregular ovulation, the ovaries continue to put out estrogen every day, and this estrogen can stimulate the lining of the uterus to thicken. If ovulation does not take place, the lining of the uterus gets thicker and thicker. Areas of it finally outgrow their blood supply and start sloughing out, producing irregular bleeding patterns. In a woman who ovulates regularly, the ovary starts releasing

progesterone into the body at the moment of ovulation. This progesterone changes the lining of the uterus so that two weeks after ovulation the entire lining will shed at one time—a normal period.

Theoretically, all an otherwise normal girl needs to have regular periods is production of estrogen from her ovaries most of the month and adequate progesterone in her body ten to fourteen days each month. Whether this progesterone comes from her own ovulation or from progesterone pills does not matter to the uterus.

If your daughter's bleeding is caused by irregular ovulation, a common symptom in young women, the doctor may prescribe progesterone, often given in the pill Provera, to establish regular bleeding. This is fine in theory, but I have found that Provera often does not produce consistently good periods. Girls on Provera often have long periods or will bleed between periods.

Birth-control pills may be required to establish regular periods. They seem to contain the best balance of hormones for controlling a girl's periods. They also are a very safe medication.

I always question a girl, however, before prescribing birth-control pills. If she indicates to me that being on them might make her more likely to have premarital sex, I encourage the use of Provera instead. (See Q. 116 regarding the use of birth-control pills by young women.)

---

82 Is it normal for my daughter to have severe cramps? Is it normal for her to have no cramps?

Yes, both are normal. It is also normal for her to have mild or more moderately severe cramps. One of the most common reasons for a young woman in her teenage years to see a gynecologist is because she has severe cramps. Generally, the girl's mother will be afraid that her daughter has endometriosis (see Q. 851). Though endometriosis rarely is the cause of severe cramps in a young woman, I do think it is good for a girl with severe cramps to be examined to make sure she does not have this problem.

Most of the time menstrual cramping, or dysmenorrhea, is a result of the normal function of the girl's body. This normal cramping is called "primary dysmenorrhea." "Secondary dysmenorrhea" is cramping caused by physical abnormalities, such as a cervical opening that is too small to let menstrual blood out, abnormality of the uterus, or endometriosis. Most menstrual cramping, however, is primary dysmenorrhea.

The changes in a girl's body that cause primary dysmenorrhea are probably due to the following sequence of events:

1. Secretion of progesterone from the ovaries starts as soon as ovulation occurs, and it continues until the menstrual period begins.
2. When the ovarian progesterone production stops, the breakdown of the endometrium starts, seen as menstrual flow.
3. The degenerating lining of the uterus then begins releasing prostaglandin hormones into the bloodstream. Prostaglandins are hormones normally produced by the inside lining of the uterus (endometrium) during the time of the period (they are also produced by other tissues in the body at other times).
4. Prostaglandins cause menstrual cramps. Research physicians who injected pure prostaglandins into women found that all the symptoms of menstrual cramps resulted: uterine cramping, diarrhea, vomiting, headache, irritability, difficulty with concentration, and dizziness.

The prostaglandins produce uterine pain by causing the uterus to contract just as it does when a woman is in labor. Such contractions come and go. During a contraction blood circulation through the uterus is slowed to a trickle. This lack of circulation deprives the uterine muscle of oxygen, causing it to hurt. This pain is sensed as cramping.

Pressure measurements of contractions during a period in some women have been found to be as high or even higher than similar measurements done on women in labor. If you know someone who has severe cramps with her periods, show compassion; she is in real pain.

As mentioned, prostaglandins can affect various other body organs. For instance, they can affect the colon and cause diarrhea, or they can affect the brain and decrease the ability to concentrate. If a young woman has these symptoms and they are severe, she should see a doctor to be sure that no abnormality of her female organs is producing secondary dysmenorrhea. If she is normal on exam, she can be fairly sure that her bad cramps are a result of the normal functioning of her body.

If a girl's cramping is not due to a medical problem, it is safe to treat with pain pills. If this does not give adequate relief, birth-control pills can be used. They are often the most effective treatment, being safe and relatively inexpensive. I do recommend their use for severe dysmenorrhea. Generally young women feel well when they take oral contraceptives.

If cramps are severe and unrelenting and treatment does not help, further diagnosis may be necessary, even if the pelvic exam is normal. A diagnostic laparoscopy (see Q. 810) will occasionally be necessary. It is possible for a physician using the laparoscope to cut the uterosacral ligaments that carry nerves into the uterus and/or the presacral nerves or to perform a sacral neurectomy. Have these procedures done only by a doctor who is familiar with the technique, and remember that these work only about half the time.

Childbirth is not more painful for a girl or woman who has severe dysmenorrhea. There is no relationship between the pain of menstrual periods and the discomfort of childbirth. Also, if a girl or woman does not have endometriosis and her pelvis is normal, severe cramps will not interfere with her future fertility.

83 What can be done about dysmenorrhea?

There are several methods of treatment available. (See Q. 678 for discussion.)

84 What can be done about heavy menstrual bleeding?

If a girl has very heavy menstrual periods, birth-control pills are the best treatment. They are safe, relatively inexpensive, and usually very effective.

For one very heavy bleeding episode that is getting dangerous, estrogen injections every four hours may be needed. These injections will usually stop heavy bleeding within twelve to twenty-four hours.

If very heavy bleeding persists, Amicar, a drug not often used in the United States, might be used. This drug can occasionally be effective in stopping life-threatening uterine bleeding that might otherwise require a hysterectomy.

A dilatation and curettage (D&C) may stop bleeding, although doctors ordinarily do not like to do this procedure on young women. It is usually not particularly effective in stopping menstrual bleeding, and it is certainly better if drugs can be used for such bleeding in a young woman. If a young woman is having bleeding this severe, she needs evaluation by a specialist for problems such as a blood-clotting abnormality. (See the discussion about bleeding and D&Cs in Q. 673, 698–699, 702–705.)

If a girl is having heavy periods, or if she has had an episode of heavy bleeding that needs treatment as suggested above, it is important that she take an iron supplement. Most teenagers do not get enough iron in their diets, and taking a supplement will help prevent anemia. An inexpensive, one-a-day iron pill is all that is necessary.

Special Health Considerations during Adolescence

85 Will menstrual periods affect athletic performance of young women? Is it safe to exercise?

Dr. Quadagno and his associates reported in *Physician and Sports Medicine* (March 1991, 19:121) that though many women and their coaches think that athletic performance is worse during menstrual periods or at some time before menstrual periods, studies show that a woman's athletic performance is not affected by the menstrual cycle. Studies in weight lifting and in sprint-swimming speed were conducted during various phases of the menstrual cycle. No difference in performance was identifiable. It is not unhealthy for a woman to exercise, including swimming, during her period.

86 When should a girl start having pelvic examinations?

A young woman should start having annual examinations when any of the following occur:

There is a problem with, or question about, her female organs
She becomes sexually active
She is going to be married
She is in her late teens or early twenties, even if none of the other situations apply (just a routine exam)

Most young women are nervous about their first examination. This is normal. If your child is nervous before the exam, she should talk to the doctor so he or she can reassure her. The doctor can tell how the exam is done, how long it will take, and that it will not hurt much. It certainly is not a comfortable exam, but it should not entail more than just a little discomfort. If the pain bothers a patient too much, the doctor can and should stop. If the hymen is too tight, a first-time exam can be completed with the patient under a general anesthesia to dilate the hymen just a little bit to allow an easier examination. This can be done as an outpatient procedure.

In the chapter on reproductive health I discuss exactly how the examination is done.

87 Are tampons safe, especially for young women?

Most doctors feel that tampons are the best technique for handling menstrual flow for both adolescents and older women. This is especially true in hot, humid climates, since external pads can cause the retention of moisture and heat around the vulva, increasing the chance of vulvar irritation and infection.

Tampons have the following advantages over external protection (see also Q. 597):

Better vulvar hygiene. As mentioned above, they keep the vulva from retaining moisture and warmth.

Greater freedom. A woman can swim, exercise, and so on, more conveniently and confidently when using tampons.

Better body knowledge. A girl who uses tampons is quite familiar with the location of her vaginal opening; she also knows how deep her vagina is and what direction in her body it takes. This knowledge and familiarity makes a young woman's first pelvic exam easier and initial intercourse less frightening.

Detection of hymenal abnormalities. If a girl cannot insert a tampon, she knows that something may be wrong. By trying to use tampons, she could, therefore, detect an abnormality of the hymen, see a doctor, and have it treated before it would become a problem with intercourse after she is married.

Tampons have the following disadvantages:

Vaginal ulceration. Occasionally vaginal ulcers can result from improper tampon insertion. Women are not normally aware that this has occurred and learn of it only when they have abnormal vaginal bleeding or during a routine examination by a doctor. This problem is easily resolved by not using tampons for a while until the ulcer heals and then, when resuming tampon use, changing the method of insertion. (This is a rare problem.)

Toxic shock. Although associated with the use of tampons, toxic shock also occurs in women who have never used tampons and has even occurred in men. Most gynecologists feel that it is safe for a girl or woman to use tampons. However, if a girl is particularly worried about toxic shock but wants to use tampons occasionally, she may use them during the day and use pads at night, or use pads and tampons alternately. Toxic shock is infrequent, and most doctors feel that the possibility of toxic shock does not warrant discontinuing tampon use. (See Q. 630–631 for more on toxic shock.)

88 My daughter has grown an excessive amount of body hair. Why has this happened, and what can be done about it?

Most girls who have more hair growth than they think they should have, or who have hair on parts of their bodies where they do not want it, are still "normal." Because such hair growth is often embarrassing to a teenage girl, she is often convinced that it is abnormal. Roughly 90 percent of patients who consider their hair growth excessive have that heavy hair growth either because it is a family characteristic or because it is their own personal body pattern.

One fairly reliable guide is that if a girl has heavier-than-average hair growth but normal menstrual periods, her hair growth is probably "normal" for her and is not due to an abnormality or disease. In spite of this, if you or your daughter think that she has an abnormal amount of hair, or that she has excessive hair growth in areas where she should not have it, you should take her to a physician for evaluation.

89 What hair growth is considered normal?

Hair growth on the upper lip, the sides of the face, around the nipples, and from the pubic hair up to the umbilicus (navel) is normal as long as it is not excessive. A girl can compare her hair growth with that of other members of her family. If her mother or father or other members of the family have heavy hair growth, her hair-growth pattern is probably inherited.

If a female of any age has a sudden increase in hair growth, she should see her doctor for evaluation. It could indicate a medical problem.

90 What abnormalities can cause excessive hair growth?

There are at least five abnormalities that may cause excessive hair growth (hirsutism). If the physician is concerned, he/she may want to test your daughter for these:

Ovarian abnormalities. The most common hormonal abnormality causing excessive hair growth is the "polycystic ovarian syndrome." (See Q. 830–831.) This condition is not dangerous, but in addition to producing hair-growth problems and irregular periods, it can cause some fertility difficulties. About 70 percent of women with very irregular periods develop excessive hair growth because of the hormone imbalance related to polycystic ovaries. Tumors of the ovary can cause production of increased amounts of male-type hormones, but this is rare.

Adrenal gland abnormalities. Excessive production of hormones by the adrenal glands can cause hirsutism. This is caused by overactivity of the adrenal glands or by a tumor in these glands.

Thyroid abnormalities. Hypothyroidism (low thyroid) can cause excessive hair growth. This growth is usually on the upper lip and on the back.

Drugs. Male hormones, anabolic drugs unwisely taken for body building, some synthetic female hormones, and Dilantin can cause increased hair growth on a woman's body.

Anorexia nervosa. This condition has various effects on a young woman's body, one of which is excessive hair growth. (See Q. 117.)

Other. Chromosome abnormalities. One example is testicular feminization.

91 How is excessive hair growth treated?

The first step in the treatment of excess body hair is to take care of any existing medical problem.

Abnormal ovarian function. Use of birth-control pills will suppress the ovaries' production of male-type hormones (androgens). Other drugs may also be used along with contraceptives to provide the best control of hair growth. Since this problem is usually a result of polycystic ovaries, which also results in irregular periods, birth-control pills are a perfect treatment. They will cause the periods to be regular and also slow the growth of hair.

If the ovarian problem is due to a tumor, that tumor will need to be removed by major surgery. (See Q. 722–755 for a complete discussion of ovarian problems.)

Adrenal disease. If the adrenal glands are overactive, they must be treated with medication to suppress their activity. If the adrenal problem is caused by a tumor, that tumor will need to be surgically removed.

Thyroid disease. If the thyroid is underactive, thyroid medication should be administered.

Drugs. If the young woman is developing excessive hair growth because of Dilantin, her doctor may be able to find a substitute anticonvulsant for her. Other drugs that can cause hirsutism, such as male-hormone medications and anabolics, should not be taken by young women unless there is some unusual medical problem that makes such drugs necessary.

Treatment of this type of hair growth is complicated by the fact that once it has occurred, treatment of the disease that caused it rarely results in lessening of the hair growth already developed. Treatment can prevent the growth from becoming worse, however, and this is the main reason for seeing a doctor as quickly as possible if a problem is suspected.

Though treatment of the disease that caused the hair may not make the hair growth better, there are some techniques to directly treat the hair and make it better.

Birth-control pills should be taken if possible; if not, medroxyprogesterone acetate (Provera 150 mg) can be used. This is given as an intramuscular injection every three months.

A drug called spironolactone can be taken along with birth-control pills or Provera. The combination can be very effective in decreasing hair. This can be started at 200 mg once a day, and possibly lowered to 25–50 mg a day. Other drugs such as cimetidine sometimes help.

If a girl or woman is dissatisfied with the amount of hair that remains after twelve months of treatment with oral contraceptives or medroxyprogesterone acetate and spironolactone, she can add electrolysis to the regime. Electrolysis is a medically sound method of removing unwanted hair. Many people dismiss the use of electrolysis because of its reputed expense and discomfort. However, over a period of time electrolysis can be quite effective, and it is not very uncomfortable. Its expense and discomfort are almost always worth the good results that are usually produced.

If your doctor does not outline a plan for both treatment of the underlying problem and decreasing the hair, you may need to see an endocrinologist.

92 My husband and I are tall and our daughter is afraid she is going to be "too tall." Is there anything we can do to prevent this?

It is possible to predict fairly accurately a person's height as an adult. This can be done with a set of tables called "Bayley-Pinneau Tables for Girls." It will be necessary for the doctor to take an X-ray of your daughter's hand and wrist for bone age to determine which set of tables to use.

If your doctor is unfamiliar with Bayley-Pinneau tables for height prediction, he or she can find them on page 432 in the book, *Clinical Gynecologic Endocrinology and Infertility,* 4th ed., by Leon Speroff, Robert H. Glass, and Nathan G. Kase (Baltimore: Williams & Wilkins, 1989).

Whether or not to treat a girl for this predicted height attainment is primarily up to the parents, because treatment must be started *before* she begins her menstrual periods for it to be successful. At this young age, most girls would not be able to participate knowledgeably in the decision. "Late" treatment, begun after the menses have started, may be able to eliminate up to one inch of growth, however.

The treatment is safe. It consists of the use of estrogen tablets taken by mouth. This hormone treatment will cause regular periods but will stimulate the bones to complete their growth and the bones' growth centers to close, preventing the girl's height from attaining its predicted level. If your gynecologist is uncomfortable with this therapy, you may want to take your daughter to a gynecologic endocrinologist for consultation.

93 Can tumors of the female organs develop in children and teenagers?

Although they are rare, tumors do develop in young people, and both parents and physicians should be alert to this.

Since almost half of the pelvic tumors discovered in children have the possibility of being malignant, it is important that such tumors be discovered early. It is unfortunate that parents and doctors often discount the probability of a pelvic tumor in an adolescent. Any time a girl develops any of the warning symptoms listed by the American Cancer Society, it is important that she be taken to a doctor for examination. (You can get a list of these warning signs by calling your local American Cancer Society or by calling the National Cancer Institute at [800]-4-CANCER.)

In addition, if a girl develops abdominal swelling or pain, or even abdominal fullness or discomfort, she should be taken to a doctor for evaluation. The same advice applies if a girl has vaginal discharge or passes blood erratically from her vagina, or if she has an ulcer or a sore around the opening of her vagina or on her labia. As previously mentioned, if your daughter shows signs of sexual maturation before the age of eight, she should also see a physician. (See Q. 67–71.)

Tumors of the female organs are rare in children, especially those below the age of sixteen, but almost any type of tumor seen in adults can also occur in children. Tumors, benign and malignant, can develop in the vagina, on the cervix, in the uterus, and in the tubes and ovaries. Ovarian tumors are the most common tumors to develop in a girl sixteen years or younger. For more information on these tumors, see chapter 10.

94 What type of female-organ infections can an adolescent develop?

From puberty on, a girl may have the same genital infections as an adult woman. These infections are diagnosed and treated the same way as in an adult.

If an adolescent girl has vaginal discharge and itching, she needs to see a gynecologist or a knowledgeable physician to have the problem diagnosed and treated. If she has had intercourse and has developed symptoms that might be due to a sexually transmitted disease, she will also need to consult a physician. A young girl is more susceptible to sexually transmitted disease than an adult. If an adolescent is sexually active, she should also have an annual Pap smear. For a complete discussion of sexually transmitted diseases, see chapter 13.

95 Is it harmful for my daughter to masturbate? Should I encourage her to masturbate as a means of releasing sexual tension?

Masturbation does not produce any physical damage to a person's body. It does not cause warts, insanity, loss of hair, infertility, or blindness.

Masturbation can cause anxiety on the part of both children and parents. If you know that your daughter is masturbating, reassure her that it will not damage her body physically and also that she is not perverted or evil for having done so. However, if she is involved in pornography or is compulsively masturbating, she may have an emotional problem. This could even be a sign that she has been sexually abused. If these problems seem present, she needs to see a counselor for evaluation. I would not suggest masturbation to my child as a means of relieving sexual tension. It is probably better for her to expend her energies in sports, school, etc.

One of the best statements that I have read concerning teenage masturbation was written by Dr. James Dobson in his book, *Preparing for Adolescence* (Ventura, Calif.: Vision House, 1978). He states (pp. 86–87):

> Unfortunately, I can't speak directly for God on this subject, since His Holy Word, the Bible, is silent at this point. I will tell you what I *believe*, although I certainly do not want to contradict what your parents or your pastor believe. It is my *opinion* that masturbation is not much of an issue with God. It is a normal part of adolescence which involves no one else. It does not cause disease, it does not produce babies, and Jesus did not mention it in the Bible. I am not telling you to masturbate, and I hope you won't feel the need for it. But if you do, it is my opinion that you should not struggle with guilt over it.

96 I think my daughter is lesbian. What should I do about that?

If you have reason to believe your daughter is homosexual, I suggest that you first go to a counselor alone. A very important reason for you to aggressively investigate this possibility is that a recent report stated one-third of teenagers who think they might be homosexual will attempt suicide. Obviously all youngsters who have questions about their sexual orientation have tremendous anxiety.

Choose a counselor with extreme care. You will want a counselor who is knowledgeable, has good suggestions, and agrees with your moral values. Then you can leave your daughter in the privacy of the counselor's office with confidence. Appropriate counseling at this fragile time in your daughter's life can spare her tremendous unhappiness in the future. It can also help develop a healthy relationship between parent and child as well as wholesome future adult relationships. Remember that in the early adolescent years it is normal for both boys and girls to develop very close relationships with children of the same sex. Children need reassurance that this is normal and in no way means they are homosexual or lesbian.

There is absolutely no reliable scientific evidence that a female is born genetically as a lesbian. Homosexual orientation seems to be psychological, not physical. Also, since lesbian sex can lead to infection with sexually transmitted disease, it would be well to encourage sexual abstinence for an adolescent who feels that she is homosexual.

Sexual Molestation and Abuse

97 What should I tell my daughter about rape and sexual molestation?

The discussion you have with your daughter depends on her age. It is best to bring up this subject when the child is small and continue to add to her knowledge in this area as she matures. As you talk to your daughter, remember that 85 percent of episodes of child sexual abuse are committed by someone whom the child knows and trusts. Such persons include relatives, baby-sitters, or family friends. It is uncommon for child sexual abuse to be forcible and violent and it often does not even include vaginal or oral penetration. It is much more likely to be subtle, with no physical force, partly because child sexual abuse often develops gradually over a long period of time. Though it may be subtle and not include penetration, the damage it can do to a child's future emotional development is enormous (see Q. 99).

The following suggestions may help with your discussion of this topic with your child:

1. Teach your child a sexual vocabulary, so that she will know what area of her body you are referring to when you talk about sexual contact.
2. Reassure her that her body is her own and that no one has a right to touch it or handle it except herself, parents, medical personnel, or her husband when she is married.
3. Teach your child that her feelings count. If someone talks to her or touches her in a way that makes her uncomfortable, she should realize that her discomfort is legitimate and that she should tell you about it.
4. Teach your child that she has a right to and should say no. Often children feel that they must do what adults tell them to do. Children should be taught that they should not allow adults to take advantage of them.
5. Explain to your child that if someone tries to touch her genitalia or wants her to look at or touch his or her genitalia, she should say no and run away as fast as she can.
6. Teach your child to tell someone about any unsettling experience. A most important part of a child's avoiding a problem of sexual abuse is to know that it is okay to talk to a trusted adult. She should know that she can talk to you, a relative, a teacher at school, her minister, or her Sunday school teacher, and be believed. Help your child develop sound relationships with people she can

trust so that she can feel free to talk to them about personal matters.
7. Be sure she knows that you will protect her from such undesired, immoral, and uncomfortable episodes.

By forewarning your child about such things, she will be reassured that you are not afraid or ashamed to talk about these matters and that she should not be either. This type of discussion also allows the child to have a ready answer to someone who tries to fondle or otherwise abuse her sexually. Remember that indecent exposure is also sexual abuse. Your child should be warned about this form of harassment.

The most important aspect of the situation is that your child be reassured that if someone has already abused her sexually, or is currently abusing her, she is free to talk to you about it and you will believe her and be supportive. Emotionally healthy children are unlikely to lie about being sexually abused. If your child tells you that this is going on, believe her and contact someone to help you decide what to do, even if a loved one or close friend is implicated.

This is a good life lesson for her to learn. Unfortunately she could become a battered woman in later years. This could happen before she is married or in marriage. You can help her learn now that if this happens there is always someone she can turn to for help and that it is never appropriate for a male to hurt her physically and usually not appropriate for him to hurt her emotionally. If, however, you or your daughter do need to talk to someone in regard to being a battered woman, a hotline is available at (800) 799-7233.

98 How widespread is the problem of sexual victimization of children and adolescents?

Sexual abuse can involve rape, sodomy, oral sex, exhibitionism, fondling, masturbation, intercourse, or physical injury. Often the activity involved is "dry intercourse" in which there is no penetration of anus or vagina but rather a rubbing of the attacker's penis between the thighs and against the anus of the victim, who of course cannot tell whether or not penetration was involved. No physical mark is left and the victim is therefore thought to be lying about being abused.

According to the Texas Department of Human Resources, one person out of four experiences some degree of sexual abuse in his or her lifetime. Girls are victims 90 percent of the time. Other studies show that at least one in seven women has been approached sexually by an older male at some point during their childhood or adolescent years, and that only one in ten girls who are sexually abused ever report it to authorities. The Centers for Disease Control has shown that 20 percent of college coeds have experienced forced sexual intercourse.

To a significant extent child sexual abuse does involve middle-class Americans. It is quite common for the adults involved to be highly respected citizens.

99 What effect does sexual abuse have on its victims?

The effect of sexual victimization on the physical and emotional health of its victims is inestimable. Of course, girls who have started their menstrual periods may become pregnant as a result, and they are subject to contracting sexually transmitted diseases. The emotional effects of sexual abuse, however, can be even more devastating. A woman's memory of sexual abuse as a child can make it extremely difficult for her to adjust sexually in marriage. In addition, since it is so often a person the child trusts who inflicts the abuse, the victim may feel that there will never be anyone in the world she can ever trust again. This belief not only colors her relationships with other people but may also affect her relationship with God.

It is appropriate here to point out to any person who is abusing a child or who is contemplating initiating such abuse that harming a child is dealt with quite strongly in Scripture: "But whoso shall offend one of these little ones which believe in me, it were better for him that a millstone were hanged about his neck, and that he were drowned in the depth of the sea. Woe unto the world because of offenses!" (spoken by Jesus, as recorded in Matt. 18:6–7 KJV).

Another effect of sexual victimization is that as the victims grow older, they may experience unwarranted guilt, thinking that they were responsible in some way for having been molested. This creates self-doubt, which, combined with the bitter hatred they may feel, intensifies other destructive emotions that have resulted from past experiences. One common result is that girls who have been sexually abused will often become sexually promiscuous or develop anorexia and/or bulimia later in life.

A major effect of such abuse, however, is one that is almost impossible to believe: Women who were abused often become abusers of their own children. This abuse is usually physical rather than sexual. The fact that this problem "passes along" in families makes it imperative that it be stopped whenever it is found.

100 Why don't little girls report sexual abuse more often?

Because sexual abuse is often a middle-class problem, when children do get the courage to tell someone that their father, a close friend, or a family acquaintance has abused them, they are often not believed. Many times a child is accused of lying because the accused is so often a "nice person," known as moral, modest, and upright. This rejection may reinforce the child's opinion that no one can be trusted, and it can cause the child's feelings of worthlessness to grow.

When a girl's father abuses her, the problem is especially difficult. A little girl may not only fear that her mother will not believe her if she tells what is going on, but she may also be worried that if she reports her father's abuse, he will be taken to jail or will leave home, thereby hurting the entire family.

One of the major reasons more child abuse and sexual victimization is not reported, however, is the fear of retaliation. Children are often threatened by their abusers so that they will not tell anyone what is going on.

101 What can be done to prevent the tragedy of sexual molestation in my family?

There are a number of actions that you can take.

Marry a man with strong moral and emotional health. For example, if you marry a man who is continuously rebelling against authority, including his parents, he may be more susceptible to the temptations of incest, especially if he has a poor moral base for interaction with the world.

Choose healthy contacts for your child. Use the same guidelines in selecting baby-sitters, including nurseries and preschools, that you use to choose a husband. If you have any question at all about the morality and emotional stability of any of these people, including relatives, do not allow them to stay alone with your child, no matter at what age or how convenient it might be. Do not allow such persons to hold your daughter in their laps or to caress her excessively, even in your presence.

Talk openly to your child. All children should be taught about the possibility of sexual assault. They should be given rules to make the probability of sexual assault less likely. Do not wait until your children ask. Give them the necessary information now, before it is too late. (See Q. 97.)

102 What should I do if I think my child might have been sexually abused?

Take your child to a kind, sensitive, gentle physician for examination. (See Q. 184–194 about rape.) Generally, such a doctor would be an obstetrician/gynecologist or a family physician. Of course, if you suspect that a rape has occurred, you would want to take the child immediately to an emergency room. Most emergency rooms these days have physicians who have been trained in the evaluation of a child or woman who has been raped. The specific conditions of the event will dictate the type of tests that should be done. Of course, if rape has occurred or is suspected, the child would be tested for sexually transmitted disease and a search for sperm would be conducted.

If you suspect that long-term sexual abuse is going on, the doctor would examine the child for evidence of this abuse.

An important part of the physician's care would be to explain clearly the result of the examination. If there is sexually transmitted disease, the child would be treated for that. If there is no evidence of sexually transmitted disease, no pregnancy, and no damage to the female organs, the doctor can reassure you and your child that there is no possibility of lingering physical damage. Children who have been sexually abused often carry into adult life the fear that something is wrong with them. The reassurance by a physician that there is no physical damage can help such victims drop that load of worry and not carry it into their adult lives where it might interfere with the sexual relationship with their husbands in marriage.

If sexual abuse is strongly suspected or is proven, contact the proper authorities for their counsel about what to do with the one who did the sexual abusing of the child.

103 Where can I get further information on child abuse?

Several organizations can give you help.

> Your local police department.
> Your local county sheriff's department.
> Your county health or social-welfare department.
> Child Help, USA, Pasadena, CA 91370. Telephone: (800) 4-A-CHILD.
> Child Abuse Hot Line (800) 252-5400.

In addition, there are several books that might be helpful.

> *Carol's Story* by Chip Ricks (Tyndale House, 1981).
> *A House Divided* by Katherine Edwards (Zondervan, 1984).
> *My Very Own Book About Me* by Jo Stowell and Mary Dietzel (available from the Lutheran Social Services, 7 South Howard, Spokane, WA 99204). This book distinguishes between "good" and "bad" touching and does

an excellent job of explaining the right not to be touched in any way a child does not like (including tickling and wrestling). This is for young children through third grade.

Child Sexual Abuse: Hope for Healing by Maxine Hancock and Karen Mains (Harold Shaw, rev. ed., 1997).

Helping Victims of Sexual Abuse by Lynn Heitritter and Jeanette Vought (Bethany, 1989).

Sex Talk for a Safe Child by Domenna C. Renshaw (American Medical Association, 515 North State Street, Chicago, IL 60610) helps parents find a way to talk comfortably and accurately about normal and abnormal sex practices.

Check with your local public or church library or bookstores for additional titles.

104 What should I do if I was once sexually abused and have never worked through that experience?

It is normal to respond to the trauma of sexual abuse with major emotional and psychological problems. This is just as normal as it is for the body to respond with scars as a result of severe injury in an automobile accident. If you have been the victim of sexual abuse and feel you have problems resulting from the experience, it is important that you seek counseling. Just as you would want your daughter to confide in someone if she had been abused, so it is important that you tell someone if you have been sexually victimized in the past.

Unmarried Adolescent Sexual Activity

105 What should I do if my adolescent daughter has started having intercourse, or if I believe

she may be contemplating sexual activity?

If you have reason to believe your daughter is having or planning to have intercourse, the situation needs to be dealt with openly. Both you and your daughter need to be aware of the health hazards to any girl who begins having intercourse in her teenage years.

Not only is sexually transmitted disease (STD) common among sexually active teenagers, but also many girls become pregnant and either carry their pregnancies or have abortions.

Once unmarried teenagers start having intercourse, they are more likely to have multiple sexual partners in their lifetime. The Centers for Disease Control study on premarital sexual experience among adolescent females from 1970 to 1988 (*Morbidity and Mortality Weekly Report*, 1991: 39:929–32) reported that of the girls who became sexually active before the age of eighteen, 75 percent had had two or more partners, and 45 percent had had four or more. The earlier these adolescents had initiated sexual intercourse, the more sex partners they were likely to have had.

The more sexual partners a woman has had in her lifetime, the more likely she is to have sexually transmitted disease (STD) and pregnancy out of wedlock. In March 1991, Dr. Nancy Lee reported in *Obstetrics and Gynecology* (March 1991, 73.3:425) that women who had four or more sexual partners were over three times more likely to be hospitalized for PID (pelvic inflammatory disease). There is an 11 to 25 percent chance that a woman will be sterile if she has one episode of PID.

AIDS is a real threat to teenagers. "The prevalence of AIDS has been escalating in the adolescent population and estimates indicate that the number of teens with HIV infection doubles every fourteen months." (Gennis and Gennis, "Orgasm without Organism," *Clinical Pediatrics* [January 1996]). It is now estimated that 25 percent of all people who have become HIV infected were below the age of twenty-two when they got their infection.

Don't rely on your school's sex education to protect your child from the dangers of sexually transmitted diseases, pregnancy, and risky sexual practices. A report by the National Campaign to

Prevent Teen Pregnancy called "No Easy Answers" showed that the dominant sex education programs taught in America since 1980 have shown very little success in altering the age of onset or the frequency of adolescent sexual activity, or of increasing contraceptive use, or of preventing unplanned teenage pregnancy. Modern teenagers have more information about sex than any group of young people in the world, but sex education programs have not prevented teens from engaging in sexual activity, from having out-of-wedlock babies, or from becoming STD infected.

Because of the potentially devastating effects of sexual activity among teenagers today, it is not enough to say to a classroom of adolescents, "If you are going to have sex, at least be responsible and use a condom." No! Sex education in the classroom is setting the standard expected for students. The standard that will help protect young people the best is "no intercourse until marriage." What is more, it is impossible to teach something so private as the use of condoms in a classroom.

In addition to encouraging abstinence until marriage, sex education should, at the appropriate age, teach how often contraceptives fail. For example, this education should emphasize that condoms do not protect against the sexual transmission of HPV (a virus that causes more than 90 percent of cervical cancer). Also, condoms give very unreliable protection for a girl's fertility. Whether she uses condoms or not, she has the risk with unmarried sexual activity of becoming sterile.

The message given youth in school sex education is important. The most important message, though, needs to come from you, the parents. I recommend that you have a discussion with your child if he or she is having sex or is contemplating sexual activity. The discussions you have with your daughter (or son) may be unpleasant, even stormy, but scientific fact and truth (and love!) are on your side.

1. Warn the child that if she does start having sex before she gets married, she is entering a very dangerous lifestyle that can end all her hopes of ever having a child. This lifestyle can cause her to get pregnant when she does not want to be. It could lead to death from AIDS. Encourage her to read the section in this book on sexually transmitted disease (or read it to her). Encourage her to read the information about teenage pregnancy and about abortion in this and other books. Explain that abortion can damage her female organs and cause her to be infertile. It can also cause her serious, long-term physical, emotional, and spiritual problems.

2. Tell her that no matter what her friends or boyfriends may say, they are wrong if they want her to have sex before she gets married. The staggering increase in sexually transmitted disease, teenage pregnancies, and teenage abortions is evidence that they are wrong. The horrible epidemic of STD in our society today is one result of teenagers having sex.

3. Have her read the information on sex education in this chapter. Explain to her that the education she might have received about "safer" or "safe" sex is wrong. She cannot protect herself adequately against sexually transmitted disease and pregnancy in the years before she gets married. Condoms and birth-control pills fail teenagers too often. If she participates in the casual sex lifestyle, she will almost always get a sexually transmitted disease, even if she uses condoms.

4. Tell your daughter that it is morally wrong to have sex outside of marriage. It is wrong to do something that hurts her own body or another person's body. Tell her that you are asking her to abstain from sex for her present and future physical and spiritual health.

5. If she refuses to follow your recommendation, it may be necessary for you to apply some principles of "tough love." You can talk about this with a psychologist or psychiatrist who agrees with you.

6. Tell her how wonderful it is to save herself as a virgin for her husband in marriage, and that this choice will give her a better opportunity for health and happiness in the future.

7. Through all of this, reassure your daughter or son that you are giving this advice and requiring these things for their own good and because you love them, not because you are

trying to be legalistic or mean. Your child's future health, happiness, and marriage and home depend on a positive response to this message. It is important that your child feel that you are not helpless in this situation. It is important for you to not "just give in." Children need the firm guidance of adults who love and care about them. Studies clearly show that one of the strongest influences on the choices young people make in this area is what their parents believe and teach.

106 I feel such pain over my daughter's choices. What did I do wrong?

When parents have done their best to raise a child the way they feel is right and that child then turns against all that she has been taught, they may feel great despair. This is one of the most difficult times for parents and their children.

Hopefully, your daughter is merely going through a period of rebellion in an attempt to establish her independence and maturity. On the other hand, she may be starting down a path that will lead her away from you and your moral values for many years. She may never return to the beliefs that you hold and have taught her as she was growing up, and there is no way you can make this happen. However, if you have provided her with a caring, nurturing, loving home—and you have not been overly legalistic in your approach—the situation is probably only temporary.

It is a good idea to counsel with your pastor, a psychologist, or a psychiatrist who can help you handle the situation. In addition, there are some excellent books that you could read.

Parents in Pain by John White (InterVarsity Press).
The Wounded Parent by Guy Greenfield (Baker Book House).
No Time for Fairy Tales by Fred Grimm (Impact Books).
Hold Me While You Let Me Go by Rich Wilkerson (Harvest House).

What's the Matter with Christy? by Ruth Allen (Bethany House Publishers).
Easing the Pain of Parenthood by Mary Rae Deatrick (Harvest House).

When your family and your child have gone through a time of intense emotional struggle, there may be some scars of pain, resentment, and bitterness left behind. For help with these problems from the spiritual dimension, I strongly recommend Dr. Neil T. Anderson's books, *Victory Over the Darkness* (Regal Books) and *The Bondage Breaker* (Harvest House). Dr. Anderson also gives seminars that are helpful in healing the scars of life. (For further information, write Freedom in Christ Ministries, 491 East Lambert Road, LaHabra, CA 90631.) Problems of this kind involve the physical, emotional, and spiritual aspects of life. It is important to address all these in the process of healing.

Teenage Pregnancy

107 What are the statistics on teenage pregnancy in the United States?

The statistics are startling. Four out of every ten girls in the average high school classroom will be pregnant before their twentieth birthday. Approximately one million teenage girls become pregnant each year, and nearly 70 percent of these pregnancies occur outside of marriage. About 40 percent of teenage pregnancies are terminated by abortion. Nine out of ten teenage mothers who deliver their babies keep them. Finally, six in ten teen mothers who deliver before they are seventeen become pregnant again before they are nineteen.

The most common reason for hospitalization of teenage girls in the United States is for childbirth. These pregnancies represent a tremendous cost both to society and to the individuals involved. There is a high risk of birth complications for the young mothers and frequent health problems for their babies. These girls are more likely to have medical complications during pregnancy because they do not have the wisdom, discipline, or money to get good medical care, and because they may have a sexually transmitted disease. The children of teenage mothers statistically have a greater chance of dying or of having serious illnesses during their developmental years. Babies born to teen mothers often have low birth weight; this correlates closely with the higher incidence of neurological defects, retardation, epilepsy, and cerebral palsy in these babies.

The personal and public economic drain is tremendous, frequently resulting in poverty and the need for public support, for both health and social reasons. These young mothers drop out of school and frequently do not return. If they have jobs, they often lose them or leave because of problems connected with the care of their infants. The children raised in these homes with young mothers and no fathers are much more likely to be involved in criminal activity.

108 What should my attitude be if my teenager gets pregnant?

To deal with her problem, you must also deal with yours. You will feel violated, as if your teenager has defiled your trust and all that you have taught her. To dwell on those feelings, however, can ruin your relationship with your daughter.

It certainly is appropriate for you to let her know that you are disappointed in her actions, but you must also communicate to her that you love and accept her as a person. I have often seen parents, after clearly expressing their disapproval, continue to berate their children for their misconduct. This can damage the future relationship between the parents and child.

The relationship between parent and child is far more important than whether or not the daughter has committed an act that is repulsive and disappointing to the parent. Most girls learn adequately from the pregnancy itself, without having their parents inflict more harsh lessons on them by misdirected and unloving attitudes.

Your daughter will go through a great deal of trauma, no matter how lovingly you care for her. It seems prudent, therefore, that you treat her with as much love and acceptance as you can. In this way you should be able to maintain a loving and caring relationship with her, allowing the trust between you to grow and allowing her to mature from her experience instead of having it permanently damage or destroy her. Her life is not over just because she has become pregnant. Neither is her relationship with you. She will continue to need your parenting the rest of her life.

109 Should I suggest—or insist—that my daughter have an abortion?

In your distress and anxiety, do not hastily advise abortion. I do not believe abortion is a good choice for an adolescent. (See Q. 174–183.)

The risks of both emotional trauma and physical damage from an abortion do exist, especially for a teenager. In addition, there is the possibility of developing a pattern of activity for the future. Without wise counseling, a girl may believe that she can misuse contraception and sex, become pregnant again, and repeat the pregnancy/abortion process with no adverse effects. That is not the case. I have seen many older women who had repeated abortions when they were young and who are now unable to get pregnant. There is a statistically greater chance of infertility as well as a higher incidence of emotional problems in patients who have had abortions in the past.

110 How should my unmarried daughter's pregnancy be handled? What if she chooses to keep the child?

It is vital that your daughter have good medical care during her pregnancy, to enable her to stay healthy and to have a greater chance of delivering a healthy baby.

The importance of good medical care for a teenager during pregnancy is shown by the fact that a teenager who is pregnant is about three times more likely to have toxemia of pregnancy than a mature woman. An adolescent is twice as likely to have a premature baby than a mature woman and is more likely to produce a baby with

The Female Body in Change

congenital abnormalities. Her baby will have a greater chance of dying before or right after delivery and a higher risk of developmental problems in the future, including cerebral palsy, mental retardation, or epilepsy. In addition, a teenager is more likely to have trouble delivering a baby. There is a greater chance that she will need a cesarean section and have a longer labor than would an older woman. The chance of most of these problems is lessened with good medical care. Even if problems do develop, good care can decrease the likelihood of the mother or baby being permanently hurt.

It may be best that your daughter contact an adoption agency that has domiciliary care. Such an agency provides a place for her to live during part or all of her pregnancy. If you are not familiar with this type of agency in your area, you might write to an organization such as The Gladney Center, 2300 Hemphill, Fort Worth, TX 76110, (817) 926-3304. They can help you make contact with a similar home in your area.

Loving and Caring, Inc., 1905 Olde Homestead Lane, Lancaster, PA 17601, phone (717) 293-3230, has some excellent material on decision making, relationships, and options for unwed mothers. A counselor's manual and a series of workbooks handle the situation with insight and sensitivity.

I feel that adoption is usually the best answer for the teenage mother and her baby. My opinion stems from the fact that a great deal of my practice time is spent helping infertile women. About 10 or 15 percent of married couples are unable to have children. If unmarried women carried their pregnancies to term and offered their babies for adoption, those couples who were unable to become pregnant would be able to adopt children into a stable, two-parent home.

Another fact to consider is that there is more child abuse and neglect among teenage mothers than the general population. Due to her immaturity, a teenage mother initially may want to keep a child because of the excitement and fun of having a baby of her own. She cannot fully comprehend the challenge and responsibility (financial and otherwise) of motherhood. Later, when the child

causes problems, a teenager is more likely to mistreat her child than would a more mature mother.

There are other factors. If a teenage girl decides to keep a child, her relationship with her parents is permanently changed now that she has a child to care for. Furthermore, the child can create problems in a later marriage or can end the girl's attempt to gain a higher education.

If a teenager does decide to keep her child, it is important that family, friends, and church help her with what will be a big job.

Sex Education

111 **I am confused about sex education for my child. What is the best approach?**

Sexual activity for an unmarried teenager is dangerous physically, emotionally, and spiritually. I will be focusing on the physical dangers, but keep in mind that damage to one's moral and spiritual self can be more destructive than physical damage.

Teenagers are more susceptible to the physical damage of STDs than are adults. First, if single teenagers start having sex, they will almost always change sexual partners before they marry. The Centers for Disease Control states (*Morbidity and Mortality Weekly Report*, January 4, 1991, vol. 39): "The initiation of sexual intercourse early in life is associated with an increased number of sex partners and a greater risk for sexually transmitted disease." The same study showed that adolescents who "had sexual intercourse earlier in life reported greater numbers of sex partners."

We should ask ourselves, "Is it wise for unmarried teenage young people to have intercourse?" Almost every responsible adult will say, "No!" It is just not worth the risk for the teenager to start having intercourse and to take the "Russian roulette risk" of pregnancy and sexually transmitted disease.

Do we conclude that the present sex education programs are not working? An article by

James W. Stout, M.D., and associates in *Pediatrics,* the primary journal for pediatricians in America, stated: "There is little or no effect from school-based sex education on sexual activity, contraception or teenage pregnancy" (1989, 83: 375–79). Obviously, the $3 billion Americans have poured into traditional sex education has been, for the most part, wasted. Thomas M. Vernon, M.D., of the Colorado Department of Health in Denver, stated in the *Journal of the American Medical Association:* "The failure of such general education is particularly discouraging" (1988, 260:22). The situation has not improved, as is shown by a comprehensive literature review of sex education programs published by the Department of Policy, Strategy, and Research of the United Nations NUAIDS agency. This 1997 report showed that although some sex education programs had some theoretical (statistical) success, they have actually protected only a tiny number of teens.

Increased promiscuity, increased pregnancy rates, and increased rates of sexually transmitted disease correlate directly with the amount of money spent on the traditional sex education programs nationwide. The more money that has been poured into these programs, the more sexual activity, pregnancies, abortions, STDs, there are. The dominant sex education of the past fifteen years, which says be abstinent if you can but if you have sex use a condom, has not dramatically decreased sexual activity and its problems, and there is some evidence it has increased the problem.

What is the answer then? What kind of "sex education" works? (See Q. 112.)

112 What do you mean by "character-based sexuality education programs"?

Character-based sexuality education encourages young people to develop a foundation of good values, including respect, responsibility, etc. With this foundation, young people then have the strength of character to avoid risky behaviors, including sexual activity before marriage. This choice is based on the fact that sex outside marriage is unhealthy and unwise, both physically and emotionally, and it hurts both individuals involved. Further, these sex education programs

- are based on the fact that adolescents do not use adult reasoning and, therefore, need guidance to make right choices. The advice is directive, just as the "just say no" drug program is. These programs flatly state to a young person, "It is harmful to you to have sex before marriage."
- seek to involve parents because they have the strongest influence on the future sexual choices their children make and, ultimately, any program for teenagers will fail without parent involvement.
- explain anatomy and physiology appropriately and without arousing the desire to experiment sexually.
- present abstinence as the norm and as being both obtainable and positive. Young people are told that the sex drive is something that can be controlled, just as the appetite for food can be controlled.
- emphasize the fact that despite all the talk among peers about sexual escapades, 50 percent or more of students in high schools are not having sex—they are choosing to remain virgins. Teens are beginning to hear the message of the new sexual revolution.

The goal of abstinence sex education—abstinence until marriage—is attainable, and many knowledgeable professional people are strong advocates. One of them, Dr. James L. Fletcher Jr., M.D., of the Department of Medicine, Medical College of Georgia in Augusta, stated, "Sex education promoting safer sex with condoms and sex education promoting abstinence are mutually exclusive. Implicit in safer sex programs is the well-worn maxim that adolescent coitus is inevitable and inexorable. It is important, therefore, that parents and schools make a decision about which type of sex education they want to have available for their students. It must be one or the other" (*Southern Medical Journal,* December 1990, 83: 12).

113 How does character-based sexuality education differ from traditional sex education? Is "safer sex" a tenet of both programs?

Basically, character-based sexuality education says to young people, "There is no such thing as 'safe sex.' Make a decision to avoid sex until marriage because sex before marriage is harmful both physically and emotionally." Mixed message "safer sex" education programs say, "Since you are probably going to have sex anyway, be prepared to have 'safer' sex by taking birth-control pills or having condoms available." There is a world of difference in the messages teens receive from these two approaches.

As an example, let me share what a young woman told me about an episode in her local high school. A physician who participated in sex education came to the school and told the girls he would prescribe birth-control pills for any of them in case they ever did decide to have intercourse. The young woman told me that she could name at least two dozen friends who began taking the pills in high school "just in case." What is so unfair and so incompetent about this advice is that though pregnancy for a teenager is a problem in some ways, the greater problem for a teenager is STD. The birth-control pills those girls started taking made them feel "safe." The doctor, however, did not tell these teenagers that about 8 out of every 100 teens become pregnant just in the first year of using birth-control pills. He also did not tell them that birth-control pills provide no protection against sexually transmitted disease. Even worse, the physician undermined the commitment to abstinence many of them may have had when they first came to his class.

This so-called authority's advice and birth-control prescriptions may have kept some of these girls from becoming pregnant, but who knows how many of them still became pregnant or are now sterile from STD, or have AIDS, because of this physician's counsel.

But even if this doctor had told these women to have sex only if their boyfriends used condoms, he would not have helped them much

more because condom failure rates for teens in protecting against STD are so high.

For all of the advice and information given in the traditional approach to sex education, studies rarely show that more than 25 percent of any age group of people use condoms consistently. The Centers for Disease Control made some startling statements in its 1997 "CDC Update." It said "consistent means 100 percent of the time—no exceptions" about condom use. Then it said that if condoms were not used in this way, they did almost as little good as if they were not used at all.

Robert C. Noble, M.D., in a commentary in *Newsweek* (April 1, 1991), states:

> Condoms don't hack it. Passing them out to teenagers is futile. . . .
>
> I'm an infectious-diseases physician and an AIDS doctor to the poor. Passing out condoms to teenagers is like issuing them squirt guns for a four-alarm blaze. . . .
>
> Smart people don't wear condoms. I read a study about the sexual habits of college women. In 1975, 12 percent of college women used condoms when they had sexual intercourse. In 1989, the percentage had risen to only 41 percent. Why don't college women and their partners use condoms? They know about herpes. They know about genital warts and cervical cancer. All the public-health messages of the past 15 years have been sent, and only 41 percent of the college women use condoms. Maybe your brain has to be working to use one. In the heat of passion, the brain shuts down. You have to use a condom every time. *Every time.* That's hard to do. . . .
>
> "Condoms may be more likely to break during anal intercourse than during other types of sex. . . ." Condoms also break in heterosexual sex; one study shows a 4 percent breakage rate. "Government testing can *not* guarantee that condoms will always prevent the spread of sexually transmitted diseases." That's what the government pamphlet "Condoms

and Sexually Transmitted Diseases—Especially AIDS" says. Condoms are all we've got. . . .

What am I going to tell my daughters? I'm going to tell them that condoms give a false sense of security and that having sex is dangerous. *Reducing* the risk is not the same as *eliminating* the risk. My message will fly in the face of all other media messages they receive. . . .

There is no safe sex. Condoms aren't going to make a dent in the sexual epidemics that we are facing. If the condom breaks, you may die.

There is one major failure of condoms that is often overlooked—they provide almost no protection against human papilloma virus (HPV) infection, which is the most common STD in the United States (even condom educators agree with this). HPV is a dangerous infection causing more than 93 percent of all precancer and cancer of the cervix, which kills about 5,000 American women a year. There is also strong evidence that condoms do not protect a woman's fertility if she has years of sexual exposure with several sexual partners.

114 Do character-based sexuality education programs really work?

Yes, they do. A program called Best Friends (2000 N. Street N.W., Suite 201, Washington, D.C. 20036) has had a total of 1,000 girls enrolled from its start until the present. The girls enter in the fifth grade and continue through high school graduation. The program fosters self-respect and promotes responsible behavior by helping the girls understand the value of postponing sexual activity and rejecting drug use. In January 1996 they reported a 1.1 percent pregnancy rate among their girls. Girls in the same school environment who were not a part of Best Friends had a 26 percent pregnancy rate. This is the effect we want sex education to have on our children—a dramatic decrease in sexual activity, in STD, and in pregnancy.

Another study, done in the Teen Services Program of Grady Memorial Hospital in Atlanta, Georgia, by Marian Howard, Ph.D., of Emory University School of Medicine, showed the same positive results. The study was reported in an article "Postponing Sexual Involvement Among Adolescents" (The Society of Adolescent Medicine, 1985). Dr. Howard's program was "adapted from the model used in the smoking field to help adolescents thirteen through fifteen years of age postpone sexual involvement, thereby curtailing negative health outcomes (STDs and premature pregnancy)." The assumptions that guided the development of the program were:

1. Adolescents under the age of sixteen are not mature enough to handle the consequences of many of their actions.
2. Adolescents under the age of sixteen are often pressured into behavior they do not really want to engage in.
3. Adolescents need to be given skills to be able to resist pressure.
4. Adolescents respond well when information about what to do and how to do it comes from peers.

The results of the study were quite positive. "When asked if they had actually been able to resist becoming sexually involved, 47 percent indicated that they had not had an opportunity to become sexually involved. Of the 53 percent who had an opportunity to become sexually involved, nearly ⅚ had been able to resist the pressures while roughly ⅙ had sexual intercourse."

There were other significant findings reported in a study by Dr. Howard and Dr. McCabe published in *Family Planning Perspectives* (January–February 1990, 22.1: 21–26). It showed that abstinence-based sex education programs lowered sexual activity and pregnancies among the participating students. (Though PSI does give contraceptive information, the strong emphasis is on abstinence.)

I believe it is time for us to realize that the millions of dollars that have been spent on the dominant sex education programs of the past fifteen years has largely been wasted money. It is time to make a dramatic change to help the young people of our society who are being devastated by sexually transmitted diseases and teenage pregnancies.

Character-based sexuality education programs seem to offer the only hope, just as abstinence-based teaching about drugs proved the only hope we had for teaching our young people to avoid drug use.

Virginia governor Douglas Wilder, the first African American in U.S. history to be elected to a state governorship, sums up the question of sexual responsibility in a speech reprinted in *Reader's Digest* ("Straight Talk on Black Families," July 1991, p. 99):

> Precautions should be taken by the young and unmarried, those who are not remotely ready for the unending responsibilities of parenthood. If these young men and women want to have a future, it is imperative that they embrace the ultimate precaution: abstinence.

115 Should I try to get character-based sexuality education programs into my schools? Are they religious in nature? How do I approach school personnel about these programs?

Because the character-based sexuality education programs are so important—and so effective—I encourage you to do all you can to get these programs introduced into your school systems. I recommend that you contact the Medical Institute for Sexual Health for information concerning getting character-based abstinence education into your schools. Their address and phone number are: Medical Institute for Sexual Health, 2600 Dellana Lane, Suite 100, Austin, TX 78746, phone: (512) 328-6268.

116 What about contraceptives for teenagers?

If teenagers are having intercourse, it is very important to encourage them to talk with their parents and to tell them that they have begun relating to a person of the opposite sex in a very dangerous way. Very rarely does a teenage sexual relationship outside of marriage become a permanent sexual relationship. If they have begun having sex with the person they are currently dating, they will probably have sex with the next person, and the person after that.

It is important to encourage teenagers to stop having sex with the person they are dating. If they will not do that, encourage them to plan now not to have intercourse with the next person they date when their current relationship is over. I am talking to an increasing number of young women who are choosing not to have sex when they get out of a current sexual relationship. They greatly increase their chances of staying healthy by abstaining from sex in future relationships with men. This is called "secondary virginity." This is a powerful concept. It means they have a second chance—a chance to start over. That hope is important to a young person. Physically it offers hope. The greatest risk of a person being infected with a sexually transmitted disease is having more than one sexual partner. The more sexual partners in one's lifetime, the more risk of STD.

If a girl is having sex at this point and will not stop, I would suggest two mechanical methods of birth control. I encourage the girl to use vaginal foam and her partner to use condoms *every* time they have intercourse. This does not totally prevent all sexually transmitted disease, but it will at least decrease the chance of a person becoming infected with sexually transmitted diseases for a short period of time. During this time the young person can consider more realistically her risky behavior and spend time talking to her parents. I always warn my patients that if they fail to use this protection even one time, they can become infected with sexually transmitted disease and the girl can become pregnant. If a couple will use these two methods of birth control every time, they have a very small chance of getting pregnant over a short period of time.

I do not recommend birth-control pills alone for sexually active teenagers because they offer no protection against sexually transmitted disease. You will occasionally see some so-called experts recommending the use of both birth-control pills and condoms. This is absolutely illogical. Studies show that of teens on birth-control pills, only about 20 percent also use condoms. Because teenagers are so susceptible to STD, if they are going to refuse to be abstinent they should at least use contraception that can provide some STD protection.

Though I do not think birth-control pills are best for an unmarried teenager, studies have conclusively shown that if a girl has matured enough to have regular menstrual cycles, the birth-control pills will not harm her. Even for a young teenager, oral contraceptives will not affect future fertility or her hormones. Nor will taking the pills affect her ultimate height, since if a girl has developed regular menstrual periods, she has already had her major growth.

The IUD should not be used by a teenage girl. An IUD significantly increases the chances of infection in a girl's uterus, tubes, and ovaries (PID). This dramatically increases her chances of becoming sterile. Since a teenager has all of her childbearing years ahead of her, it is best to avoid even a small chance of becoming sterile because of an IUD-caused infection. As a matter of fact, I do not recommend that any woman use an IUD until she has finished having all the children she ever wants to have.

Norplant and Depo-Provera are different forms of progesterone. Norplant involves the insertion of six small Sylastic tubes under the skin. I feel very strongly that this is a terrible method of contraception for a single teenager to use. Certainly it is an effective contraceptive technique, but the problem is that because a teenager knows she cannot get pregnant with it, she will feel "safe" to have intercourse. Norplant, however, leaves her wide open to be infected with sexually transmitted germs. Depo-Provera (depo medroxy progesterone acetate [DMPA]), given as an injection every three months, has the same drawbacks. Sexually transmitted disease is as much a risk for a teenager as pregnancy.

Above all, parents should counsel teens about their sexual choices whether the teen is abstinent or has become sexually involved. New studies show that parents are the strongest influence in the lives of teens who are avoiding risky behavior.

Bulimia and Anorexia

117 **My daughter seems to be overly concerned about her weight. She is very thin and yet constantly talks about how fat she is. Her eating habits are strange. Could she be developing an eating disorder?**

If your child is becoming excessively thin, or seems to be gorging food and not gaining weight, you may correctly suspect that something is wrong. She may have anorexia if she is exercising excessively and compulsively, withdrawing from friendships, becoming irritable, has developed unusual attitudes toward food, and is losing weight.

If a girl is not gaining any significant amount of weight but is obviously overeating, she may have bulimia. This is especially true if she is storing empty food containers in hidden places, confiscating and eating food belonging to associates, spending a lot of money on food, missing chores, and spending excessive amounts of time in the bathroom after meals.

Both anorexia nervosa and bulimia often include the compulsive use of laxatives, diuretics, diet pills, and caffeine.

Bulimia and anorexia nervosa are two diseases of a group of problems called "eating disorders." Some experts feel these disorders should be included in a group of diseases called "addictive disorders," which includes alcoholism and drug addiction. Girls with a certain personal psychological framework (similar to people who become drug addicts or alcoholics) seem to be susceptible to an eating disorder and may become bulimic or anorexic without meaning to when they "flirt" with distorted eating habits. These young women do not realize that they are dancing on the thin crust of an abyss of quicksand that at any moment can crack open to engulf them—and, quite literally, kill them.

Bulimia (bingeing and purging) and anorexia (starving) may be due in part to our society's abnormal preoccupation with food, dieting, and weight, especially among high school, college, and

The Female Body in Change

young professional females. Experts estimate that half of the coeds at many colleges in the United States regularly use self-induced vomiting to control their body shape and weight. It is not unusual for young women to go several days without eating to keep themselves thin.

Bulimia and anorexia nervosa often originate from what seems to be an innocent and well-intended attempt to control weight. Unfortunately both disorders are now epidemic among young women in our society. It is estimated that 13 percent of college coeds are true bulimics. One in 150 white females between ages twelve and eighteen have anorexia nervosa, and the incidence of anorexia nervosa is much more common than previously thought. The great majority of people with this problem are female (95 percent), but a growing number of men are developing anorexia, especially jockeys, wrestlers, gymnasts, and actors.

Characteristic Family Traits

The victims of anorexia and bulimia do not generally come from troubled, distorted homes, but rather usually have confident parents who feel that they have done a better-than-average job of raising their children. They may be described as good, directed, ambitious parents.

The families of victims of anorexia and bulimia have few sons, with two-thirds of them having only daughters. Girls with this problem often come from upper-middle-class or upper-class families where financial achievement and social position are often high. The relatively few homes of lower-middle-class or lower-class families that produce children with eating disorders are usually upwardly mobile and success-oriented.

These families usually average about three children per family, and the age of the parents at the birth of their children is often rather high.

Usually the mothers of these girls are career women who gave up their careers when they married. They are often submissive to their husbands but do not truly respect them. The fathers, despite social and financial success, feel in some sense "second-best."

These mothers are usually preoccupied with physical appearance, admire fitness and beauty, and expect proper behavior and achievement from their children. These mothers tend to be weight-conscious and preoccupied with dieting. Some can be obsessively preoccupied with any flaw in their bodies.

Not only do the parents often feel that they have done a good job as parents, but the children themselves often feel that their parents have been good parents and that their home has been happy. This perception of their homes may sometimes be an outright denial of facts. These girls are often afraid of being put in a position of having to say something critical. It can also be an expression of overconformity—what the parents say is always right—and the daughters blame themselves for not being "good enough" for such "perfect" mothers and fathers.

Generally these families expect too much in the areas of appearance, good behavior (politeness is emphasized), and academic achievement. Teachers often have commented throughout the school years that the anorexic child was a joy to have in class—cooperative, reliable, and a hard worker.

Although no one knows what actually causes these diseases, children with the following characteristics seem to have the emotional framework on which to hang bulimia or anorexia nervosa:

> They are judgmental of others, feeling that they are too immature and not serious enough.
> They are especially hardworking and markedly helpful to less advantaged friends.
> They are *very* responsible, always desiring to please, and compliant at home and at school.

Bulimia

Bulimia, the more common of the two eating disorders, is also known as the "binge-purge syndrome." The *Diagnostic and Statistical Manual of Mental Disorders* (American Psychiatric Association, 1990) gives this definition of bulimia:

> Recurrent episodes of binge eating (rapid consumption of a large amount of food in a short period of time).

A feeling of lack of control over eating behavior during the eating binges.

The person regularly engages in either self-induced vomiting, use of laxatives or diuretics, strict dieting or fasting, or vigorous exercise to prevent weight gain.

A minimum average of two binge eating episodes a week for at least three months.

Persistent preoccupation with body shape and weight.

Victims of bulimia feel dominated by the disease and become desperate for help. They are occasionally even suicidal.

Bulimics can develop physical problems. Menstruation can be erratic or absent even though weight is normal. This does not permanently damage one's body, but pregnancy is often impossible during this time. The poor nutrition that results from such abnormal eating habits can result in hair that is of poor texture, or even in partial hair loss. The complexion, too, can deteriorate.

Bulimics who have abnormally low weight can develop electrolyte (the body's salts) disturbances that can result in weakness, muscle spasm, kidney problems, and death. In addition, stomach acid that washes across the teeth during repeated vomiting episodes can dissolve the enamel of the teeth and can, if prolonged, cause the teeth to literally rot out of the mouth.

A dangerous practice sometimes tried by bulimics is the use of Ipecac. This drug causes vomiting. If Ipecac is used excessively, it can cause major problems, including muscle damage (even to the heart muscle) and death.

Though the bulimia problem usually starts in adolescent years, it can begin in early adulthood. For many people, the problem of bulimia carries over from the teenage years into their middle adult years. Most bulimics are women, but there are a growing number of bulimic men. Bulimia is much more common than anorexia, but often a person will practice both bulimia and anorexia (called bulimiarexia).

Anorexia Nervosa

Anorexia nervosa is widely known because the skinny bodies that are the result of the disease are so publicly obvious and because it more commonly results in death than does bulimia. Even with treatment, various studies show that from 5 percent to 15 percent of people die from anorexia nervosa.

The *Diagnostic and Statistical Manual of Mental Disorders* (American Psychiatric Association, 1990) gives the following definition of anorexia nervosa:

> Refusal to maintain body weight over a minimal normal weight for age and height, e.g., weight loss leading to maintenance of body weight 15 percent below that expected; or failure to make expected weight gain during period of growth, leading to body weight 15 percent below that expected.
>
> Intense fear of gaining weight or becoming fat, even though underweight.
>
> Disturbance in the way in which one's body weight, size, or shape is experienced, e.g., the person claims to "feel fat" even when emaciated, believes that one area of the body is "too fat" even when obviously underweight.
>
> In females, absence of at least three consecutive menstrual cycles when otherwise expected to occur (primary or secondary amenorrhea). (A woman is considered to have amenorrhea if her periods occur only following hormone [e.g., estrogen] administration.)

Victims of anorexia nervosa starve themselves, and this starvation results in noticeable and excessive weight loss. People with this disease often exercise compulsively, in spite of their inadequate diet, accelerating their weight loss. In addition, they will frequently use laxatives, diet pills, diuretics, and excessive coffee to help them lose weight.

Family or friends tend to either ignore or praise the victim's weight loss until the scarecrow-like body forces them to admit that something is dreadfully wrong. Then, typically, they respond with too simplistic advice, such as, "Just *eat*. You know you're too thin," or, more destructively, by trying to force their loved one to gain weight.

The medical problems that result from anorexia nervosa are numerous. Menstruation stops even before the person's weight is low enough to have caused such absence. The hormone problem that causes irregular periods can also cause osteoporosis that does not easily reverse to normal even after an anorexia patient gains her weight back. The complexion and hair suffer, and there is occasional head hair loss or abnormal growth of hair on other body areas. Electrolyte disturbances can develop, and these imbalances in the amount of fluids and "salts" in the body can be life-threatening.

Anorexia nervosa is considered a form of suicide by most specialists. Although many victims threaten suicide, few patients actually commit violent suicide in the midst of their anorexic process. Studies do show suicide rates up to 5.3 percent.

Treating Anorexia and Bulimia

First of all, before there is any indication of an eating disorder parents should be knowledgeable. If your family has some of the characteristics mentioned earlier, or if your child has some of the character traits mentioned, I encourage you to read the following books:

The Golden Cage by Dr. Hilde Bruch (Random House, 1979).

Starving for Attention by Cherry Boone O'Neill (Dell Books, 1982).

The Monster Within by Cynthia Joye Rowland (Baker Book House, 1984).

These books may give you the insight that will enable you to change some things for the future well-being of your children.

If you suspect that a child or a friend may have bulimia or anorexia nervosa, one approach would be to get professional help to set up an intervention session with that person and those who are close to her. Observations and concerns should be communicated, along with love and support. If parents of the victim are unaware of their child's condition, they should be contacted because their involvement is vital to healing the disease.

The victim should immediately contact a psychologist, psychiatrist, or counselor familiar with the treatment of these problems. The longer the disease is allowed to exist without treatment, the more entrenched it becomes and the more difficult to cure.

If a person refuses to admit she has a problem, and she refuses to get help, you should contact a psychologist or psychiatrist familiar with these problems to determine the appropriate next step.

Proper therapy for these patients is absolutely vital. It is the unfortunate experience of many bulimic and anorexic patients to find that many physicians, psychologists, and psychiatrists do not understand or know how to treat these diseases. Professional care for these problems should be similar to that which is discussed in the books by Bruch, O'Neill, and Rowland.

Generally, hospitalization is best at the beginning of treatment if any of the following criteria exist:

Rapid loss of more than 25 percent of body weight in less than four months

Fatigue (If a person had been strenuously exercising but has now stopped and is constantly fatigued, she is very sick)

Fainting and/or irregularity of the pulse; abnormally low blood pressure, pulse, or temperature; abnormality of the electrolytes (the body's salts)

Failure to get well with previous therapy

Suicidal

Family situation is bad

Admission being the only way to get the patient into treatment

Other significant medical or psychiatric problem complicates bulimic condition

If the care of the patient seems to differ from the approach described above, you may want to contact one of the organizations mentioned at the end of this section or a specialist mentioned in one of the books to get a second opinion on the type of care being offered. Remember, care must be aggressive and good; do not be reassured when your child says that her anorexia or bulimia is not much of a problem. These victims are experts at deception and denial.

Even with proper treatment, success is not guaranteed. For example, good treatment of anorexia nervosa results in a 50 percent cure rate and 30 percent improvement rate. Approximately

20 percent of these patients remain chronically ill and chronically troubled by their disease.

During the past several years, I have had contact with many young women suffering from anorexia and bulimia. Those troubled young women are bright, intelligent, and gifted, but they have been blinded to the gifts God has given them. They are frequently confused about spiritual things, which can often be a root of their problem.

Because these young women do not believe that they have value and worth, they try to feel good about themselves by dieting or bingeing. It is vitally important that they realize they are people of great worth and that they are deeply loved and appreciated.

I recommend that those with anorexia and bulimia (and their families and friends) become familiar with the work of Dr. Neil T. Anderson, founder of Freedom in Christ Ministries. Two of his excellent books, *Victory Over the Darkness* (Regal Books) and *The Bondage Breaker* (Harvest House) are available in Christian bookstores. Both his books and his seminars have been extremely helpful to people with eating disorders.

Emotional problems can both contribute to and result from eating disorders. Counseling with a psychologist or psychiatrist may be helpful. It is vital that such a counselor be an expert in the care of people with eating disorders. Much time and money can be wasted if they are not.

If a person with bulimia or anorexia is desperately ill, hospitalization may be necessary. Because of expense, this is much less common than in the past. Most communities no longer have special eating disorder units available in local hospitals. If a person is desperately ill, he/she may be admitted to a general psychiatric floor for care. This can be a lifesaver. So please use this option if necessary.

If your child has an eating disorder, you probably are having an agonizing experience. I encourage you to find other parents in similar circumstances. Don't try to go it alone. You don't need to broadcast your problems, but discussing your situation with other parents whose child has had an eating disorder can be of tremendous help.

Organizations You Can Contact for Help

"Eating Disorders," a video produced by the American College of Physicians, may be borrowed without charge by calling (800) 222-0025. In New Jersey, call (201) 628-9111.

American Anorexia/Bulimia Association
418 East 76 St.
New York, NY 10021
Phone: (212) 734-1114

Anorexia Nervosa and Related Eating
Disorders (ANRED)
P. O. Box 5102
Eugene, OR 97405
Phone: (503) 344-1144

National Anorexic Aid Society (NAAS)
1925 E. Dublin-Granville Road
Columbus, OH 43229
Phone: (614) 436-1112

National Association of Anorexia Nervosa and
Associated Disorders, Inc. (NAANAD)
P. O. Box 7
Highland Park, IL 60035
Phone: (708) 831-3438

Overeaters Anonymous
Box 420962
San Francisco, CA 94142
Consult your telephone directory for information regarding local chapters. (This organization offers help for all types of eating disorders.)

Remuda Ranch
P.O. Box 2481
Wickenburg, AZ 85358
Phone: (800) 445-1900
(provides in-patient and out-patient care)

An Afterword

We have discussed some difficult and heartbreaking situations in this chapter, but these things are not the norm. Most females have absolutely no major health problems during childhood and adolescence unless they become sexually active. Young girls who develop problems can benefit from the wealth of medical knowledge and treatment available today.

If you have problems with your child—medical, emotional, or spiritual—don't hesitate to seek help. Contact a physician, a psychologist or psychiatrist, or get counsel from your pastor. It is important for both you and your child to know that you are not helpless and alone.

Pray a lot, whether or not you are having problems! If your child does well, you should realize that you have a great deal for which to be thankful. If your child has problems, you are not totally responsible for those problems, but you are an important part of the solution. There is no way that you were totally responsible for the good results, or the bad. I believe the best way for loving parents to raise mature, self-confident, well-directed, and loving children is with the help of God!

The following self-evaluation form, designed by K. Kim Lampson, Ph.D., 550 16th Ave., Suite 301, Seattle, Washington 98122, © 1982, can help a person decide if she needs help.

Are You Dying to Be Thin?

The following questionnaire will give you an indication of whether or not you are living a lifestyle that indicates anorexic and/or bulimic tendencies. Anorexia nervosa (key symptom: extreme weight loss due to self-starvation) and bulimia (key symptom: bingeing followed by purging) are becoming more and more openly acknowledged as publicity increases public awareness and understanding.

Answer the following questions honestly. Write the number of your answer in the space at the left.

_____ 1. I have eating habits that are different from those of my family and friends.
  1) Often   2) Sometimes   3) Rarely   4) Never

_____ 2. I find myself panicking if I cannot exercise as I planned for fear of gaining weight.
  1) Almost always   2) Sometimes   3) Rarely   4) Never

_____ 3. My friends tell me I am thin but I don't believe them because I feel fat.
  1) Often   2) Sometimes   3) Rarely   4) Never

_____ 4. (Females only) My menstrual period has ceased or become irregular due to no known medical reasons.
  1) True   2) False

_____ 5. I have become obsessed with food to the point that I cannot go through a day without worrying about what I will or will not eat.
  1) Almost always   2) Sometimes   3) Rarely   4) Never

_____ 6. I have lost more than 25% of the normal weight for my height (e.g. 30 lbs. from 120 lbs.)
  1) True   2) False

_____ 7. I would panic if I got on the scale tomorrow and found out I had gained two pounds.
  1) Almost always   2) Sometimes   3) Rarely   4) Never

_____ 8. I find that I prefer to eat alone or when I am sure no one will see me, thus am making excuses so I can eat less and less with friends and family.
  1) Often   2) Sometimes   3) Rarely   4) Never

_____ 9. I find myself going on uncontrollable eating binges during which I consume large amounts of food to the point that I feel sick and make myself vomit.
  1) 3 or more times per day   2) 1–2 times per day   3) 1–2 times per week
  4) Rarely   5) Never

_____10. I use laxatives as a means of weight control.
  1) On a regular basis   2) Sometimes   3) Rarely   4) Never

_____11. I find myself playing games with food (e.g. cutting it up into tiny pieces, hiding food so people will think I ate it, chewing it and spitting it out without swallowing) telling myself certain foods are bad.
  1) Often   2) Sometimes   3) Rarely   4) Never

_____12. People around me have become very interested in what I eat and I find myself getting angry at them for pushing food on me.
1) Often   2) Sometimes   3) Rarely   4) Never

_____13. I have felt more depressed and irritable recently than I used to and/or have been spending increasing amounts of time alone.
1) True   2) False

_____14. I keep a lot of my fears about food and eating to myself because I am afraid no one would understand.
1) Often   2) Sometimes   3) Rarely   4) Never

_____15. I enjoy making gourmet, high-calorie meals or treats for others as long as I don't have to eat any myself.
1) Often   2) Sometimes   3) Rarely   4) Never

_____16. The most powerful fear in my life is the fear of gaining weight or becoming fat.
1) Often   2) Sometimes   3) Rarely   4) Never

_____17. I find myself totally absorbed when reading books about dieting, exercising and calorie counting to the point that I spend hours studying them.
1) Often   2) Sometimes   3) Rarely   4) Never

_____18. I tend to be a perfectionist and am not satisfied with myself unless I do things perfectly.
1) Almost always   2) Sometimes   3) Rarely   4) Never

_____19. I go through long periods of time without eating anything (fasting) as a means of weight control.
1) Often   2) Sometimes   3) Rarely   4) Never

_____20. It is important to me to try to be thinner than all of my friends.
1) Almost always   2) Sometimes   3) Rarely   4) Never

Add your scores together and compare with the table below:

Under 30   Strong tendencies toward anorexia nervosa
30–45   Strong tendencies toward bulimia
45–55   Weight conscious, not necessarily with anorexic or bulimic tendencies
Over 55   No need for concern

If you scored below 45, it would be wise for you to (1) seek more information about anorexia and bulimia and (2) contact a counselor, pastor or physician, to determine what kind of assistance would be most helpful for you. Anorexia nervosa and bulimia are potential life-threatening disorders which can be overcome with the proper support and counsel. The earlier you seek help, the better, although it is never too late to start on the road to recovery.

4

The Reproductive Years

The reproductive years are those years in a woman's life from the time she starts having her menstrual periods until the time they stop. These are the years when her reproductive organs work the hardest, are the busiest, and are the most subject to disease. They are the years when the female hormones surge, producing characteristic ups and downs in a woman's physical and emotional self.

Because the time span of the reproductive years extends from adolescence to middle age, it occupies center stage in a woman's life. The changes that occur between the beginning and the end of this period are enormous and multiple.

The excitement, joys, opportunities, and challenges of this period of life can be exhilarating. The disappointments, heartaches, and pain can, at times, be overwhelming. It is so often in this period of life that a woman goes from one extreme to another. Her body blossoms and then matures. Having sex may go from being uppermost on her mind to being the least of her concerns. She welcomes children into her life and watches them leave. She may both find her mate and lose him—all in this period of transition from little girl to mature woman!

Other parts of this book are devoted to specific aspects of the reproductive period of a woman's life (conception, pregnancy, labor and delivery, contraception, and sexually transmitted disease). This chapter includes these vital topics:

Annual routine examination
Surgery on female organs
Endometriosis
Low abdominal and pelvic pain
Bladder infections
Premenstrual syndrome (PMS)
Diethylstilbestrol (DES)
Abortion
Rape and Sexual Assault

Many of the subjects discussed in this chapter are included because they involve more than just one of the female organs and therefore would not properly fit into the chapter on diseases of the reproductive organs; some subjects are included because it is during this reproductive phase of life that these situations are most likely to be bothersome, even though they may also occur before or after this age span. Other topics, such as rape and abortion, are included because it is during the reproductive years that they are most likely a consideration.

Routine examinations are discussed in this chapter because it is during this time that you establish the habit of going to a physician. Often the doctor you go to early in your reproductive years is the one you still consult when you reach menopause! Hopefully you have already chosen a doctor, as outlined in the introduction.

Although I am not a urologist, I am including a brief discussion of bladder infections in this book. The reason for this is that women usually call their gynecologist, or the doctor who does their annual exams and Pap smears, for treatment of their bladder infections. Also, since bladder infections can be so intimately involved with a woman's genital function, it seems appropriate to answer here some questions you might have about this medical problem.

The Annual Routine Examination

118 **Is it necessary to have an annual examination?**

I believe that it is. The American Cancer Society recommends that Pap smears be done annually. At least 5 percent of abnormal Pap smears will worsen so rapidly that, in one or two years' time, the cervix can develop dangerous invasive cancer.

Some doctors encourage patients to have examinations every six months, especially at menopausal age. This seems unnecessary unless a woman has a health problem that needs to be watched closely. True, there is a greater possibility of breast cancer as one grows older, but seeing a doctor twice a year instead of annually will not significantly increase the chance of finding a breast

Routine Medical Tests Often Included in an Annual Physical Examination

Test	Purpose
Blood pressure measurement	Detect high blood pressure
Neck and thyroid exam	Detect infection or primary tumors
Breast exam	Detect any lumps or other abnormalities
Pelvic exam	Visual and manual examination of vagina, cervix, and other female reproductive organs
Pap smear	Microscopic examination of cells shed from cervix
Digital rectal	Manual examination of rectum
Fecal blood	Detect microscopic blood in stool samples
Urinalysis	Detect sugar, albumin, or germs in urine
Mammography	X-ray exam of breast, occasionally between ages 35–40; every other year after 40; yearly after 50

cancer early. Breast cancers are usually detected by mammograms or by breast self-examination, not by seeing the doctor twice a year.

119 What is included in an annual gynecological examination?

The routine examination varies from physician to physician, but the following guide suggests minimum expectations for the usual checkup.

Every year. From the time the routine exam is started, it should include an examination of the neck, breasts, abdomen, and pelvis, including a digital rectal examination; a blood pressure check; urine testing for albumin (for nephritis), sugar (for diabetes), and germs (for infection of the kidneys or bladder); a Pap smear; and a weight check.

Beginning at age forty. In addition to the usual checks, the exams after age forty should include a mammogram every other year until age fifty.

After age fifty. In addition to the above, a woman should have a mammogram every year from the age of fifty on. (See Q. 756–787 for further information on breast care.) She should also have a proctoscopy or similar test. I also think it is wise for a woman to have a bone-density test at this age to see if she has any sign of osteoporosis.

120 What should I do if my doctor finds a problem during my annual examination?

If your doctor finds an abnormality and recommends that you come back to the office for any reason, comply with this recommendation. Take any medication prescribed, in exactly the way the doctor tells you, and please take all of it. If you have any questions about how to take your medicine, call your doctor or ask your pharmacist.

In addition, reading is a good way to find out all you can about a problem. I hope this book serves you well in that respect. If something your doctor says does not make sense to you, consult with another physician before complying with the original suggestion. Remember, a doctor can almost always say what has to be said in terms you can

Bimanual Pelvic Examination

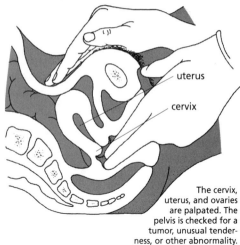

uterus

cervix

The cervix, uterus, and ovaries are palpated. The pelvis is checked for a tumor, unusual tenderness, or other abnormality.

understand. If you cannot understand what he or she is trying to tell you, your doctor may be confused or unsure and may be "putting up a smoke screen" so you will not know about his/her confusion. If what your doctor has to say does not "add up" in your mind, or if you cannot get an adequate explanation, get a second opinion.

If your doctor suspects some type of cancer, and you cannot find another source of good information, call the National Cancer Institute's Cancer Information Service for information and confidential answers to your questions about cancer. The number is (800) 4-CANCER.

121 Is it wise to have an examination by an internal-medicine specialist in addition to my annual gynecological exam?

If you are feeling fine and your regular doctor does the exams and studies listed in Q. 119, you probably do not need to see an internal-medicine specialist in addition to your gynecologist. If your gynecologist finds a medical problem that is outside his or her field of expertise, you will be referred to another physician. For instance, if you have pneumonia or high blood pressure, you will be referred to a family practitioner or to an internal-medicine

Pap Smear

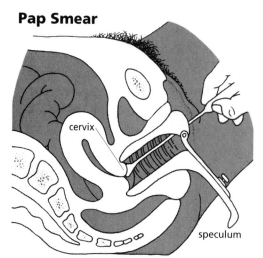

The cervix is examined and cells are scraped from the surface, smeared on a glass slide and sent to a lab for microscopic examination.

specialist. If a significant breast lump is found, you will usually be referred to a general surgeon. (See Q. 756–787.)

But even when your gynecologist has found nothing wrong, if you want to see an internist or family practitioner for a more complete examination, you certainly should do so. If your doctor's exam has been thorough, however, it is unlikely that an internist would find a disease on performing a more detailed exam.

Surgery on Female Organs

122 What types of surgery do gynecologists do?

Gynecologists perform numerous operations, and I will not try to outline them all. However, most do the following procedures:

D&C (dilatation and curettage of the uterus for women having miscarriages or abnormal uterine bleeding). Contrary to rumors you might have heard, this is not an outmoded procedure.

Vaginal and abdominal hysterectomies

Vaginal repairs

Endometriosis surgery

Infertility surgery

Operations for complications of pregnancy, including cesarean sections and operations for ectopic pregnancies

Sterilization procedures on women (urologists and general surgeons do vasectomies on men)

123 Can doctors other than gynecologists do surgery on the female organs?

Since many surgical procedures of the female organs are considered "fairly easy," general practitioners, family practitioners, general surgeons, and gynecologists all do female-organ surgery. However, because of their training and expertise, gynecologists are the only physicians whom you should allow to perform surgery on your female organs unless you have no other choice.

I am obviously biased, but my biases are a result of the problems I have seen produced by ill-thought-out, poorly timed, or poorly done "easy" operations performed by nongynecologists.

Here are some examples:

D&Cs done on patients who had supposedly miscarried, but who were actually still carrying normal pregnancies. Such procedures terminated pregnancies that these women wanted to continue.

Hysterectomies done for fibroid tumors on women who had not had all the children they wanted. Most of these hysterectomies could have been avoided by a gynecologist who would simply remove the fibroids from the uterus, leaving the uterus intact so the woman is able to bear children.

Both ovaries removed from young women who had ovarian tumors, leaving them permanently sterile and having to take hormones daily for years to come. A gynecologist will at least attempt to "shell" tumors out of the ovaries in this situation. Leaving some ovarian tissue present in such a patient can probably enable her to get pregnant in the future. It can also keep her from having to take hormones every day for many years.

Sterilization procedures done with large, four- or five-inch incisions in the abdomen, when the same thing could have been accomplished by simple laparoscopy or mini-laparotomy, with very small incisions.

While the surgical procedures of gynecology seem fairly simple and straightforward, the judgment involved in deciding when to do the surgery, and what to do during the operation, is why gynecologists spend four years in specialty training following the completion of medical school. This training makes a difference for patients, and patients should avail themselves of a gynecologist's expertise.

The one exception is when a C-section is necessary during pregnancy. If a general or family practitioner is well trained in obstetric care, I have no qualms about such a doctor doing a cesarean section. The operation is a fairly easy procedure. The difficult part is the decision about when to do it.

124 What is a hysterectomy?

Hysterectomy refers to removal of the uterus. The cervix is part of the uterus; the fallopian tubes and the ovaries are not. Removal of the uterus can be accomplished through an incision in the abdomen or through the vagina. The decision of which method to use is not based on the surgeon's personal preference or a flip of the coin. There are definite reasons for doing either procedure.

In addition, it may be necessary to remove the tubes and ovaries along with the uterus. Most women think of this as a "complete hysterectomy" but that is not the correct term. A complete hysterectomy involves removal of the uterus only. When the tubes and ovaries are also removed, the procedure is called a "complete (or total) hysterectomy *and* bilateral salpingo-oophorectomy." It is no wonder the term *total hysterectomy* has been adopted by laypeople to mean "they got it all!"

It is important to note that your vagina will not be open at the upper end after your hysterectomy. When the cervix is removed from the upper vagina, the front and back walls of the vagina are sewn together, closing it completely. When a doctor looks into your vagina after a hysterectomy, it looks the same as it did before, except that there is no cervix at the upper end.

A man cannot normally tell at intercourse whether or not a woman has had a hysterectomy. If anything, the woman's upper vagina is likely to be a little tighter after a hysterectomy than before.

Briefly, the different operations and their impact on the body are:

Hysterectomy. This is removal of only the uterus, but both parts of the uterus—the body of the uterus and the cervix. The tubes and ovaries are left in place. The term *total abdominal hysterectomy* means removal of the uterus with its cervix through an incision in the abdomen. *Total vaginal hysterectomy* means removal of the uterus and cervix through the vagina. A hysterectomy means that there will be no more periods, no more pregnancies, no possibility of ever having cancer of the uterus or cervix, and no hormone change. The ovaries will continue functioning as they always have until menopause. Sexuality is unaffected and a woman will feel no different after this form of hysterectomy has been done, except that any medical problems she had with her uterus will be healed and her PMS may be gone (not guaranteed unless the ovaries are removed).

Supracervical hysterectomy. This term means a hysterectomy in which only the upper part of the uterus is removed, leaving the cervix in place. This operation is much simpler to do than a regular hysterectomy, and even doctors who are not well trained in gynecologic surgery can do it quite easily. It was used a great deal many years ago by doctors who were not specialists. Today there are only three situations that call for a supracervical hysterectomy: first, if a patient is having massive uterine bleeding and the doctor must remove the uterus in a hurry; second, if a woman has ovarian cancer in her pelvis that would make it unwise for the doctor to remove the cervix at the time of the hysterectomy; and third, if a woman has a terri-

Types of Hysterectomies

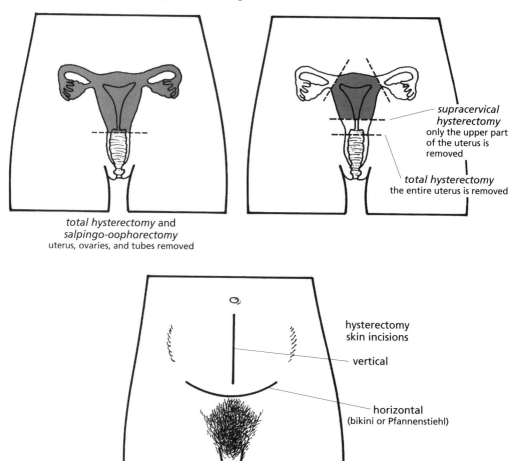

total hysterectomy and
salpingo-oophorectomy
uterus, ovaries, and tubes removed

*supracervical
hysterectomy*
only the upper part
of the uterus is
removed

total hysterectomy
the entire uterus is removed

hysterectomy
skin incisions

vertical

horizontal
(bikini or Pfannenstiehl)

ble scar in her pelvis that would make a total hysterectomy dangerous. If there is massive ovarian cancer in a woman's pelvis and the cervix is removed at a hysterectomy, the ovarian cancer can sometimes more easily grow down into the vagina, causing bothersome bleeding and discharge. A supracervical hysterectomy will mean no menstrual periods, no pregnancies, no hormone change, no change in sexuality, and no possibility of uterine cancer in the future. It is still necessary to have a Pap smear once a year, however, because there is still a possibility of cervical cancer, since the cervix is still in its original position.

Hysterectomy with removal of tubes and ovaries.

Physicians call this "total abdominal hysterectomy and bilateral salpingo-oophorectomy" (or "panhysterectomy"). This surgery means no more periods, no pregnancies, and no possibility of cancer of *any* of the female organs except the vagina or vulva. Because the ovaries have been removed, there will be no female hormones being produced in the body. This usually necessitates taking supplemental hormones if the woman has not already gone through menopause at the time of the hysterectomy. (Actually, a minimal amount of both female and male hormones is always being produced from the adrenal gland, but not enough to supply a woman's hormone needs.)

90

125 Is it true that many unnecessary hysterectomies are done?

It is true that more hysterectomies than any other major operations are done in America, and that 25 percent of all women will eventually have their uterus removed. This is not an indication that doctors are doing "too many" hysterectomies, however. If you question this, take a poll of your friends who have had hysterectomies and ask them if they regret having had the procedure done. I expect that you will find that they are almost unanimously glad that they had a hysterectomy and appreciate the beneficial changes in their bodies.

The few patients who are unhappy with having had a hysterectomy are usually those who had some medical problem that made their hysterectomy necessary before they could complete their family. These women, though, would not be counted in the number that some experts say represent "unnecessary hysterectomies."

The truth is that many doctors who write articles about so-called unnecessary hysterectomies are in academic environments and do not have to deal with patients on an everyday basis. They would probably even say that many of the situations that most doctors agree definitely warrant hysterectomies would be unnecessary indications. If their guidelines were followed, women would have to live with female organ problems that cause their quality of life to be worse than it needs to be.

Furthermore, hysterectomy is perhaps the safest major operation done today. Patients rarely have any complications during the operation or during recovery. It is for this reason that a hysterectomy can be done for problems that are not life-threatening and that some doctors might label "unnecessary."

In saying this, I am not advocating that you have a hysterectomy "at the drop of a hat," but if you have a problem that is significantly affecting your quality of life, and you and your doctor think a hysterectomy will solve the problem, I do not think you need to wait till you have a dangerous situation to have the hysterectomy.

126 In general, when should a hysterectomy be done?

A hysterectomy should be performed when a woman, regardless of age, is having enough "female trouble" or disease associated with her uterus that it needs to be removed or that she wants it removed. Fortunately most of the uterine problems that occur in younger women are not ones that demand a hysterectomy. Women can normally delay a hysterectomy until they have had all the children they want.

Many women delay a hysterectomy unnecessarily, however. I had a patient who finally had the needed surgery, after delaying it for years. She came back to my office feeling significantly better and questioning why she had put it off so long. She made an interesting statement: "I felt that since I was so young, I should have a uterus, even if it was diseased!"

Doctors occasionally tell patients they should have a hysterectomy to avoid ever developing cancer of the cervix or uterus. Fear of having cancer in the future should ordinarily have little influence on your decision to have a hysterectomy now. A hysterectomy should generally be done for specific problems, not for what might develop in the future. Besides, cervical and uterine cancer can often be discovered by your doctor before they become dangerous. One of the few exceptions to this is a hysterectomy with removal of the ovaries for a woman who has several close relatives with ovarian cancer—a legitimate procedure.

I tell my patients that there are hysterectomies that (a) *must* be done and those that (b) *can* be done if a woman feels her problems are serious enough. Examples of both situations are discussed in the next two questions.

127 What situations definitely require a hysterectomy?

Hysterectomies must be done in the following situations. A complete discussion of these disorders is found in chapter 10.

Cancer of the uterus
Severe precancerous changes in the uterus

Severe pelvic infections that do not respond to antibiotics. Such infections, if allowed to progress, can result in death.

If a hysterectomy is not done in these situations, major health problems or even death may result.

128 What are the situations in which a hysterectomy can legitimately be done if the woman chooses to have one?

Hysterectomies can be done, if a woman is bothered enough by a problem, in the following situations:

Early precancerous changes in the uterus

Prolapsed uterus or prolapsed uterus with looseness of the vaginal walls (bladder wall looseness is called cystocele; rectal wall looseness is called rectocele)

Looseness with intercourse

Enough difficulty having a bowel movement to necessitate a woman using her fingers to press on her tissues (either in the vagina or just above the anus) to have a bowel movement

Excessive loss of urine with coughing, sneezing, or laughing

Fibroids that are causing pain

Pelvic pain originating in the uterus

Heavy bleeding with periods

Certain low-grade infections

Severe premenstrual (PMS) or menstrual problems

Severe endometriosis with large pelvic masses made up of endometriosis tissue

Severe bleeding that produces anemia and is not corrected by other treatment

Fibroid tumors the size of a three-month pregnant uterus or larger

Pain when deep penetration occurs during intercourse with no other abnormality present

Some physicians might argue with my suggesting a hysterectomy for severe PMS, severe cramps, or severe headaches that may occur just at the time of menstruation. There are some women, however, who have had all the children they intend to have and whose lives are wrecked by these symptoms. If such a woman is having debilitating problems and has been unable to get relief from her symptoms any other way, a hysterectomy will sometimes help. She would want to proceed only after consultation with a competent gynecologist, so that she can know that her chances of cure from such a procedure are good. To assure a good response to such surgery, it is sometimes necessary to remove the ovaries too.

A woman can tolerate any of these problems and not have a hysterectomy, and many women prefer to do just that. The choice is an individual one in most cases.

I suggest that you check the Index for a complete discussion if you are bothered by any of the problems listed above. The majority of this information is in chapter 10.

129 What are the advantages of having a hysterectomy?

Having a hysterectomy can result in these advantages:

It can be lifesaving in certain situations.

It can improve your enjoyment of life by removing a nagging and troublesome problem.

It means no more menstrual periods; not a reason to have a hysterectomy, but a pleasant side benefit.

It usually means no more premenstrual tension and the end of symptoms caused by the rise and fall in hormones. Most women stop having these symptoms even if they do not have their ovaries removed, but PMS *may* continue if ovaries are left intact.

It means no more pregnancies and no need for contraception.

Furthermore, if you ask, your doctor can remove your appendix during an abdominal hysterectomy, which means you will never have appendicitis. If you have already gone through the menopause or are older than about forty at the time of hysterectomy, you may want your doctor to also remove your ovaries, permanently eliminating the risk of ovarian cancer. (See Q. 131.)

130 What are the disadvantages of a hysterectomy?

The drawbacks of a hysterectomy are:

1. *No more pregnancies:* A woman should not have a hysterectomy unless it is mandatory for life and health if she wants to have children in the future. (A woman whose ovaries are left in at hysterectomy could later have an in vitro fertilization procedure with a surrogate mother carrying the pregnancy. I personally do not recommend this because of the problems associated with a surrogate.)

2. *Pain:* There is some discomfort the first three or four days after a hysterectomy, although pain medication generally makes this tolerable. Patients should ask for pain medicine as often as it is allowed, normally every three hours. A machine called "Patient Controlled Analgesia" (PCA) allows patients to give themselves an injection of pain medication whenever they want it without waiting for a nurse. The machine is set so a patient cannot get too much medication. Also, some anesthesiologists will give patients a continuous epidural (see section on obstetric anesthesia). This is a great technique when it works, and it usually does. With an epidural, women can move their legs, walk, and have some feeling in their legs but feel no pain from surgery till the epidural is removed two or three days later. This not only keeps them from feeling tense during the first few days after surgery but will actually allow them to feel better sooner than if they let themselves hurt.

3. *Complications:* Although complications from hysterectomies are extremely rare, all surgery carries some risk, and this is no exception. For example, complications and even death can occur from the anesthetic.

(In 31 years of surgery, I never had this occur.) Bleeding during or after surgery that would require transfusions from which one *might* get AIDS or hepatitis is a risk from all types of surgery. Other possible complications from a hysterectomy are a hole between the bladder and vagina (vesicovaginal fistula), ureteral damage (involving the tube carrying urine from the kidney to the bladder), a bowel obstruction, or infection in an ovary. These complications are extremely rare. Studies show that a hysterectomy is the safest major operation a woman can have.

131 Does a hysterectomy make a woman "different"?

Many myths surround hysterectomy. Such myths include:

The vagina becomes "just like a sack" for the man during intercourse. I have not had a single patient whose husband could tell that she had had a hysterectomy by the way her vagina felt to him during intercourse. Actually the upper vagina is somewhat more snug after a hysterectomy because of the way the top of the vagina is sewn together and heals.

It is normal for a husband to be afraid of having intercourse for many weeks after his wife has had a hysterectomy. He can picture his penis pushing right out through the top of his wife's vagina. However, once a woman's vagina is healed and the doctor says it is permissible, intercourse is okay, no matter how deep or vigorous the vaginal penetration. This is usually possible six weeks after surgery. Common sense says for a couple to take it easy at first, but only for the sake of the wife's comfort.

Many women ask what happens to the space in the body where the uterus was after the uterus is removed. To understand the amount of space involved, remember that the uterus is about the size of a small orange, approximately three to four ounces in weight. When it is removed the intestines merely fall into the space where the uterus was. This repositions the intestines so that the abdomen flattens out just enough to take up the place where the intestines were. Even if the uterus is fairly large, this repositioning of the abdominal contents is not enough to make much difference in the flattening of a woman's abdomen or in how much a woman weighs. (Sorry!)

Menopause will come sooner if a woman has had a hysterectomy. This is not true if the ovaries are still intact. The ovaries are independent of the uterus and feed their hormones to the body through the bloodstream. The uterus seems to have no effect on the way the ovaries function.

Women who have their ovaries removed have to take hormones the rest of their lives. Women who are forty years old or older but still not past menopause can choose to have their ovaries removed at the time of a hysterectomy to eliminate the future possibility of having ovarian cysts, ovarian growths, ovarian cancer, or ovarian surgery. They should then start taking estrogen as described in Q. 215, 218 because young women who are without estrogen in their bodies are more likely to develop osteoporosis. When they reach the average age for menopause, about fifty, they will be no different from other postmenopausal women and can then decide if they wish to continue taking estrogen. I recommend that all women take estrogen from the age of menopause on unless they have a medical problem that makes hormones unwise.

A woman's sexual interest will decrease after a hysterectomy. Studies have shown quite clearly that a woman's sexual interest and responsiveness are not related to her uterus, tubes, and ovaries, once her sexual responsiveness has been established. There is no change in a woman's sexuality after a hysterectomy unless she develops a psychological hang-up about it. If a woman thinks that she might have some emotional problem from a hysterectomy, she should see a counselor before she has the hysterectomy.

There is less sexual feeling with intercourse. A woman's sexual feelings are primarily located in the undisturbed portion of her vagina and vulvar tissues, not in the uterus. Her feelings during intercourse and orgasm, therefore, will not be disturbed by a hysterectomy.

Women get fat after a hysterectomy. There is no relationship between the female organs and the body's metabolism. Therefore, women do not get fat after hysterectomies *because* of the surgery. It just so happens that women often gain weight in their forties and fifties, and this is when they most often have hysterectomies. This holds true even if a woman has her ovaries removed (if she takes estrogen). This lack of impact on a woman's weight was once again confirmed by a study published in the *Journal of the American Medical Association* in 1996.

There is no lubrication with intercourse. Some women seem to have a little less vaginal moisture than before a hysterectomy. This may occur because the cervix does produce some secretions into the vagina that can increase the moisture around the opening of the vagina. If this decrease in lubrication is bothersome, a couple can use a vaginal lubricant with intercourse. Some excellent "more natural" lubricants are now available: Maxilube, Replens, Lubrin, and others. They don't leave bodies and clothes greasy and are more like natural body moisture than older lubricants.

132 I am afraid I will feel "castrated" if I have a hysterectomy. Is this feeling unusual?

This is not an unusual thought for a woman to have, in spite of all the reassuring information she might read. She should remember, though, that it *is* just a "thought" problem and not a physical one. A hysterectomy does not seem to change a body in any undesirable way. The uterus is, after all, a "passive" organ whose primary jobs are letting its lining get ready for a pregnancy, shedding its lining if no pregnancy occurs, and holding the baby if pregnancy does happen. Except for releasing prostaglandin hormones (that cause cramps) into the body just before and during menstrual periods, the uterus is a receiver of hormones from the ovaries and the rest of the body. It would be best for you to see a psychologist, psychiatrist, or other counselor if you need a hysterectomy and are worried excessively. If you have had a hysterectomy and you now feel a sense of loss, regret, or castration, don't dwell on it or deny it. Talking to a counselor or a friend will often help a great deal.

Vaginal/Abdominal Hysterectomy

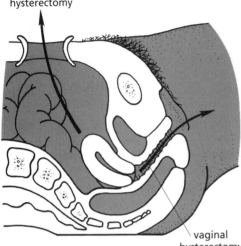

abdominal hysterectomy

vaginal hysterectomy

133 Which is best: a vaginal hysterectomy or an abdominal hysterectomy?

Medical conditions usually dictate whether your hysterectomy should be done through an incision in the abdomen or through the vagina. Both are sound procedures. A vaginal hysterectomy is not done "blind." The doctor can see the area quite well while he or she performs the surgery. There is almost always plenty of room for good visualization during vaginal surgery if there are no significant adhesions or growths. The advantages of vaginal surgery include less pain, shorter hospitalization, quicker recovery, no abdominal scar, and no chance of infection or hernia of an abdominal wound. It is also important to note that the vagina is not "stretched" in the process of a vaginal hysterectomy as many people assume.

Occasionally the supporting ligaments of a woman's uterus hold the uterus so high that a doctor cannot remove it through the vagina. Of course, if the surgeon doing a vaginal hysterectomy finds blood vessels he or she cannot get to through the vagina, or adhesions are fusing the pelvic organs together, the surgery may have to be finished by doing an abdominal incision. This is not a "complication," but rather a turn of events that is always possible when a doctor is doing vaginal surgery.

If you strongly prefer a vaginal procedure but your doctor insists on doing it abdominally, you can get a second opinion. Your doctor may *prefer* to do an abdominal hysterectomy because he or she is not well trained nor comfortable doing vaginal surgery. However, it may be that the vaginal procedure is truly not the best one for you.

Generally, I would suggest that you agree to the technique your doctor recommends if you like and trust your doctor. If you question his or her recommendations based on the information in the next two questions, you might want to get a second opinion.

134 What medical situations would best be handled by an abdominal hysterectomy?

An abdominal hysterectomy is best in these cases:

Uterine growths are too large to be removed through the vagina. Once a uterus is the size of a two-month pregnancy or larger, it is best that it be removed through an abdominal incision because of difficulty in getting it out through the vagina.

Ovarian growths are present. If you are having surgery for ovarian growths, and you are going to have a hysterectomy at the same time, it must be done through an abdominal incision unless the doctor is able to deflate the ovarian growth with a laparoscope early in the operation. It may be difficult or impossible to remove enlarged ovaries through the vagina, and if cancer is present, more extensive abdominal evaluation and surgery must be done.

Pain is the indication for a hysterectomy. When surgery is being done because of pelvic pain, it is usually best that it be performed with an abdominal incision, so that the doctor can evaluate the entire pelvic abdominal area. Occasionally the pain is coming from some part of the body other than the uterus. It is best, therefore, to have the entire abdomen explored at the time surgery is performed for pain, because the doctor cannot see much of the abdomen above the level of the uterus, tubes, and ovaries when operating vaginally.

Some doctors will do a laparoscopy to see if there is an abnormality in the abdomen causing pain, after which he or she will do a vaginal hysterectomy. If the pain is not very significant this may be satisfactory, but a laparoscopy does not allow a complete evaluation of all abdominal organs. Therefore, an abdominal exploration and hysterectomy when pain is present is usually best.

The uterus is infected. If you are having a hysterectomy because of infection, it must be performed through an abdominal incision. When infection is or was present, it can cause the organs inside the body to stick together as though glue had been poured on them. The bands of scar tissue that hold the internal organs together in this situation are called adhesions. A doctor operating through the vagina would not be able safely to cut adhesions and remove the uterus. In trying to cut adhesions, the surgeon might cut into the bladder or bowel.

135 What problems are best handled by a vaginal hysterectomy?

A vaginal hysterectomy can usually be done when the following situations exist:

Bleeding. If you are having a hysterectomy because of bleeding problems, and your uterus is not too large, it can most easily be done through the vagina.

Pelvic relaxation. If you are having a hysterectomy because your uterus is prolapsed, or because your vaginal walls are relaxed and a hysterectomy is necessary to repair the problem, this is best accomplished through the vagina. (Both the hysterectomy and vaginal repairs can be done in the same surgery and the ovaries can usually be removed vaginally if you and the doctor decide it would be best to take out the ovaries.)

Uterine growths that have not enlarged the uterus too much. A uterus with fibroids that have not enlarged past the size of a two-month pregnancy can often be removed through the vagina. If your vagina is too tight, the doctor might have to finish the operation with an abdominal incision.

Precancerous changes in the lining of the uterus or of the cervix. Generally these conditions can be successfully taken care of by a vaginal hysterectomy.

136 Will you describe normal hospitalization procedure for a hysterectomy?

The hospital procedure for a hysterectomy is basically the same as with other major surgery.

Before surgery the following things are routine:

Blood tests are taken to be sure there is no significant anemia.

Urine is collected for a urinalysis to be sure there is no infection, kidney disease, diabetes, etc.

Your medical history will be taken.

You will sign a permission form for the surgery.

The anesthesiologist will talk to you.

You will often be given an enema and an antiseptic vaginal douche.

You will be given nothing to eat or drink after midnight the night before surgery because any food in your stomach might be vomited up into your lungs during the administration of the anesthetic, an extremely dangerous situation. If you cheat on this rule, be sure to tell your anesthesiologist or your doctor so they can delay your surgery for a day. This can be a life-or-death matter.

About an hour before surgery you may receive an injection to relax you. The shot will not usually put you to sleep. An antibiotic is often given before surgery. This helps prevent infection from the surgery.

Following surgery the common procedure is:

You will receive fluids in your veins for one or two days. If you start eating immediately after surgery, before your intestines start working, the fluid and food can puddle in your intestines and cause severe bloating and gas pain. (Blood transfusions are not usually necessary following a hysterectomy.)

You will normally stay in the hospital about two to four days after surgery. Generally you will be allowed to go home when you feel well enough.

Pain medication will be provided. You should not hesitate to take it if you are uncomfortable. You will not have more pain if you have had uterus, ovaries, and tubes removed than you would if only the uterus had been removed.

If you have had a vaginal hysterectomy with no vaginal repairs, you will probably have less discomfort than with an abdominal operation. You should be able to go home a day or two earlier than if you had had an abdominal operation, perhaps as early as the first or second day after surgery. Some physicians, myself included, occasionally do vaginal hysterectomies (without repairs) as outpatient surgery. This means that a woman could have surgery early in the day and go home the evening of the same day or at least the next day. The primary advantages of this are less expense and less hospital time.

You will usually have a catheter in your bladder when you wake up from surgery. If you have not had a vaginal repair, this catheter will usually be removed the day after surgery. If you have had vaginal repairs done, you will have either a regular Foley catheter or a suprapubic catheter in your bladder. The suprapubic catheter is inserted through the skin above your pubic bone into your bladder. This is more convenient and comfortable for you, because you will not have a catheter in your urethra. When you begin voiding urine again, the suprapubic tube measures how much urine is left in your bladder. When you first start urinating, you will probably be able to pass only a few drops of urine (or none at all). As the days go by and the swelling lessens inside, you will be able to void more and more urine. When you are emptying your bladder completely, the tube can be painlessly removed. If you have a Foley catheter, you will normally have it removed five days after surgery to see if you can void. If you

cannot, the catheter will be reinserted and taken out again the next day or two. This procedure will be repeated until you are able to empty your bladder.

I warn my patients who are having bladder repairs done that they may not be able to urinate normally for as long as two months after surgery. Most patients are able to have their catheter or suprapubic tube removed within one or two weeks of leaving the hospital. Remember, though, being unable to void normally for two or three months after vaginal surgery is not a complication. It merely means that a good, tight bladder repair was done and can even mean that there is less chance of developing urinary incontinence later.

137 What will my recovery at home be like after a hysterectomy?

I give my patients the following suggestions as they leave the hospital to go home after a hysterectomy.

The first two weeks. Let someone else do the cooking and housekeeping. If you go home and assume the responsibilities of running the household, it often takes months to recover from the resultant tiredness and fatigue. If you go home and take it easy for two weeks, you'll feel better more quickly, with less lingering tiredness. As soon as you get home you can climb stairs slowly, take leisurely walks, and ride in a car. You can drive a car as soon as you know you can hit the brake in an emergency.

Resuming normal activities. You should not plan on resuming normal activities, including going back to work, for six weeks after surgery. However, after three weeks you can resume many normal activities. If you don't feel like it (and you may not), you should wait up to three more weeks, or until you feel up to it. (Occasionally patients do not feel truly normal for up to six months. I encourage such slowly recovering patients to start an exercise program of walking six weeks after surgery. This will usually make them feel better.)

Exercise. Do not begin exercising for six weeks after surgery, and then start back slowly with an exercise program. If you start immediately doing sit-ups, jogging, and other vigorous exercise, you will strain ligaments and muscles that have gotten weak from inactivity. However, starting six weeks after surgery, a gradually accelerating exercise program will help you feel better than if you do not exercise.

Bleeding from the vagina. Two or three weeks after a hysterectomy or vaginal repairs, as the sutures absorb out of the vagina, you may have some bright red vaginal bleeding. This is nothing to worry about unless it becomes heavier than a normal menstrual period. If that happens you should call your doctor. It is also just as normal for this *not* to occur.

Two or three weeks after surgery, you may notice a few dark strings falling out of your vagina. These are sutures that have completed their job and are absorbed. It does not mean that the tissues are separating.

Intercourse. Before resuming intercourse after a hysterectomy, you should be checked by your doctor to be sure you are healed. Patients are normally healed well enough to have intercourse about six weeks after surgery, but this is not always the case. Intercourse may be mildly uncomfortable for up to a year following vaginal repair. Scar tissue is hard and takes a while to soften up. Until it does there may be discomfort with intercourse. The eventual improved sexual enjoyment, good urine control, absence of bowel problems, and elimination of pressure and pain in the pelvis more than make up for the temporary discomfort.

Granulation tissue. Granulation tissue, often called "proud flesh," is commonly found in the vagina along the incision lines after a hysterectomy. It is comparable to the bright red tissue that is visible when a scab is knocked off a sore.

The vagina heals by forming granulation tissue but in the vagina no scab forms. This can cause bleeding, spotting or discharge, and pain with intercourse. If this happens, the doctor will have you come back every week or two to have silver nitrate applied to the granulation tissue to burn it off until you have total healing. This may require from one to five or more treatments. This type of treatment causes essentially no pain and is quite effective.

Follow-up exams. After the granulation tissue has been successfully treated and you are feeling well, your doctor will want you to come back for annual exams as usual. Most doctors will want you to have a Pap smear at least every three years after a hysterectomy because vaginal cancer can be detected with a Pap smear.

Endometriosis

138 What is endometriosis, and what should be done if I have it and do not want to have any more children?

For a definition of endometriosis see Q. 849. If your endometriosis is causing significant discomfort and you do not want more children, you probably should have a hysterectomy. Consider carefully these facts.

Your doctor could be wrong about your having endometriosis. A doctor cannot definitely diagnose endometriosis without seeing it at surgery or laparoscopy.

If you have pain that is bothersome enough to require investigation, or if your doctor finds a pelvic growth at your pelvic exam, you need to make sure you do not have ovarian cancer or some other significant medical problem. You can have the doctor do an exploratory operation with a large incision with the plan to proceed with removal of your uterus and, if necessary, your tubes and ovaries. You could, however, have a laparoscopy. With laparoscopy, the presence of endometriosis can be confirmed. Then, if you are not too uncomfortable, you can choose to leave it alone, take birth-control pills to keep it from progressing, or use Danocrine (as discussed in Q. 852) or a GnRH agonist such as Lupron or Synarel to suppress it so that the symptoms will stop. If endometriosis is present but not too extensive, the laser can be attached to the laparoscope to get rid of the endometriosis without making a larger incision.

A large incision may be necessary if the endometriosis is too extensive to remove at laparoscopy. If the endometriosis is widespread, however, it will probably grow back later. Therefore, you would probably be better off with a hysterectomy, including removal of the ovaries and tubes, if you do not want children in the future. After a hysterectomy, endometriosis almost never recurs, even when a woman starts taking estrogen.

If your uterus, tubes, and ovaries are removed for endometriosis, you should take estrogen. Your doctor will normally have you take something like Premarin (0.625 mg every day of the month along with Provera 2.5 every day). If a woman does not have endometriosis at the time of surgery, she does not need Provera after hysterectomy. If endometriosis was present, however, adding Provera to the daily medication can decrease the possibility of endometriosis returning.

139 If I have endometriosis and want to have more children, what should be done?

See Q. 852–860.

140 If I have not had all the children I want, but my doctor says my endometriosis is too extensive for fertility surgery, what should I do?

First, be certain that you are in the hands of a doctor who is enthusiastic and knowledgeable about fertility surgery. It is far easier for a doctor to do a hysterectomy than it is to do surgery for removal of only the endometriosis. If your doctor is skilled in treating fertility problems and still recommends a hysterectomy, it is likely that your female organs have been damaged so extensively that a fertility-type operation would be useless.

If it is worth it to you to take the risk of repeat surgery to maintain your fertility, you can ask your doctor to do fertility surgery, with the under-

standing that you will not allow a hysterectomy. I do recommend, though (provided your doctor is a capable fertility specialist), that you give your permission for a hysterectomy if the surgeon finds that he or she is unable to leave any normal ovarian tissue. In this situation you should accept the fact that both you and your doctor have done your best and should have no regrets in the future. It is possible now for a woman who has no ovaries to become pregnant with an embryo from a donor egg and her husband's sperm—if she still has her uterus. So if you would be interested in this fertility procedure, get consultation about it before having your uterus removed. (See the discussion of assisted reproductive technology in Q. 867–876.) A second opinion might be helpful. You might prefer that your surgery be done by a gynecologist who is a fellow of the American Society of Reproductive Surgeons of the American Society of Reproductive Medicine. Though there are many excellent fertility surgeons who are not a part of this group, you can be more sure you have a good surgeon if yours is a member. For more information about endometriosis contact the Endometriosis Association, 8585 N. 76th Pl., Milwaukee, WI 53223, (800) 992-3636 in the United States and (800) 426-2363 in Canada.

Low Abdominal and Pelvic Pain

141 What is meant by "low abdominal and pelvic pain"?

The type of pelvic pain we will be discussing in this section is not a sudden, acute, severe pain. That type of pain is usually easier to diagnose and does not require the observation and testing that the persistent, long-term pain involves.

Low abdominal and pelvic pain varies from mild to moderately severe. It is rarely disabling, but it may include pain with intercourse, severe or unusual pain related to menstrual periods, or severe and abnormal pain at the time of ovulation.

142 What causes pain on skin surfaces in the abdominal or vulvar areas?

Patients occasionally experience pain on skin surfaces, either in the low abdominal area or on the vulva. This discomfort is usually due to herpes if on the vulva or to shingles (herpes zoster) if on the low abdomen or vulva. Pain from these two problems is usually not difficult to diagnose and is not usually confused with the pelvic pain we will discuss in the next few questions. Obviously, other skin problems can cause discomfort. A dermatologist can be of help for discomfort in the vulvar area if the gynecologist is not sure what the problem is.

143 What causes low abdominal and pelvic pain?

Low abdominal and pelvic pain is a problem for both patients and their doctors. It is not only difficult to diagnose, but it can also be just as difficult to treat. Many well-qualified physicians believe that 50 percent of the pelvic pain that women experience is not due to physical abnormalities. The implication is that the pain is often psychological in origin. Although I do not doubt that some pelvic pain is due to emotions, my experience has been that this is uncommon. When pain is caused by emotion, the emotion often causes true physical pain that can be treated (such as irritable colon). When the physical pain is alleviated, a woman's emotional problems can be evaluated and treated more easily. If a patient and her doctor pursue pain evaluation, the cause can almost always be found and treated. Some physical causes of this type of pain are discussed in the following questions.

144 What symptoms might indicate a pain problem that is related to my female organs?

If the pain you have gets worse at the time of your menstrual periods or during the time of ovulation, and it goes away at other times during the month, its origin is probably your female organs. If your pain is not affected or is affected only a little by the regular monthly menstrual cycle, you probably do not have a problem of your female organs. You more likely have a problem related to your urologic or intestinal system. (See Q. 147–148.)

One standard action I take in the event of pelvic pain is to remove an IUD if one is being used. Even if a woman does not think her problem is caused by the IUD, it must be removed because it could be the cause of pain in the back, side, upper abdomen, and upper legs. The only way to know for sure that a pain is IUD-caused is to remove it and see if the pain disappears. (See Q. 906–910.)

145 What problems of the female organs might cause low abdominal and pelvic pain?

There are several gynecologic problems that can cause low-grade but persistent pelvic pain. (Also see Q. 143.)

Endometriosis (See Q. 138–139.)
Adenomyosis (See Q. 692–693.)
Pelvic-congestion syndrome (See Q. 694–695.)
   This is a condition in which the tissues of a woman's pelvis have become swollen and sensitive. Occasionally the veins in the woman's pelvis will be enlarged (like varicose veins). This is not a dangerous situation, but sometimes a hysterectomy is the only solution.
Pelvic relaxation. If the vaginal tissues are relaxed and the uterus is prolapsed, a woman can experience pelvic discomfort, usually felt as a "bearing down" or "bottom falling out" feeling.
Pelvic inflammatory disease with adhesions. Women occasionally have low-grade infections with no fever. Although the pain may be present some months and not present other months, typically this PID pain will be present with each period. Chlamydia infections of the tubes and ovaries are a common cause of low-grade persistent or recurrent pelvic pain.
Ovarian growths. A growth on an ovary will sometimes cause pain.

Ovarian torsion. Occasionally an ovary will twist on its supporting ligaments, cutting off its own blood supply, causing pelvic pain. This can be difficult to diagnose because the ovary and tube can untwist and look totally normal at laparoscopy, and then twist back again a few days later.

Retroverted uterus. (See Q. 382 and 671.) A retroverted (tilted) uterus can cause pelvic pain occasionally, usually only during intercourse. This normal situation is rarely a problem, however. One-third of all women have a "tilted" uterus and there is generally nothing abnormal or unhealthy about this condition. Occasionally a woman will have a markedly retroverted uterus causing pain, but this is usually associated with pelvic congestion (see above).

146 If my pelvic pain is not related to my menstrual cycle, what is the procedure for diagnosis?

If your pain comes with ovulation and then disappears in two or three days, or if it comes with your period and disappears after the period, the pain is obviously related to your cycle and may be coming from an abnormality of your female organs. If the pain comes any time during the month and the time of its appearance is unrelated to your cycle, the pain is usually not caused by an abnormality of your female organs. For that reason, with pain unrelated to the woman's cycle, I usually do not recommend testing at the time of the first visit. If there is no abnormality with a thorough pelvic exam, a woman should see a gastroenterologist (intestinal specialist) and, if he or she finds nothing, a urologist (bladder and kidney specialist).

I would definitely recommend a patient see a gastroenterologist (GI specialist) if she has any of the following symptoms and a normal pelvic examination.

Abdominal bloating
Nausea
Diarrhea

Constipation
Pain that increases on eating or drinking
A history of intestinal disease, such as an irritable or spastic colon

I definitely recommend a patient see a urologist if she has a normal pelvic exam and has symptoms related to the urologic tract, such as:

Burning with urination
Unusual frequency of urination
Inability to hold urine when the bladder is the least bit full
Blood or pus in the urine
History of urologic problems, such as stones or infection

Before a woman sees the consultant, I recommend vaginal ultrasound scan (sonogram) of the woman's pelvis. This procedure, which is painless, safe, and relatively inexpensive, can show growths and other abnormalities that could be missed on a regular pelvic exam.

147 What would the GI specialist do, and what might be found wrong?

The gastroenterologist would ask questions about the nature of your pain and would be especially interested in the problems listed in Question 146 in reference to the intestines. He or she might do some colon studies, depending on your age and the nature of your problem. These studies could include an X-ray (barium enema) or a direct exam of the colon with a proctoscope or using a newer technique called "flexible sigmoidoscopy."

These exams are not as terrible as you may have heard! Although they are not *comfortable*, they usually are not *horrible* tests. Any discomfort should be weighed in light of the importance of the tests, which can detect such things as polyps and cancers before they become dangerous.

The gastroenterologist will often find irritable or spastic colon in a woman who has abdominal pain. Let me warn you though that doctors *often* do not think of this problem. I have had many patients through the years who have been treated by gynecologists for PID when there was no PID or for endometriosis when there was none; the real problem was irritable colon. Some women have had unnecessary hysterectomies for pain that was actually caused by their colon. (Unfortunately these patients still had pain following unnecessary hysterectomies.)

Let me encourage you to think of irritable colon yourself if your problem has the following characteristics:

1. *Variation in pain:* Your pain may come and go all month. It may be a little worse during your menstrual time, but it is definitely present at other times during the month. (You also may be free of the pain at times.)
2. *Constipation:* You may not think you are constipated, but if you are not having one or two bowel movements every day, you are having mild constipation, even if your stools are not hard. (You can have irritable colon syndrome without constipation also.)
3. *Diarrhea:* If you have a little diarrhea every one to two weeks, or even every one to two months, it may be a sign of irritable colon.
4. *Nausea:* If you become nauseated when the pain comes, you may have a colon problem. This is much less common with pelvic pain from other causes. (Nausea is not always present with irritable colon, however.)
5. *Pain in low abdomen:* The pain of irritable colon is low in the abdomen. People usually complain that they are having "pain in the ovaries." When I hear that, I usually "know" they have irritable colon if their pelvic exam is normal.
6. *Pain on pelvic exam:* Women with irritable colon syndrome are usually tender on pelvic exam because the colon is down in the pelvis just as the uterus and ovaries are.
7. *Pain with intercourse:* If you have pain with intercourse, it may be caused by the penis hitting against the irritated colon, which is down in the pelvis.

Irritable colon is a common problem. If you suspect you may have irritable colon syndrome, see an intestinal specialist even if your gynecologist is not enthusiastic about the idea. (You can always go back to the gynecologist and have surgery later!)

Treatment for irritable colon is usually very simple. It often does not even require medication. A patient is usually put on a high-fiber, low-sugar diet. If these suggestions are followed the pain will almost always go away.

An occasional patient will have chronic appendicitis that flares up periodically. The pain from this is normally more severe and occurs less often than the pain of an irritable or spastic colon. The gastroenterologist would be the doctor to diagnose this but would then refer the patient to a general surgeon for an appendectomy.

148 What would a urologist do, and what might he or she find wrong?

A urologist would usually want a urinalysis and a urine culture; he or she would also look into a woman's bladder with a cystoscope to check for signs of inflammation of the urethra or of the bladder, if this was necessary. The urologist may also take a kidney X-ray, called an IVP (intravenous pyelogram), in which a special dye is injected into a vein. X-rays of the kidneys are then taken as the dye collects in them.

An irritated bladder, urethritis (irritation of the urethra), or cystitis (infection of the bladder) can cause persistent pelvic pain. If you have cystitis, antibiotics will be used. If the urologist believes that your bladder is merely spastic, you might be put on Ditropan, or a similar drug, to relieve the spasms. If you have urethritis, the doctor will often dilate your urethra. This compresses the small glands of the urethra, squeezing out the pus so that the infection will go away. Antibiotics may also be prescribed. Urethral irritation is a fairly common cause of pelvic discomfort in women, but it is often hard to diagnose. See a good urologist if you have persistent pelvic pain.

Interstitial cystitis is a fairly common cause of bladder pain. Be sure your urologist evaluates you for this if you are having burning with urination, frequency of urination both day and night, and a feeling of incomplete emptying of the bladder, pelvic pain, and pain with intercourse. A patient with all these symptoms with no sign of infection in the urine may have interstitial cystitis. This problem can be missed even by good urologists. Try to see a urologist interested in this problem if you are having these symptoms.

For further information on this subject, contact the Interstitial Cystitis Association at: P.O. Box 1553, Madison Square Station, New York, NY 10159, phone (212) 979-6057.

149 What other problems might produce low abdominal or pelvic pain?

A few of the problems that can cause pelvic pain are:

Hernias. If you notice a bulge in the groin when you strain or have bowel movements, you probably have a hernia. Hernias in women are sometimes difficult to find. If you have persistent pain in the groin, and the doctor does not find any abnormality, including no enlarged lymph nodes, he or she may order a CT scan (see glossary) to see if there is a bulge, a telltale sign of a hernia. If the CT scan is negative, your pain is almost certainly not a hernia but could be a problem with the ligaments in the pelvic area. In this case you could see an orthopedist for evaluation of those ligaments and bones.

Hematomas of the abdominal wall. In both young, athletic women and in older women, tears of the rectus muscles, the muscles of the central part of the abdominal wall, can cause bleeding into these muscles. This causes pain and a thickening that can feel like a growth in the pelvis. If your pain increases when you lift your head and goes away when you put your head down, you may have a hematoma of the abdominal wall. Occasionally, in a relaxed position, you can actually "pick up" part of the muscle in your fingers and feel the knot in it where the blood has accumulated. This accumulation of blood is a clot, but it is not the dangerous kind that can break loose and go into your lungs or heart, nor does it require surgery. The blood will absorb out of the area. A heating pad to the area and pain pills are usually all the treatment needed.

Enlarged lymph nodes. Lymph nodes can become enlarged in the groin area and cause pain. If these nodes remain for several weeks, you need to have them evaluated.

150 If no one is able to find the cause, but my pain persists, what should I do?

If pelvic pain persists after evaluation by other specialists, a patient should return to her gynecologist for a more thorough evaluation. The first thing I would do for persistent pain after doing another pelvic examination would be a laparoscopy. (For a description of this procedure, see Q. 810.) The laparoscopy will occasionally show some adhesions, some mild inflammation of the tubes, or some other abnormality that was not suspected from the history and examination.

At the time a laparoscopy is done, a hysteroscopy and an endometrial biopsy can also be done to show whether or not there are abnormalities inside the uterus that might be causing pelvic pain. A hysteroscopy is a simple procedure that can be done at the same time as the laparoscopy. A pencil-sized telescope is inserted through the cervix into the uterus. It allows the doctor to view the interior of the uterus. If there are polyps or tumors inside the uterus, they can be seen during this procedure. An endometrial biopsy can also be done at the time of laparoscopy. It involves scraping the inside wall of the uterus and sending the tissue to a pathologist to check for infection. This can identify a mild infection that could cause pain.

If these two procedures have identified no abnormality, the process of elimination has narrowed the possibilities of physical problems down to two probable choices: pelvic congestion syndrome or adenomyosis. (See Q. 692–695.) These problems will normally get worse at the time of the menstrual period and get better afterward, but not necessarily. When diagnostic procedures have been exhausted and no physical cause of the pain has been discovered, the possibility that the pain is of emotional origin must be considered.

151 If the gynecologic and related evaluations fail to find a cause for my pain, what else can be done?

If you have gone through the complete evaluation process and are still having pain, you can be sure that there is nothing seriously or dangerously wrong and that you have nothing to worry about, even though you may still have discomfort. Empiric treatment can now be tried. This is treatment with a technique that might stop the problem, although there is no specific indication for the treatment. Empiric treatments for pelvic pain may include:

Birth-control pills. If a patient has pain in her female organs, birth-control pills are sometimes useful in eliminating it. They essentially put the female organs to sleep and can cause endometriosis and adenomyosis to become inactive. Unfortunately, if a woman has pelvic-congestion syndrome, birth-control pills can occasionally make that worse.

Danocrine. If a doctor suspects adenomyosis, Danocrine can be tried. (See Q. 852.) Danocrine can cause adenomyosis to clear up, and if that has been the problem the patient's pain will lessen. A patient can stay on Danocrine for only six months. However, if her pain recurs after one round of treatments, Danocrine can be tried again. But if pain persists after a second round, most physicians recommend that a woman discontinue using Danocrine because it obviously is not going to be a permanent cure. A hysterectomy might then be indicated if a woman does not desire fertility.

GnRH agonist (Lupron, Syneral). If the pain seems to be from the female organs, there is a third choice for treatment—a drug called gonadotrophin-releasing hormone (GnRH) agonist. An agonist in this situation is a drug that is similar to a naturally occurring hormone. GnRH agonist medication is more potent than a person's natural GnRH. (See Q. 61–65 for an explanation of the female hormone cycle.) This extra potency causes overstimulation that literally shuts down the pituitary's production of gonadotrophins (FSH and LH). When this happens, the ovaries are no longer stimulated by these hormones. They stop producing eggs, es-

trogen, and progesterone. Everything in the woman's pelvis goes into "hibernation," much like a temporary menopause. Menstrual periods stop, the menstrual cycle stops, the vaginal tissues start thinning and becoming dry, and hot flashes develop.

If a woman's pelvic pain is caused by a problem in the female organs, it will usually stop with this treatment. If the pain is from the pelvic muscles, the bladder, etc., it will continue because these organs are not affected by this treatment.

GnRH agonists must be stopped after six months because a woman starts losing bone just like she would if she had gone through the menopause. If pelvic pain then returns, she and her doctor will know for sure that the pain is from the female organs. Other treatment can be considered at that time, such as presacral neurectomy or hysterectomy.

Psychiatric consultation. Women do occasionally have pain in pelvic organs that stems from an emotional disturbance. If you have been physically evaluated to no avail, and you know that you are under significant emotional stress, have your doctor refer you to a good psychologist or psychiatrist. Such a specialist can often help you rid yourself of not only the burden of pain but also of the underlying problem that produced it.

Surgery. Presacral neurectomy (see Q. 853–854), cutting the nerves whose pathways go near the cervix (paracervical uterine denervation), and D&C are procedures that can occasionally help a woman with pelvic pain.

If the quality of a woman's life is affected by her pain, and she has been unsuccessfully and thoroughly evaluated for every other cause—and the pain seems to be from the female organs—then hysterectomy is useful. My experience, and the experience of many other gynecologists, has been that this procedure does stop patients' pain if thorough evaluation has preceded such surgery.

Doctors opposed to hysterectomy for pelvic pain will say that the patient's pain was "emotional" to start with and that she will, a few months after the hysterectomy, begin feeling pain in some other part of her body. This may occasionally be true, but in the patients I have thoroughly evaluated, found no other problem, and who felt better with three months of GnRH agonist, all have benefited from a hysterectomy.

Bladder Infections

152 What causes bladder infections, and why do they occur more often in women than in men?

Bladder infections (cystitis) are caused by germs that invade and infect the bladder. These germs cause the lining inside the bladder to become red and inflamed, just as your throat does when it gets infected. Since pus cells and germs from the infection are passed in the urine, it is often easy to diagnose a bladder infection by urine tests.

Bladder infections occur frequently in women because the urethra, the tube through which the urine leaves the bladder and empties to the outside, is so short (one and one-half to two inches long). This makes it easy for germs from the vulva to get up through the urethra to the bladder.

Germs can be massaged into the bladder with intercourse, and most women do not have bladder infections until they start having intercourse. Poor toilet habits can also introduce germs into the bladder. For this reason a woman should wipe her vulva from front to back after urinating or having a bowel movement.

153 What are the symptoms of cystitis or bladder infection?

A bladder infection usually comes on suddenly. A burning sensation when urinating and the need to urinate frequently are common symptoms. Other symptoms are blood in the urine and pain in the lower abdomen, behind the pubic bone. When she first notices these symptoms, a woman should immediately call her doctor and get medication, whether it is night or day. If she does not, she can quickly get extremely uncomfortable.

154 What is "honeymoon cystitis"?

Honeymoon cystitis is a term applied to a bladder infection that develops after a woman first starts having intercourse. This type of cystitis is often merely an irritation in the urethra, but sometimes it is an irritation of the bladder caused by the penis thrusting against it. Many times this is not a true infection of these tissues, and all that is required is a drug to soothe the bladder and urethra. I recommend that a bride who is a virgin take antibiotics and Pyridium on her honeymoon just in case she develops this problem.

Honeymoon cystitis can also occur when a woman resumes intercourse after several months of abstinence. It does not necessarily occur immediately, but sometimes develops several weeks or months after resuming or starting sexual activity.

155 Are there other things related to sexual practices that might encourage cystitis?

There are two sexual practices that might contribute to bladder infections: oral sex and anal sex. If your husband stimulates your clitoris and vulvar areas with his mouth and tongue, he may be contaminating the area with germs. For most women, oral stimulation by their husbands is not a factor in their cystitis and is generally a normal, healthy sexual activity. If you have a frustrating problem with recurrent bladder infections, you might try stopping this practice for a few months to see if it makes any difference.

The same applies to anal, or rectal, intercourse. If you do have anal intercourse, gynecologists recommend that you not allow your husband to insert his penis into your vagina after it has been in your rectum because this puts germs from your rectum into your vagina. If you practice anal intercourse and are having a major problem with bladder infections, you should stop this practice completely even if your husband does not go back into your vagina after rectal intercourse. If you notice that this helps clear up your bladder infection, you should discontinue anal intercourse.

One other sexual practice that may contribute to cystitis is the penis entering the vagina from the rear. If you feel that you get a great deal of poking on your bladder from your husband's penis with this or any sexual position you normally use, change that technique if you continue to have problems with cystitis and see if it makes any difference.

156 How is cystitis treated?

Treatment for cystitis is classified into three categories.

First cystitis episode. You should call your doctor immediately when you have symptoms of cystitis. If it is inconvenient for you to take a urine specimen to a laboratory—for instance, if the problem develops at night or while you are out of town—the doctor will probably prescribe medications anyway. The medications might be Pyridium to soothe the bladder, and an antibiotic such as Septra, Macrodantin, or Ampicillin to kill the germs. Pyridium will color your urine orange. Since this can stain your clothing, you need to carefully avoid getting this colored urine on clothes that you value.

With this type of medication, the burning will usually stop within twelve hours. It was once thought that women needed to be treated with antibiotics for ten or twelve days, but it has recently been found that treatment with an appropriate antibiotic for five days, or even for one day, will get rid of most bladder infections. However, it is important that you take all the medication your doctor prescribes.

Repeat episodes of cystitis. It is common for cystitis to return, even though it has been treated properly. Most doctors want a urine culture done if a woman calls back with another infection within a month or two of the first infection. This is done to determine which germ is causing the infection and which drug is most likely to cure it. (If the germs responded to the drug previously used, the same drug may be given again.)

This time, though, the doctor may encourage you to drink cranberry juice and take vitamin C. This promotes an acidic urine in which germs grow poorly. Drinking more water will promote flushing of the bladder. You should also urinate after each act of intercourse to wash any germs from your bladder and urethra, and to keep stagnant urine from staying in your bladder.

Recurrent cystitis infection. If you continue to have bladder infections, you should see a urologist. The infection may actually be coming from germs that have infected the kidney and are coming down in the urine to infect the bladder. Of course, the reverse could happen: Continued presence of germs in your bladder could eventually result in your kidneys becoming infected.

Recurrent bladder infections may be caused by a stricture of the urethra, a condition in which the opening of the urethra is so tight that it prevents complete emptying of the bladder. Stagnant urine can provide excellent culture media for the growth of germs.

If you have recurrent infections and you see a urologist, he or she will normally check to be sure your urethra is not too small. The doctor may also look inside your bladder by cystoscopy to make sure you do not have a growth that might be causing the infection, and will often order a kidney X-ray (IVP) to make sure your kidneys do not show signs of chronic infection. You will then be treated and kept under the urologist's care for repeat treatment of your bladder or kidney problems if that is necessary. Call the urologist (rather than your gynecologist) when symptoms recur.

There are many patients on kidney machines today because their kidneys were destroyed by neglected kidney disease. There is no need for you to risk this.

Premenstrual Syndrome (PMS)

157 What is premenstrual syndrome (PMS)?

Premenstrual syndrome (PMS) is the name used for a variety of physical and/or emotional problems that occur prior to a woman's menstrual period. Symptoms of PMS may occur only one day or as long as two full weeks before the period starts. A woman may have only one symptom of PMS, or she may have many.

Because it is the production of progesterone at the time of ovulation that seems to be associated with the onset of PMS, PMS can only occur during the time from ovulation until the menses begin (about fourteen days). Occasionally PMS symptoms may persist until the period is over. Problems that occur at other times during the month cannot be PMS.

Up to 90 percent of all women who menstruate have premenstrual tension of some degree. For most it is not severe, but for 20 to 30 percent of women, PMS is a major problem that may interfere with relationships, increase alcohol consumption, make them feel suicidal, or cause them to miss work or school.

If you experience PMS (as defined by the previous question and the ones that follow), you should get help from your physician. If your physician tells you that your symptoms are all "in your head," find a physician who understands PMS and will help you.

158 What are the symptoms of PMS?

The symptoms of PMS can best be divided into two groups: physical symptoms and emotional symptoms. Some women will have only physical symptoms; some will have only emotional symptoms; some will have both. Some women will have only one symptom; some women may have as many as twenty or thirty symptoms.

Women with PMS typically experience the feeling of being out of control, which may cause them to withdraw from family, friends, and activities. Tension from PMS may cause them to lash out at those around them, and they frequently refer to themselves as "mean" during that time. The physical discomfort of abdominal bloating and breast tenderness may cause further irritability.

While as many as a hundred symptoms may be associated with PMS, no one of them is unique to the syndrome. The symptoms may also indicate thyroid disease, anxiety, hormone imbalance, etc.

The key to determining whether or not a symptom indicates PMS is whether or not it occurs primarily during the two-week period before the menstrual period begins.

PMS may include the following physical and emotional symptoms:

Physical symptoms

abdominal bloating
fullness in the lower abdomen
aching in the lower abdomen
generalized swelling of the body
tightness of rings
tightness of shoes
tingling in the fingers (parasthesias)
carpal tunnel syndrome (numbness of the hands related to swelling in the wrists)
breast tenderness
headaches
acne
skin rashes
irritation of the eyes not caused by infection
outbreaks of herpes (including fever blisters of the lips or herpes of the vulvar area)
sinus congestion (due to increased fluid production from the sinuses)
increased vaginal secretions (causing a woman to suspect a vaginal infection)
increased problems with preexistent epilepsy
increased problems with asthma (not a cause, but symptoms may worsen)
backache
muscle spasms and pain in the arms and legs, especially the joints
fainting episodes (syncope)
tiredness and fatigue
dizziness
lack of coordination
clumsiness
heart palpitations
poorly fitting dentures
easy bruising
increased problems with hypoglycemia or with symptoms of hypoglycemia
increased problems with ulcerative colitis
increased problems with preexistent heart disease
ulcerations of the mouth

Emotional symptoms

tension
irritability
depression
anxiety
mood swings
outbursts of temper
shouting
throwing things
paranoia
forgetfulness
self-blaming
desire to withdraw from others
suicidal feelings
compulsive activity
change in sexual interest (usually increased at
    time of ovulation and decreased after)
aggression
lethargy
sleeping disorders
insomnia
nightmares or unusual dreams
unnatural fears
increased use of alcohol and other mood-
    altering drugs
argumentativeness
inability to initiate activities or accomplish
    work at the usual pace
indecisiveness (or making poor decisions)
marital conflict
food cravings
increased appetite
difficulty in concentrating

159 **If I have PMS, does it mean that there is something wrong with my body, that I am just "emotional," or that I am spiritually out of touch with God?**

On the contrary. It is important that you realize that PMS is not a sign that your body is abnormal but evidence that the hormones in your body are working just the way they are supposed to work. (See Q. 62–65 for a further discussion of this.) If you have PMS, you do not need to worry that you have a disease in your body that is going to be dangerous for you. Rather, you can concentrate your efforts on doing things to make yourself feel better.

The irritability, anger, depression, and other psychological changes associated with PMS do not mean that a woman is weak or unstable, or that she has lost touch with God. These changes are a result of physical changes, not a sign of emotional or spiritual weakness. While it is certainly appropriate to pray about these feelings, if they affect a woman's relationship with her husband, her children, or her friends, she should also seek medical help.

There is no doubt that PMS is a physical problem, evident by the fact that all of the symptoms disappear either before the period starts or by the first or second day of the period.

160 **How can I know if I have PMS?**

Make a calendar like the one shown and keep a record for three months. If, according to the calendar, your symptoms always occur after ovulation and tend to go away at the time your menstrual flow starts, you probably have PMS. If your calendar does not show that you are free of PMS symptoms for at least a week after your menstrual period, you do not have PMS. Or, at least all your symptoms are not due to the premenstrual syndrome.

When you keep a PMS calendar, *record only your three worst symptoms.* Otherwise your chart may be almost unreadable. If this charting indicates PMS, you may be able to control your PMS symptoms by using some of the suggestions offered in the answer to Question 162. If the things you try at home do not work, you may want to take your calendar to your physician and talk about further evaluation and therapy. Your doctor will want to be sure your symptoms are not a sign of some other medical problem. He/she will probably want to test you for thyroid disease, diabetes, or other illnesses. He/she will also talk to you to see if there are any unusual stressors in your life that may be making mild PMS more severe. (This is a common problem.) When the evaluation is complete, you can continue with treatment.

161 What is the treatment for PMS?

Even though doctors are not sure exactly what causes PMS, they have found some ways to control it. These methods can be divided into two groups. The first includes commonsense, nonmedical changes in your life, which may alleviate your problem if you do not have severe PMS. The second group includes medical treatments, which are often helpful only if nonmedical lifestyle changes are followed also.

162 Which nonmedical changes might help control PMS?

There are several nonmedical measures you can adopt to control your PMS.

Adjust your life to your cycle. Live with your menstrual cycle; don't fight it. In her book, *The Joy of Being a Woman* (Harper & Row, 1975), Ingrid Trobisch suggests that women should be aware of when they will have their premenstrual symptoms and reserve that time for the quiet activities of life, such as reading and doing things that do not require much interaction with other people. If a woman works, she can concentrate on work-related duties that require less intensity. A woman should not plan big dinner parties or a household move at the time of her premenstrual symptoms if she can avoid it. Obviously no woman can control these things completely, but it does help to remember to schedule the events in your life around your cycle.

Talk about PMS. Discuss your PMS with your family and, if appropriate, with close friends. This will help them be aware of what is going on. It would certainly be appropriate for you to warn those you are closest to as soon as you sense the onset of PMS symptoms.

I suggest that a husband keep up with where his wife is in her cycle so that her PMS symptoms may be anticipated. A husband will usually find that doing "something nice" for his wife during that time will be greatly appreciated. It is helpful if the husband dispenses hugs and kisses and shows his wife tenderness during the time of her PMS. This should be the type of physical closeness that does not demand intercourse as a reward.

Many women do not hug their husbands as often as they want to at this time because they "know what will happen" if they do, and they are often not interested in sex at this time of the month.

Cut calories and eat more frequently. Decrease your intake of calories, not just at premenstrual time but all month long. This helps control body weight, decreasing the swelling during the premenstrual days. Cutting calories can also lessen the symptoms of hypoglycemia during this time, and any hypoglycemia can aggravate PMS symptoms. Almost all Americans get too much sugar, and the extra sugar can be a problem for PMS sufferers.

Eating more frequently can also help decrease hypoglycemia, resulting in help with PMS. Try eating some cheese or a small meal every three hours during the time of your PMS, whether or not you have hypoglycemia. Such meals should include a minimum of sugar.

Increase physical activity. This too should be done all month long. It will not only decrease body fat but will also improve your health and general sense of well-being. I believe that women who do not exercise adequately are rarely able to get their PMS under control no matter what else they do (including taking medication). Thirty minutes of walking three to six times a week can be adequate. Some women find that more exercise makes them feel even better.

Cut salt intake. Follow a low-salt diet, especially during the premenstrual time. This helps decrease swelling and bloating.

Discontinue use of caffeine. Avoid the intake of caffeine during PMS time because caffeine may increase your level of agitation. This means drinking caffeine-free coffee, tea, and colas and not eating chocolate.

163 What medical treatments can help alleviate PMS symptoms?

Before discussing medical treatment for PMS, I must emphasize the importance of two things. First, once you have determined that you do, indeed, have PMS (based on a doctor's diagnosis or by your keeping a PMS calendar), your goal should

PMS Calendar

Name _____

Baseline Weight on Day 1: _____ lbs.

	1	2	3	4	5	6	7	8	9	10	11	12	13	14	15	16	17	18	19	20	21	22	23	24	25	26	27	28	29	30	31	32	33	34	35	36	37	38	39	40	41	42	43	44	45	46	47	48	49
BLEEDING																																																	
Day of Menstrual Cycle	1	2	3	4	5	6	7	8	9	10	11	12	13	14	15	16	17	18	19	20	21	22	23	24	25	26	27	28	29	30	31	32	33	34	35	36	37	38	39	40	41	42	43	44	45	46	47	48	49
Month: Date:																																																	
WEIGHT CHANGE																																																	
SYMPTOMS																																																	
Irritable																																																	
Fatigue																																																	
Inward anger																																																	
Labile mood (crying)																																																	
Depressed																																																	
Restless																																																	
Anxious																																																	
Insomnia																																																	
Lack of control																																																	
Edema or rings tight																																																	
Breast tenderness																																																	
Abdominal bloating																																																	
Bowels: const.(c)/loose (l)																																																	
Appetite: up↑ down↓																																																	
Sex drive: up↑ down↓																																																	
Chills (c)/Sweats (s)																																																	
Headaches																																																	
Crave: sweets, salt																																																	
Feel unattractive																																																	
Guilty																																																	
Unreasonable behavior																																																	
Low self-image																																																	
Nausea																																																	
Menstrual cramps																																																	
LIFESTYLE IMPACT																																																	
Aggressive toward others — Physically																																																	
Aggressive toward others — Verbally																																																	
Wish to be alone																																																	
Neglect housework																																																	
Time off work																																																	
Disorganized, distractible																																																	
Accident prone/clumsy																																																	
Uneasy about driving																																																	
Suicidal thoughts																																																	
Stayed at home																																																	
Increased use of alcohol																																																	
LIFE EVENTS																																																	
Negative experience																																																	
Positive experience																																																	
Social activities																																																	
Vigorous exercise																																																	
MEDICATIONS																																																	

Used by permission of Robert L. Reid, M.D.

INSTRUCTIONS FOR COMPLETING THIS CALENDAR

1. On the first day of menstruation prepare the calendar: Considering the first day of bleeding as day 1 of your menstrual cycle, enter the corresponding calendar date for each day in the space provided.
2. Each Morning: Take weight after emptying bladder and before breakfast. Record WEIGHT CHANGE from baseline.
3. Each Evening: At about the same time complete the column for that day as described below.

   BLEEDING: Indicate if you have had bleeding by shading the box about that day's date■; for spotting use an X

   SYMPTOMS: If you do not experience any symptoms, leave the corresponding square blank. If present, indicate severity.
   MILD: 1 (noticeable but not troublesome)
   MODERATE: 2 (interferes with normal activity)
   SEVERE: 3 (temporarily incapacitating)

LIFESTYLE IMPACT: If the listed phrase applies to you that day enter an X

LIFE EVENTS: If you experienced one of these events that day enter an X

Experiences: For positive (happy) or negative (sad or disappointing) experiences unrelated to your symptoms specify the nature of the events on the reverse side of this form.

Social Activities: Imply events such as a special dinner, show, or party, etc. involving family or friends.

Vigorous Exercise: Implies participation in a sporting event or exercise program lasting more than 30 minutes.

MEDICATION: In the bottom 3 rows list medications if any and indicate days when taken by entering an X be to do all you can to alleviate the symptoms of the problem. Rather than using the diagnosis as an "excuse" to be irritable or sick, use it as a motivation to do all you can to control the problem.

Second, I must emphasize again the importance of the nonmedical treatments discussed in the previous question. The foundation treatment for PMS is limiting salt, sugar, and caffeine and exercising. If you do not do these things, it is unlikely that any drug will solve your PMS problem. Only after these changes in your lifestyle fail to bring complete relief should you try medication.

Over-the-Counter Drugs

Drugs marketed as treatment for PMS can be purchased without a prescription at your local pharmacy. Most of these drugs contain a mild diuretic for swelling, an antihistamine for tension and cramps, and acetaminophen (such as in Tylenol) for pain. These drugs may significantly help with PMS symptoms. If they work for you, there is no reason for you to see a physician for stronger drugs.

Nonprescription Drugs

Vitamin B6 (pyridoxine). A few years ago, vitamin B6 was the most popular medication for PMS. I found that it failed to help my patients very often, and studies have shown that, scientifically, it gives no relief. If you want to try vitamin B6, do not take over 250 mg a day. (Dosages higher than that have been shown to produce neurologic damage, such as numbness in the feet, hips, hands, and face.)

Magnesium and calcium. Because chocolate is high in magnesium, some physicians thought that craving it (common with PMS) indicated a deficiency of magnesium. There is nothing harmful about trying magnesium supplements. The best amount seems to be 250 mg a day, taken throughout the month. A dose of 500 to 1,000 mg of calcium daily is healthy for any woman to use to prevent future osteoporosis. If at the same time it solves a present problem with PMS, that is an added benefit.

Evening primrose oil (Efamol). This was very popular a few years ago for treating PMS, but most women found that it was not very helpful. If you

want to try it, the usual dosage is two 0.5 gram capsules of Efamol, twice a day from the time of ovulation till your PMS time is over. You can take as much as eight capsules a day without risk, though it can cause stomach upset.

Prescription Drugs

(These require that you see a physician.)

Prostaglandin synthetase inhibitors. This is a big word for drugs like ibuprofen. I normally start with this when I give a patient a prescription for PMS. The drug I usually prescribe is Ponstel, 250 mg, two capsules initially, followed by one every six hours. You may prefer to try over-the-counter ibuprofen, taking 800 mg every six or eight hours. (Ibuprofen usually comes in 200 mg tablets, but four can be taken at once every six or eight hours.) If ibuprofen doesn't work for you, a stronger prostaglandin inhibitor, such as Ponstel, may be needed.

Do not take these drugs if you are pregnant. If these drugs are taken regularly for PMS, adequate birth-control methods must be used.

Natural progesterones have been recommended for many years for women with PMS. Until just a few years ago, they were available only as vaginal suppositories, rectal suppositories, rectal oil, or injection. Oral micronized progesterone is now available. The usual dose is 100 mg a day, but it can be increased to 300 mg a day or more.

Progesterone produces a sedative effect, which may be its major contribution in helping PMS symptoms. Several research studies have shown that progesterone does not benefit PMS sufferers, but most physicians have found it helps some patients a great deal. I think it is worth a try if other things do not work.

Antianxiety agents. Antianxiety agents and tranquilizers may be useful for treating PMS. I prescribe these mostly for a woman who has only two or three days of trouble with the emotional symptoms of PMS. I usually start with Xanax, 0.25 mg, three or four times a day, to be used for two or three days. If her PMS lasts longer than this, I hesitate to prescribe a tranquilizer because of the possibility she will become emotionally dependent on it. If she and her doctor are careful, however, I see no problem with longer use.

Diuretics. If swelling is a problem during the PMS time, a mild diuretic may be useful. I often prescribe Aldactone, 25 mg, three times a day. (This should not be taken while pregnant, therefore use a good contraceptive if you take it.)

Although this very mild diuretic is used primarily to relieve the problem of swelling, it seems to help with the emotional symptoms of PMS too. If the swelling is not relieved, a stronger diuretic can be tried.

Oral contraceptives. Birth-control pills often provide relief of PMS symptoms for women who can tolerate them and who do not want to become pregnant. They are effective for about one-third of women with PMS. Unfortunately, about one-third of the women find their symptoms of PMS worsened by oral contraceptives. If they work for you, they are certainly a convenient method of treatment for PMS.

Parlodel. This drug can be very useful for breast pain and tenderness, although it can cause nausea. The usual dose is 2.5 mg, twice a day, but smaller amounts often help. (Parlodel can also help relieve breast pain that is not a PMS symptom but occurs all month.)

Psychiatric drugs. If you are having tremendous mood swings, suicidal thoughts, and depression, you may need to see a psychiatrist for evaluation and specific drug therapy. These drugs have been studied and do often help people who have severe PMS.

Drugs that stop the function of the ovaries. PMS is so bad for some women that stopping ovarian function is the best solution while getting consultation, being reevaluated, and determining a proper course of therapy for treatment. There are two drugs that are useful for this purpose.

One of these drugs is danazol, 200 mg, twice a day, continuously. It can be used for no more than six months, as it can cause excessive hair growth, voice change, and decreased breast size. It is very important not to get pregnant while taking this drug. Therefore a woman must use a mechanical, barrier-type contraceptive while on it. One problem with it that can be very bothersome is that it can cause weight gain.

A new drug, GnRH agonist (Lupron and Syneral) (see Q. 858), can also stop the function of the ovaries. Most women can tolerate this drug better than danazol. This drug, too, should be used for only six months.

If danazol or GnRH agonists are successful in stopping the symptoms of PMS, a woman has good proof that her symptoms are true PMS and that permanent interruption of her natural hormone cycle will solve her PMS problem. Women who have completed their families may want to consider having a hysterectomy (removing uterus, tubes, and ovaries). This should only be done after careful evaluation, and in my opinion, usually only after having used a drug like danazol or a GnRH agonist to prove that PMS symptoms will disappear when the ovaries are inactivated.

Other forms of treatment. Since the cause of PMS is not known, finding "the cure" is not yet possible. Many things are being tried. As with other chronic problems, such as cancer and arthritis, new forms of treatment are mentioned in newspapers and magazines almost every month. Some of these "PMS cures" that have been proposed are antibiotics, calcium, thyroid, estrogen, opiate antagonists (Naltrexone), estrogen and progesterone, Clonidine, tryptophan, and others. If the medications your physician has given you have not helped, you may want to ask him or her to look into other, less common treatment methods.

Diethylstilbestrol (DES)

164 What is diethylstilbestrol (DES)?

DES is a synthetic compound that produces the same effect in a woman's body as estrogen. DES can be used interchangeably with estrogen compounds in certain situations, such as for women who need estrogen after menopause. *Except for use during pregnancy,* DES is in no way more dangerous or unhealthy than any other estrogen-type compound.

Starting in 1941, studies indicated that DES helped decrease the chance of a woman having a miscarriage. Subsequent studies showed that DES was also useful if a pregnant woman had diabetes or toxemia of pregnancy. Because of these findings, doctors felt that a woman who had bleeding with a pregnancy, had a previous miscarriage, had diabetes, or had toxemia with a previous pregnancy would benefit by taking DES during a subsequent pregnancy. Since 20 percent of all pregnancies end as miscarriages, and since any patient who had previously had a miscarriage was supposed to be helped by DES, one can easily see why such a large number of women received DES while pregnant.

The dangers of taking DES while pregnant were exposed in 1971, at which time doctors stopped prescribing it for pregnant women. Eight to ten million people were exposed to DES in their mothers' wombs between the years of 1941 and 1972. Since the drug is no longer being used during pregnancy, we can expect no more people to join this group. Because many women's lives have been affected by DES, we should discuss this topic.

The youngest girls born after exposure to DES were born in 1972. Therefore, the only women in our society who have been exposed to DES before birth are, at the time of this publication, in their twenties up to their late fifties. The problems connected with DES are generally much less severe than was first feared when the dangers of DES were exposed. Knowing this should help those who are concerned about it to relax and not worry so much about their DES exposure. It should also help those women who took DES while pregnant to feel less guilty about having taken a drug that might have affected their offspring.

165 Did DES use in pregnancy always cause abnormalities?

If women used less than 1.5 mg of DES a day during pregnancy, their babies were not affected. Likewise, if a woman did not take DES until after the twenty-second week (fifth month) of her pregnancy, her child was not affected.

166 What abnormalities are seen in women who were DES-exposed while in their mothers' wombs?

All of the DES-caused abnormalities in women are seen in their female organs: the vagina, the cervix, the uterus, and the breasts. The abnormalities may have been present at birth, but because of the nature of the abnormalities most were not discovered until much later in life.

It is not known exactly how DES caused its damage, but the most logical theory is that it went through the placenta and into the baby's body during its early developmental stages. Once in the fetus, DES competed with the mother's and the baby's natural estrogen, effectively blocking the normal growth of the baby's vagina, cervix, and uterus at a critical time in their development. There is no other time in a person's life when that particular setup exists again. Consequently, outside of the early few months of fetal life, DES cannot in any way be more dangerous than any other estrogen-like drug. Studies have shown that DES-exposed women may have a slightly greater chance of developing breast cancer in later life. Therefore they should carefully examine their breasts monthly and have them checked by a physician regularly and follow the routine American Cancer Society mammogram guidelines. (As of 1994, though, there is still no confirmed increased breast cancer in DES-exposed mothers.)

Abnormalities that have been attributed to DES have been:

A. Vaginal

1. *Adenosis.* The vaginal lining may develop adenosis, a condition in which the vaginal lining (squamous epithelium) is replaced in spots by the type of lining that covers the inside of the cervix (columnar epithelium). This "substitute lining" is a type of glandular epithelium that is normal for some parts of the body but, in this situation, was caused to be in the wrong place. This tissue is not dangerous, and it should not be treated unless it is causing a great deal of mucus secretion.

2. *Cancer.* Doctors were tipped off to the effect of DES by a rare cancer of the cervix and vagina called "clear-cell adenocarcinoma." Prior to the use of DES in pregnancy, this type of can-

cer was almost unknown. Of the patients who were exposed to DES while in their mothers' wombs, more than 360 cases of clear-cell adenocarcinoma have now been found. The encouraging thing for those who have been exposed to DES is that most of the patients who have had clear-cell adenocarcinoma already had it the first time they were examined by a doctor. This means that patients who have been exposed to DES usually do not develop clear-cell adenocarcinoma of the vagina as the years go by. The chance of developing this cancer later in life is very low, but even if you did not have it when you were first seen by your doctor, you still need yearly exams.

3. Cervical intraepithelial neoplasia and vaginal squamous cell cancer. Precancerous and cancerous growths of the cervix develop about twice as often in DES-exposed women as in those not exposed.

B. Cervix

Smaller-than-normal cervix

Ridges of tissue, sometimes called "cervical collar"

Irregularities that make it appear that polyps are present, although true polyps are not actually present

A protrusion of the upper part of the cervix, sometimes called a "cockscomb"

C. Uterus

Almost half the women who have had DES exposure in the womb have an abnormal shape to the inside or the outside of their uterus. The most common abnormality is found by an X-ray of the uterus, a hysterosalpingogram (HSG, see Q. 808). Instead of the normal triangular-shape, about one-third of the women who have been DES-exposed will have a T-shape to the inside cavity of their uterus.

Other abnormalities that may be found, either by HSG or laparoscopy, may vary from a uterus that is smaller than normal, an irregular-shaped inner cavity, or a too-wide lower uterine cavity. These abnormalities can result in fertility problems. However, half of the women who were exposed to DES have no abnormalities and their fertility is unaffected, so far as researchers know now.

If a woman is found to have an abnormality of her uterus as a result of DES exposure, the probability of her having a premature baby increases. One study showed that if a woman had an abnormal uterus from DES, she had only a 51 percent chance of carrying a pregnancy to term and giving birth to a live infant.

If a woman has a DES-type uterine abnormality, it may be best for her to have a purse-string suture put around her cervix (called a cerclage) in early pregnancy to keep the abnormal uterus from aborting her pregnancy or to keep it from causing a premature delivery. (See Q. 557.)

Tubal ectopic pregnancies occur more often in DES-exposed women who have an abnormal uterus. Approximately 6–10 percent of the pregnancies in this group end up as tubal pregnancies, whereas only about 1 percent of the DES-exposed women with a normal uterus will have tubal pregnancies.

167 Were the sons of women who took DES while pregnant affected?

One study showed that about 30 percent of the DES-exposed sons had some abnormality of their genital tract. In spite of these abnormalities, however, DES seems to have no effect on a man's fertility or sexual function, nor on his age of puberty, first ejaculation, first intercourse, hormone levels, sperm count, or sperm quality.

Abnormalities that have been seen are mild abnormalities of the penis, the testes, and the epididymis. The most common abnormality is epididymal cysts (an insignificant finding) present in 20 percent of the males who were exposed to DES while in the womb.

No cancer has been found to be more common in men who were DES-exposed than in other men.

168 Where can I get more information about DES exposure?

The best source of information about DES is the National Cancer Institute. It has an ongoing study, the DESAD Project (Diethylstilbestrol and Adenosis Project). Institutions participating in this study are:

Massachusetts General Hospital
Harvard Medical School
Boston, MA 02114
Dr. Ann Barnes and Dr. Stanley J. Robboy

University of Southern California
Los Angeles, CA 90024
Dr. Duane E. Townsend

Baylor College of Medicine
Houston, TX 77030
Dr. Raymond H. Kaufman

Mayo Clinic
Rochester, MN 55905
Dr. David G. Decker

Your own physician may have information about DES, and there is a lay group, DES Action USA, which is publishing information for DES-exposed men and women. Their address is 1615 Broadway, Suite 510, Oakland, CA 94612.

Another source of information is:

Registry for Research on Hormonal Transplacental Carcinogenesis
The University of Chicago
5841 S. Maryland Ave.
Chicago, IL 60637
(312) 702-6671

Abortion

169 What does the word *abortion* mean?

Abortion is a medical term that refers to the ending of a pregnancy, for whatever reason, before the baby is mature enough to survive outside the mother's uterus. Physicians usually use the term

when a pregnancy ends before the twentieth week. After that time, or if the baby weighs more than about one pound, the loss of the pregnancy is considered to be a premature delivery. A birth is considered premature until delivery within two weeks of the due date for the pregnancy.

Most people call the spontaneous loss of a pregnancy a miscarriage rather than an abortion. When abortions were legalized in our country in January 1972, even doctors began using the term *abortion* for the pregnancy that a woman terminated and the term *miscarriage* for a pregnancy that she lost spontaneously. Although this helps avoid confusion, technically any loss of pregnancy before the twentieth week is termed an abortion.

Doctors use these terms to define abortion:

Spontaneous abortion (miscarriage). This term describes the spontaneous loss of a pregnancy before the twentieth week.

Missed abortion. This refers to a loss of pregnancy before the twentieth week of growth but—because the contracting mechanism of the uterus did not start working when the baby died—the dead tissue inside the uterus was not delivered. Once doctors are certain that a woman has had a missed abortion, a D&C or a suction curettage is done to remove the dead or remaining material from the uterus.

The ultrasound machine (sonogram) allows doctors to determine much earlier now than in the past that a baby has died and that a miscarriage will occur. We call these miscarriages "missed abortions" because the pregnancy is still in the uterus but the mother has had no contractions and either very little or no bleeding.

If these pregnancies are not disturbed, many of them will eventually miscarry. Most doctors and most patients prefer to proceed with a D&C when they know the baby is no longer alive. This can avoid the bleeding and cramping of a miscarriage that often leads to an emergency D&C. This also helps prevent the possibility of dangerous complications from a miscarriage, such as uterine infection or excessive uterine bleeding.

Miscarriage. This is the spontaneous loss of a pregnancy before the twentieth week. It is a lay term and is not actually a part of the medical vocabulary.

Elective (voluntary) abortion. This refers to the termination of a normal pregnancy at the decision of the mother or a guardian.

Therapeutic (medical) abortion. A therapeutic abortion is one done because of medical problems that might make pregnancy dangerous for the mother, or because of problems that might cause grave physical abnormalities or mental retardation of the baby. Pregnancies that result from rape or incest are also considered by many physicians to be an indication for therapeutic abortions.

Although these abortions are called "therapeutic," they are still elective for the mother. The decision to have (or not to have) a therapeutic abortion is hers alone. There is no law that says a woman must have an abortion because the child might be born with abnormalities or because the mother's health would suffer if she does not have an abortion. A woman whose doctor tells her that she must have an abortion because the baby might have Down syndrome or because of her own health should consider changing doctors if she does not want to have an abortion.

---

170 When does a baby become a human being?

Life clearly begins at the moment of fertilization. It does not matter at what stage of development from that point on a pregnancy is terminated; a life is destroyed and a person no longer exists.

From conception on, a baby's growth and development are continuous. The birth itself does not change a person from one type of organism into another. Birth is merely one of many significant events that occur in a person's life. Some oriental cultures seem to understand this better than our own: When a baby is born, it is considered to be one year old.

A baby's total dependence on its mother before birth does not make it less a person than it is after birth, nor does it mean the baby is merely an appendage to the mother's body. There is a change in the form of dependence that a baby has on its mother, but there is no less dependence after birth than before birth. An astronaut, for example, is no less a person when he or she is confined to a space suit and dependent on a life-sustaining "umbilical cord" for all life functions than when walking on the ground, free of the need for that cord.

Studies have shown normal human functions are detectable in a baby's body very early in pregnancy.

EEG studies. Electroencephalograms have shown brain activity in the baby after six or eight weeks of development. The brain activity shown is much like that of a sleeping adult. This brain activity does not change abruptly at the time of birth.

Heartbeat. After only two weeks from the day of conception, the baby's heart contracts occasionally. Thirty-one days after conception the heart has begun the normal, rhythmic contractions it will have for the rest of its life.

Hormones. By the sixth week of life in the uterus, the baby's adrenal and thyroid glands are functioning. These glands continue to function for the rest of that person's life.

Physical identity. By the twelfth week of intrauterine life, the baby's fingerprints have developed. He or she can be identified as an individual from that point until death by those same fingerprints.

Activity. By the marvel of ultrasound viewing, the baby can be seen moving its arms and legs, sucking its thumb, and turning somersaults. Fetal movements have been recorded on film as early as the thirty-sixth day (fifth week) of development inside the uterus. By the sixth or seventh week of intrauterine life, the baby is developed enough to respond to touch. Later the unborn baby can be seen to be urinating, holding on to the umbilical cord, and doing all the things you would expect a baby to do. Ultrasound allows us to appreciate the fact that "a baby is a baby," whether inside or outside the uterus. This emphasizes the fact that birth is only an event in the baby's life, not an act that turns a baby from a nonhuman to a human.

Feeling. Fetuses that had needles inserted into their abdomens to draw blood showed evidence that it was a stressful event. The British doctors who did the study in 1994 encouraged doctors to use painkillers when performing invasive procedures on unborn babies (*The Washington Times,* July 8, 1994).

171 Do doctors believe that a fetus is a human being?

Most doctors who perform abortions know that they are killing babies. Doctors have enough scientific orientation to know that the signs of the humanity of the fetus cannot be ignored.

A few years ago doctors did not have the evidence we have today. There were no instruments accurate enough to measure the signs of life in a young fetus. But as these tests became available, some physicians who did abortions realized the implications of what they were doing. The many facets of this complicated problem led Bernard N. Nathanson, M.D.—former director of what was the largest abortion clinic in the world at that time—to state in the *New England Journal of Medicine* (November 28, 1984): "I am deeply troubled by my own increasing certainty that I have, in fact, presided in over sixty thousand deaths. There is no longer serious doubt in my mind that human life exists within the womb from the very onset of pregnancy, despite the fact that the nature of the intrauterine life has been the subject of considerable dispute in the past."

172 Does the Bible speak about the baby inside the uterus as a human being?

Yes, in many places and from many perspectives:

Psalm 51:5, NIV. Surely I have been a sinner from birth, sinful from the time my mother conceived me.

This is not the place for a theological discussion about sin. The point is made here that the baby in the uterus is considered to be more than just living tissue.

Psalm 139:13–16, NIV
For you created my inmost being;
You knit me together in my mother's womb.
I praise you because I am fearfully and wonderfully made;
Your works are wonderful,
I know that full well.

My frame was not hidden from you
When I was made in the secret place.
When I was woven together in the depths of the earth,
Your eyes saw my unformed body.
All the days ordained for me
Were written in your book
Before one of them came to be.

Genesis 25:22, NIV. The babies jostled each other within her, and she said, "Why is this happening to me?" So she went to inquire of the Lord.

This verse speaks of the conflict between Jacob and Esau. They were twins who began their conflict with each other *even before they were born*, causing their mother, Rebekah, to inquire of God before she delivered them why they were fighting each other inside her uterus.

Luke 1:41, NIV. When Elizabeth heard Mary's greeting, the baby leaped in her womb, and Elizabeth was filled with the Holy Spirit.

John the Baptist, *while in his mother's uterus*, leaped for joy when his mother was in the presence of Mary, the mother of Jesus, while she was pregnant with Jesus.

Jeremiah 1:5, NIV. Before I formed you in the womb I knew you, before you were born I set you apart; I appointed you as a prophet to the nations.

These words were spoken by God to Jeremiah. God had a plan for Jeremiah from before the time he was born.

Based on these and other similar passages, I believe that God created every person and that he knows every person from conception to death. (See also chapter 6, especially the introductory paragraphs.)

173 How are abortions performed?

The method of abortion is determined by how far along a woman is in her pregnancy.

Abortions done during the first twelve weeks of pregnancy

1. Dilatation and Curettage (D&C). This procedure is the same one that is done when a woman has a D&C for bleeding problems or a miscarriage. The cervix is dilated enough to allow the insertion of an instrument that can scrape the uterus, to kill and remove the baby. Usually done with a paracervical anesthetic in an office, this procedure has now been replaced by suction curettage for most early abortions.

2. Suction curettage. If a woman is in her first two months of pregnancy, a suction technique is normally used. The suction is applied through the end of a thin tube, called a cannula. If an abortion is done very early in pregnancy, a straw-sized cannula can be used. If the pregnancy is more advanced, a larger cannula is necessary and the cervix must be dilated slightly to allow the cannula in.

After the twelfth week the developing baby's body is so large that it will clog even the largest cannula that might be used to suck out the baby.

Once the cannula is pushed up into the uterus, powerful suction is applied and the baby, with its placenta and membranes, is pulled apart and sucked through the cannula into the collecting bottle.

A paracervical block is usually used for pain relief and is moderately effective.

3. Dilatation and Evacuation (D&E). This can be done during the first twelve weeks of pregnancy. The procedure involves dilating the cervix and removing, with various instruments, the parts of the baby's body and the placenta. The doctor may use suction to pull out some of the tissue, but if the suction becomes stopped up by some of the baby's body parts, instruments may be inserted into the uterus to grab pieces of the baby and pull them out. A paracervical block is usually used for this type of procedure. This is the typical abortion done in an abortionist's clinic or office.

Abortions done from the thirteenth week of pregnancy

Abortions done in this stage of pregnancy are much more dangerous for the mother. Attempts have been made to reduce the number of mid-trimester abortions, but in the U.S. there are still more than 100,000 abortions a year done on women who are thirteen or more weeks pregnant. Various techniques are as follows.

1. Dilatation and Evacuation (D&E). The cervix must be dilated adequately to allow insertion of the necessary instruments into the uterus. This dilatation is sometimes accomplished by using a "laminaria" (or similar device), which is put into the cervical canal a few hours before an abortion. The device absorbs fluid, which causes it to swell and produce a gradual, less traumatic, dilatation of the cervix.

Instruments are inserted into the uterus to scrape, suck, and pull out the parts of the baby and the placenta. Because the pregnancy is so far along, large instruments must be used and great care must be taken not to tear the cervix (a problem that often occurs anyway) because this can affect future pregnancies.

Great care must also be taken to remove all parts of the baby's body. An ultrasound (sonogram) may be used to determine that the uterus has been completely emptied.

If the pregnancy is past the twentieth week, the baby's head is so large that it is difficult to remove, although all the other parts of the body may have been pulled out. It is for this reason that a modification of the D&E abortion was developed by abortionist Martin Haskell, M.D. at the National Abortion Federation meeting in Dallas, Texas, September 13, 1992. He calls it D&X (more properly termed a "partial birth abortion." See number 4 in this section.)

One study showed that D&E was the most commonly used method of abortion at thirteen to fifteen weeks of gestation, accounting for 67 percent of such abortions. It is actually used by some doctors until the twentieth week.

2. Intrauterine installation of abortifacient agents. Uterine contractions can be produced by the injection of certain materials into the fluid that surrounds the baby in a pregnant uterus. These agents may be a prostaglandin hormone (PGF2a), saline, or urea. These compounds usually kill the fetus, but many babies are born alive during this type of abortion. Some studies show live birth of fetuses as high as 7 percent with the use of urea or prostaglandins. Because of this, physicians prefer using saline because it kills most babies before they are born.

With this procedure, either salt water, urea, or prostaglandins are injected into the amniotic fluid. After a few minutes or up to twelve hours, the uterus begins contractions, stimulated by the injected drugs. These contractions cause the expulsion of the baby and the placenta (afterbirth). Occasionally the placenta does not come out when the baby is expelled. A D&C is necessary in that event.

This procedure has become less popular primarily because of the embarrassing problem of babies occasionally being born alive.

3. Hysterotomy and hysterectomy. The uterus can be opened up and emptied of the live baby and its placenta and membranes. (The baby dies, of course.) This is called a hysterotomy. A hysterectomy involves removing the entire uterus, with the baby and the placenta and membranes. (This also kills the baby.)

Hysterotomies are normally done only when a pregnancy is more than sixteen weeks along, and then only when other methods have failed or there is some reason that they cannot be used. Hysterectomies can be used at any stage in pregnancy. They are normally done as an abortion procedure only when a woman is planning to have a hysterectomy anyway. The abortion only serves as a reason for her to go ahead with the surgery.

For both hysterectomy and hysterotomy, a major incision in the abdomen is necessary. This requires a general anesthesia, a spinal, or an epidural, and the usual four or five days of recovery in the hospital.

One study showed that only 1 percent of second trimester abortions were done by hysterotomy and hysterectomy. This is fortunate because the *American College of Obstetricians and Gynecologists Technical Bulletin* (October 1987, no. 109) stated, "Because of their prohibitively high morbidity and mortality, hysterectomy and hysterotomy should be used as primary abortion methods only in unique circumstances."

4. Partial Birth Abortion (D&X). Dr. Haskell describes the procedure this way: " . . . the surgeon grasps and removes a nearly intact fetus through an adequately dilated cervix—it can be used successfully in patients 20–26 weeks in pregnancy." With this procedure the cervix is widely dilated over a two-day period. Then he inserts a grasping forcep into the uterus and while watching with the ultrasound, grasps the baby's leg and pulls it out of the cervix. Then the other leg is pulled out. Next, the surgeon "forces the scissors into the base of the skull—introduces a catheter into this hole and evacuates the skull contents. He applies traction to the fetus, removing it completely from the patient." The irony of this event seems lost on Dr. Haskell. He is killing a baby while it is still in its mother's uterus at the same stage of life that—if it were born alive—it would be cared for in an attempt to keep it alive in an intensive care newborn nursery. (This is why this procedure is more properly termed a "partial birth abortion.")

174 What complications can result from abortions?

There are numerous complications of abortions, and the further along a woman is in her pregnancy, the more likely they are to occur. Many physicians who perform abortions do not discuss the possible complications with their patients. I feel strongly that they should, especially with young women. Women below the age of twenty often are not aware of the medical complications that can result from abortion.

These complications may include:

Uterine hemorrhage. A patient may bleed heavily after any D&C, but if she is pregnant when the procedure is done, there is an increased risk of heavy bleeding. If a woman is more than thirteen weeks pregnant at the time of abortion, there is a significant risk of bleeding heavily.

Perforation of the uterus. The instruments used for doing an abortion can make a hole in the wall of the uterus. It is difficult for a doctor to feel the difference between the fetal tissue and the tissue that makes up the wall of the uterus. In trying to retrieve all the tissue of pregnancy, the doctor may push the instruments through the wall of the uterus. When this perforation occurs, bleeding into the abdominal cavity and/or infection may result. There have been instances in which a portion of a woman's intestines were sucked out of her abdomen by a suction cannula that had perforated her uterus. Occasionally a major operation may be necessary to take care of complications of abortions.

Injury to the cervix. In any abortion procedure, the cervix can be damaged. Cervical trauma is a common and potentially serious complication of abortion. The damage includes tears, scars, and stenosis, scarring so extensive that the opening of the cervix is made too small for fertility or, if future pregnancy does occur, for normal delivery. The more abortions a woman has, the greater the risk of this occurring.

Embolism. Amniotic fluid or air can be forced into the mother's blood vessels during the abortion procedure. They can cause brain damage or death if passed to the brain.

Infection. After an abortion, the inside of the uterus is raw. Since the instruments that were inserted inside the uterus can carry germs, infections can occur. Infertility or death can result from this. Infections happen often enough that most doctors recommend that women having abortions be given antibiotics.

Other problems. Other problems have been known to develop following abortion. These include later menstrual irregularities and infertility, but also more frequent spontaneous abortion, tubal pregnancies, and premature deliveries in the future.

175 Why do I read in newspapers and magazines that abortion is a "safe operation" if all these things can occur?

Those who favor abortion often state that there are fewer physical risks in having an abortion than in carrying a pregnancy to term and delivering the baby. They also mention the fact that few women are made infertile or sterile by an abortion. The number of women in our country who have been physically damaged by an abortion, however, runs in the thousands. Generally the statistics for pregnancy refer to teen pregnancy risk. Good health care can lower pregnancy complications for teens and therefore decrease such justification for abortion.

The unifying facts in this puzzling maze of information have to do with numbers. If physicians perform an operation that has a low percentage chance of complications, they consider it a low-risk procedure, and abortion definitely has a low possibility of problems. But abortions are done so often in the United States that physicians and even medical organizations have lost sight of how many individuals have been hurt or killed by abortion. The chart on page 121 describes potential risks of these abortion procedures.

When we realize how many abortions are done in our country, and how many women are having more than one abortion (a great risk factor), we comprehend the damage that is being done to women: how many women are being made sterile, or how many have loss of later desired pregnancies. The sad thing is that one-fourth of those who are being damaged are teenagers who usually have not yet had their families and who do not realize the implications of being made infertile by the abortion of the only pregnancy they might ever have.

While those who favor abortion would like us to believe otherwise, there are frightening statistics about damage and death to women who have abortions. As with any operation, there can be serious consequences. Abortion is especially dangerous for a woman who has had more than one of these procedures.

In an article published in *Contemporary OB/GYN* (February 1990), the statement is made by Hani K. Atrash, M.D., and his coauthors:

> Although the abortion related mortality rate decreased for all women from 1972 through 1978 to 1979 through 1985, blacks and others continued to have a higher risk of death from abortion than did whites. The

Complications from Legal Abortions Performed Annually in the United States[1]

1,300,700 women, one-third of whom were teenagers

Complication	Number of Women Damaged	Percentage of Women Who Had Abortions
Death	7	
Pelvic Inflammatory Disease (PID)[2]	50,730	3.9
Damage to cervix from suction curettage (can cause spontaneous abortions or premature babies)	104,061	8
Risk increases to 16–24% in repeat abortions[3]		
Risk rate doubles for teenagers below 17 (15% of all aborted women)[4]	3,317	1.7
Hysterectomy[5] (1 in 20,000 abortions)	65	
Major complications in teens having suction curettage[4]	52–156	.1–.3
Major complications in teens having saline abortion (4 or more months pregnant, 6–12% of teenage abortions)[4]	338–676	1.3
Loss of later pregnancy due to 2 or more abortions[3,6]		2–3 times greater than normal

1. Based on statistics gathered by Centers for Disease Control—admittedly underreported.
2. From E. Quistad et al, "Pelvic Inflammatory Disease Associated with Chlamydia Trachomatis Infections after Therapeutic Abortions: A Prospective Study," *British Journal of Venereal Diseases,* 59:189–192, 1983.
3. 23% of women having abortions are having their second or more abortion.
4. Figures on teenage abortions are from W. Cates Jr. et al, "The Risks Associated with Teenage Abortion," *The New England Journal of Medicine,* 309:621–627, 1983.
5. From J. E. Hodgson, "Major Complications of 20,248 Consecutive First Trimester Abortions: Problems of Fragmented Care," *Planned Parenthood,* 9:52, 1975.
6. From A. Levin et al, "Association of Induced Abortion with Subsequent Pregnancy Loss," *Journal of the American Medical Association,* 243:2495–2497, 1980.

relative risk among blacks and others increased from 2.4 for the earlier period to 2.9 for the later one. [Relative risk means the number of deaths per 100,000 abortions.]

Abortions performed during the second trimester continue to carry a markedly increased risk of death. For 1972 through 1985, the risk of death after abortion performed at thirteen to fifteen weeks was 4.6 times greater than that for abortion performed at twelve weeks gestation or earlier. Women who had abortions performed at sixteen weeks gestation or later had a 14.3 times greater risk of death than did those whose abortions were performed in the first trimester.

It is important to remember that for the past few years there have been about 1 to 1.5 million abortions done per year in the United States. The relative risk number, therefore, must be multiplied fifteen times to get the actual number of deaths per year produced by abortions. For instance, for the period 1979 through 1985, 2.9 black women out of 100,000 who had abortions died because of their abortion. If we assume a death rate of two per 100,000 for blacks and whites we can say that each year thirty women die from having abortions. This means that in the last ten years approximately 300 women have died from having this supposedly safe operation.

Other articles point out the serious nature of the complications of abortions. For instance, the *Australian and New Zealand Journal of Obstetrics and Gynecology* (1990, 30:347–50), points out that dangerous, postabortion pelvic infection developed in 11½ percent of women who had abortions and who also had chlamydia in the cervix.

A report by George R. Huggins, M.D., in *Fertility and Sterility* (October 1990, 54.4) points out that scarring of the uterine cavity, which is a result of a D&C with preexisting intrauterine infection, has been underreported. This problem is called Asherman's syndrome. When a woman has Asherman's syndrome, she cannot get pregnant

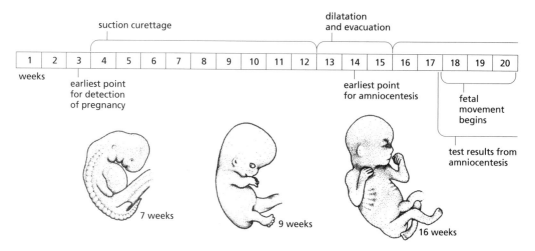

suction curettage

dilatation and evacuation

| 1 | 2 | 3 | 4 | 5 | 6 | 7 | 8 | 9 | 10 | 11 | 12 | 13 | 14 | 15 | 16 | 17 | 18 | 19 | 20 |

weeks

earliest point for detection of pregnancy

earliest point for amniocentesis

fetal movement begins

test results from amniocentesis

7 weeks

9 weeks

16 weeks

until this uterine scarring is corrected by surgery, if even then.

A report in *Obstetrics and Gynecology* (March 1990, 75.3: pt. 1) discussed fifteen women who had uterine perforations at the time of second trimester abortion by dilatation and evacuation (D&E). "All patients required laparotomy" (a major operation, opening the abdomen for repair of damage done by the abortion). "Two-thirds had bowel injuries and two required hysterectomy. Errors in estimating gestational duration, inadequate cervical dilatation, and failure to use sonography characterize these complicated cases."

An article in *Obstetrics and Gynecology* (July 1990, 76.1) by E. Hakin-Elahi, M.D., and his associates, reported on the hospitalization of 121 patients who had abortions. They were admitted because of suspected perforation of the intestines, ectopic pregnancy, hemorrhage, infection, or incomplete removal of the pregnancy. They reported that 8.46 women per 1,000 who had abortions had various "minor complications," which included mild infection, resuctioning on the same day of surgery, resuctioning later than the date of surgery, cervical stenosis, cervical tearing, underestimation of gestational age, and convulsive seizure.

Although the doctors reporting termed the complications "minor," I believe most patients would consider these "major" if they happened to

them, especially if they produced infertility and premature deliveries later in life.

These doctors were reporting on 170,000 first trimester abortions done in three free-standing clinics of Planned Parenthood in New York. The statistics given did not include the complications from abortions done after the twelfth week of pregnancy when the more severe complications increasingly occur.

With so many abortions being done, it is impossible to do a truly adequate follow-up on them all. Patients who are embarrassed about having an abortion can easily go to a hospital saying that their "complications" were caused by a miscarriage. This happens frequently when women do not want their families to know they have had an abortion.

One study showed that 50 percent of women having abortions later denied having one. This finding alone casts a great deal of doubt on the statistics about the ill effects of abortion. It means that all of the studies about the medical and psychological complications of abortion may be vastly underestimated.

In a book titled *Aborted Women* (Loyola Press), David C. Reardon makes the point that though legal abortion may have made abortion marginally safer, "the huge increase in the total number of abortions has led to an increase in the total number of women who suffer."

Method Selection

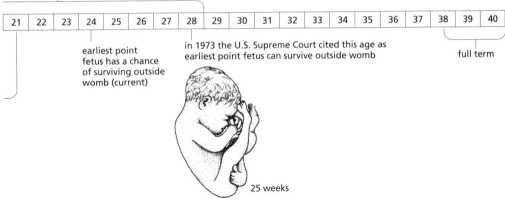

induced labor
or dilatation and evacuation

| 21 | 22 | 23 | 24 | 25 | 26 | 27 | 28 | 29 | 30 | 31 | 32 | 33 | 34 | 35 | 36 | 37 | 38 | 39 | 40 |

earliest point
fetus has a chance
of surviving outside
womb (current)

in 1973 the U.S. Supreme Court cited this age as
earliest point fetus can survive outside womb

full term

25 weeks

If only 1 percent of abortions result in medical or psychological complications, then at a rate of 1.5 million abortions a year, 150,000 women would suffer negatively. (This would amount to a total of more than 2.25 million women since *Roe* v. *Wade* was passed in 1973.)

Few, if any, health issues have sown so much harm and potential harm for so many women as has abortion.

176 How significant is the emotional trauma of abortion to the women and men involved?

Many studies show that women suffer from emotional trauma after abortion. For example, one study by David Reardon (see previous question) showed that nearly one-third of women who had abortions drank more heavily after their abortions. Forty percent said that after their abortions they began to use, or increased the use of drugs. In another study, 60 percent of women reported increased use of alcohol.

In the *OB/GYN News* (March 1–14, 1989), Vincent Rue, Ph.D., of Sir Thomas More Clinics of Southern California at Downey, found that "women who elected abortions were at greater risk for adverse psychological sequelae than were those who carried to term." In the same interview,

Dr. Rue stated that "participation in 'intentionally caused human death experience' [abortion] is sufficiently traumatic to cause significant . . . symptoms of re-experience. . . . Psychic numbing is also common and may substantially impair relationships. . . . Secondary symptoms also occur: sleeping and eating disorders, substance abuse, depression, suicidal ideology."

In his book *Aborted Women* (Loyola Press), David Reardon quotes a study reported in the *American Journal of Psychiatry* in which, at the time of a second interview, 10 percent of women who had had abortions were "suffering serious psychiatric complication."

The Psycho-Social Aspects of Stress Following Abortion by Ann Speckhard (Sheed & Ward, 1987) reports that abortion compounded women's stress by estranging them from their important loyalties. "Fearing that their sexual activity and pregnancy would strain their parents' loyalties beyond the breaking point, they confided neither in them nor in any friends they thought might tell their families. Thus these women underwent both the crisis and its aftermath isolated from their closest natural supports. . . . Many subjects reported that friends who had been enthusiastic supporters of the abortion decision were unwilling to listen to any accounts of the stress produced by the abortion."

Many women do have an emotional response

to abortion. The psychological reaction varies from individual to individual, but almost all patients who have had an abortion remember the experience as being unpleasant, both physically and emotionally. Many women seem to have no regret, others seem to have a lingering sadness. Patients who have had abortions, even those who do not feel guilty, often fail to mention an aborted pregnancy when they list all previous pregnancies for their physician. It seems that they are trying to forget the event. Patients who subsequently have problems with fertility, especially if damage to pelvic organs resulted from the abortion, often experience regret for having had the abortion.

I advise my patients not to have abortions. Although they may think they will not feel guilt or regret if they have an abortion done, they can for the rest of their lives carry in their minds, emotions, and bodies the memory of a most unpleasant experience.

A book called *Men and Abortion: Lessons, Losses and Love*, by Arthur Shostak, Gary McLouth, and Lynn Sing (Praeger, 1984), states that most men whose wives or girlfriends had abortions felt isolated, angry at themselves and their partners, and fearful of the physical and emotional damage done to the women. One of the many men surveyed stated, "It is a wound you cannot see or feel, but it exists." This is from the man's perspective, and he is not the one whose body is pregnant and undergoes the abortion.

177 When are abortions considered necessary?

There are several problems for which most physicians recommend medical, or therapeutic, abortions, but less than 5 percent of abortions in the United States are done for those reasons.

Medical problems of the mother. Medical problems can exist that endanger the life of the mother if the pregnancy continues. These include severe heart disease, disseminated lupus erythematosus, severe hypertension (including severe toxemia), and cervical cancer. An abortion or induction of premature delivery may be necessary in these situations to save the life of the mother.

Contrary to what many people think, this is not a choice between the life of the mother and the life of the child. If the mother is so gravely ill that an abortion is necessary, both she *and* the baby would probably die if she did not have an abortion. If you have been advised to have an abortion because of a health problem, and you do not want one or feel it is unnecessary, get a second opinion, and even a third. Some doctors use abortion as an easy way out of a complicated situation. If the doctors involved are convinced that your life is in danger, however, I suggest you follow their advice and have an abortion.

Abnormalities of the fetus, incompatible with life. Certain abnormalities of the fetus are totally incompatible with life. One example of this type of problem is a baby who has no brain development (anencephaly). Terminating such a pregnancy is killing a baby that could not have survived outside the uterus. The decision about whether or not to have an abortion in this situation is a personal one. I can understand why a couple would decide to have an abortion in this situation, since the baby will die within minutes or hours of its birth, even if it is born at full term. I can also understand the feelings of the couple who chooses to continue to a term delivery under these circumstances. They may prefer to wait for as normal a delivery as possible and to hold their child in its dying moments.

The couple should make the decision they feel is right for them. They need feel no guilt for whichever path they choose to take.

178 Are there other medical reasons for abortion?

Other reasons for abortion are not absolute indications for abortion, although many physicians and laypeople may recommend them. Whether you have an abortion for one of these reasons depends on your personal morality as it relates to abortion.

Genetic/chromosomal problems. Some couples will decide to abort if they know she is carrying a child with a disorder such as Down syndrome. There is much help now available for children suffering from this disorder. No longer does the presence of this and other syndromes necessarily provide justifiable reasons for an abortion. (See Q. 455–464 for more information on genetic/chromosomal problems.)

Incest. Generally, if a girl is old enough to become pregnant, she is old enough to deliver a child. Delivering a child is a normal, sexual function, and even a young woman can accept that as a natural part of the function of her body. Abortion, however, is *not* natural, and it can leave adolescents and young women with tremendous emotional and physical scars.

Rape. Rape only infrequently results in pregnancy. Studies in Pennsylvania and Minnesota have shown that as many as five thousand rapes have occurred without a single pregnancy resulting. When a pregnancy does result from rape, however, a mother must realize two things: Half of that baby is from *her*, and no matter how it was conceived, the baby is still a baby. If an abortion is done for this reason, there is always the danger that a mother's emotional and psychological makeup may be even further damaged. Two wrongs cannot make a right or correct the first wrong.

German measles (rubella). If a mother develops German measles during the first three months of pregnancy, there is a 15–50 percent chance of having a baby with a major abnormality. This means that if an abortion is done because of German measles, there is a 50–85 percent chance that a *healthy, normal* child has been aborted. (See Q. 328–331.) This is a totally preventable dilemma. If you are in your reproductive stage of life, and have not had a rubella immunization, get your shot now.

There are obviously a few valid reasons for which doctors and laypeople advocate abortion. Unfortunately, however, it is commonly recommended because it is an easy solution to a problem or worry.

179 Are babies still alive when they are aborted?

Sometimes a baby is delivered alive after an abortion. Doctors in most states are not legally bound to perform abortions only in early pregnancy. Consequently, there are babies being aborted today who are the same size and maturity as many premature babies being successfully cared for in intensive-care nurseries.

Because abortions are common during the second trimester of pregnancy, we occasionally see headlines such as appeared in the *Dallas Times Herald* (AP) on March 23, 1983:

Six Live Births After Abortions
Cause Furor

Madison, Wisconsin—The live births of six babies whose mothers had abortions at Madison hospitals in the past ten months have shocked residents and become a rallying point for abortion foes.

The births also have prompted one hospital to drastically curtail the surgical procedure.

All six babies died within twenty-seven hours of birth, four at Madison General Hospital and two at the University of Wisconsin Hospital.

This problem is one reason abortionists developed the "partial-birth abortion" technique. With this technique, the baby is killed just before delivery of its head, eliminating the worry about a live abortion.

180 What advice do you have for women considering abortion?

A woman should not let anyone push her into having an abortion. The relationship a pregnant woman has with the baby she carries is too personal for her to let the baby's father, whether or not he is her husband, her parents, or anyone else convince her to kill her baby.

My advice is:

Don't take the easy way out. Many examples in life show us that the easiest way is not necessarily the best way. For example, exercise is important in maintaining a body that will do what we want it to do. It is not easy to exercise, but the "hard" way is best.

Since most abortions are performed because of the inconvenience of the pregnancy and not because of medical reasons, abortion can be considered in this same light. Though an abortion may seem to be the easiest way out of a difficult situation, it may be the worst choice. There are some issues to consider if you are thinking about an abortion.

1. Some would argue that a woman has total rights to her own body; that argument is not correct. For our own good—and society's—some government regulation of what we do with our bodies is necessary and desirable. This is evidenced by laws against suicide, prostitution, and use of illegal drugs.

Our rights end where another person's "nose begins," and the baby inside the mother's uterus is another person. It has a totally different chromosomal makeup from its mother, and it is even of a different sex half of the time. The baby is alive and growing from conception on. If it were not, it would not have to be killed to stop its growth.

When a woman's right to her body is discussed, the euphemistic term *choice* is often used. I agree that reproductive "choice" is important, but I believe the choice should be made earlier—before the pregnancy begins. A woman can choose abstinence until marriage (and subsequent desired pregnancy), or she can use contraceptive techniques very carefully and usually not get pregnant.

2. I believe that the only reason abortions are allowed is because they take place "out of sight," in the dark of a woman's uterus. If the babies were taken out of the uterus, for instance, and their little heads were crushed in public, our society would immediately put a stop to such killing. (I don't believe we would even allow televised public killing of kangaroo fetuses, which could easily be pulled from their mother's pouches.)

3. Physicians who care for pregnant mothers know that they are caring for two patients—the mother and her unborn child. The only time people rationalize that the unborn child is not a person is when they want to kill it by abortion.

I received the following letter from a patient who came to me in early pregnancy, planning to have an abortion. After we talked for a while, she decided not to have the abortion.

Dear Dr. McIlhaney,

If you have a woman come in and wants to abort or her husband wants her to, as mine did . . . please show her this picture and tell her I almost made the biggest mistake of my life and had it done to this beautiful boy. Maybe it might save a life . . . it is a life . . . anything that can make you that sick (when pregnant) has got to be a life.

Thank you for bringing two of the most precious children in the world into this world and into my life.

Name Withheld

Be realistic. A woman should not be naive when she considers an abortion. Abortionists often picture it as a simple, straightforward procedure. Most women who have an abortion report that it was a very traumatic experience. Many women complain of being handled "like cattle" in abortion clinics and compare an abortion with rape—as a procedure that leaves a woman feeling violated.

Be prepared for guilt. For many women, guilt following abortion is inescapable. This procedure is one that a woman will never forget, and one that she may regret for the rest of her life.

Expect possible infertility. Physicians who treat women with infertility problems often have patients who have been pregnant in the past, had that pregnancy aborted, and since then have been unable to become pregnant.

Don't base an abortion on finances. Don't let your worry about money cause you to make a bad situation worse. Almost no one feels that she can really afford adding a baby to her family. However, just like millions of other parents in America, you will, somehow, be able to provide for your child. The baby needs primarily your *love*, not material things. Besides, the baby would prefer life to death.

There is a great deal of rhetoric about abortion from both sides of the issue. I encourage you to read and give honest consideration to the information in this chapter. Consider the consequences of a decision to end a human life.

181 What advice do you have for a woman who has had an abortion?

It is possible that you will never regret having had an abortion, but many women do. If you are one who does have such regrets, it is important that you not let these regrets dominate your life. You can do several things to help keep a past mistake from weighing on you for the rest of your life.

If you are having a major problem with guilt and self-blame, see a counselor (pastor, psychologist, or psychiatrist). Choose a counselor whose viewpoint is compatible with your own. Otherwise he or she can cause you even more frustration.

If you find yourself blaming your husband, boyfriend, or parents, you must realize that blaming others will not accomplish anything. If you cannot overcome the anger toward the people who may have influenced you in your decision, talk to a counselor.

Ask for God's forgiveness, accept it, and then forgive yourself. It is helpful to remember examples of God's forgiveness. King David, for example, got Bathsheba pregnant and then, to cover his tracks, had her husband killed. When Nathan, God's prophet, confronted David with his sins, David thought God would not forgive him. His response was not a mere statement, "I have sinned." He was truly sorry and expressed his repentance to God, whose response was complete forgiveness. God will do the same for you. When God forgives you, you must forgive yourself so that guilt does not ruin the rest of your life.

Become a "counselor" for those who are considering abortion. Those who have the best insight into the abortion problem are those who have had one. If you have decided, since your abortion, that abortion is not the best solution to a problem pregnancy, you could serve as a helpful counselor for someone who finds herself pregnant and is considering abortion as a solution.

182 What is RU-486 (Mifepristone)?

Mifepristone, the much-heralded new French abortion method, is a synthetic hormone called an antiprogestin. It works by blocking the effect of a woman's natural progesterone on her uterus.

Progesterone is absolutely necessary for a baby to grow in a woman's uterus. When it is inactivated, the lining of the uterus (on which the baby is dependent for oxygen and nutrition) degenerates. This causes the baby and his or her placenta to be deprived of oxygen and nutrition, bringing about its death and abortion.

The drug RU-486 was developed during the 1980s and became available for abortions in France in 1988. At the time of this writing (1998), the drug had no other confirmed medical use, but studies are being conducted.

When RU-486 is used with a synthetic prostaglandin-like drug to produce contractions of the uterus and given within the first forty-nine days of the last menstrual period, abortion occurs 95 percent of the time. The process is not simple and straightforward, however.

Visits to the doctor are necessary before the medication is administered. A synthetic prostaglandin drug is given along with the RU-486 to make it work better. After that, the baby dies and the woman starts to bleed. This bleeding, which is more excessive than a menstrual period, may last up to two weeks, and most women experience a great deal of cramping. Ten percent of patients will require a D&C to complete the process.

The president of Roussel-Uclaf, the drug company which manufactures RU-486, states that an RU-486 abortion is an "appalling psychological ordeal. A woman must live with her abortion for two weeks."

Roussel-Uclaf has found that the drug requires such careful medical monitoring that it must be used only in clinics that follow their strict guidelines. In other words, it requires a high degree of medical sophistication for use. Because of this, the company will not allow RU-486 to be used in undeveloped countries, nor have they made it available to the general population or to general OB/GYN specialists in France where the drug has been studied most extensively. It is released only to special clinics that are trained in its use.

RU-486 is not a "morning after" pill. According to the manufacturers, even if RU-486 is used the morning after unprotected intercourse, a high percentage of women will still become pregnant.

Obviously, RU-486, despite what has been said

in newspaper and magazine articles, is not the answer to a quiet, private, simple, inexpensive, and safe abortion.

A new combination of drugs can cause an abortion early in pregnancy. This combination is cytoxan plus an antiprostaglandin. Not all pregnancies will abort with either this combination or with RU-486. If the pregnancy continues, the resulting baby could be damaged by the drugs.

183 Where can I go for counseling about a pregnancy that has the potential for causing me problems?

Talk to a family member, a friend, or a pastor who would be more objective than you can be about the best solution to your problems. If any of these people suggest abortion, remember that they are recommending what seems to be the "easy road." They are not thinking about your long-range physical and emotional health, but only about the immediate, comfortable solution to the "problem."

In his book, *Aborted Women*, David Reardon discusses the experience women have had with their friends and family. He found that "eighty-three percent of the women surveyed indicated that they would definitely have chosen against abortion if their husbands, boyfriends, abortion counselors, doctors, and family members had suggested and encouraged alternatives." Social and family pressures were generally in favor of the abortion, so much so that "fifty-five percent of respondents felt that they had been very much forced to abort by others."

If the people you talk to seem to be pushing you to have an abortion, I suggest you contact a Crisis Pregnancy Center. These centers, staffed by qualified volunteers who can counsel you about your pregnancy, are available all over the United States. They will explain to you that the child you are carrying is already a baby, and they will show you what it looks like. They will be honest with you about what you are getting into if you have an abortion, including medical and emotional dangers. More importantly, they will offer you help with finances, clothes, and a place to stay if you

need it during your pregnancy. They will also help you after you deliver your child.

If you are not sure where a Crisis Pregnancy Center is in your area, call CareNet at (800) 395-HELP or (703) 478-5661.

If you would like to have information about how a baby develops and what it looks like at different stages of pregnancy, contact the Human Development Resource Council, Inc., 3916 Holcomb Bridge Road, Suite 200, Norcross, GA 30092. The phone number is (404) 447-1598. This organization has information about pregnancy, including videos, booklets, and other written material that might help you with your pregnancy.

Do not rely on the counseling you might receive at a local abortion clinic. Such clinics make their money doing abortions, and if, after counseling, you choose not to have an abortion, you have eliminated part of their income. Although a very distraught woman might be counseled to "wait" before having her abortion, most women will be advised by these clinics to abort immediately. These clinics will almost never offer financial support, a home, and clothes so that a woman can carry her pregnancy.

Rape and Sexual Assault

184 What is the definition of rape?

According to the dictionary, rape is the crime of forcing a woman to submit to sexual intercourse. The technical definition, however, does not do the word justice, because the word *rape* evokes such horror, fear, and dread in a woman that mere words cannot express it. Those powerful emotions are due, no doubt, to the fact that rape is not just an act against a woman's body, but an act against the very essence of her womanhood.

Even the most powerful emotions must sometimes be reduced to legalities, however, and rape and other sexual crimes are no exception. There has recently been a change in the legal terminology used in reference to sex crimes. Most states and most police departments now use these new terms. Old terms such as *rape, statutory rape,* and *aggravated rape* have been replaced by:

Sexual assault. Forced sexual activity, which includes rape and intercourse with someone incapable of giving knowledgeable consent. This term does not apply to a child under fourteen years of age. Sexual assault is a second-degree felony offense.

Aggravated sexual assault. Forced sexual activity that includes the involvement of a weapon; or serious bodily injury; or intercourse with a girl under the age of fourteen, even if she consents to such activity. Aggravated sexual assault is a first-degree felony offense.

Attempted sexual assault. Activity that indicates by words, acts, or deeds that a person intends sexual assault but who does not, for some reason, have the opportunity to carry through with his or her intent. This is a third-degree felony offense.

Indecent exposure. This terms refers to an act in which a person exposes his or her genitals to another person. An example would be a man exposing himself to a woman while masturbating. This is a Class B criminal offense.

Indecency with a child. If a man or woman exposes himself or herself to a child under seventeen years of age, it is referred to as "indecency with a child." Other acts are included under this heading: putting the mouth on a girl's breast, or touching a child's genitalia (both of these are second-degree felony offenses). This is a third-degree felony offense.

185 What do statistics reveal about the act of rape?

Rape is the fastest-growing violent crime in the United States. Some facts concerning this horrible crime are:

At least ten times as many rapes occur as are ever reported to authorities.

Fewer than 50 percent of the rapists who are caught are ever brought to trial, and very few of those are convicted.

One woman in four will be the victim of rape or attempted rape or sexual abuse during her lifetime.

About 85 percent of women who are the victims of rape are also beaten or threatened with physical force.

Roughly half of all rapes occur in the homes of the victims.

Rapists sometimes choose their victims according to their appearance or age. Every woman is a potential victim. One in four rapists has a preference for a certain type of female (age, appearance, and so on). Seductive attire and behavior are given by many rapists as factors in their selection of a victim and as a self-justification for the act.

The incidence of rape in women over sixty has increased by 800 percent during the past twenty years. However, the highest risk group is still women in their twenties.

About 50 percent of rapists have committed prior crimes.

Students constitute 11 percent of rapists.

Over half the victims who report rapes know their attacker.

Over half of convicted rapists are married and have "normal" sex lives.

Almost three-fourths of arrested rapists will repeat the crime at some time in the future.

Rape is not usually spontaneous. Over 70 percent of all rapes are planned and victims and place are chosen ahead of time.

Rape is a crime of violence, not "passion."

186 What can I do to protect myself and my daughters from rape?

First, learn all you can about rape and teach what you learn to your daughters. Next, practice precautions against rape and teach your daughters to do the same. The often-used saying, "It's better to be safe than sorry," is extremely applicable in this case.

If at all possible, take a self-defense course. Being able to react quickly and effectively may give you the advantage you need to repel an attacker and get away from him.

Further suggestions include:

Secure your home so that visitors can enter only when you admit them. When you are alone at home, never allow anyone inside unless you know that you can trust him or her completely. Insist on identification even from "authorized" service personnel.

Never walk in an unsafe or secluded area. Avoid eye contact with strangers. If you must be in areas where you will be alone, carry a loud whistle or take a dog with you.

Travel only in a well-maintained automobile on major roads or highways. Do not travel alone if you can avoid it, especially at night. Keep your car doors locked and never give rides to hitchhikers or stranded motorists. You can always offer to call for help for them. If you are stranded, do not accept a ride with a stranger.

Be cautious in parking lots. Park so you do not have to get in or out of your car in an isolated area. Attackers can hide under your car, grab your legs, and pull you under. Don't get out of your car if a van with dark windows is next to your car. An attacker could drag you into a van, abduct, and rape you. Do not go alone to bars or public dances. Go with a man or woman for protection.

187 What should I do if I am attacked by a rapist?

Fighting, screaming, and running are not always possible nor the best tactic. When your life is threatened if you do not submit to an attacker's demands, you must decide whether to endure the sexual demands of the rapist or risk serious injury or lose your life.

If you are attacked, you may be able to avoid rape by the right reactions. Rapists often say that they are more likely to rape a woman if she shows no emotion and stays quiet. Therefore you must try to do the following:

React strongly and physically. Kick the man in the genitals; poke at his eyes with a comb or pen; scratch, tear, and bite.

Make all the noise you can, scream as loud as you can.

If you can throw the attacker off guard, run. The idea of using self-defense is to get him off guard so that you can get away without being hurt.

There is no cut-and-dried answer that fits all situations or all women. Some women, for instance, would rather die than submit. Others are able to deal with the horror of rape by realizing that they at least preserved their life.

188 What should I do if I am raped?

If your attempts at preventing an attack fail, and you become the victim of rape, the following suggestions may help.

Do not alter your surroundings, your appearance, or your body in any way. The best evidence of what has happened to you is the physical changes of your surroundings and your body. For example, do not straighten up the room or the area; leave any torn clothes where they were thrown by your attacker; do not wipe off any secretions; do not change clothes; do not urinate or have a bowel movement; do not douche; do not shower or bathe.

If you are physically injured, phone for help. Call the 911 emergency number if available in your area; call your local emergency medical service; or call an ambulance, a hospital, or a doctor.

Also call the police, the sheriff, or some other law enforcement official immediately.

Have a medical examination as soon as possible.

189 What will the medical examination following rape be like?

Whether or not you plan to bring charges against your assailant, it is important that you go immediately to a doctor or an emergency room if one is nearby. Most emergency rooms have established procedures for evaluating and treating rape victims.

At this time, testing is done for evidence, not for treatment. Police are interested in testing for STDs primarily with minors or abstinent women, since an STD with no previous history of sexual activity would be evidence of assault.

The doctor and nurse will talk to you and record in great detail what has happened to you. In addition, they will ask what contraceptive technique you have been using and when your most recent episode of intercourse prior to the rape took place. The physician will also want to know if you have bathed or douched or changed clothes since the assault.

A complete physical examination will be done. The physician will record your emotional state, note any bruises or cuts or broken bones, and look for bruising, cuts, and swelling of your female organs.

The doctor will attempt to get specimens from your body to confirm the rape. Some of this material may be stored by the police department for future identification and comparison with the perpetrator's own body materials. This evidence may require:

Combing your pubic hair to remove any hair or thread that might be from the assailant.

Obtaining small specimens of your own pubic hair to differentiate it from the attacker's pubic hair.

Obtaining vaginal secretions that would be tested for the presence of sperm and acid phosphatase. There is a high concentration of this chemical in semen. If the man has had a vasectomy there would be no sperm, but the presence of this chemical can confirm that he ejaculated.

The doctor will also obtain blood from you to check for syphilis and AIDS and order a culture of your vaginal secretions to make sure the attacker did not pass gonorrhea or chlamydia germs to you. If there is any question of your being pregnant at the time of the attack, the doctor will obtain a serum pregnancy test to determine whether or not this is the case.

After a medical examination and testing, if you are able, you will be taken to the police station to give a statement that will be used as the basis for a complaint. After the statement, the police do not talk with you or see you again until a trial, unless they need you to make either a photo identification or lineup identification. The prosecutor's office will stay in contact with you while the police investigate. Some victims stay in touch by phone to monitor the progress of the police investigation.

After giving your statement, if you have not already contacted the local Rape Crisis Center, someone from the center will see you while you are still at the police station. The people from the Rape Crisis Center are usually very helpful. They can give advice, encouragement, and support during this terrible time. I encourage you to talk to them. There is much helpful information in the book, *The Dancer*, by Susan Lee (Grand Rapids: Baker, 1991). Susan, herself a rape victim, gives a compelling account of her journey to healing.

190 What medical treatment might be necessary because of rape?

If you have had injuries from a rape attack, these will be treated by the doctor with traditional therapy. In addition, you will probably be given antibiotics to prevent gonorrhea, chlamydia, or syphilis.

If you have not been using contraception, and the attack occurred at a time when you might get pregnant, your doctor may recommend that you use birth-control pills twice a day for two or three days as a morning after pill. Sometimes this technique does not prevent a pregnancy. You will have to decide this for yourself after discussing it with your physician.

191 Is any follow-up treatment necessary?

If pregnancy as a result of the rape is a possibility, you should see a physician in two or three weeks. By that time a serum blood test for pregnancy could be positive.

You should also have a vaginal culture for

chlamydia and gonorrhea and another blood test for syphilis and AIDS twelve weeks after the assault, to be sure that you did not contract a sexually transmitted disease. Of patients who were raped and not treated at the time of the first medical exam, 3 percent developed gonorrhea and 0.1 percent developed syphilis. Although the chance of your becoming HIV-infected from one sex act is very small, it is normal to be worried about AIDS at this time. Be sure to get follow-up testing so you can be relieved of this worry.

192 Is counseling important for rape victims?

Counseling is very important, and I encourage you not to hesitate to get it. You should not feel abnormal if you respond to rape with deep emotional upheaval. All rape victims are left with some degree of fear, and there is often a reaction of helplessness. A woman feels that she no longer has control over her own life and destiny.

Women who do not get counseling after rape often find that the greatest damage from the rape has been emotional rather than physical. It is important to undergo counseling to keep these emotional problems from becoming deep-seated and permanent.

In addition to formal psychological or psychiatric counseling, Rape Crisis Centers can be useful. Counseling there is usually free, and it will often involve not only the victim but her family as well. In addition, these centers can help a woman through the legal procedures necessary for bringing charges against her attacker. Support groups, which can be very helpful, are also available at most Rape Crisis Centers.

193 Is it really important to file charges against a rapist?

Although you may feel strangely guilty and/or embarrassed about being raped, you should not let this keep you from filing charges against your assailant. People who work with rape victims are often discouraged by the failure of these women to

press charges. It is important to remember that almost three-fourths of arrested rapists will repeat the crime. All of us should do whatever we can to keep these men from having an opportunity to commit rape again.

194 Where can I get further information about rape?

Because rape is the fastest-growing violent crime in the United States, it is important that we all become better informed about it. All women should learn how to protect themselves from rape, and both men and women must learn how to protect their children from it. Information about rape is available from these sources:

If your physician does not have information about rape for you, it is available from the state or county medical society or from the state department of health.

Emergency-room personnel often have information about rape or will know who has such information.

Almost all large cities in the United States have a Rape Crisis Center. You can probably find the phone number in the phone book, or call information. If you live in a town that does not have such a center, call the Rape Crisis Center in the nearest large town. They can send you information or can help you if you have been a rape victim.

Rape is a crime. Your local law enforcement agency has dealt with rape victims many times. The agency's personnel will have information not only for rape victims but also for those seeking to learn more about rape. They are vitally concerned with reducing the incidence of rape as are the thousands of other men and women around the country who are sickened by this horrible crime.

National Organization for Victim Assistance (NOVA)
1757 Park Road NW
Washington, D.C. 20010
(202) 232-6682

National Criminal Justice Reference Service
   (NCJRS)
Box 6000
Rockville, MD 20850
(301) 251-5500
(800) 851-3420

National Center on Child Abuse and Neglect
   (NCCAN)
330 C Street, SW
Washington, D.C. 20201
(202) 245-0586, Clearinghouse (703) 821-8955

National Maternal and Child Health Clearinghouse
8201 Greensboro Drive, Suite 600
McLean, VA 22102-3810
(703) 821-8955

Children's Defense Fund
25 East Street NW
Washington, D.C. 20001
(202) 628-8787

National Coalition against Sexual Assault
   (NCASA)
P.O. Box 21378
Washington, D.C. 20009
(202) 483-7165

National Center on Women and Family Law
Room 402 – 799 Broadway
New York, NY 10003
(212) 674-8200

National Legal Aid and Defender Association
   (NLADA)
1625 K Street, N.W.
Washington, D.C. 20006
(202) 452-0620

The National Crime Prevention Council
1700 K Street, N.W.
2d Floor
Washington, D.C. 20006-3817
(202) 466-6272

195 What is date rape, and how can I avoid it?

While date rape has no absolute definition, it is usually considered to be rape that occurs in a social situation when a man becomes sexually aggressive and forces intercourse against his date's will.

Most people think of rape as something that is done by a stranger with violence and injury, but rape can also be committed by an acquaintance or a date. Rape occurs whenever a woman is forced to have intercourse against her will—even if a woman is unconscious from having had too much to drink or if she submits to intercourse from fear of injury by the man. This problem is appallingly common. The Centers for Disease Control reported its survey of college women in early 1998, which showed that 20 percent of college women have been forced to have sexual intercourse against their will.

A study done by Mosher et al. at the University of Connecticut and reported in the *Journal of Research and Personality* (1988, 20:77) showed that most of 175 middle-class, nineteen-year-old student males had used force or exploitation to gain sex from dates. Two out of three reported getting a woman drunk to have sex with her, and more than half had arranged to come into a date's apartment "so I could get her where I wanted her." In addition, more than 40 percent had sought to intimidate their dates with verbal manipulation ("I have told a woman that her refusal to have sex with me was changing the way I felt about her") or angry rejection ("I have gripped a woman tightly and given her an angry look when she was not giving me the sexual response I wanted"). Almost 20 percent had actually forced a date to have sex or had frightened her into compliance with displays of violence.

Playing games with a male can light a fire of expectation in him that can result in a woman being forced into sex. In an article by N. Denney et al. in the *Archives of Sexual Behavior* ("Sex Differences and Sexual Needs and Desires," 1984, 13.3), it was reported that "a large majority of men said that physical affection should always eventually lead to intercourse and orgasm." Some of the comments of these men include these:

Affection, touching, hugging, talking, kissing are all meaningless and uninteresting unless there is at least some hope that they will eventually lead to sex.

Affection is important in the early stages of life, but as far as affectionate sex, that is childish. Sex is not meant for affection. It is a release of pressure, and every man has his own level of how much pressure he needs.

This means that many men expect a woman to have sex with them. If she teases or encourages a date, he may take this as a sign that she wants to have intercourse. He might then refuse to stop even if the woman says no, even if she meant to stop intimacy prior to intercourse.

It is absolutely wrong for a man to force himself on a woman in this fashion. Every woman who is raped should go immediately to a hospital emergency room for an exam and then file charges of rape against the man.

To every dating woman I give a little advice: Though it is right to file charges of rape, it would be better if the act had never taken place, both for you and for the man. I encourage you to decide before you date a man that you are not going to have sex with him until he marries you. Let him know that is the basic requirement you have for dating him: no intercourse until marriage. If he is interested only in your body, he will not come back. If he is interested in you as a person, he will call again and will probably not be the kind of man that would rape you.

The decision you make before you date a man is the key. It can help free you from worry.

The other decision that can help insulate you from date rape is the decision to not take drugs or drink alcohol while on a date. Statistics on date rape show that it almost always occurs when the woman has been drinking. Avoid drinking alcohol on dates and it is unlikely you will ever experience date rape with its horrible consequences.

An Afterword

During the reproductive years, a woman's body is working hard and it requires good care. If a woman maintains a healthy lifestyle during this important period of her life, her body will usually serve her well during the reproductive years and in the years beyond. A woman should keep herself in good condition, have regular health checkups, and get good medical care for any problem that she may have. Hopefully, this chapter provides the information a woman needs to maintain and preserve her health and vitality.

Many of the topics discussed in this chapter also affect other aspects of a woman's life and are discussed in different parts of this book. Please use the index to locate related discussions so that you can be fully informed on these topics

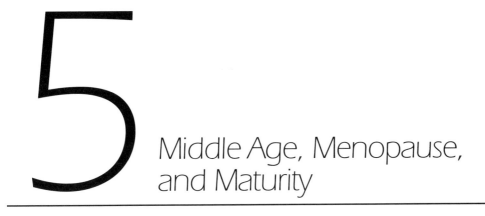

5

Middle Age, Menopause, and Maturity

The poet Robert Browning expressed a possibility that most of us do not consider when we are younger:

> Grow old along with me!
> The best is yet to be,
> The last of life, for which the first was made.
> Our times are in his hand
> Who saith, "A whole I planned,
> Youth shows but half;
> Trust God: see all, nor be afraid!"

Youth is only half a life; the other half is lived as a middle-aged or older person and it can be the best part.

The Book of Isaiah speaks of God's care for us as we get older:

> I will be your God through all your lifetime,
> Yes, even when your hair is white with age.
> I made you and I will care for you.
> I will carry you along and be your Savior
>
> Isaiah 46:4 LB

How gracious of God to assure us that he will carry us along in our old age, and to remind us that he made us and has been with us since our youth. If we are assured of God's care in our later years, how can we dread the years of maturity?

There is much more going for midlife, menopause, and maturity than mere survival, but misinformation and fear of change often cause young women to look with dread on midlife years. While change is always difficult, the anticipation and dread of change are even worse. I hope this chapter will help not only those who are already in the midlife and mature years but also those who are younger. A clear understanding will enable young women to enter the best of life "for which the first was made" without fear or dread.

Young women seem to dread middle age and the mature years for fear that they cannot be as physically active and healthy, as mentally alert, or as physically attractive as they once were. One goal of this chapter is to introduce to younger women the idea that if they live healthy lives in their youth and carry these good health habits into their middle years, they can be healthier, freer from disease, and more mentally alert in old age than they ever thought possible. And because of the glow of good health and the charisma of a sound mind and happy heart, their physical attractiveness will be maximized.

The goal is the same for those women who are already middle-aged or older. If they do not have well-established good health habits, they should understand that much of the deterioration they are experiencing is due to poor health habits, not to the inevitability of age decline. A program begun now for improving their health will pay off in feeling better and being healthier both now and in later years.

Some older people have apparently done nothing to care for their bodies or minds, yet seem to be alert, healthy, and active. A visit to a nursing home, however, will show many whose health has declined. Why take a chance? The better you care for yourself now, the more likely you are to be healthy in the future.

Good health should not become an obsessive goal or the god of your life. Doing whatever is necessary to insure and maintain your health, however, will enable you to attain your life's goal and to reach your maximum potential for serving God until he calls you home.

Some Basic Definitions

196 What is the meaning of the various terms that are used to refer to this particular time of life?

The definitions of these various terms and the ages at which they occur tend to blend into each other and overlap. The following definitions and ages are generally accepted.

Midlife. The years between the ages of forty and sixty are considered the middle age of life. This term has nothing to do with menopause except that it usually occurs during the midlife years.

Climacteric. This term applies to the period of life that starts when the ovaries begin having decreased estrogen production. It includes the menopause, continues for several years, and ends when all the estrogen-sensitive tissues in the body have thinned out (atrophied) as much as they ever will. The entire climacteric period can last for thirty years.

Premenopause. This period extends from the time a woman's ovaries have begun producing less estrogen until she has her last period. This is the first phase of the climacteric.

Menopause. Menopause is actually the name given to a woman's last menstrual period. In our society the term *menopause* is usually used, even by medical personnel, when they are talking about the climacteric. The menopause occurs in most women from the age of forty-eight to fifty-five, with the average age being fifty-one. This is the second phase of the climacteric.

Postmenopause. This term describes the time from the last menstrual period through the rest of life. A woman is postmenopausal when the menopause is totally over. Normally, menopause is considered to have occurred when twelve months have elapsed without a menstrual period.

Midlife to Maturity Age Ranges

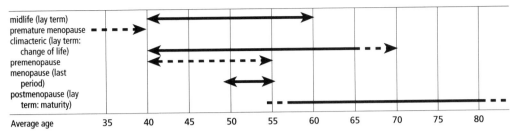

midlife (lay term)										
premature menopause										
climacteric (lay term: change of life)										
premenopause										
menopause (last period)										
postmenopause (lay term: maturity)										
Average age	35	40	45	50	55	60	65	70	75	80

Change of life. This nonmedical term usually applies to the time from the first changes in a woman's body due to decreased estrogen, through the last menstrual period, or menopause. It is often used to refer to the few years after menopause during which, as a result of her climacteric, a woman has hot flashes or trouble sleeping. This period of time roughly corresponds to the climacteric. Most laypeople use this term in reference to the symptoms of the climacteric.

Mature years. The years from about sixty until death encompass the years of a woman's "maturity."

General Health Care in Midlife

In 50 A.D., the philosopher Seneca said, "Man does not die; he kills himself." Because of the way we live, many of us will not live long enough to die a natural death.

You can make the necessary changes in your life to insure that you are doing all you can to live long enough to die a natural death.

The diseases that cause so many deaths are not always inevitable. Your lifestyle determines, to a greater degree than was imagined years ago, the quality of life you will have in years to come. You can make choices that enhance your health and enjoyment of life in the future. Making the right choices will give you the optimum possibility of being healthy, alert, and happy as the years go by.

Most of us are going to live years longer than our family members of previous generations, due

largely to the fact that Americans as a whole have access to better medical care and to better year-round nutrition than did our ancestors. To a large degree, however, we have not "adjusted" to the reality of living into our late eighties and nineties. If we really comprehended such longevity, surely we'd take the best care of ourselves possible so that those latter years could be lived to the fullest.

The National Institute on Aging provides interesting information about life expectancy:

> A baby boy born in the U.S. in January, 1890, could expect to live to the ripe old age of 42, and a baby girl born that same day could expect to live to 45.
>
> Today, life expectancy has increased by at least thirty years. The average American man will live at least 72 years and the average American woman will live nearly 79 years.
>
> By the year 2050, it is estimated that a million Americans will be at least one hundred years old.

You have a choice. You can live those years feeling good and being alert, independent, and healthy. Or you can live those years as an invalid, having a stroke, heart attack, broken hip, and all the things we associate with old age.

Getting older is inevitable, but much of the *aging process* of the mind and body can be dramatically slowed down. The body will gradually look older, but it can often be kept fairly healthy into old age. A healthy body is not as likely to develop the problems and diseases we commonly associate with growing older. It is never too late to change harmful habits and to incorporate new, healthy ones into your life.

197 How is exercise related to growing older?

Many women get into a vicious cycle as they enter midlife. First, in the back of their minds they believe they are supposed to slow down. Then, at a picnic or on vacation, they perform some unusual physical activity and strain a ligament or muscle, confirming in their minds that they really do need to slow down. As a result they engage in even less activity. This downward spiral causes these women to do less and less physical activity, assuming that this is normal for the human body.

This attitude and approach to physical activity from the middle-aged years on is absolutely wrong. Women should continue exercising until the day they die if they can. Even if they have a physical problem, they can have a local health and fitness center custom design an exercise program to get around that problem.

There are many good books about exercise and how much exercise a woman should have.

A wonderful study published in the *Journal of the American Medical Association* (1990, 236:22) showed that it is never too late to exercise for good health. In this study, ten frail, nonagenarian, institutionalized volunteers did eight weeks of exercise with weights. The research by Maria A. Fiatarone and her associates found that weight training, even in these ninety-year-old men and women, led to significant gains in muscle strength and size. If exercise can restore functional mobility to frail residents of nursing homes, think what it can do for you!

Most women are concerned about gaining weight after going through the menopause, and there is basis for that fear. A study done by Dr. Wing and associates in the *Archives of Internal Medicine* (1991, 151:97–102) showed that after menopause women do have a weight gain of about five pounds, and those women who gain weight after menopause have an increased risk of cardiovascular disease.

This weight gain occurs even in men and women who are runners, Paul T. Williams reported at the American Heart Association scientific session in 1995. As years went by weight increased even if exercise continued. Exercise had to be increased to keep weight stable. He also found

that as weight increased, so did blood pressure and cholesterol. Dr. Williams found that for the purpose of health, the more exercise the better.

A study done by Sforzo and reported in the *Journal of American Geriatrics Society* (March 1995, 43:209) showed that interruptions in an older person's exercise for up to five weeks did not cause them to lose their muscular fitness. They therefore should not be discouraged if illness causes them to temporarily stop exercising.

Studies have shown that poor vision and lack of exercise cause the majority of falls in elderly people. Ophthalmologists can usually take care of the visual problems, but the responsibility of exercising is up to you. Start this habit today!

198 What major health hazard should be avoided by women seeking optimum health in later years?

Smoking! Studies show over and over again that smoking is the worst health hazard for Americans in general, and that it is particularly detrimental for the woman who is growing older.

Many studies have demonstrated that cigarette smoking causes menopause to come earlier. More importantly, smoking causes the estrogen produced in a woman's body to be relatively inactive compared to that produced by the ovaries of a nonsmoker. These two things combine to increase the smoking woman's chance of having osteoporosis and the dangers that entails.

Besides increasing the wrinkling of skin and making a woman look older, smoking increases the incidence of lung cancer and is responsible for the fact that lung cancer is now more common than breast cancer in women. Smoking greatly increases a woman's chance of having heart disease, strokes, and poor circulation, and it limits the amount of oxygen distributed from the lungs to the rest of the body, decreasing energy and making a woman less likely to exercise. All of these effects are devastating to a woman as she grows older.

Studies are beginning to confirm that if a woman stops smoking, she is more likely to remain a nonsmoker if she exercises regularly.

Smoking women are more likely to lose their teeth because the bone that holds the teeth gets weak. So, if you don't want to be a toothless old woman, stop smoking!

199 Is a yearly physical still important once a woman is past reproductive age?

Yes! You should have an annual physical examination for the rest of your life. It is very important for women who are going through menopause to have a physician whom they trust, who will listen to them, and who is knowledgeable about climacteric women's health. So many questions arise during this time about important issues: irregular periods, the possibility of pregnancy, whether or not to take hormones, etc. So many health problems are common to women over fifty: cancer of the uterus (most likely to occur between ages fifty and seventy), elevated blood pressure, etc. A complete examination every year is important *for the rest of a woman's life*, both to find problems and to provide opportunity for ongoing consultation about these issues. This exam should include a blood pressure check, a blood count, a urinalysis, and a Pap smear. The doctor should, at minimum, check your thyroid, your breasts, your abdomen, and your pelvis. This basic examination will detect most abnormalities that an otherwise healthy woman might not know she has. In addition to the annual exam, if you have pain, discomfort, or other symptoms, you should go to the doctor for that. (See Q. 118–121 for a more complete discussion of the annual exam.)

Colon cancer is so common in our society that routine testing is worthwhile. The American Cancer Society recommends that every person over forty years of age have a digital (with the finger) rectal exam every year. An examiner can feel a cancer growing in a patient's rectum if it is within reach of his or her finger. In addition, since a colon cancer will usually bleed into the intestines even when it is very small, a simple test for blood in the stools will often detect the presence of a colon cancer quite early. You can get a small inexpensive test packet to check your stools from your doctor, your local cancer society, or your pharmacy. The American Cancer Society recommends that you check your stools every year from age fifty on. Because this test is so cheap and easy to do, I feel that a person might as well do it from the age of forty on.

In addition, the American Cancer Society recommends that a person who is age fifty or over have a proctoscopy or flexible sigmoidoscopy done, followed by another one a year later, and then one every five years.

Proctoscopy (or sigmoidoscopy) requires that a doctor insert a tube through your anus into your rectum and colon to see if any growths are present. These procedures are not done by gynecologists. They are usually done by gastroenterologists (intestinal specialists), internal medicine specialists, general surgeons, and family practitioners.

In May of 1989 Gilda Radner died of ovarian cancer. She began having symptoms in January 1986, but the cancer was not diagnosed until October 1986. Her book about the experience, and her subsequent death, have made women very aware of the dangers of ovarian cancer.

The best protection against ovarian cancer is to have your annual examination. If your doctor suspects a growth in your pelvis, he or she will probably want you to have an ultrasound examination. In addition, there is a blood test, called CA 125, that will sometimes be elevated if a woman has ovarian cancer. (Because CA 125 can be elevated with endometriosis, pelvic infection, menstrual periods, and from other causes, no expert recommends a CA 125 as a routine part of a yearly exam. See Q. 728–755 for more information on the subject of ovarian growths and diseases.)

Menopause

200 What causes menopause?

Menopause comes when the ovaries no longer manufacture enough estrogen to produce menstrual periods. The ovaries stop producing estrogen when the ovarian follicles—small cysts that contain egg cells—die. When all these egg cells with their follicles are gone, the ovaries no longer produce estrogen, and a woman can no longer have periods. When this occurs the ovaries are essentially dead. Over the next few years they shrink, becoming small nubbins of fibrous tissue no more than one-half inch in diameter in the eighth and ninth decades of life. They unfortunately do still have enough live cells to be a possible source of cancer for the rest of a woman's life.

201 At what age does menopause normally occur?

Menopause usually occurs between the ages of forty-eight to fifty-five, the average age being fifty-one. It is also normal for women to go through menopause as early as forty or as late as sixty. About 30 percent of women will have had menopause by the time they are forty-five and 98 percent will have had menopause by the time they are fifty-five.

There are variations.

Premature menopause. If a woman has menopause before the age of forty, she is said to have "premature menopause," and even adolescent girls can experience this. The medical term is "premature ovarian failure." This is a permanent condition, and there is nothing that can be done to make the ovaries begin again to produce eggs or hormones. Obviously a woman with premature menopause cannot become pregnant.

It is vitally important that a woman begin taking estrogen immediately if premature menopause occurs. Women who have early menopause have a much higher rate of osteoporosis, fractures of their bones, strokes, and heart attacks, than women who go through menopause at the usual age.

Surgical menopause. A woman is said to have "surgical menopause" if she has her ovaries removed by surgery. She will not go through "natural" menopause because her menopause is over in one act of surgery. If she starts taking hormones immediately following surgery, she will never experience any symptoms of menopause. Meno-

pause will not result from the removal of one ovary if the other ovary is functioning normally. In fact, the remaining ovary will increase its production of estrogen and eggs to allow normal function and near normal fertility.

Menopause after the age of sixty. This is a reasonably common occurrence among American women. If a woman continues to have periods after the age of sixty, most doctors feel that she should have an endometrial biopsy, or scraping of the inside of the uterus, to make sure that cancer is not present. If a woman's periods persist into her sixties, she is more likely to have endometrial cancer than if her menopause had occurred earlier. If you are such a woman, make sure your doctor does an endometrial biopsy, or a D&C, every year or two.

202 Are women having menopause later in life now than they did in the past?

The age at which a woman goes through menopause has not changed through the years. It only seems that more women today are having late menopause because women are living to an older age than they did in the past.

Menopause is apparently fixed in a woman's genes at birth and is unaffected by diet or any other factor. A woman's menopause is unrelated to when her periods started and has nothing whatsoever to do with her having taken birth-control pills or fertility drugs in the past.

203 How will I know that I have gone through menopause?

When you have gone six to twelve months without a period—and your female organs are otherwise normal—you have probably gone through menopause.

A blood test for FSH (follicle-stimulating hormone) will positively indicate whether or not you have gone through menopause. If your ovaries are no longer functioning (menopause is a result of the ovaries no longer functioning), your pituitary will increase its production of FSH in an effort to force the ovaries to produce follicles, eggs, and estrogen. An FSH blood test will detect a significantly elevated level. If your FSH level is elevated to the postmenopausal level (40 mIU/ml or more), you cannot get pregnant and do not have to worry about contraception anymore!

204 How will I feel before and after menopause, in other words, during the climacteric?

Several changes in your body may occur during this time.

Changes in menstrual pattern. As the ovarian production of estrogen decreases and the ovaries stop putting out eggs regularly, your periods may change. You may have decreased or increased menstrual flow. Your periods may be irregular and you may have spotting between them.

Unfortunately, it is impossible for you or your doctor to know whether spotting between periods and/or unusual bleeding is due to premenopausal changes or to uterine cancer. Because uterine cancer is so much more likely to occur from the age of forty on, doctors will usually recommend a D&C or endometrial biopsy and/or hysteroscopy (see Q. 704) if a woman in that age group has unusual bleeding.

After menopause, a woman should not have any more vaginal bleeding unless she is taking hormones. If she is not on hormones and has bleeding, she almost always needs a D&C or a thorough endometrial biopsy and/or a hysteroscopy to be sure she has no uterine cancer.

Hot flashes and sweating. A hot flash has been described as being "a welling up of heat inside that begins in the chest and moves up into the head." A woman may perspire and turn red in the face with a hot flash, but most of the time a woman feels much redder in the face than she really looks! These flashes may last from only a few seconds to an hour and may occur rarely or every ten minutes, and it is common for hot flashes to occur at night.

Trouble sleeping. Because hot flashes often occur at night and may wake a climacteric woman, she often does not sleep well. This insomnia leaves her continually in need of sleep and constantly tired.

Joint aches. Patients who are going through the climacteric often have aching of the large joints of their body or of their back. This may be due to calcium changes in the body from decreased estrogen.

Thinning of the estrogen-sensitive tissues of the body. This problem is primarily noted as the vagina thins out, causing dryness and discomfort with intercourse. Tissue atrophy can also affect the bladder, producing pain with urination and later a relaxation of the bladder tissues that causes a leakage of urine when a woman coughs, sneezes, or laughs. (See Q. 612–615.) In addition, a woman may notice that her breasts are becoming thinner and droopier at this time of life.

Other problems. Lack of estrogen can produce depression and irritability in some women. Others will have headaches and decreased interest in sex.

205 Do all women have symptoms of inadequate estrogen after menopause?

No. Some women go through menopause with no symptoms at all, and they are almost surprised when they remember that it has been a year since their last menstrual period. Other women have severe symptoms. At least half of the women who go through menopause find that some type of medical treatment for their symptoms is helpful.

Three factors seem to be associated with the degree of problems that menopause can cause. Drs. Speroff, Glass, and Kase state, in their excellent book *Clinical Gynecologic Endocrinology and Infertility* (Williams & Wilkins), that the three factors associated with the severity of a woman's symptoms are:

The amount of estrogen depletion and the rate at which estrogen is withdrawn.
The collective inherited and acquired propensities to succumb or withstand the impositions of the overall aging process.

The psychological impact of aging and the individual's reaction to the emotional implications of a change in life.

The woman who will probably have the most trouble with menopausal symptoms is the one whose estrogen levels drop suddenly, whose body is so made that it readily senses these changes, and who, because of her psychological makeup, reacts more emotionally to the changes in her life than other women do.

206 What causes hot flashes and how long do they last?

Hot flashes are a real physical symptom of menopause and are definitely related to physical change in a woman's body. Many other symptoms during this time may be due to the psychology of midlife.

Hot flashes are not a result of *no* estrogen; they are a result of *change* in estrogen levels. This explains why a woman can have hot flashes even though she is still having menstrual periods. In that case, she is still producing estrogen or she could not have any menstrual bleeding.

About 75 percent of women who undergo natural menopause will have hot flashes, and one-third of these women will experience severe hot flashes. The more severe the symptom is, the greater the change in estrogen levels. Half of the women who have hot flashes have them once a day; one-fifth of women with hot flashes will have more than one "attack" daily. Hot flashes usually last from one to two years, but rarely more than five years.

If a woman is thin, or below her ideal body weight, she is more likely to have hot flashes than if she were heavier. This is because there is some estrogen production from the fatty tissues of a heavier woman that keep her estrogen levels from changing dramatically as menopause occurs. This also explains why women who are overweight have less osteoporosis following menopause than thin women.

Hot flashes are a result of an increased flow of blood through certain parts of the body. This increase seems to be due to instability of the autonomic nervous system, the part of the nervous system that controls the degree of dilation of blood vessels, the amount of sweat that is put out by sweat glands, and sexual lubrication. This instability is termed "vasomotor instability" and usually produces heat, redness, and sweating of the face, neck, and upper chest. Studies show that the woman's blood vessels and temperature do not return to normal for about thirty minutes after a hot flash.

There are those who believe hot flashes are caused by hormones from the pituitary gland trying to make the ovaries work. In other words, they think the increased amount of FSH in the body causes the hot flashes. This is not the usual mechanism, however, if indeed it is part of the cause of hot flashes at all. Women who do not have pituitary glands can have hot flashes.

Estrogen after Menopause

207 Should women take estrogen after menopause?

Yes! Although there has been a great deal of controversy about this in the past, there is almost no controversy now. Estrogen is so important for your health during the entire last half of your lifetime that if your doctor will not prescribe estrogen for you, when there is no medical reason for your not taking it, you should change doctors.

Taking estrogen after menopause will not make a woman ovulate or become fertile. Menopause means the ovaries stop functioning and nothing will reactivate them.

Also, taking estrogen probably does not increase the risk of developing breast cancer. (See Q. 212 in this chapter.) Or if it does, it is such a tiny increased risk it is almost undetectable by scientific studies.

208 Why should a woman take estrogen after menopause?

There are several reasons a woman should take estrogen:

Osteoporosis. This thinning of the bones, which begins when the estrogen levels in some women's bodies start decreasing, makes the bones weaker. Therefore, when a woman's ovaries stop producing estrogen her bones become more susceptible to fractures. Experts estimate that 25–50 percent of white females will experience some degree of osteoporosis unless they take estrogen.

Reduction of heart disease. Premenopausal women have a lower risk of heart attack than men of the same age. Postmenopausal women who do not take estrogen soon begin having heart attacks at the same rate as men. Recent studies show that if a woman will start taking estrogen immediately after menopause, she can lower by 50–75 percent her risk of having a stroke or a heart attack. This fact is one of the most significant reasons for using estrogen after menopause.

Symptoms of climacteric. If a woman is having annoying symptoms of inadequate hormones, estrogen will relieve those symptoms and help her feel "normal" again.

Symptoms after menopause. Estrogen helps to keep the vagina from becoming dry (allowing comfortable intercourse) and prevents the vaginal tissues from weakening, thus helping to decrease the possibility of hysterectomies and vaginal repairs later in life.

Psychological and physical symptoms. Estrogen helps provide a sense of psychological well-being. It will usually prevent irritability, headaches, anxiety, and depression.

209 What effect does estrogen have on the symptoms mentioned above?

Estrogen is without question the best treatment for these pre- and postmenopausal symptoms. Excellent studies show that when women with menopausal symptoms are given estrogen, the symptoms almost always cease to be a problem.

If a woman cannot take estrogen (see next question), the use of progesterone is the next best thing. Progesterone, however, requires high doses to stop hot flashes. One worry with the use of progesterone alone is that it can increase the bad cholesterol (LDL) in a woman's bloodstream and increase her chance of a stroke or heart attack. (It is also expensive.) Twenty milligrams of Provera in pill form a day will usually stop hot flashes. A less expensive, but just as effective, way to take progesterone is through an injection of 150 mg of Depo-Provera every three months.

Other drugs that can help prevent hot flashes are Bellergal, Symmetrel, Catapres, and Aldomet. It is possible that Depo-Provera may have some effect on delaying osteoporosis. The other drugs are not hormones and do not prevent osteoporosis.

210 Who should not take estrogen?

There are several groups of women who should not take estrogen.

Women who have tumors that might be stimulated by estrogen. The most common of these is breast cancer. Estrogen will not cause breast cancer but can make an already present cancer grow faster.

Women with liver disease. An internal medicine specialist can determine if liver disease is too severe for taking estrogen.

Women who have a tendency to form blood clots. Your doctor can determine if your tendency to blood clotting is severe enough to keep you from taking estrogen. If it is, it may be possible to take anticoagulants so you can take estrogen.

Women who have problems when they take estrogen. For example, women who have had migraine headaches will sometimes start having them again when they take estrogen. Some women will bleed from the uterus excessively if they take even small doses of estrogen. Other women just do not feel well if they take it.

If you cannot take estrogen for alleviation of bothersome menopausal symptoms, you may want to ask your doctor to prescribe one of the other drugs that has been found effective for the relief of these symptoms.

See Q. 225 about endometriosis.

211 Should I take estrogen if I have fibrocystic breast condition?

Because breast cells are sensitive to hormones and fibrocystic breast condition is thought to be caused by overreaction of breast tissue to these substances, women who have fibrocystic breast condition with bothersome pain and increased nodularity may have more breast problems if they take estrogen. However, this does not cause an increased chance of breast cancer. It is so important that a postmenopausal woman take estrogen that even if it does make her breasts tender, it is worth it. There are several things a woman can try to help stop the tenderness so she can continue her estrogen. She can try taking vitamin E, 400 mg a day, and decreasing (or cutting out altogether) caffeine. If those measures don't provide relief, a drug called Parlodel may help. Also, a three- to six-month course of Danocrine may diminish the breast pain to the point where she can take estrogen. It is wise to resolve problems associated with fibrocystic breast condition so that a woman can take estrogen after menopause. Again, taking estrogen will not appreciably increase the risk of developing breast cancer even in a woman with fibrocystic breast disease.

212 Before you tell me about how to take estrogen, I want to know if taking estrogen after menopause will cause me to get breast cancer.

This is the most common question I get when I start talking about estrogen and menopause, and I always reassure my patients that breast cancer does not seem to be caused by taking estrogen after menopause. I say "does not seem to be caused by estrogen" because there are some studies that seem to indicate that there may be a little increased risk of breast cancer if a woman takes estrogen after menopause.

Two definitive studies published prior to 1990, however, showed that there is no increased risk of breast cancer if women are taking estrogen for their menopausal symptoms. Another study published by the *Archives of Internal Medicine* (1991, 151:67, Dr. William DuPont of Vanderbilt University) showed that there is no increased risk of breast cancer from taking estrogen.

Finally, there was an excellent study by Newcomb P.A. et al. *American Journal of Epidemiology* (1995, 142:788–195) that showed no hint of an increased risk of breast cancer in women on estrogen even if they continued taking estrogen for years. The risk of breast cancer was not increased if a woman was also taking progesterone as most women do in the postmenopause.

It is important to realize that there is a slightly increased risk of breast cancer as women age, which may account for the increased risk that some researchers attribute to estrogen.

You may hear that women who have breast cancer are told that they must stop taking estrogen, but this does not mean that it was estrogen that *caused* the cancer. Perhaps an analogy that I use for my patients will illustrate. Logs in a fireplace do not cause fire, but if a fire is already burning, adding more logs to the fire will keep it burning. Similarly, if a woman has no cancer in her breasts, estrogen will not start cancer, but if she has breast cancer, adding estrogen might keep the breast cancer growing. (Some studies now indicate that it does not, but, at this point, we do not know for sure.)

Breast cancer accounts for 1.7 percent of the deaths of women over the age of sixty-five; heart and cardiovascular disease account for 66 percent of the deaths of women over age sixty-five. In 1989, for instance, there were 440,000 deaths of women in the U.S. from heart attacks; there were 43,000 deaths from breast cancer. In terms of relative risk, cardiovascular disease is much more dangerous to women than breast cancer, *and up to 60 percent of heart attacks in women can be prevented by the use of estrogen.*

Another statistic (confirmed by three good research reports) presents the surprising fact that women with breast cancer who were taking estrogen at the time their breast cancer was found had a higher survival rate than women who were not.

Even if there is a slightly increased risk of breast cancer, it would be worth the risk to take the estrogen. The primary reason for taking estrogen after menopause is that it dramatically lowers the risk of strokes and heart attacks. This occurs for two reasons. First, it increases the good cholesterol (HDL) in the body. HDL acts as a cleaning agent, actually cleaning cholesterol off the walls of the blood vessels, which keeps them from becoming hardened and narrowed. Second, estrogen has a direct beneficial effect on keeping blood vessel walls healthy that is independent of the activity of HDL. Not only is there a decreased risk of death, but women who take hormones after menopause have significantly increased health.

In conclusion, my recommendation for postmenopausal women is to take hormones, practice breast self-exams, and have regular mammograms (and do the other things we mention in this chapter).

213 Is osteoporosis really a serious enough problem to warrant taking estrogen for the rest of my life?

Yes, it is. The following statistics show the problems that osteoporosis produces in women in our society.

Bone loss for women begins at about age thirty-five and continues at the rate of .5 percent annually until menopause. After menopause bone loss increases dramatically. Ten years after menopause women have lost from 15–20 percent of their bone mass and, at that point, can begin having fractures. Most of the time, however, a fracture indicates a loss of about half of the bone mass of a woman's body. Many women who have a fractured vertebra have lost two-thirds of the bone of their body. If you have suffered a fracture of any of your bones since menopause, you have probably already lost a considerable quantity of your bone mass. You should use that as a warning and consider the advice in this section even more seriously than the average woman.

By the age of sixty, 25 percent of all women have compression fractures of the vertebrae of the spine. This explains why they get shorter and have humped backs. Fractures of the vertebrae are the most common fractures of osteoporosis. By the age of seventy-five, 50 percent of women have had fractures of bones somewhere in their body.

About 40 percent of white women have a fractured hip by the time they reach ninety, and 15 percent of these women die within six months of that hip fracture. Those who do not die are often left invalids.

In a study about hip fractures in the *Journal of the American Medical Association* (August 1982), it was reported that of a group of 108 patients who were treated for hip fractures (all over fifty years of age), 41 percent were discharged to nursing homes. After one year, nine (8 percent) had died and the majority of these patients were still in nursing homes. Fewer than 25 percent ever regained their previous independence. Seventy-five percent of those who had hip fractures were permanently affected in some way. Obviously, prevention is far better than all the wonderful hip operations that can be done.

Dr. Bill Creasman of Duke University calculated that a woman has a one in sixty chance of dying of a hip fracture or of its complications if she lives past the age of seventy.

About 40 percent of women over sixty will lose their teeth because of loss of bone from the jawbone. This is an osteoporosis problem. Women who have osteoporosis between the ages of fifty and sixty are three times as likely to need dentures as women who do not have it.

Ten years after menopause, women have ten times as many arm fractures as men of the same age if the women are not taking estrogen.

214 Is estrogen really effective against osteoporosis?

If a woman starts estrogen right after menopause, she will not usually lose significant bone mass and will not be subject to the risk of fractures. The routine that is used by most physicians includes progesterone. Recent studies have shown that the combination of estrogen and progesterone not only keeps a woman from losing bone but can also actually increase existing bone mass.

If you use estrogen for a few years and then stop taking it, you will lose bone mass faster than

Effects of Osteoporosis

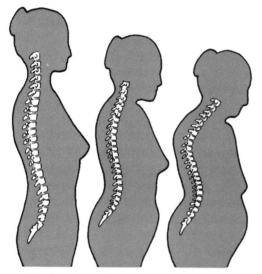

The effects of osteoporosis. When 30–40 percent of bone loss occurs, the vertebrae start to collapse and as much as five to eight inches in height can be lost, all from the upper part of the body. The lower spine curves inward and the abdomen protudes.

is usually normal—until the weakness of your bones is, within about four years, where it would have been if you had never taken estrogen. Therefore you have the benefits of estrogen as long as you take it, but when you stop taking estrogen, the benefits soon evaporate. The only thing that would change this course of treatment would be if some better treatment were discovered before the time of your death, or if you develop a medical problem that makes it unwise for you to take estrogen.

215 Are there women who are more likely to develop osteoporosis and, consequently, bone fractures?

Yes, there are several groups of women who are more likely to have problems with osteoporosis. These women face a magnified risk for future fractures if they do not take estrogen.

Women who exercise so excessively that their menstrual periods cease. Such women probably need to start taking estrogen and proges-

terone as though they were postmenopausal (very common in those who run marathons, do ballet, or who are anorexic).

Women who have had their ovaries removed surgically before the menopause occurs or who start menopause early.

Smokers. Women who smoke are more likely to have early menopause and will lose bone faster. (Even taking estrogen does not "catch up" with the osteoporosis effect of smoking, but it will, perhaps, help some.)

Diabetics.

Women who have taken cortisone for a long time.

Inactive women (or women who have been immobilized longer than three weeks).

Tall women.

Thin women.

Women who have been exposed to minimal amounts of sunlight. Such women have inadequate vitamin D in their bodies and have probably not been absorbing adequate calcium from their diet.

Heavy alcohol consumers.

Women who have never had a pregnancy. Studies show that they are at greater risk than women who have been pregnant.

Women who take in excessive caffeine.

Women who use long-acting benzodiazepines (certain tranquilizers).

216 If I am not in any of the categories listed above, can I wait to see if I develop osteoporosis before I start taking estrogen?

If you wait, it may be too late. Once bone loss has occurred in your body, it is difficult to make those weak bones strong again. If a woman waits until she begins having health problems of *any* kind, measures to repair damage are not nearly so effective as preventive measures would have been. Estrogen is in this category. Early use will help prevent later problems.

If you cannot, or will not, take estrogen, don't wait until you have a fracture to do something. Get a bone density test now. This test can be done

The Female Body in Change

for moderate expense and is totally painless and safe. There are several techniques used, the most common one being the use of a dual energy bone densitometer.

A bone density test will show if you have lost a significant amount of bone density. If you have, you are more likely to experience a fractured hip or vertebra, or some other complication of osteoporosis. I actually recommend that a woman do this by the age of forty-five to know what to expect about her bones.

Knowing you have decreased bone density might motivate you to take estrogen; it could encourage you to explore the possibility of taking etidronate (or the newer alendronate—see Q. 217); and it could encourage you to eliminate any unhealthy habits, such as smoking, drinking too much, and failing to exercise.

217 Are there other things I can do to help prevent osteoporosis?

There are several things a woman should do to help prevent osteoporosis. None of these will take the place of estrogen, but each is good and should be practiced along with taking estrogen.

Enter menopause with good heavy bones. Reliable studies show that the strength of your bones when you are thirty-five has a great deal to do with whether or not you will develop osteoporosis after you reach menopause. (Men are less likely to have osteoporosis because they are more likely to have strong bones when they are in their thirties.) It is important to start using calcium when you are thirty-five. My recommendation is 500 mg of elemental supplement every day from the age of thirty-five on, in addition to some milk, cottage cheese, cheese, or yogurt every day.

Take calcium. Although many women want to try to take enough calcium so that estrogen is not necessary, enough calcium to keep the bones healthy would cause kidney stones and would often still not work. Before menopause, women need to have about 1,000 mg of calcium a day; after menopause without estrogen they need 1,500 mg daily. If a postmenopausal woman is taking estrogen, she should have 1,000 mg of calcium daily.

A normal diet contains about 400 to 500 mg of calcium a day. A woman, therefore, needs to take enough supplemental calcium to make up the extra calcium needed. She can take one or two 250 mg calcium pills with breakfast and one or two with the evening meal.

Vitamin D is included in many calcium preparations but is not necessary for most women. The majority of women get enough vitamin D from everyday exposure to the sun. If a woman is exposed to adequate sunlight, her body will manufacture enough vitamin D for its needs.

The intake of more than 1,000 units of vitamin D a day may actually cause bone loss, so do not overdo the intake of vitamin D (usual dose 400 units/day). Vitamin A can also cause bone loss if taken in dosages larger than 5,000 units a day.

There are several forms of calcium available on the market. An excellent study of the use of calcium was reported in the *New England Journal of Medicine* (1990, 323:13). This study showed that healthy older, postmenopausal women could decrease their bone loss significantly if they took enough calcium. The study showed that women who were taking less than 400 mg of calcium had significant bone loss, but this loss slowed considerably when they increased their calcium intake to 800 mg a day. The most effective calcium seemed to be calcium citrate, rather than calcium carbonate. Calcium citrate is probably the best form of calcium to take, but it is more expensive and some women have intestinal upset from it. Calcium carbonate is probably fine for most women.

Exercise. Next to estrogen and calcium, exercise appears to be the most important technique for preserving bone. Exercise actually stimulates the formation of new bone in a woman's body. Some studies indicate that adequate exercise on a regular basis stops bone loss, even if a woman is postmenopausal!

Exercise seems to work by making the muscles stronger. The muscles pull on the bone, and this causes the bone to thicken and become stronger. This means that you do not necessarily need to do weight-bearing exercises. Swimming is excellent, for instance, in preventing osteoporosis and strengthening bones.

Exercises that involve the use of the entire

body are the best for this purpose: walking, jogging, bicycling, swimming, and jumping rope. Exercise done now is very beneficial in helping avoid bone loss in the future. It is good to get in the habit of exercising now, so it will be a natural part of your life as you get older. Remember, these exercises need to be started before the damage is done, not after bone loss has already developed. Once a woman has developed significant osteoporosis, she should avoid activities that involve strain to her bones, such as running or jogging, but she still needs—vitally needs—to exercise. Walking (or swimming) can be ideal exercises.

I do not recommend that a woman depend on exercise exclusively for maintenance of her bone mass as an alternative to taking estrogen, but if she cannot take estrogen, exercise may help much more than we thought in the past if it is done adequately, week after week, year after year.

Don't fall down! Falling can cause a fractured bone even in a person who has strong bones. An excellent study reported in the *New England Journal of Medicine* (1991, 324:19) points out that many things contribute to falls that cause older people to break a bone. These include poor vision, neurologic problems, medication, etc.

Other means of maintaining healthy bones. There has been a new and exciting development in the treatment of osteoporosis—a group of drugs called biphosphonates. There are two forms of these drugs now available, etidronate (Didronel) and alendronate (Fosamax) and others will be available soon. Studies clearly show that these drugs cause an increase in bone density of the patients treated.

The treatment schedule for Didronel is 400 mg of etidronate taken once a day for fourteen days, two hours before or after a meal. This schedule should be repeated every thirteen weeks. Fosamax is simpler to take—one 10 mg pill daily all the time.

Both of these drugs are already commonly used by physicians in the United States for women with osteoporosis. They seem very safe, and currently there have been no significant adverse effects detected in any of the women who take them.

A woman should consider using Fosamax if she cannot take estrogen. If a woman has developed osteoporosis because she did not begin taking estrogen when she went through menopause, she can begin taking both Fosamax and estrogen to stop—and even reverse—the development of osteoporosis.

If you have osteoporosis and your physician does not mention these drugs to you, ask him or her to prescribe them for you. This can save you a hip fracture or other devastating effects of osteoporosis.

You might be interested to know biphosphonates appear to work by preventing the normal absorption of bone that occurs every day. Cells called "osteoclasts" are constantly resorbing bone. This resorption is normal. If you get a fracture or dent of your bone, the damaged part is "resorbed" so that new bone cells can deposit new bone in its place and smooth the bone out. Biphosphonates inhibit that normal bone breakdown. (In the future it may be that people who take them will have more *bumpy* bones, but at least they will have strong bones that do not fracture easily!) No other osteoporosis treatment seems to be very acceptable. Although some doctors advocate the use of fluoride to keep bones healthy, at least one-third of patients who take fluoride in adequate dosages for this purpose have side effects from it. In addition, the bone formed when a person takes this drug is not normal bone. It is less elastic and possibly more fragile than normal bone. (Studies are in progress.)

A drug called calcitonin, which has an effect similar to calcium, has been approved by the FDA for treating osteoporosis. It may be useful in maintaining bone integrity or in helping women with osteoporosis develop healthy bone again. Its primary use now is for people with bone pain from a fracture. Since it is now available as a convenient nasal spray (Miacalcin), it can be used for osteoporosis more easily.

A long-acting progesterone, Depo-Provera, in large dosage not only stops hot flashes and reverses vaginal atrophy but also has positive effects on the bone if a patient takes enough calcium by mouth.

218 What type of estrogen should I use?

A dose of estrogen equal to 0.625 mg of conjugated estrogen (Premarin) is enough to take after menopause to reverse the symptoms of menopause and to prevent osteoporosis and vascular disease. Another advantage to taking Premarin may have been found by Dr. Brinton of the Department of Molecular Pharmacology and Toxocology at the University of Southern California. He reported in 1996 that one component of Premarin called equilin was found to cause growth of neurons in a laboratory setting. The neurons were derived from brain tissue. When this brain tissue was cultured with equilin (derived from Premarin) it was found that these nerve cells grew much better than when they were not in the presence of this form of estrogen. This may explain why women who do not take estrogen after menopause have a greater chance of developing cognitive dysfunction, have more likelihood of developing stress response, and more likelihood of developing Alzheimer's disease. Micronized estradiol (Estrace) 1 mg, estrone sulfate (Ogen) 2 mg, ethinyl estradiol (Estinyl) 5 to 10 micrograms, and Estraderm 0.05 mg, all are probably equivalent in protection for a woman after menopause.

The protection given by estrogen shots or estradiol pellets under the skin has not been studied as long as the above mentioned oral estrogen, but they probably give as good protection as Premarin, Estrace, or Ogen. The main thing is for a woman to find an estrogen that she feels good with and that she will use. If she cannot remember to use a tablet but can remember to use a skin patch, that is fine. If she cannot remember to put a patch on and prefers a shot, that, too, is fine.

It is so important for a woman going through menopause to take estrogen that she should be encouraged to use whatever method she is comfortable with.

219 Will I keep having menstrual periods if I take estrogen?

This is the second most common question I hear when I talk to a woman about estrogen after menopause. (The first one is about estrogen and breast cancer. See Q. 212.) If you take estrogen in the traditional way—taking it for the first twenty-five days each month, with the addition of a progesterone pill the last thirteen days followed by a few days off of hormones—you may keep having menstrual periods for several (perhaps many) years. This "traditional" way is safe and is a good schedule to follow. It protects your blood vessels and bones, and it stops your symptoms of menopause.

If continued menstrual periods are a concern for a woman, there are several choices:

1. A new method of taking hormones (discussed in the following question) will stop almost all menstrual bleeding after one year for 90 percent of women.
2. An endometrial ablation could be done. This procedure consists of using either laser or cautery to remove the lining of the inside of the uterus. When there is no uterine lining to shed, there is no bleeding. See Q. 705 for further information about this minor operation.
3. Hysterectomy is another option. Some women will bleed no matter what their use of estrogen is. If they prefer a hysterectomy to endometrial ablation, that is fine. Most physicians who treat women after menopause feel that a hysterectomy is "worth having" if that is what it takes to keep a woman on estrogen.

This may seem fairly aggressive to some women, but I encourage you to review the information about the benefits of estrogen before you dismiss the idea of an operation (a hysterectomy or ablation) to stay on hormones.

220 What is the new method of using hormones?

The new method of using estrogen, which I think will become the standard way, is as follows: a woman takes an estrogen pill (such as Premarin) and a progesterone pill (such as Provera) every day of the month, all month long, all year long, and from now on. I usually recommend 0.625 mg of conjugated estrogen (Premarin) and 2.5 mg of medroxy progesterone acetate (Provera).

Most women will have some bleeding intermittently during the first few months of this treatment, but 90 percent of women will stop all bleeding after one year.

The advantages of this are multiple. The most important advantage to women is the end of their monthly periods. This fact alone will keep most women taking their hormones.

The second advantage is that it is simple. If a woman knows that she is supposed to take two pills every day, she is less likely to forget to take them.

Third, taking two pills every day becomes a normal part of her life so that she does not have to think about "hormones and menopause" all the time. Having to remember which days to take what pills, as with the old method, is bothersome.

If a woman continues to bleed almost every day while she is on this regimen, she can return to the traditional method of taking estrogen. After a few years, the uterus of most women becomes a little less sensitive to hormones, and the woman can again try the continuous combined estrogen/progesterone therapy.

If a woman has any unusual bleeding with her hormone therapy, her doctor may want her to have an endometrial biopsy. This type of medical care is standard for any woman past the age of forty who has abnormal bleeding, whether or not she is on hormones.

221 Is it necessary to take progesterone with the estrogen?

It is best to take both progesterone and estrogen. First, taking progesterone lowers the possibility of you having cancer of the uterus below the percentage you would have if you were not taking any type of hormones. In other words, progesterone protects your uterus against uterine cancer.

Second, the progesterone can keep you from bleeding if you use it every day as described in the "new" treatment schedule. If you use the old se-

quential treatment schedule (taking it only with the last thirteen estrogen pills), bleeding will occur at the end of each month and you will not have spotting or bleeding all month long.

If you are using the old traditional schedule of taking progesterone, most physicians still recommend that you use 10 mg of medroxy progesterone acetate (Provera), but if you experience symptoms of PMS (bloating, breast tenderness, depression), it is probably okay to drop the progesterone to 5 mg or even, if necessary, down to 2.5 mg a day. Most studies done with progesterone for protection of the uterus against cancer have used 10 mg for thirteen days. Current studies have not identified the lowest dose of progesterone that will protect against uterine cancer, but 2.5 mg of Provera for thirteen days each month seems to be safe.

If you are using the new schedule of daily estrogen and progesterone, 2.5 mg of Provera is usually adequate. Some women experience bleeding and need to increase it to 5 mg. Many women, though, will feel bloated and have breast tenderness on that dosage. A substitute for the Provera would be 0.35 to 0.7 mg of norethindrone. A newer progesterone called oral micronized progesterone can be used by some people who cannot use other forms of progesterone. This is a more natural form of progesterone. Physicians will usually recommend 100 mg per day of this type of progesterone. Some women don't feel well on one progesterone but do on another.

Today most physicians recommend that progesterone be taken for at least thirteen days each month. This seems to provide the best protection against uterine cancer. If your doctor has prescribed only eight to ten progesterone pills a month, you are probably safe, but recent studies seem to indicate that thirteen progesterone pills a month increases protection against uterine cancer.

Some patients feel terrible on any kind of progesterone. For these women, I prescribe estrogen for the first twenty-five days of every month and eliminate all progesterone. I do insist, though, that these women have an endometrial biopsy or a D&C of the uterus every three years to make sure they have no precancerous changes and are not developing cancer of the uterus. Studies have shown that a woman who takes estrogen alone has a slightly increased risk of uterine cancer. When it does occur, the cancer is usually not serious and is almost always cured by simple hysterectomy.

222 If I have had a hysterectomy, how should I take estrogen?

If you have had a hysterectomy before menopause and have become menopausal, you can now start taking Premarin (conjugated estrogen) 0.625 mg daily. (Of course, you can use a similar dosage of one of the other estrogens.) I tell my patients to take their estrogen every day, all the time, for the rest of their lives, just as they would if they still had a uterus. (If any of them experience breast tenderness, I advise them to stop taking the estrogen for one week whenever that tenderness bothers them too much.)

Women often ask if they should take estrogen after having their ovaries removed. I always recommend that if a woman has her ovaries removed before menopause, she take estrogen until the age of menopause, which is about fifty. This will eliminate hot flashes, osteoporosis, and avoid a feeling of being not quite well. So she should take estrogen from the time her ovaries are removed until the time she would probably have naturally gone through menopause. At that time, she can decide whether or not to continue taking estrogen, just as she would have to decide about taking estrogen had she not had a hysterectomy. (I strongly urge that she continue to take the estrogen for the rest of her life.)

A young woman who starts estrogen may need more than the 0.625 mg dosage of estrogen to feel healthy and normal. If a woman is younger than menopausal age, she may need to take 1.25 mg of conjugated estrogen or 2 mg of micronized estradiol (Estrace) to feel healthy and not have hot flashes.

Some past studies indicated that taking progesterone decreased the chances of breast cancer, but more recent studies have not confirmed that. Currently, my patients who have had a hysterectomy take only estrogen. If, as years go by, it can

be demonstrated that taking progesterone does, indeed, decrease the chance of breast cancer, I will change my policy, but your "bad" cholesterol levels may be the most optimal if you take no progesterone.

If you prefer to take both progesterone and estrogen, it is certainly permissible.

I do recommend that a woman who has had a hysterectomy for endometriosis take daily both estrogen and medroxy progesterone acetate (2.5 mg tablet). Some women have developed cancer of endometriosis. Taking progesterone would perhaps decrease the chance of getting cancer in any endometriosis remaining after a hysterectomy and may prevent endometriosis from recurring.

223 I continue to have vaginal dryness even though I take my hormones. What should I do?

Even though a woman is taking enough estrogen by mouth to stop her other menopausal symptoms, vaginal dryness and resulting discomfort with intercourse may still be a problem. In this case a woman needs to use vaginal estrogen cream in addition to the hormones taken by mouth.

An application of vaginal cream three times a week for several weeks will normally stop vaginal discomfort. Some women, though, must use the vaginal cream for up to nine months before the vaginal lining becomes as thick and tough as it was when she was twenty or thirty. Once the problem is under control, a smaller amount of cream used less frequently, perhaps half an applicator once or twice a week, is usually adequate to keep the vagina from becoming sensitive.

An added benefit of the use of the vaginal cream is that if a woman has gone through menopause and begins leaking urine when she coughs or sneezes, the vaginal cream may strengthen her tissues enough to stop such a loss. (See Q. 612–615.) For many women hormones may not be adequate to stop such urine leakage, and then surgery might be necessary. There is also an estrogen-containing vaginal ring that can be used for this purpose. Because it is less messy some women may prefer it.

Whether a woman is using estrogen only by mouth, only vaginal estrogen cream, or a combination of the two, it seems important that she take a 10 mg Provera tablet ten to fourteen days every month to help prevent any chance of developing uterine cancer.

It has been found that women who have intercourse after menopause have healthier vaginas with thicker vaginal linings. It is important for a woman to realize that intercourse is healthy for the vagina just as physical activity is good for her body in general.

224 Aren't hormones dangerous?

No. Circulating in your body are literally hundreds of different types of hormones, without which you would die. Further, if your body had not begun producing estrogen, a hormone, you would not have developed as a woman. Hormones are normal and extremely important for your overall health.

All hormones cannot be lumped together. You should not confuse hormones in birth-control pills with those used for menopause. The dose of estrogen used for treating menopausal and post-menopausal symptoms is the same amount of hormone that you have been producing in your own body, with your own ovaries, all your reproductive life! The amount of hormones in birth-control pills is many times higher than that which you would take for menopause and is used for a different purpose.

Also, the birth-control estrogen is different from the more natural estrogen used for menopause. The chemical makeup of the hormones used in birth-control pills makes these pills much more potent than those needed for alleviation of menopausal symptoms.

I am frequently asked by patients if taking hormones will increase their blood pressure, and I assure them that the hormones doctors prescribe following menopause or hysterectomy are only replacing those that their bodies lost when their ovaries ceased functioning. Studies have shown that women who take hormones have no greater risk of hypertension than those who don't take them.

Some internal medicine specialists seem not to understand this. They may tell a woman to stop taking hormones if she develops hypertension. Since hypertension makes a woman more likely to have a heart attack or a stroke, hormones may actually be beneficial if a woman is hypertensive. They can make the blood vessels of a hypertensive woman healthier and less likely to become blocked.

In summary, studies have shown that a woman is more likely to be unhealthy and more likely to have an early death if she does not take hormone pills than if she does take them after menopause.

A study done by Paganini-Hill et al. in *American Journal of Epidemiology* (1994, 140:256–61) showed that women who took estrogen after menopause had a lower incidence of Alzheimer's disease. Even better news was that the longer they had used estrogen the less was their chance of having Alzheimer's.

225 Are some pelvic problems aggravated by taking estrogen?

Some women with endometriosis cannot take estrogen because estrogen increases that problem; other women have fibroid tumors of the uterus (see Q. 680–686) that become larger if they take estrogen. In these cases there are two choices. One is not to take any estrogen; the other is to have a hysterectomy so that estrogen may be taken.

Consideration of the information we have just reviewed would suggest that as a woman grows older it would be healthier for her to have a hysterectomy, so that she can take estrogen, than not to take estrogen. This, of course, would be a personal decision for you to make with your doctor's professional guidance. But certainly if you have any of the high-risk factors mentioned in Q. 215, making you more likely to have osteoporosis, or if you are at high risk for vascular disease, you should strongly consider proceeding with a hysterectomy.

226 I am still having periods, but I am also having an occasional hot flash and other menopausal symptoms. What should I do?

Symptoms of this type may indicate the need for supplemental estrogen. You might start with a small dose, such as 0.3 mg of conjugated estrogen once a day, beginning on the fifth day of your menstrual period and stopping when the next period begins. If this seems to help, but you still do not feel as well as you would like, you can double, triple, or even quadruple this dose. If the pills give no relief, then your symptoms are not due to menopause, but are more likely due to the stress of the midlife time that you are in.

Adjusting to Midlife Change

227 My doctor says that I am not having symptoms of the climacteric, but I am depressed, irritable, and do not have any interest in intercourse. I tried estrogen and it didn't help. Is my doctor right?

True symptoms of the climacteric are caused simply by a lack of estrogen, and estrogen intake will reverse them. Symptoms that are "left over" after you have started taking adequate amounts of hormones are not due to the menopause but to other causes, such as "midlife crises."

It has been aptly stated that "menopause chooses a bad time to come!" It is difficult sometimes to decide whether midlife pressure or decreasing levels of estrogen are causing you to feel miserable. The best way to determine this is by taking some hormones for a few months to see if your symptoms go away. If you take progesterone with your estrogen, the progesterone can make you feel bad, so try taking estrogen by itself for two to three months to see if you feel normal. Then work out a hormone

regimen with your doctor that allows you to stay off progesterone.

If your symptoms do not go away, they are probably due to your being in a stressful time of life. Sometimes your physician can help you deal with this stress. Occasionally it is helpful to get away from your daily pressures for a vacation, and sometimes it is advisable to see a counselor, such as your pastor, a psychologist, or a psychiatrist.

Many things are going on during midlife that can cause stress.

Your children are leaving home, making you feel that your primary job in life is over. Or this may be creating financial strain due to college and living expenses, and so on.

Your husband may have become more involved in his work, making you feel that he is less interested in you.

Your body is changing. Wrinkles and gray hair begin to appear. Perhaps "middle-age" spread has set in.

Your parents are getting older. There is often great stress in taking care of sick, elderly parents, and severe stress in facing their deaths.

Sexual monotony may be a reality. It is during midlife that many couples fall into predictable patterns in their sexual relationship. This can lead to boredom and dissatisfaction. Medications commonly prescribed at this time in life, especially those taken for hypertension and irregularities of the heart, can affect sex drive and orgasmic response.

228 My spouse died and I am devastated. Is that a normal response?

Most people assume that menopause automatically includes depression, deterioration, and limited activity. This is not necessarily true. David D. Youngs, M.D., reported in *Obstetrics and Gynecology* (May 1990, 75:5), that most studies actually show a decline of depression among postmenopausal women.

In another study reported in the *Medical World News for Obstetricians and Gynecologists and Urologists* (May 14, 1987), Dr. Alvar Svanborg said that people over the age of seventy who have goals or enjoy particular activities, sedentary or not, tend to cope better than others. He showed that social interaction and physical activity contribute to the well-being of the elderly because any interest that challenges physical, mental, and emotional resources improves vitality and function.

One exception to the otherwise accurate and positive picture of aging is the death of a spouse. Dr. Robert N. Butler, chairman of Geriatrics and Adult Development at Mt. Sinai Medical Center, reported in 1987 that the death of a spouse can be a devastating blow to the elderly. He found a dramatic increase in mortality among those aged seventy to seventy-four during the three months following a mate's death compared with men and women in the same age bracket who had not lost a spouse (48 percent higher in men and 22 percent higher in women).

Dr. Butler says, "The physician whose older patient has lost a spouse has to be alert to the hazard and encourage the patient to reach out." He suggests that physicians can direct such patients to support groups such as the American Association of Retired Persons or Widow(er) Program. I mention this one particularly terrible problem for older people so you will know that this is a real problem. If your spouse dies, or you have a relative or friend over seventy who has lost a spouse, be sensitive to the devastating effect of this event. Help a survivor to become active and involved immediately after the death of a spouse.

Dr. Richard C. Halverson, former chaplain of the U.S. Senate, publishes a biweekly devotional letter called *Perspective*. In the January 17, 1990, edition, he said, "For years, the following quotation has held profound significance to me personally as a new year began. It is as real approaching 1990 as the first time I read it many years ago. May I commend it to you for your blessing and assurance."

> I said to the man who
> stood at the gate of the year:
> "Give me a light that
> I may tread safely
> into the unknown."
> And he replied:

> "Go out into the darkness
> and put your hand
> into the hand
> of God.
> That shall be to you
> better than light and
> safer than a known way."

If you have lost a spouse, or if you know someone who has, perhaps that quotation will be a blessing. The death of a loved one is, certainly, the threshold of a new stage of life.

---

229 Are there any health problems of the female organs that are specifically related to the post-menopausal time?

There are no problems that are entirely confined to this age in life, but I have many suggestions for the care of your female organs. (For a more complete discussion, see chapter 10.)

Breasts. Regularly do a breast self-examination (BSE), and have a mammogram every year from age fifty on. If there is any question about a breast problem, see your doctor without delay.

Ovaries. After menopause your ovaries shrink to about one-half inch in diameter. Unless you are extremely thin, your doctor cannot feel them. If the doctor is able to feel an ovary, it means that it is enlarged and may have a tumor. You should allow the doctor to operate if he or she thinks it is necessary, because there is a 50 percent chance of ovarian cancer if there is a growth on an ovary after menopause.

Uterus. After menopause the uterus rarely causes any problems. It can develop cancer, but this does not happen frequently. If you have any bleeding after menopause, you should immediately see a physician, who will probably recommend a D&C. If you are taking hormones regularly, it is common to have irregular bleeding occur, but, even if you are taking estrogen, if bleeding occurs at an unusual time, you should notify your physician immediately and anticipate that a D&C or an endometrial biopsy or a hysteroscopy will be required.

Cervix. An annual Pap smear is important, even

after menopause. There is rarely a reason to have a Pap smear more often than once a year after menopause.

Vagina. The vagina can become loose after menopause, causing loss of urine when a woman coughs, sneezes, or laughs. The vagina can also seem very loose during intercourse.

An additional problem can be a bulging of the back wall of the vagina with bowel movements. This bulging can be so marked that a woman must push with her fingers in her vagina, or just above her anus at the opening of the vagina, to help the stool be expelled. Gynecologists call this "rectal splinting." Surgery can be performed to correct these problems.

Occasionally estrogen vaginal cream will help such problems. At times it takes both the estrogen cream and surgery to solve a problem of vaginal looseness, loss of urine with coughing, or problems with bowel movements. Gynecologists lump all these conditions together in the term *symptomatic pelvic relaxation.*

In addition, the vaginal lining can become so thin and sensitive after menopause that intercourse is uncomfortable. If a couple then has intercourse less often, the vaginal lining can thin out even more, causing additional pain with intercourse. A vicious cycle has developed that results in the couple no longer being able to enjoy intercourse, even though they would like to. If this happens see your doctor. Estrogen can reverse this process and allow normal, comfortable intercourse.

The vulva. If an area of your vulva itches persistently, or if you have a small growth on it, you should insist that your doctor biopsy it. Such a biopsy can usually diagnose a cancer of the vulva long before it becomes dangerous.

230 If a woman in her late forties or early fifties is afraid of getting pregnant, can she use birth-control pills?

It has only been in the last few years that physicians felt comfortable about women in this age group taking birth-control pills, because research is now reassuring about the safety of taking them. If a woman does not smoke, her cholesterol is normal, and she is not diabetic, she can take birth-control pills till menopause. (This is assuming that there is no other reason to stay off birth-control pills. See Q. 897 in the chapter on contraception.)

A study done in 1983 showed that women who had used birth-control pills in the past had a lower than average chance of having hardening of the arteries as they aged. This seems to be true because birth-control pills contain estrogen, and estrogens are protective against cardiovascular disease.

If you are concerned about the possibility of becoming pregnant during the time of menopause or premenopause, taking birth-control pills can relieve that worry. True, the chance of your getting pregnant during these years is very small, but if you do get pregnant during that time it can be a startling, significant, and sometimes undesired event in your life. Protect yourself against pregnancy if you do not want it to happen.

231 What about sex during my later years?

It is normal for people to have intercourse right up until the day they die of old age! One warning, though: If you have not enjoyed a healthy and happy sexual relationship with your husband when you were young, you are less likely to have a happy sexual relationship as you get older.

Masters and Johnson were the first to show that men and women in good health should be able to continue to function sexually for as long as they live. In a study done in 1983, Consumer's Union (well-known evaluators of everything from cars to toasters) interviewed elderly people concerning their sexual activity. The majority of respondents reported that they were leading happy sexually active lives. A large number of them claimed that although frequency and passion were diminished somewhat, the overall quality of sex had improved as they got older.

If you are on birth-control pills and you turn fifty years of age, your doctor will probably do a blood test for FSH. If the level is greater than

40 mIU/ml, you are past menopause, will not get pregnant, can stop taking the oral contraceptives, and begin taking estrogen and progesterone pills.

A study done at Duke University Medical Center in 1982 revealed that of 278 married couples over forty-six years of age, 52 percent reported having intercourse at least once or twice a week, and 9 percent had intercourse three times a week. Only 38 percent had intercourse less than once a week.

There are advantages to sexual relations after menopause.

First of all, you do not have to worry about getting pregnant, and many women find this increases their sexual interest. Many couples also report that they become much more relaxed and comfortable with each other as time goes by. This, plus the increased mutual sexual understanding that time can produce, greatly heightens the sexual experience for many couples.

Since the children are not around any longer, you can have intercourse whenever or wherever you like without worrying about being seen or heard!

Sex in the later years can be a major part of "communication" between you and your spouse. You should anticipate its having great importance in your relationship in the years to come.

232 What changes in sexual responsiveness occur in men as they get older?

Masters and Johnson found that the four phases of sexual responsiveness change in men as they get older. If a man understands that his sexual function will undergo changes at about the age of fifty, he will take this into account and change his lovemaking accordingly. If he is not prepared for these changes in responsiveness, he can become so scared that he becomes impotent on a purely emotional basis.

The excitement phase of intercourse, which is the phase during which foreplay occurs, usually takes longer from middle age on. The man takes longer to develop an erection, and the erection is not as hard when it first develops. The actual likelihood of a man's developing or not developing an erection remains the same, no matter what his age (unless there is an unusual medical problem).

During the plateau phase, which is the period during which the husband usually has his penis in the vagina, he will often find that he is able to maintain an erection without the need to ejaculate for a much longer time than when he was younger. It is the discovery of this fact which allows many couples in their midlife period or beyond to have more satisfactory sex than they have ever had.

Orgasms for the man of fifty years or older are usually shorter and produce less semen volume than ejaculations of previous years. The expulsion of the seminal fluid is also less forceful for the older man than for the younger man. As a man gets older, he may even find that he does not need to ejaculate to be satisfied and can therefore bring his partner to satisfaction and then stop the sex act without having to ejaculate, if his ejaculation is coming unusually slowly.

The phase of resolution is usually much shorter for a man from fifty on. After ejaculation his penis usually becomes totally flaccid within a few seconds. He also may not be able to have another erection for many hours; whereas when he was younger he was able to develop another erection, either immediately or within an hour or two.

Obviously a man's body is designed to have intercourse until the day he dies. If he will realize that slower arousal during foreplay allows the advantage of better control during intercourse, he will not begin to question his ability to achieve an erection. Once he begins questioning this ability, he tends to become an observer of his own performance, watching to see whether or not his penis will become erect. When he becomes a spectator he has taken the first step on the road to impotence.

It is important that a man accept the changes in his body as improvements and recognize that for the last half of his life he will probably find it easier to satisfy his wife, especially if her response has always been slower than his own.

233 What if my husband and I have reached midlife and are having sexual problems?

If you and your husband have sexual problems, I suggest a thorough reading of chapter 14. If you continue to have problems in spite of trying some of the suggested techniques, see your gynecologist and urge your husband to see a urologist because physical problems can affect sexual responsiveness.

If both you and your husband are healthy and yet are unable to make love physically to your mutual satisfaction, I suggest that you see a sex counselor so that you can develop a healthy sexual relationship.

If you do choose to see a sex counselor, choose that person wisely. It is my opinion that he or she should pattern counseling after the Masters and Johnson techniques. If your counselor is a good one, you and your husband should make progress within just a few weeks in developing a healthy sex life that will bring you pleasure the rest of your life.

Sex counselors should not recommend "kinky" or immoral things, and if they recommend practices that are counter to your own ethics, they are probably not legitimate counselors. If they recommend divorce or separation as an answer to your problems, they are not to be trusted. I suggest that you find another counselor. I have seen marriages among my patients almost destroyed by bad sexual counseling.

If you or your husband has had a stroke or heart attack, you can usually resume sexual relations after recovery. Sometimes fear of another attack will keep a spouse from initiating sex. If your partner seems disinterested in having sex, this may be the reason. It is important that the two of you talk to your doctor about this problem.

234 Will testosterone help me be more interested in sex?

I am often asked if testosterone will help a woman's sexual responsiveness. Testosterone is the primary male hormone, but women's bodies normally have low levels of it produced by their ovaries. Testosterone does not seem to be necessary for a woman's sexual responsiveness once she has established a responsive pattern to sex. Currently there is a lot of publicity about the possibility of using low doses of testosterone to help women alleviate their problems with poor sexual responsiveness. Reliable studies have not documented benefit from postmenopausal testosterone therapy, but if you are bothered by this condition, you may want to ask your doctor to treat it with testosterone briefly to see if it helps.

Heavy dosages of testosterone can make a woman have a very uncomfortable abnormal interest in sex. Such dosages also can cause her body to develop abnormal hair growth, cause her voice to get lower, and cause partial baldness. The dosage of this medication therefore must be kept low. If my patients want to try estrogen with testosterone, I will let them try it in proper dosages. It is usually not the answer. Other problems need to be taken care of for good sexual responsiveness to take place.

235 What can I expect during the postmenopausal years?

The postmenopausal years can be extremely fulfilling and rewarding in many ways. In fact, you can anticipate a growing satisfaction with life. Most women in the postmenopausal age develop a serenity about life and an acceptance of the situations that they cannot change. This is maturity.

You can expect a lot of company! In 1982 there were over 26 million Americans over age sixty-five. By the year 2020, there will be 52 million. By that same year, there will be more than 6.7 million Americans over age eighty-five.

In your older age you can look forward to having time to do things that you have never had time for before. You might be able to go back to school and earn a degree. There may be time to do things for your church or to develop some skills that you never had, such as painting, writing, or tennis.

An Afterword

As a closing thought for this chapter, I'd like to share this appropriate prayer:

Seventeenth-Century Nun's Prayer

LORD, thou knowest better than I know myself that I am growing older and will someday be old. Keep me from the fatal habit of thinking I must say something on every subject and on every occasion. Release me from craving to straighten out everybody's affairs. Make me thoughtful but not moody; helpful but not bossy. With my vast store of wisdom, it seems a pity not to use it all, but thou knowest, Lord, that I want a few friends at the end.

Keep my mind free from the recital of endless details; give me wings to get to the point. Seal my lips on my aches and pains. They are increasing, and love of rehearsing them is becoming sweeter as the years go by. I dare not ask for grace enough to enjoy the tales of others' pains, but help me to endure them with patience.

I dare not ask for improved memory, but for a growing humility and a lessening cocksureness when my memory seems to clash with the memories of others. Teach me the glorious lesson that occasionally I may be mistaken.

Keep me reasonably sweet; I do not want to be a saint—some of them are so hard to live with—but a sour old person is one of the crowning works of the devil. Give me the ability to see good things in unexpected places, and talents in unexpected people. And, give me, O Lord, the grace to tell them so. *Amen.*

Part Two

Bearing a Child

6

Conception

The most exciting, mysterious, and complex events of your entire life took place in the darkened, hidden recesses of your mother's abdomen. The events occurred without applause, without recognition, without appreciation.

You were completely unaware of your debut into the human race. And even your mother was unaware of the entirety of the miraculous superdrama being enacted within her body.

God, however, knew. The one who masterminded the creation of all life from the beginning was also responsible for yours.

Your beginning was not merely an accidental accumulation of matter. You were created by God with a distinct value and purpose—from the moment of conception. This fact that we were meant to be is the source of true self-esteem for all of us.

Conception is not a trivial event. Although its occurrence might seem routine, it is truly a miracle of the highest order. There is no better illustration anywhere of God's handiwork than the delicate, fascinating, awe-inspiring event of conception.

One edition of Webster's dictionary describes life as "the form or quality of existence that distinguishes animals and plants from inorganic or inanimate things." The definition states further: "There are four characteristics of life that are shared by all living organisms: growth, reproduction, metabolism, and the capacity to respond to stimuli."

According to that definition, there is no doubt that the first minuscule collection of cells created by conception is already "life."

However, it is more than mere life itself, for the personhood of the newly created life is instantly established when egg and sperm unite. The new person has already been programmed—created with a definite pattern—for life.

At the moment of conception many things are determined by your genetic makeup, including your sex, your physical appearance, and many aspects of your personality.

At the point of conception you are unique; the only "you" that has ever been or ever will be again.

And the entire process is absolutely fascinating.

This chapter will explain as simply as possible a truly complex, fascinating process. It begins with the first moment of your life and the steps leading up to that moment; then it looks at the reason why you developed into a female rather than a male. It showcases the most unique aspect of womanhood: the ability to conceive and carry a new life.

The Marvel of Conception

236 Where do the egg and the sperm meet, and how do they get there?

The meeting of the sperm and egg usually occurs in the outer half of the fallopian tube, the half farthest away from the uterus.

Sperm reach the meeting place via a journey from the vagina, up through the cervix and uterus, and into the tube. This is accomplished by swimming, with their progress being aided by contractions of the uterus and fallopian tubes. Tubal contractions are called peristalsis, the same activity used by the intestines to propel food. The entire trip takes only about ten to twenty minutes.

The egg cannot swim. It is expelled from the surface of the ovary where it briefly floats passively

and freely in the abdominal cavity. This freedom is short-lived, for the egg is quickly taken in by the fallopian tubes.

The fallopian tubes do not connect the ovary to the uterus, as many people imagine. This explains how an egg can be produced by one ovary, cross to the tube on the other side, pass down that tube into the uterus, and grow into a normal pregnancy. This has happened to women who have had an ovary removed on one side and a tube on the other side.

The egg is captured and brought into the tube by small tentacles called fimbriae on the end of the tube. These tentacles are active. They sweep over the surface of the ovary, and when the egg escapes, the fimbriae capture it. This action starts the egg on its passive journey to the womb.

This procedure has been photographed in animals. Richard Blandau, M.D., Professor Emeritus, University of Washington, has used time-lapse photography to produce some enthralling films that show fimbriae catching eggs and sweeping them toward the openings of the fallopian tubes, where the tubes suck in the eggs like miniature vacuum cleaners.

The egg's trip is aided, as is the sperm's, by the muscular activity of peristalsis. It is further helped along by small hairlike structures, the cilia. These line the inside of the fallopian tubes and are also present on the fimbriae. They are beating constantly, physically sweeping the egg, which is sticky, into and through the tube.

The cilia also cause a small current of fluid to flow through the tubes and into the uterus. This current helps draw the egg into the tube.

237 Do the egg and the sperm unite immediately when they meet in the fallopian tube?

Neither the egg nor the sperm is capable of fertilization at that point. Both must go through a cleansing process termed "capacitation" before they can become fertile. This fact, and the parallel sequences that must take place prior to fertilization, make the act of conception just that much more fascinating.

As the egg passes into and through the fallopian tube, it is scrubbed clean of material that has clung to it from the ovary. When the sperm and the egg meet, the egg is further cleansed by "hyaluronidase," an enzyme produced by the sperm.

A sperm, however, is unable to produce the hyaluronidase until substances that prevent its production are removed from its surface during the journey through the uterus and tubes. This is accomplished by the sperm's exposure to uterine and fallopian tube secretions.

Recent research indicates that the woman's eggs may actually draw sperm toward themselves. A study published in the *Proceedings of the National Academy of Science USA* (1991, 88:2840), showed that samples of fluid released with the egg during ovulation attract sperm. The samples of this fluid that attracted sperm most strongly were associated with eggs that were fertilized the most successfully in test tubes later. This type of communication is not too much of a surprise since studies have shown that other types of cells communicate with each other. If this chemical "homing signal" in the fluid could be isolated, it might be of great use in infertility treatment and also in contraception. If this recent study is confirmed, it would show why so many sperm are drawn to one egg.

Many sperm, all now capable of producing hyaluronidase, work together to change the surface of the egg until it is finally possible for *one sperm* to penetrate the egg. Once fertilization occurs, the surface of the egg becomes impervious to all other sperm.

238 What happens after fertilization of the egg?

The fertilized egg remains in the fallopian tube for about three days. If it were to get into the uterus earlier, it would be too immature to adhere to the uterine wall and would pass on out of the uterus as a very early miscarriage, even before the mother would miss a menstrual period.

The tube acts as a preincubator, allowing the fertilized egg (embryo) to grow to just the right degree of maturity for its start in the uterus. Scientists think that the hormones of the normal menstrual cycle cause this tightening and loosening of a tube's opening into the uterus.

Upon its entrance into the womb, "home" for the next nine months, the baby has grown to be about twelve cells in size. The embryo, though, is still too premature to stick to the wall of the uterus. It floats around in the uterine cavity for about two more days before it has grown surface cells that will stick to the uterine wall. When it does adhere to the uterine wall, it begins to draw life-sustaining oxygen, fluid, and nourishment from the mother's tissues instead of from the fluid in which it had been floating. This is called implantation.

239 What happens to an unfertilized egg and the sperm that did not fertilize an egg?

An unfertilized egg lives about twelve to twenty-four hours. Sperm have a useful life of about forty-

Fertilization and Cell Division

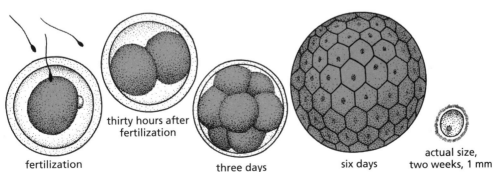

thirty hours after fertilization

fertilization

three days

six days

actual size, two weeks, 1 mm

Fertilization and Conception

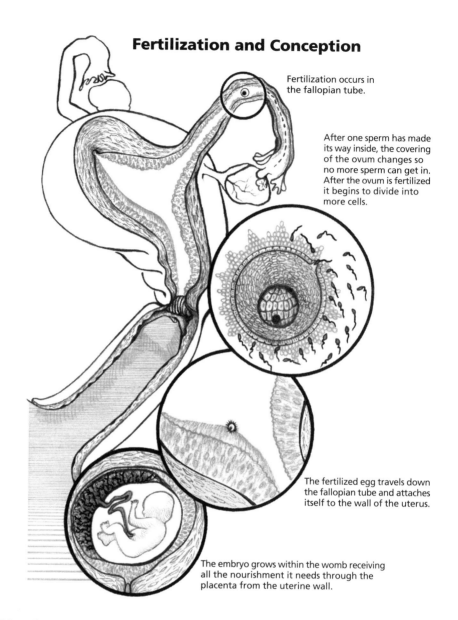

Fertilization occurs in the fallopian tube.

After one sperm has made its way inside, the covering of the ovum changes so no more sperm can get in. After the ovum is fertilized it begins to divide into more cells.

The fertilized egg travels down the fallopian tube and attaches itself to the wall of the uterus.

The embryo grows within the womb receiving all the nourishment it needs through the placenta from the uterine wall.

eight hours, although they may live four or five days.

If an egg has not been fertilized, it either disintegrates and is absorbed (it is just a tiny bit of protein) or passes on out of the uterus into the vagina. In a normal, healthy female, the process will be repeated again in another month, when another egg is produced, released from the ovary, and begins its journey through the tube.

Sperm are usually deposited by the millions into the vagina but only one of them will produce fertilization. When the sperm are deposited into

the vagina, they swim out of the semen, which consists mainly of mucus, into the cervical mucus. Some sperm immediately pass on through the uterus into the tubes, some swimming into one tube, some into the other. Some never make it into the cervical mucus and drain with the semen from the vagina.

Excess sperm that do make it into the tubes help cleanse the egg and prepare it for penetration, but those not accepted merely swim right on through the tubes and out into the abdominal cavity where they are absorbed by the body.

Bearing a Child

Sperm, which live much longer than an egg, have been found in the uterus and tubes up to sixty hours after intercourse. Though they may live that long, they are usually fertile only the first twenty-four to forty-eight hours of their life.

240 What are the chances for fertilization to occur?

Fertilization depends on many factors, such as the abundance and health of the sperm, the time of intercourse, and the health of the partners (see chapter 11).

Even if everything is functioning properly and the act of intercourse is timed perfectly, there is only a 25 percent chance of pregnancy occurring each month. Within a year's time, however, 85 percent of couples actively trying to conceive will be successful. Often couples come to me for infertility counseling when they have been trying to conceive for only four or five months. I encourage them to wait until they have been trying to get pregnant for one year to start infertility evaluation. I explain that it is normal for couples to take up to a year to get pregnant. My exceptions to this are couples over age thirty-five who have tried unsuccessfully for six months to get pregnant or couples who know they have had a medical problem that could cause infertility. I suggest to these couples that they start a modified infertility evaluation because of the age factor or because of their medical history after only six months of attempting to get pregnant.

A recent study showed that couples who have intercourse every day for the four to five days before ovulation are the ones who become pregnant the soonest of couples trying to become pregnant.

It has been estimated that 30 to 50 percent of human pregnancies are aborted naturally. Most of these are very early pregnancies, and most of the time the woman is not even aware that she had conceived and has not even missed a period.

Many of these spontaneous abortions occur because the conceptions are abnormal. Something has gone wrong in the fertilization process and the resulting fetus could not develop normally. This high percentage of miscarriage has led some people to say that human reproduction is inefficient. But there is some good in this. It is estimated that 7.5 percent of all human conceptions are chromosomally abnormal, and yet only 1 in 200 babies are born with chromosomal abnormalities. The high miscarriage rate keeps many abnormal babies from being born.

Fertilization is obviously a difficult and exacting procedure. When successfully accomplished it is further proof of the miracle of conception.

XX and XY Chromosomes

241 What determines the gender of a fertilized egg?

It is the chromosomes within the egg and sperm that determine both a baby's gender and many other characteristics. A chromosome is a microscopic piece of protein, several of which are present in the nucleus of every living cell. Each chromosome is made up of hundreds of smaller units called genes. These are responsible for your (and your husband's) ability to transmit to your child such characteristics as small feet, curly hair, and blue eyes.

Each cell has forty-six (twenty-three pairs) chromosomes. Out of those twenty-three, one pair (the "sex chromosomes") carries the sex determinants.

The remaining twenty-two pairs are called autosomes and have little to do with determining sex, although they carry hundreds of genes that guide the growth of the rest of the body.

Geneticists are able to identify and number individual chromosomes. Sex chromosomes, however, are not numbered but are labeled XX or XY.

The male's sperm carry the sex chromosomes that determine the sex of the offspring. All eggs always carry X chromosomes, while sperm may carry either X or Y chromosomes. Whether or not the child is a boy or girl depends on which sperm—an X chromosome or a Y chromosome—fertilizes the egg.

Every normal baby is conceived with either XX (female) or XY (male) sex chromosomes. Every cell in a person's body will have one of these chromosome pairs making each of us totally male or totally female, no matter what is done to our sex organs or what kind of hormones we take.

Technically, there is a fifty-fifty chance of producing a boy or girl when the egg is fertilized. Two simple addition problems will explain what happens:

$$
\begin{array}{ll}
\text{Egg} & \text{with X chromosome (all have this)} \\
\underline{+\ \text{Sperm}} & \text{with X chromosome (half have this)} \\
=\text{GIRL} & \text{(XX sex chromosomes)}
\end{array}
$$

$$
\begin{array}{ll}
\text{Egg} & \text{with X chromosome (all have this)} \\
\underline{+\ \text{Sperm}} & \text{with Y chromosome (half have this)} \\
=\text{BOY} & \text{(XY sex chromosomes)}
\end{array}
$$

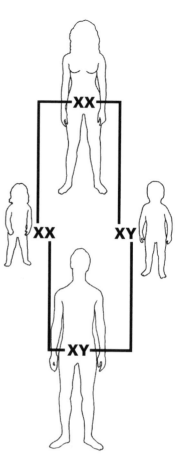

242 How does an XX chromosome create a woman and an XY chromosome create a man?

XX chromosomes cause a baby to develop ovaries, whereas XY chromosomes cause a baby to develop testicles. Beyond this statement lies a combination of theory and fact. Further research may prove some of the following information wrong, but, as it is understood today, here is a brief look at this fascinating process.

243 Is my baby going to be a boy?

The sex-chromosome pair for a boy is XY and is determined at fertilization by the type of sperm that fertilizes the egg.

After five weeks of growth, two little nubbins of tissue are developing in the male embryo, one on each side of what will become his abdomen. These are sex organs, or gonads, which at that point look as if they could become either ovaries or testes. The baby is only about one-fourth inch long at this time.

The Y chromosome begins to stimulate the small "neutral" gonads to become testes instead of ovaries. This appears to be all the Y chromosome does. It does not seem to make any further detectable difference in the development of male characteristics in the child.

Researchers had wondered for years how the Y chromosome produces its effect on the testicle. In the 1980s, they found that the Y chromosome has a special gene called the "testes determining factor gene" (TDF gene) on the short arm of the Y chromosome (Ulrich Muller, *Contemporary OB/GYN*, April 1990). The protein this gene produces is called *testes determining factor* (TDF). This protein reacts with the DNA and RNA in other parts of the embryo's body, turning it into a male. As Drs. Speroff, Glass, and Kase say in *Clinical Gynecologic Endocrinology and Infertility* (1989), this makes the gene the "master switch for male differentiation by its capacity to react with genes elsewhere on X, Y, and autosomes, as well as their diverse gene products." TDF is, therefore, responsible for organizing the gonad into a testicle.

The gonads are now true male organs, and they begin their work of changing this seemingly sexless little fetus into a male being by doing three things.

The first duty of these male organs is to suppress the cells in the body of the fetus that would have developed into female organs (müllerian cells). They accomplish this by secreting a compound termed "müllerian inhibiting factor."

The secretion of this compound is the very first hormonal function of these new male hormone glands called testicles. It takes place in the seventh week of pregnancy.

With the production of the müllerian inhibiting factor in the little boy's body, most of the female cells are suppressed into inactivity. A few, however, do persist. Instead of becoming female organs as they would have done had this baby been a girl, they help form part of the connection to the testicle (the vas deferens), which will transport the sperm out of the testicle in later life. The suppression process is complete by the end of the third month of pregnancy.

The second duty of the testicles began even before the müllerian cell regression was complete. The production of the major male hormone testosterone by the testicles began during the ninth week of pregnancy. Testosterone "stabilizes" the cells of the fetus's body (wolffian duct cells) that will form the seminal vesicles, the vas deferens, and the epididymis. This allows these organs to begin their development properly and to form completely, under continued testosterone stimulation.

The third function of the fetal testicle is to produce the enzyme "5x reductase." This enzyme causes some of the fetus's testosterone to change into dihydrotestosterone. The male fetal body requires this altered form of testosterone to form a penis, a scrotum, and a prostate gland.

The remainder of the pregnancy, as it relates to the boy, merely provides the important time that is necessary for his male sexual organs to grow and develop, a process that includes the descent of his testicles into the scrotum.

244 Is my baby going to be a girl?

The sex-chromosome pair for a girl is XX. This is also determined at fertilization.

After four weeks of growth, the girl's gonads, or sex organs, have developed in the area that will eventually be her abdomen. These little ovaries begin producing small amounts of estrogen, the major female hormone, when the fetus is about two months old.

Over the next seven months, estrogen is responsible for the development of the girl's female organs, which include a complete uterus by eighteen weeks of pregnancy and a complete vagina during the last three months of pregnancy.

An interesting fact to consider in the development of a female baby is that although she is producing small amounts of estrogen, her mother's body has a huge amount of estrogen constantly bathing the fetus. No one knows how much influence the baby's own estrogen has on its development and how much effect the mother's estrogen has, because a human fetus has never yet developed outside a mother's body and away from the mother's estrogen.

A male fetus is subjected to the same bathing of maternal estrogen, but the Y chromosome and subsequent events keep the male baby from becoming female. It has been shown, however, that if a fetus does not receive "normal" sex chromosomes at the time of fertilization and does not have a Y chromosome, it will always develop female sex characteristics.

It appears that the development of the fetus as a female may be in part a passive process, aided by the mother's hormones.

This entire process is much more complicated. For instance, although XX and XY chromosomes are the most important ones in sexual development, at least nineteen other genes are involved in the development of the sexually normal adult man and woman.

245 At what age can the gender of a miscarried baby be determined?

If a pregnancy is two and a half to three months along, and the baby has continued normal growth up until the miscarriage, the doctor can probably determine the gender. At that point the baby would be about three inches long.

246 What techniques might I try so that I can increase my chances of choosing my child's gender?

There do seem to be some ways to improve your chances of choosing your child's gender, but there is no technique that will give you your choice 100 percent of the time.

The first widely read, modern book on the subject of gender determination was *Your Baby's Sex: Now You Can Choose*. This was written by David M. Rorvik and Landrum B. Shetles, M.D., and was published by Bantam Books in the 1960s. The ideas advocated for gender selection in this book have now been generally discarded.

In a book, *Boy or Girl?* (New York: Bobbs-Merrill, 1979), Dr. Elizabeth Whelan reports that if you follow her suggestions, you will increase your chance of having a boy from about 50 percent to 60 percent, and your chances of having a girl from about 50 percent to 57 percent. Briefly, here is a summary of her suggestions, most of which require determining carefully which day you ovulate. This can be done by:

Watching for *Mittelschmerz*. This is a pain in the low abdomen that some women feel at the time of ovulation.

Watching the calendar. Most women ovulate about fourteen days prior to the start of their next period.

Taking your basal body temperature. Ovulation usually occurs twenty-four to forty-eight hours prior to the sustained rise in temperature, as recorded the first thing in the morning before getting out of bed.

Observing changes in cervical mucus. When ovulation occurs, a moderately heavy vaginal discharge may be noted.

According to Dr. Whelan, once you feel confident about predicting your ovulation date, you should then time your intercourse to improve your chance of having a child of the desired gender.

If you are attempting to have a boy, you should have intercourse on the sixth, fifth, and fourth days prior to ovulation. This is necessary because, while it is true that sperm do not have a useful life of five or six days, ovulation *may* occur earlier than expected. If you are trying to have a girl, you should have intercourse on the third and second days prior to ovulation. While Dr. Whelan points out that statistics show that this system works, no one knows exactly why it works.

Basal Body Temperature Chart

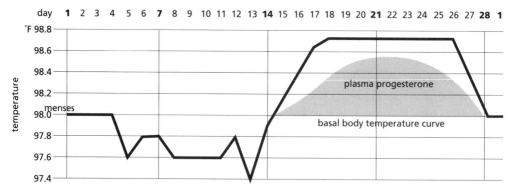

To get a basal body temperature curve, a woman's temperature is measured immediately upon awakening and charted according to the day of the menstrual cycle. The hormone progesterone, which is produced only after ovulation, makes a woman's basal temperature rise. Thus if ovulation has occurred, the basal body temperature curve will show a rise and a plateau after ovulation. The rise and fall in basal temperature somewhat parallels the rise and fall of progesterone levels.

Either way, avoid intercourse or use contraception during the other days of the cycle.

Dr. Whelan has gone into much more detail in her book. For further information on this subject, a study of the methods stated in the book may prove helpful.

The most recent techniques for gender selection that have been posed are filtration techniques. Using these methods, the man's sperm is filtered through special media to separate "female" from "male" sperm. The prospective mother is then inseminated with sperm that would be expected to produce the desired sex. A form of this procedure has been developed and patented by Ronald Ericsson, a Ph.D. in reproductive physiology. He is president of a company in Wyoming called Gametrics, Ltd., which is marketing Ericsson's technique by training individuals in the performance of the techniques, and licensing clinics around the country. His company claims a success rate of 77 percent in producing male infants. Ericsson's technique cannot be used to increase the chance of having a female child, although Gametrics and other groups are working on this too. If you would like information about Dr. Ericsson's technique, you may ask your obstetrician.

If you have an infertility problem or want to get pregnant as quickly as possible, any attempt at gender determination will only slow your attempt to become pregnant, and I would advise against trying such a procedure.

My final word on this subject is that it may not be wise to become pregnant if you are not willing to accept your child's gender and love the child without reservation. I strongly counsel you against abortion just because the child you conceive is not the gender you preferred. A better alternative would be to use reliable contraception and not get pregnant.

The major consideration in any conception should be the parents' full acceptance of the baby, not that the baby fit all the preconceived ideas the parents have as to what that baby should be like.

An Afterword

Conception is truly a miracle. Even the brief study of conception contained in this chapter fills us with wonder and delight as we consider the incredible precision, intricacy, and mystery that surrounds the creation of a new life.

7
Pregnancy

There are perhaps no three words in any language more pregnant with meaning than the words *You are pregnant!* These words have evoked the gamut of emotion—joy, pride, disbelief, fear, dismay, thanksgiving, wonder—for countless generations of men and women. Whatever your reaction to the confirmation of your pregnancy, you can be assured that you are neither the first nor only woman who has felt exactly like that!

If you have never had a baby before, you are faced with many unknowns. Your body has never been swollen with pregnancy. Will your husband like the way you look? Will you like the way you look? What will labor be like? Will you be able to nurse the baby? What will your infant look like? Whom will he or she resemble? Will your baby be normal? Will you be a good mother?

If you have already had a child, you face different problems. Your family is enlarging. Is there enough love, time, and money to go around? With a new baby you may face serious financial strain, and certainly emotional and physical pressures. Will the baby be normal? Can you handle it? Will you be a good mother to more than one (or two, or three, or more) children?

As your pregnancy progresses and each new hurdle is passed, both mother and father begin to identify with the child in the uterus. Both can feel movement, hear the heartbeat, and even "see" the baby on an ultrasound machine.

One thing seems clear to me. In spite of our advanced medical and technical knowledge, infertility clinics, in vitro fertilization programs, obstetric clinics, and home deliveries, human beings can't make a baby. It is quite obvious that the psalmist was right: "Children are a gift from God" (Ps. 127:3 LB).

Before You Try to Get Pregnant

247 Is there anything I should do before I get pregnant that will help me have a good pregnancy and a healthy baby?

Planning for a pregnancy is one of the wisest things a woman who wants to have a baby can do. A woman's health before she gets pregnant can influence both hers and the baby's health during pregnancy. I strongly recommend "preconception care." It will help insure a healthy pregnancy and a healthy baby.

"A woman's health before conception influences her ability not only to conceive, but also to maintain pregnancy and to achieve a healthy outcome," said Ronald Chez, M.D., professor and vice-chairman of obstetrics and gynecology, New Jersey Medical School (*Contemporary OB/GYN*, June 1989). His is just one of many voices that stresses the importance of preconception care.

There are many things to consider before becoming pregnant:

1. *Backgrounds:* Both husband and wife should look at their family backgrounds to check for any hereditary disease that might be present. Another important part of a "background check" is knowing whether or not the wife's mother used DES while she was pregnant with her. (See the section in this book on DES, Q. 164–168.)
2. *Lifestyle:* Both the husband and wife should stop smoking before they conceive, neither should have more than two alcoholic drinks a week, and neither should use illegal drugs of any kind. (Street drugs are not only dangerous in themselves for a developing baby, but they may also contain contaminants that can hurt the baby.)
3. *Previous pregnancies:* If the wife has had two or more miscarriages in the past, she may need an X-ray of her uterus to check for abnormalities. (She might want to consult a fertility specialist if miscarriage has been a problem in the past and her doctor does not offer good solutions for avoiding the problem.)
4. *Nutrition:* It is important that the woman maintain good nutrition. Anorexia and bulimia are fairly common now. If a woman has either of these problems, I strongly advise that she not get pregnant until she is able to practice good nutrition.
5. *Medications:* If either the husband or wife is on medication, it is important to discuss this with her obstetrician/gynecologist to see if the drugs are safe for a pregnancy. If not, they need to be changed or pregnancy needs to be delayed.
6. *Illnesses:* If either parent-to-be has a disease, this needs to be evaluated. Diabetes in the mother, for instance, can cause increased risk to the baby. If there is a possibility of diabetes, the woman should be tested before she gets pregnant to stabilize her blood sugar levels. (It is important that the couple realize that the pregnancy of a diabetic woman will require intense care.)
7. *Infections:* Parents-to-be need to understand the impact some illnesses can have on a pregnancy. If a woman has not been tested for immunity to German measles, for instance, she should be. If she is not immune, she should be vaccinated against German measles (rubella) before she becomes pregnant. Another prepregnancy evaluation is one for toxoplasmosis titer. If a woman is immune to this disease, she can more safely keep cats in her home during pregnancy. If not, she needs to be very careful about having cats around. (See questions on toxoplasmosis and other infectious diseases in this

section.) She should be tested for Hepatitis B. If she has not had this disease she could be vaccinated. If she is a Hepatitis B carrier, she would then want her child protected by vaccination after delivering. (See Q. 322.) Sexually transmitted diseases, especially herpes, need to be discussed with a physician. If a woman or her husband have ever had sex with someone else, the prospective mother could have sexually transmitted disease germs infecting her cervix. These germs, such as *Trichomonas vaginalis* and bacterial vaginosis, can cause premature birth.

8. *Birth-control pills:* Couples often ask how far in advance of trying to become pregnant they should get off birth-control pills. The general recommendation now is that a woman should stop the pills long enough to develop a regular menstrual cycle before conception so she will know when she got pregnant. (If you should become pregnant while on the Pill, don't worry. Studies have now shown that birth-control pills do not harm a newly conceived baby, even if the woman becomes pregnant while she is taking them.)

9. *Prenatal vitamins:* A study published in the *Journal of the American Medical Association* (November 1989, 262:2847) showed that taking prenatal vitamins for six weeks or longer before getting pregnant offered some protection against neural tube defects in the baby. The important element is folic acid. Over-the-counter prenatal vitamins seem to be as good as any. (The vitamin you take should contain 0.8 mg of folic acid. For more information about vitamins and pregnancy, see Q. 264.)

10. *Finances:* A couple should have some idea what they are getting into financially when they decide to have a child. Very few couples, of course, ever feel that they have enough money, adequate time, or the necessary maturity to be parents, but somehow, once the baby arrives, the things he or she needs are provided. It's probably true that if a couple waits to become pregnant until they can afford a child or have the perfect schedule for it, they'll never have one!

11. *General health:* An examination before pregnancy can be very important. It can show that there is no cervical cancer, no pelvic tumors, no breast cancer, no liver disease, and so on. See your doctor for an exam before you get pregnant.

Planning for your pregnancy with "preconception care" will not only help insure the best pregnancy—and healthiest baby—possible, but it will also make your pregnancy less stressful because you will have the assurance and confidence that you have done everything possible to make it so.

If You Think You Are Pregnant . . .

248 Are there any very early symptoms of pregnancy that I might notice?

Possibly. Some women experience early symptoms; others notice nothing out of the ordinary. In any case, the hormones of pregnancy are secreted into the body five to seven days after fertilization takes place. Although they are produced in tiny amounts, they do begin changing the body even before a menstrual period is missed.

Occasionally, even before the first missed period, some women have been able to tell that something is different. They guess, often correctly, that they are pregnant. Most of the early changes that might herald an early pregnancy, however, will not develop until after the missed period, and even then may not be noticed.

The earliest symptoms of pregnancy may include the following:

Feeling that the missed period is about to start. For most women, that a period fails to arrive on time is the first sign of pregnancy, and usually this failure of the menstrual flow to start on time is accompanied by the feeling that it is going to begin at any minute. The typical sensation is of pelvic fullness and low abdominal bloating. When that feeling accompanies the failure of a period to start, you are probably pregnant. This is especially so if you have always had regular periods.

This feeling that you are going to start menstruating at any minute is a little trick your body plays on you. Many women assume that they cannot be pregnant because they have such a strong feeling that the period is about to start. Accordingly, they delay coming in for a pregnancy check until many days after they have missed their period. This is especially true for infertility patients who cannot believe they are really pregnant!

Cramping. Cramps are common at the time the period is missed and for a few days afterward. This is a normal sign of early stages of pregnancy—accept it as such. There is no need to limit activity or do anything different because of these cramps. Bleeding with the cramping, however, may indicate the beginning of a miscarriage. If this occurs, contact your physician immediately.

Nausea. Morning sickness, as this nausea is commonly called, does not come only in the morning; it can occur at any time during the day. It usually begins just after the missed period but can start even before. The nausea may be either mild or severe and may include vomiting. (See Q. 257.)

Constipation. Mild constipation is a common, early sign of pregnancy and will often occur soon after a woman misses her period.

Breast changes. Soon after missing a period, you may notice that your breasts are more tender and full. A doctor can almost as easily detect the early state of pregnancy by examining a woman's breasts as by examining her uterus. This is not always true, but it points out that the breasts do change quite significantly and quite early in pregnancy.

Frequency of urination. You may experience more frequent urination early in pregnancy, soon after the missed period.

Tiredness and sleepiness. These symptoms do not usually start immediately, but the feelings of tiredness and a need for more sleep can occur before you miss your second period. These feelings usually disappear toward the end of the third month. If you are experiencing nausea and vomiting, the tiredness will often go away when your nausea disappears.

Fainting. It is normal for a woman to have fainting spells and/or feelings of dizziness. When and if you think you are going to faint, lie down immediately so that you do not hit your head on a sharp object.

249 What should I do if I think I may be pregnant?

The first thing to do is to get a pregnancy test. Some women will want to try a home pregnancy test; others would rather have the doctor or laboratory make the diagnosis.

Urine pregnancy tests done at home or in the physician's office are fairly accurate and easy to do. They are reliable from about the ninth day after a missed period. If a test shows negative and you still think you are pregnant, it would be wise to repeat the test a week later or get a blood pregnancy test done in your doctor's office. A positive test does not absolutely mean that you are pregnant, and a negative test that you are not, especially if you have a tubal pregnancy (see Q. 304–310).

Blood pregnancy tests (serum pregnancy tests), if done by a reliable laboratory or office, are quite accurate. They can determine pregnancy even before a missed period, as early as seven or eight days after conception. If a woman wants to know before (or at the time of) her missed period whether or

Signs of Pregnancy

Indication	First Appearance
Blood or urine contains HCG	Day 9–10
Sleep patterns change	Week 3–4
Cervical tissue softens	Week 3–4
Breasts enlarge	Week 4
Nipples darken	Week 4–5
Mild constipation	Week 4–5
Cramping	Week 4–5
Frequent urination	Week 4–5
Nausea	Months 1–3
Dizziness	Months 1–3
Uterus enlarged at exam	Week 9

not she is pregnant, because of its greater reliability she should have the blood test rather than the urine test. She can usually get this done in her doctor's office.

250 What do pregnancy tests detect?

The tests detect a hormone called human chorionic gonadotrophin (HCG), which is produced by the placenta. Trophoblastic cells (which contribute to the formation of the placenta through which the embryo receives nourishment from the mother) produce this hormone. These cells can hardly be called a true placenta only seven or eight days after conception, but that is basically what they are.

The HCG hormone is necessary for the pregnancy to stay in the woman's body. It is produced only by a pregnant woman's body, with the exception of abnormal conditions, such as tumors associated with abnormal placentas from a previous pregnancy and certain types of cancer. The ability to test for pregnancy is one of the modern medical miracles. A human body has billions of cells, yet HCG can be detected telling us there are a few hundred new cells in the body!

251 Isn't a physical examination by the physician the best way to know that I am pregnant?

When frog-and-rabbit testing for pregnancy was still in use, the physician's exam was often the most accurate way to determine pregnancy. Now urine and blood pregnancy tests and vaginal sonograms are the most accurate methods for determining pregnancy.

252 Is it possible for me to have a period even though I am pregnant?

It is possible for you to have a totally normal period and still be pregnant. If that happens, of course, you would not know you were pregnant until you missed your next period or noticed bodily changes. Then, when you are examined by a doctor, he will find your uterus larger than would be expected. He might order a sonogram to see if you are carrying twins or triplets because of your big uterus only to find that you are just further along in your pregnancy than you thought.

Although it's possible to have a "normal" period while pregnant, it is more common to have one that is somewhat abnormal. If your period is noticeably "different" (a few days later, lighter or heavier, longer or shorter), you could be pregnant.

If you suspect that you are pregnant because of this kind of a period, it is important for you to get a pregnancy test. Women who bleed in early pregnancy will usually still carry a normal baby in a normal pregnancy, but it is possible for a woman who bleeds in early pregnancy to have a miscarriage.

Bleeding during early pregnancy can also indicate the presence of an ectopic (tubal) pregnancy. Because of this possibility, I strongly suggest that if you have a late period or one that is unusual, you have a pregnancy test. (The most accurate test is done with blood, especially important in case of a tubal pregnancy.) If you are pregnant, your physician can determine whether or not there is a tubal pregnancy by doing the kind of testing discussed in Q. 308. If you do have an ectopic pregnancy, the doctor can usually remove the pregnancy by laparoscopy, a relatively minor operation with very little loss of blood.

253 If a pregnancy test at home or in the office is positive, when should I see my doctor for a physical examination?

Patients should come in for an examination after their second missed menstrual period. A pelvic exam at that time will usually confirm pregnancy—the uterus will be enlarged. At this time the doctor can usually tell whether or not the uterus is progressing normally in its growth, and if it is the size it should be in relation to the date of the last menstrual period. Occasionally the uterus will not be quite as large as would seem compatible with the last period. In this situation it is better for patients not to announce their pregnancies until the doctor examines them three weeks later to confirm that the uterus is continuing to grow, or until a vaginal sonogram is done.

If the uterus is not enlarged at that examination, it is fairly certain that the woman is not pregnant or has become pregnant only recently. If her pregnancy test was positive, but the uterus is not enlarged and she has had some bleeding, she can be fairly sure that she either is miscarrying, has miscarried, or has an ectopic (tubal) pregnancy. But before the doctor even worries a patient about these findings, he/she will get a sonogram to see what is happening.

An examination before the second missed period will not definitely confirm pregnancy. Although the uterus may be a little enlarged on examination at this time, a little enlargement or a little softening of the uterus does not always indicate pregnancy. Women who skip a period, but are not pregnant, will often have a uterus that is slightly swollen, boggy, and enlarged. In years past, I had many patients come to me after other doctors told them, incorrectly, that they were pregnant. This assessment was based on an exam that was done too early; what the doctors felt was only the swelling from a missed period. Today though, the ultrasound machine has become very important in clarifying situations like these. If there is any question about whether or not you are pregnant, about how far along you are, about whether your uterus has stopped growing, or about whether or not you have a miscarriage or a tubal pregnancy, a vaginal sonogram can help determine what is going on. (See Q. 290, 399.)

The Role of the Doctor Early in Your Pregnancy

254 What will the doctor do on my first examination?

Your physician will do a complete physical examination. This includes checking your heart and lungs, as well as doing a pelvic examination. If you have not had a Pap smear in the past year, your doctor will want to do one. This will not disturb your pregnancy. When your doctor does a Pap smear, he or she merely scrapes cells from the surface of the cervix; any bleeding that occurs comes from that surface, not from inside the uterus.

If this is your first pregnancy, or if it is the first time you have seen this doctor, he or she will examine your pelvic bones to check for any prominence or deformity that might keep you from being able to deliver a full-term baby normally. Even if such an exam shows an adequate pelvis, however, it does not guarantee that you will be able to deliver without a cesarean section. Cesarean sections are done because a pelvis is too small to let a baby through, but also for many other reasons that have nothing to do with the size of the pelvic bones.

Following the physical exam, the doctor will discuss pregnancy and delivery with you (see Q. 256), answer your questions, and schedule a return visit in three or four weeks.

255 How will the doctor determine my due date?

The formula is simple. (See the accompanying chart.) The doctor calculates from the *first* day of your *last* normal menstrual period. Conception normally occurs approximately two weeks after that day. The doctor subtracts three months from that day and then adds seven days to it to determine the day you are most likely due. Most doctors will tell patients that their due date is plus or minus two weeks from that date.

This technique is based on a pregnancy schedule of 280 days from the first day of the last period (nine months and seven days). One recent study indicated the following figures:

48 percent of babies were delivered within seven days of calculated date,

26 percent of babies were delivered between seven and fourteen days of calculated date,

Gestation Chart

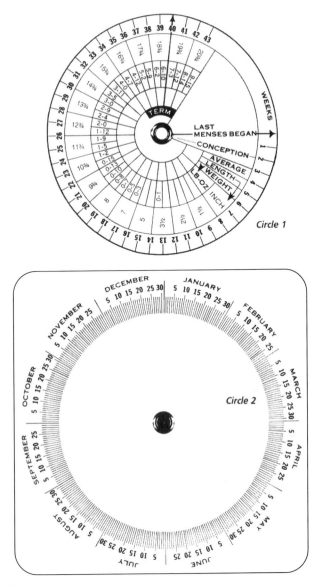

Circle 1

Circle 2

To make a gestation chart for each of your pregnancies, photocopy the two parts above, cut out circle 1 and center it over circle 2, tape the larger arrow to the beginning date of your last menstrual period, and circle the projected date of delivery at the point of the arrow in Week 40.

© 1974, Mead Johnson & Company

26 percent of babies were delivered more than fourteen days before or after calculated date (pre- or postmature).

The length of time from actual conception to delivery is normally about 270 days. This can be confusing. Some of the time your doctor will be talking about your pregnancy as though it began on the first day of your period and at other times as though it began at the time of the actual conception. You may need to listen carefully to your doctor's terms to know which gestation time (length of pregnancy) is being discussed. If you are not sure, just ask.

If there is any question about your due date, the doctor may want you to get an ultrasound (sonogram) done to get accurate dates. A reliable due date is very important. Much of the accuracy of the testing you may need later on in the pregnancy is dependent on knowing exactly how far along you are. If your dates are not accurate and you do not have an ultrasound early in your pregnancy to determine accurate dates, tests you have later could give erroneous information and cause you to think your normal baby is unhealthy.

Terminology

Weeks of Pregnancy. Counts from first day of your last period. You were not pregnant the first two weeks. Length of pregnancy is forty weeks. Doctors will be referring to this dating when they talk about how far along you are. Doctors call this menstrual age or gestational age.

Weeks from Fertilization. Counts from day of conception. Refers to the actual day you got pregnant and refers to the actual number of weeks the baby has been alive. Thirty-eight weeks from conception to delivery. Doctors call this ovulation age or postconception age.

Trimesters. First trimester is weeks one through twelve. Second trimester is weeks thirteen through twenty-four. Third trimester is weeks twenty-five through forty.

Embryo. Conception until the end of seventh week.

Fetus. Eighth week until birth.

Abortion. Loss of a pregnancy by any means whether spontaneous or done by an abortionist prior to the stage of viability—twenty weeks of pregnancy.

Late-term abortion. An abortion done by an abortionist from twenty weeks gestation on in pregnancy.

Partial-birth abortion. A lay term used to define a particular technique for aborting a baby from about twenty weeks on in pregnancy.

Miscarriage. A lay term used to refer to the loss of a pregnancy spontaneously prior to twenty weeks of pregnancy.

Preterm or premature delivery. Delivery from twenty weeks of pregnancy through thirty-seven weeks of pregnancy (counting by gestational age, which is forty weeks total pregnancy).

256 What general advice might my doctor give me during my first visit to the office?

One of the most important outcomes of the first obstetric visit is establishing a comfortable relationship with your doctor. If possible, your husband should accompany you on this visit. Not only will he learn a lot, but he will also feel like "part of the team" and be more comfortable during your pregnancy because he knows your doctor.

During this visit you will become familiar with your doctor's office routine and its physical setup; you will find out what appointment schedule your doctor prefers for pregnancy; you will find out if your doctor shares calls with other doctors, which hospital you will use, whether your doctor plans to be out of town at the time you are due, and so on.

You will also want to discuss childbirth classes. Determine which ones your doctor recommends and find out when and how to enroll.

It is important that you know what kind of expense you are facing during pregnancy and delivery. Fees vary from doctor to doctor. Hospital expenses will be determined by many factors, such as the hospital used, what kind of delivery is done, and whether there are any complications. Additional expenses throughout the pregnancy may include extra tests, such as ultrasound, or special laboratory work. Whether or not you have insurance is a major financial factor to be considered.

You need to know your physician's general suggestions for your activity. You will want to know if your doctor wants you to exercise regularly during your pregnancy. If so, what type of exercise does he or she think is best?

There are various opinions about the best diet

and the best weight gain during pregnancy. It is important that you have some idea what your physician thinks is best.

Does your doctor want you to have any particular, regular amount of rest during your pregnancy? It is important for your doctor to know if you work outside the home. If so, he or she needs to know your schedule to advise you later in pregnancy if you have some medical problems or some unusual tiredness.

If you are having morning sickness, your doctor would discuss that with you then and offer suggestions to minimize it.

You would want to discuss with your doctor any travel plans you might have during your pregnancy so you can be aware of any precautions about that.

When traveling by car it is important that you wear your seat belt even though it is uncomfortable. Studies have clearly shown that a pregnant woman and her baby are much more likely to survive an automobile accident if she has her seat belt in place.

It is important that you know how to reach your physician twenty-four hours a day. I encourage you to keep the necessary phone numbers by each telephone at home and work, and to also carry them with you.

If you can tell from the initial visit with your obstetrician that he or she will be difficult for you to communicate with, difficult to reach, or is one whom you would hesitate to "bother" with a problem or question, you should consider changing doctors. A good relationship with your physician makes for a happier, healthier, safer pregnancy and delivery.

257 What is morning sickness? Does every pregnant woman have it?

Researchers think morning sickness may be due to the high hormone levels of pregnancy (estrogen and HCG), though they do not know for sure what causes it. Recent research suggests that this nausea may be responsible for a woman avoiding foods and drugs that might be toxic to her baby in the first few weeks of pregnancy when the baby is the most susceptible. Perhaps you should be thankful for that awful nausea.

More than half of pregnant women experience nausea and vomiting to some degree early in pregnancy. Morning sickness usually appears soon after the first period is missed, and usually spontaneously disappears at the end of the third month. When the nausea goes away, the accompanying tiredness usually also leaves.

The term *morning sickness* is misleading; physicians prefer to label this normal complaint "nausea and vomiting of pregnancy." It may occur at any time during the day or night and the severity can vary greatly. The nausea may be so mild that it does not interfere in any way with a woman's schedule or diet. She may have no vomiting. Other women will have more severe nausea with occasional, or even daily, vomiting. Then there is a small group of women who get very ill from this nausea and vomiting. They lose weight and can become dehydrated from lack of or loss of fluids. Sometimes the problem is severe enough to require hospitalization and then it is called *hyperemesis gravidarum*.

The treatment of the nausea and vomiting of pregnancy depends on its severity. A woman does not *need* treatment until her nutrition and body fluids are significantly affected. She may *want* it before that occurs.

These hints may help a pregnant woman experiencing nausea and vomiting:

Nibble on toast or crackers all day. Have crackers at your bedside. Start nibbling when you awaken.

Eat smaller, more frequent meals.

Do not eat spicy food unless you know it does not upset your stomach.

Avoid foods that seem to cause nausea.

Eat foods that seem soothing to your stomach.

Do not cook if that upsets your stomach. (I learned to cook during the months my wife had morning sickness with our three pregnancies.)

Use medications if your problem is especially bothersome, i.e., if you do not seem to be able to keep much food down and are sick most of the time. (See the discussion of medications that follows.)

- Consult with a nutritionist. The hospital at which you will deliver probably has a nutritionist who would be happy to help you choose a diet that you can not only tolerate but also one that is nutritious.
- Do not take prenatal vitamins until the nausea is gone; they can aggravate nausea.

As long as you are not becoming dehydrated and are not losing weight, the problem is "awful" (my wife's word), but not dangerous. However, when your symptoms are severe and hyperemesis gravidarum results, your doctor will probably want to give you some medications. You may need to go to the hospital to get fluids in your veins. If you do go into the hospital, your doctor will want you to rest.

Medications can be helpful. Many women have a negative attitude toward taking drugs for morning sickness. As long as this attitude is not carried to the extreme, it is a healthy position. Unfortunately, I have had patients who were so afraid of such medications that they refused to use them when they should have and as a result began to lose weight and became dehydrated. At this point poor nutrition would seem more likely to hurt a developing baby than any medication a careful obstetrician might prescribe.

A drug called Bendectine was given in the past to many thousands of women for nausea of pregnancy. It helped many of them to control their nausea. (My wife used it with all three of our pregnancies.) Bendectine was taken off the market because of lawsuits, in spite of the many studies that showed the drug did not cause deformities in babies during pregnancy. The problem was that 3 to 5 percent of all newborn babies have some type of abnormality and the parents of some of these babies sued the manufacturing company claiming that Bendectine caused the abnormalities. The claims were unfounded, but the company chose to stop making the product rather than to go through the turmoil and expense of unwarranted lawsuits.

I feel that the studies are fairly conclusive that the medications in Bendectine are safe in pregnancy. Although this drug is not available, its com-

Distribution of Weight Gain during Pregnancy

Trimester	Weight Gain of Mother
1st (months 1–3)	3–5 lbs
2nd (months 4–6)	10–12 lbs.
3rd (months 7–9)	10–13 lbs.
	Total 23–30 lbs.

ponent parts are sold without a prescription. One Unisom tablet and two 50-mg capsules of vitamin B6 equal two Bendectine tablets. Daily dosage should not exceed the equivalent of four Bendectine tablets. It is probably best to take half of a Unisom and one vitamin B6 before arising and repeat the dosage later in the day. A full dose (equal to two Bendectine tablets) may be taken at night if necessary.

Other medications given for nausea that seem to be safe are Phenergan and Dramamine. The manufacturers of four other drugs, Tigan, Thorazine, Merezine, and Bonine (Antivert) say that there are no studies that show whether or not these drugs are safe in pregnancy, and they suggest using them only on a physician's advice. I agree. Although these drugs have not been shown to cause abnormalities, the manufacturers are protecting themselves by cautioning against use in pregnancy except on the advice of a doctor.

Causes of Weight Gain in Pregnancy

Cause	Pounds
Baby	7.7
Placenta	1.4
Uterus	2.0
Breasts	0.9
Amniotic fluid	1.8
Blood volume increase	4.0
Body fluid	2.7
Other (fat deposits)	3.5
	Total 24

Some doctors give patients vitamin B6 shots or prescribe vitamin B6 tablets. Be careful not to take an excessive amount of B6. More than 250 mg a day can cause nerve damage. A study reported in the *Journal of Obstetrics and Gynecology* (July 1991, 78: 1) by V. Sahakian, M.D., and associates showed that vitamin B6 did significantly reduce nausea and vomiting in some pregnant patients. Neither a doctor nor a patient knows which drug will be helpful. Keep trying until you get relief. Remember, however, it is possible that none of these drugs will relieve your symptoms. Take heart if the drugs do not help you. Usually the nausea diminishes or completely disappears after the third month of pregnancy.

258 Should I rest more while I am pregnant?

You should get an adequate amount of rest. During the early and late months of pregnancy you may feel tired; it is best to respond to your body's demands and get more rest at those times. Pushing yourself would only make you more tired. I recommend that pregnant women lie down for thirty to forty-five minutes at midday during the last two or three months of pregnancy. However, if you are particularly tired at any time during the pregnancy, lie down for thirty to forty-five minutes both morning and afternoon.

259 Should I eat differently while I am pregnant? How much weight should I gain during my pregnancy?

Actually, not enough is known about the nutritional requirements for pregnancy. A safe rule of thumb is to eat only wholesome, healthy foods. If you eat good food, in amounts adequate to gain weight, your baby should get the nutrition it needs.

Studies have shown that the development of the baby's brain is most significant around the time of birth. During the last three months of pregnancy, when the brain cells are growing and dividing the fastest, and during the first eighteen months after birth, when the brain cells are maturing, a balanced diet for mother and infant is crucial to avoid permanently affecting the baby's brain and decreasing intelligence.

Many years ago, women were advised to gain only fifteen or twenty pounds during pregnancy, but this weight gain limit had been literally "pulled out of the air." Experts now recommend a weight gain of between twenty-five and thirty-five pounds during a normal pregnancy. (Weight gain for underweight women should be in the range of twenty-eight to forty pounds; gain for overweight women should be in the range of fifteen to twenty-five pounds.)

The National Academy of Sciences Institute of Medicine did some research on weight gain in pregnancy. In addition to the recommendations above, they also suggest that a woman gain one pound a week during the second and third trimesters of her pregnancies. (If a woman is overweight at the start of pregnancy, she should gain a half pound per week during that time.)

Your weight gain during pregnancy cannot be appropriately regulated by your appetite. You may be too hungry or not hungry enough. Eat what you should eat, not what your appetite tells you to eat!

The reason for these weight gain recommendations is that when women have severe diet restrictions during pregnancy to keep their weight down, their infants may have a lower birth weight at delivery and might be less healthy.

You should not use pregnancy as a time to lose weight. Eat right and gain weight according to the recommendations given above. By the way, NutraSweet is safe in pregnancy.

260 Can I continue normal activity and exercise during pregnancy?

If you have not had a history of repeated miscarriages and seem to have a normal pregnancy with no bleeding, you probably do not need to make much change in your lifestyle. I advise all my patients to continue to do the reasonable activities they did before pregnancy. The key phrase in this sentence is "continue to do the reasonable activities they did." I do not think pregnancy is the time for a woman to take up a new sport or to begin vigorous, active exercise if she is not already conditioned to such activity.

I believe exercise is even more important to a pregnant woman than it is to one who is not pregnant. It should be done on a regular basis, generally at least three times a week.

Even if you are not in good physical shape when you become pregnant, I recommend that you start regular exercise. The best approach would be joining an exercise class for pregnant women. If this is not possible, one of the most ideal exercises during pregnancy is walking. If you will walk three miles at a time, three or four times a week, or swim or bicycle regularly, you can keep yourself in good condition. If you have not been exercising, you can start slowly and build up to a good workout.

I suggest that patients begin exercising as soon as their nausea and tiredness are diminished enough to allow them to be active. Exercise early in pregnancy will make you stronger and will make you feel better later in your pregnancy. Exercise also helps keep weight down.

Extremely vigorous exercise may cause the baby's heartbeat to speed up or even be temporarily irregular. Because of this, most physicians recommend no more than fifteen minutes of vigorous exercise or thirty minutes of aerobic-type exercise with each workout.

A guideline that might help you gauge your activity is to keep your heart rate under 140 and try not to get extremely hot or dehydrated.

A major benefit of exercise during pregnancy is that being in good shape physically can make labor easier. Labor is a physical activity and cannot be done as well by someone who is weak and in poor physical condition.

The American College of Obstetricians and Gynecologists has excellent pregnancy and postnatal exercise programs available in videocassette and audiocassette form. Check with your doctor before exercising and ask him or her where you might be able to obtain these videos or tapes. These programs were designed by health officials who understand the special needs of pregnant and postnatal women.

Some conditions in pregnancy make it unwise for you to exercise. If the baby is growing poorly (intrauterine growth retardation), you should not exercise. If your cervix tends to open (incompetent cervix), do not exercise. If your bag of waters ruptures prematurely, you will not only be unable to exercise, you will also probably be confined to bed. If you have triplets (or more), your doctor will probably advise that you not exercise. Your physician will give you further guidance about exercise and care in these situations.

There are some exercises you should not do. Scuba diving is probably safe down to thirty feet, but below that during the first trimester has been associated with some facial malformations in babies. Waterskiing is questionable because of the possibility of water being forced into the vagina during a fall.

If you have any questions about participating in a specific sport or exercise, consult your doctor. The greatest risk from sports is probably trauma from a fall or accident, for example from downhill skiing or from riding a motorcycle.

261 Is intercourse during pregnancy harmful?

There is little evidence that intercourse is harmful during any stage of pregnancy. Dr. James L. Mills of the National Institute of Health did a study involving more than 10,000 women. He found no relationship between any problem they had during pregnancy or after delivery that was associated with intercourse during pregnancy. Although there have been some studies that indicate that intercourse can be associated with problems such as infections, my feeling is that Mills's studies are correct. I tell pregnant women that unless there is a problem in the pregnancy, they may have intercourse at any time during pregnancy until the cervix dilates significantly (two centimeters or more). This usually occurs during the last month.

262 What about travel during pregnancy?

You may travel wherever and whenever you wish until the last month of pregnancy. At that time, you should stay within an hour's drive of home so that your baby can be delivered at your own hospital as planned. Babies can come prematurely and in inconvenient locations. A reasonable cutoff time for long-distance travel seems to be four weeks before your due date.

If you travel long distances by car, get out each hour and walk around a bit. This will keep you more comfortable and help circulation to your legs (to help you avoid blood clots).

Pregnant women should wear seat belts. A few years ago, women thought seat belts might damage the uterus and cause premature labor or miscarriage in case an accident occurred. Statistics clearly show that both mother and baby are much more likely to survive an accident safely if the mother wears a seat belt. One study in California, for instance, showed that in 47 percent of accidents, the baby would die inside the mother when she was thrown from a car. If she was not thrown from the car, the baby died only 11 percent of the time.

A woman may travel by airplane during pregnancy. An excellent study done on flight attendants by William Daniell and his associates (*Aviation, Space & Environmental Medicine*, 1990, 61:840) shows that they do not have an increased rate of miscarriage, premature deliveries, or abnormalities of their babies. Other studies have also shown that flying does not harm a woman or her pregnancy.

263 May I bathe while I am pregnant? Are hot tubs, saunas, and electric blankets okay during pregnancy?

Bathing or showering during pregnancy is obviously good for personal hygiene. However, during the latter part of pregnancy, take care to avoid slipping and falling in a bathtub. If you think your bag of waters has broken, don't bathe—call your doctor.

The other part of your question has to do with increasing the internal temperature of your body while pregnant. Studies (Milnnsky, *Journal of the American Medical Association*, 1992, 268:882–885) have shown that if you do expose your body to heat, it increases your chance of having a baby with a neural tube defect. (See Q. 458–462.) These researchers showed that the heat from electric blankets was okay. Saunas, hot tubs, and long, hot baths were risky for the baby, especially in the first few weeks of pregnancy. So my advice is to avoid them in pregnancy.

Some people are also worried about exposure to the electricity from electric blankets, wiring running over a bed, heated waterbeds, video display terminals, or exposure to electromagnetic fields that might be present with high-voltage electrical lines built over the homes of some people. A study done by Bracken et al. and published in *Epidemiology* (1995, 6:263–270) showed no relationship between electric fields and the health of a baby at birth. It seems, therefore, that it is safe to be exposed to these electrical fields.

264 Should I take vitamins while I am pregnant? Should I take other medications while I am pregnant?

Yes. Not only should you take prenatal vitamins while you are pregnant, you should take prenatal vitamins before you get pregnant. The most important content of these vitamins is folic acid. (See Q. 247). As mentioned in that question, it has now been proven that if a woman consumes at least 400 micrograms a day of folic acid during the first six weeks of her pregnancy, she has a 70 percent less chance of having a baby with a neural tube defect. Neural tube defects, what they are, their diagnosis, and maternal serum alpha-fetoprotein are discussed extensively in Q. 458–462.

Because of this milestone finding, the FDA has ordered that folic acid be added to fortified foods. This is the first time foods have been fortified to prevent a birth defect. This decision was made on February 29, 1996.

Most obstetricians also believe that it is good

for women to take prenatal vitamins with 800 micrograms (0.8 milligrams) of folic acid before they get pregnant. The other elements of prenatal vitamins are also beneficial.

Recently research showed that zinc was important in the growth of the baby. Goldenberg et al. in the *Journal of the American Medical Association* (August 9, 1995) showed that if a woman was lacking in zinc, then took zinc during pregnancy, her baby would have a better birth weight and better growth of its head. Therefore, it seems wise for pregnant women to be sure their prenatal vitamin has at least 25 milligrams of zinc for each day's dose.

If the vitamins cause nausea and she is eating a well-balanced diet and gaining weight, a woman can omit the vitamins until her nausea is over, except for the folic acid. She can get a prescription for just folic acid from her doctor.

Excessive Vitamin A can increase the risk of birth defects. A woman should not take more than 5,000 international units a day. Even a dose as low as 10,000 units a day may hurt the baby.

The prenatal vitamins that may be purchased over-the-counter contain almost exactly the same supplements as the prescription vitamins, and they are less expensive. Check the expiration dates on any over-the-counter vitamins you purchase. Make sure the label indicates that it meets Pharmacopeia standards. (If you are interested, write the manufacturer and ask to see lab results that will show whether or not the vitamin is absorbed well, and is a quality product.) As far as other medications are concerned, you should take as little medication as possible during pregnancy. Try to avoid taking medications when you have a common cold or mild nausea. If you are feeling sick and want medication, call your obstetrician.

Inform your obstetrician of any medication prescribed for you by another physician. For example, tetracycline or sulfa antibiotics should not be taken during pregnancy without consulting your obstetrician. Tylenol (or a similar medication containing no aspirin) should be used instead of aspirin during pregnancy. (See Q. 437–445.)

One important advantage of the preconceptual counseling discussed earlier (Q. 247) is to evaluate any medications you take on a daily basis before you get pregnant. Many questionable medications can be changed to safer ones during pregnancy.

Two books that almost all physicians have discuss the safety of drugs in pregnancy. One is *Drugs in Pregnancy and Lactation* by Drs. Briggs, Freeman, and Yaffe (Williams & Wilkins, 1986) and the other is *The Physician's Desk Reference.*

265 Should I see the dentist while I am pregnant?

If a woman is planning a pregnancy, the best thing she can do is to see the dentist before she gets pregnant. Any treatment she needs can be taken care of before the pregnancy begins.

You should see your dentist while you are pregnant if it is necessary, however. Dental work should be done during the middle three months of pregnancy. During that time the placenta is healthier and is better equipped to filter out bacteria that may be released into the bloodstream while the dentist works on your gums and teeth. An abscess or any infection must be treated.

If X-rays are needed, they should be taken after the third month and *the abdomen should be protected with a lead shield.* Cavities may be filled as needed during the middle three months of pregnancy; it is preferable that your dentist use only a local anesthetic. However, I recommend that you have as little dental work as possible done during pregnancy.

266 Are there problems common to pregnancy that are uncomfortable, but not dangerous?

Many troublesome but not dangerous problems may occur during a pregnancy.

Backache. As your pregnancy progresses, the weight of the baby can tend to make you "swaybacked." The best way to avoid this problem is to be in good physical condition before becoming pregnant and to continue exercising during pregnancy to keep your abdominal and back muscles in good condition. Resting each day will help your back muscles relax. Good posture and sitting in chairs that have maximum support will also help. If your back pain persists, tell your physician. (For more about backache, see Q. 269.)

Swelling. Swelling of the body during pregnancy is a normal response to the hormones circulating throughout the body. If you experience some swelling, don't worry, unless it is sudden and severe. Diuretics (medications that increase the amount of urine output, thereby relieving some of the swelling caused by excess fluid) are used much less frequently than in the past. If swelling is a problem, try other means of dealing with it. You could increase your water intake to three quarts a day; prop up your feet when you sit to allow fluid to drain from them; and decrease (but do not eliminate) your intake of salt. If those means do not provide relief, and the swelling causes significant discomfort, some doctors will prescribe diuretics. Obstetricians who have trained more recently will almost never prescribe diuretics, even for this problem. This is probably the best approach, so don't argue if your doctor feels it is not healthy for you to use diuretics. (See Q. 443.)

Hemorrhoids. Many women have their first experience with hemorrhoids during pregnancy. Hemorrhoids are merely varicose veins around the anus. You can help prevent hemorrhoids by adding either unprocessed wheat bran (miller's bran) or Metamucil to your diet every day. Increasing dietary fiber causes stools to be looser and softer, which means you will not have to push so hard with bowel movements. If your hemorrhoids are particularly bothersome or they are bleeding, be sure to tell your physician. (See also Q. 270.)

Varicose veins. If veins in your legs become more prominent and the skin over them bulges, you may have varicose veins. Call your physician's attention to them. These veins generally do not cause any problems except for discomfort and appearance. (If you have a history of blood clots in your leg veins, tell your doctor.)

Care of varicose veins during pregnancy is the use of elastic stockings and leg elevation. The stockings may not keep your veins from enlarging, but they can make you more comfortable. Lying down and elevating your legs both morning and night can also make you more comfortable.

Other problems. Other problems during pregnancy may include increased vaginal discharge from the increased moisture of the vagina, increased quantities of saliva, tiredness due to hormonal changes, or headache. Let your doctor know if you have a problem during your pregnancy. He or she can help you to get through your pregnancy as comfortably as possible.

---

267 May I continue to work while I am pregnant?

Continue all your normal activities during pregnancy; this includes working. An exception would be if you are in a job that might cause problems for your body or damage to the baby.

If your job requires a great deal of lifting, you should probably stop the lifting after the fifth or sixth month. Continuing to lift during the latter part of pregnancy could cause back injuries. If you work where you are exposed to strong chemical fumes, you probably should change jobs while you are pregnant.

Some reports indicate that continued exposure to high temperatures during the first months of pregnancy can damage the baby. It is therefore probably best not to be on a job that exposes you to high temperatures, although it is highly unlikely that you could tolerate working in such a situation while you are pregnant.

Radiation (X-rays, radioisotopies) can be harmful to both you and your baby and should be avoided during pregnancy.

Studies have also indicated that a large number of "questionable" work or environmental factors do not seem to be harmful to the fetus. These include video displays, TV screens, magnetic or electronic fields, noise, or ultrasound.

Other reports indicate that it is not good for a pregnant woman to be exposed to very high altitudes, or to dive to deep depths, or to experience compression or decompression more than that experienced in normal air travel. Air travel is safe during pregnancy, whether or not it is in a pressurized aircraft.

If a woman has previously had a premature baby, it might be best for her to stop working during the last three months of her pregnancy and to rest both morning and afternoon. Some studies have indicated that if a mother rests more during the latter part of her pregnancy, she is more likely to carry that pregnancy to term and to have a larger, healthier baby.

You might be interested in a study reported in the *New England Journal of Medicine* (November 11, 1990, 323:15) that studied female physicians who were in their residency training. (Residency is the time of training during which a physician becomes a specialist. The work is stressful, difficult, and requires long hours.) Mark A. Klebanoff, M.D., and his associates, found that the long hours of stressful work had little effect on the outcome of the pregnancy. It seems to me that if physicians in residency training can go through pregnancy without harm to themselves or their babies, then other stressful, difficult jobs are probably "safe" for mother and child, unless there is actual physical danger to the woman.

268 What physical changes can I expect during pregnancy?

The hormones of pregnancy are produced in large amounts, and these hormones, coupled with the growth of the baby, produce truly amazing bodily changes. Some of the major changes are as follows.

The abdomen. By the time most patients see a physician (after the second missed period), their abdomens feel bloated. Since at this point the uterus is about the size of a man's fist, obviously the uterus is not causing the bloated feeling. The feeling occurs because of the swelling effect of the hormones on all the tissues of the lower abdomen and pelvis.

Toward the end of the third month, the abdomen is a little more protuberant. At about this time the doctor, and sometimes the mother herself, will be able to feel the uterus as a lump extending about two inches above the pubic bone.

Most women could probably "hide" their pregnancy until the sixteenth to twentieth week of pregnancy, especially if it is the first pregnancy. However, it is probably going to be most com-fortable if a woman is ready to don her maternity clothes by the fourteenth or fifteenth weeks of her pregnancy. So by the end of the third month (twelve weeks) have those clothes ready for your proud coming out. By the twentieth week, the end of the fifth month, the top of the uterus is at the level of the umbilicus (belly button), and most women cannot conceal a pregnancy once it is at that stage.

As the abdomen becomes larger and larger, women often wonder how much bigger they can get. The capacity of the uterus and the abdominal wall to expand is almost beyond belief. The uterus is not limited by the rib cage and can expand forward as much as it needs to, for twins, triplets, or more babies.

Most people do not realize how miraculous is the enlargement of the uterus. It goes from a ball of muscle that weighs about two and a half ounces and can hold one or two teaspoons of fluid, to an organ that weighs two pounds and can hold two or three five-pound babies plus a placenta(s), which might each weigh one or two pounds. This is accomplished not by new muscle cells but by the stretching and enlarging of muscle cells that are present when pregnancy begins.

Breasts. During pregnancy the breasts change almost as much as the uterus does. Early in pregnancy the breasts may be tender and full. After the second month they increase in size and become nodular, or lumpy. The nodularity is due to the growing and thickening glands that are necessary for the production of milk after delivery.

Most women will find it most comfortable to start wearing maternity bras, even nursing bras, at this time. They can expand up to a point to allow for the extra growth of the breasts after delivery, during nursing.

The nipples may or may not produce a thick yellow fluid called colostrum, but its production at this point is unrelated to the ability of a woman to nurse. Don't worry if you begin having colostrum after only a few weeks of pregnancy; this is not abnormal.

A darkening of the nipples and areola (the skin around the nipples) is normal. This change in color

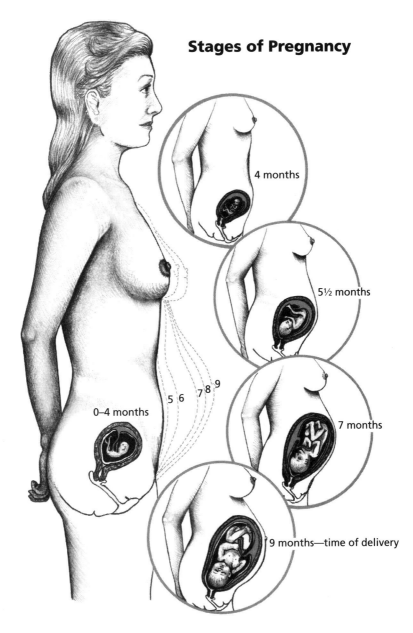

Stages of Pregnancy

4 months

5½ months

0–4 months

7 months

9 months—time of delivery

5 6 7 8 9

is due to the effect of hormones on these tissues. Also, small elevations on the areola are the so-called glands of Montgomery, oil glands that are increasing in size during pregnancy. The oil from these glands helps keep the nipple and areola from becoming dry and cracked during nursing.

Blue veins may appear beneath the skin overlying the breasts. These are normal during pregnancy. The body's blood vessels carry 40 percent more blood during the latter part of pregnancy than they normally do. It is also normal for stretch marks (see the next paragraph) to develop in the skin of the breasts.

Skin. Many people are not aware of the fantastic hormonal changes that the skin undergoes during pregnancy. The most obvious change involves stretch marks *(striae gravidarum)*, the pinkish lines that resemble scars and appear on the abdomen, breasts, and thighs of some women. These marks occur in about one-half of all pregnancies, remaining even when the skin returns to its normal position after pregnancy. Stretch marks will become lighter and less visible after the pregnancy is over.

Stretch marks are not, as commonly thought, due to stretching alone, but also to changes caused by the hormones of pregnancy. Moisturizers and lubricants may make the skin feel better, but they will not usually prevent stretch marks.

In addition to the darkening of the skin of the areola and nipples, which usually occurs with the first pregnancy, a dark line *(linea nigra)* will often develop from the umbilicus (belly button) down to the pubic hair. These discolorations usually get darker with each pregnancy.

Facial discolorations develop in many pregnant women. These various-sized brown patches *(chloasma)* are often called the mask of pregnancy. Although the discoloration usually fades after delivery, the skin does not normally return to its original color. Birth-control pills produce the same change.

Vascular spiders develop in about two-thirds of white women and approximately one-tenth of black women during pregnancy. These are small (one-eighth to one-quarter inch) red discolorations of the skin, occurring most commonly on the face, neck, upper chest, and arms. From the central spot, small red lines extend outward. The blood drains from them and they blanch when they are touched lightly. These are also known as *nevus, angioma,* or *telangiectasia.*

Redness of the palms is common in pregnancy, occurring in about two-thirds of white women and one-third of nonwhite women. This condition usually disappears after pregnancy.

Skin tags, small, flesh-colored growths of skin about the size of a small tick, often develop during pregnancy. Changes in the color of moles also will often occur. Skin tags usually go away after pregnancy; moles usually lighten but remain. Some women are afraid that such changes mean they have skin cancer. This is highly unlikely, but if there is any question, you should have your doctor check.

Arms and legs. Occasionally a pregnant woman will develop numbness of her hands. This is called the *carpal tunnel syndrome.* If a patient just has occasional numbness, nothing usually needs to be done

about it. However, if her hands become totally numb and this numbness lasts twenty-four hours or longer, I suggest that she see a neurologist, an orthopedist, a neurosurgeon, or a plastic surgeon. She may need a simple operation that will relieve the pressure on the nerves to her hands. This can prevent permanent damage to those nerves.

The veins of the legs become prominent during pregnancy because vessels are carrying much more blood than they normally do. In the latter part of pregnancy, small blood vessels are at least 50 percent larger than normal, making it possible to see small veins and capillaries that are not ordinarily visible. These veins are generally not varicosities. A varicose vein is normally one that is enlarged to at least the size of your little finger, large enough to make the skin bulge over it. For small collections of veins or small isolated veins, there is no treatment. Besides, most will usually go away after pregnancy. Your skin, though, will never be the way it was before your first pregnancy, and some of these veins will continue to be visible.

Varicose veins are normally not very responsive to any particular recommendations during pregnancy. I have not found it useful to have patients wear elastic stockings. In the southern part of the country, elastic stockings are uncomfortable to wear because of the heat. Most women choose not to wear them, but if a patient has severe varicose veins, she can have custom-fitted elastic stockings made. These are probably the only type that are significantly helpful if varicose veins are painful.

Changes in the internal parts of the body. During pregnancy remarkable changes occur in almost every system of the body. The tubes from the kidneys to the bladder (ureters) elongate and dilate in an extraordinary way. The kidneys enlarge. Each becomes about a half inch longer, and 50 percent more blood flows through them. The actual work of the kidneys also increases remarkably. The stomach and intestines change and are "displaced" by the enlarging uterus. The lungs change because the growing abdomen pushes the diaphragm up, thus reducing the volume of air in the lungs. The actual function of the lungs is not impaired by pregnancy, but certain diseases of the lungs, such as pneumonia and bronchitis, are more common in pregnancy.

One of the most dramatic changes in your body during pregnancy has to do with your heart and blood-vessel system. The heart rate increases ten or fifteen beats a minute, and the output of blood from the heart increases, especially during the first three months of pregnancy. Because of increased blood flow through the heart, a doctor may hear murmurs when he or she listens to your heart. These murmurs are usually not due to disease, and they sound like the noise household pipes make when lots of water flows through them. If your doctor is concerned, though, you will probably be referred to a cardiologist. In the past, doctors were afraid that pregnancy was hard on a woman's heart and gave stern warnings of the danger of pregnancy to women with heart disease. There certainly are some problems associated with severe heart disease in pregnancy, but these are not nearly so dangerous as was felt in the past.

Gums. Your gums may become soft and bleed easily during pregnancy. These changes seem to be related to the hormones of pregnancy and usually disappear after delivery. The best treatment seems to be good dental hygiene, which includes flossing and brushing.

A condition called *epulis* (a swelling of the gums in a specific spot that resembles a growth) can occur during pregnancy. If that happens, your dentist should check to be sure that this is merely an epulis swelling and not a tumor.

There is no truth in the old wives' tale: "The baby sucks the calcium away from its mother's teeth and causes them to decay." This does not happen.

Muscles and bones. Several things happen to your muscles and bones, the most obvious of which is a change in posture. As your uterus enlarges and grows forward, you must lean back to balance yourself. This is called *lordosis* and is one of the most common causes of low back pain during pregnancy. This is one reason women are encouraged to start exercising early in pregnancy. Exercise makes the muscles strong enough to help support the body during the latter part of pregnancy when there is more stress on it.

A woman may develop aching, numbness, and weakness in the arms. This is due to the tendency to lean back, pulling the neck forward and thereby pulling on the nerves that go down to the arms.

There is also a softening of the ligaments between joints, not only of the arms and legs but also of the pelvic bones. This relaxation seems to be what causes the bones to grate against each other, to pop, and to produce some of the discomfort that a woman feels in her arms, legs, back, and pelvis. These changes are important. X-rays reveal the amazing way that the pelvic bones separate during labor to allow the baby's head to pass through the birth canal.

269 Are there any ways to avoid or ease low back pain during pregnancy?

Suggestions for avoiding back pain, in addition to beginning exercise early in pregnancy to keep the muscles toned all along, include the following.

Resting. Lie down; don't sit. Lie on a firm surface with your knees elevated by a pillow. When you get up, roll over on your side and lower your legs to the floor without jerking your back.

Lifting things. When you lift, squat down directly in front of the object you are planning to lift. Do not bend over. Pregnant women usually do more injury to their backs when they already have one baby; their tendency to bend over and pick up that small child, with a back that is weakened by the present pregnancy, is a real problem. Be careful with your back if you already have a young child to care for.

Sitting. When you sit, avoid soft, low chairs that allow you to sink down into the upholstery. It is easy to hurt your back when you stand up. Never sit for more than fifteen minutes at a time if you can avoid it, especially late in pregnancy. Get up and move around as frequently as possible.

Driving. Push the car seat forward so that your knees are higher than your hips. Always wear your seat belt and, if possible, use a vehicle that has an air bag for the driver. If you are in an accident and hit your uterus against the dashboard or steering wheel, you can damage your unborn baby.

Standing and walking. When you are pregnant, you are naturally a little more clumsy. Be careful when you are stepping over curbs or walking on rough ground. Don't stand in the same position for more than a minute; shifting from one foot to the other occasionally will help.

Physical work. Get on your knees to do jobs that you might be tempted to do by leaning over. When your back is really hurting, don't do any physical work that will aggravate your condition.

270 What are some of the most common complaints during pregnancy?

Inevitably, because of the numerous major changes occurring in your body, there will be some discomfort or even pain. I believe these aches and pains are more easily borne if they are understood. An explanation of some of the more common problems follows.

Round ligament pain. This pain is caused by a woman coughing or moving in such a way that one (or both) of the round ligaments is pulled. These ligaments, located one on each side of the uterus, help stabilize the uterus and keep it from rotating around and cutting off its blood supply.

This type of pain is probably the most common during pregnancy. It can begin after only a few weeks of pregnancy and can occur at any time during pregnancy. The pain, which can be as severe as appendicitis, may be brief or may last for days, occurring in the lower abdomen on either side. If the pain is bad, you should see your physician. He or she can usually confirm that it is round ligament pain by merely pressing on the areas where the round ligament attaches to the uterus and finding tenderness in these spots.

Braxton-Hicks contractions. These contractions are commonly called false labor pains. Many people have the idea that they occur only as a warm-up for labor, but this is not true. The uterus contracts and relaxes all the time, even when a woman isn't pregnant. However, during pregnancy, as the uterus is being stretched, it does contract more and with stronger contractions than it does in the nonpregnant condition.

Braxton-Hicks contractions will normally become less frequent and less strong if a woman

rests, but can be intensified by physical activity and intercourse. When a woman is having discomfort with false labor pains, the best thing is to rest and to refrain from physical activity or intercourse for a short time. If a woman has strong or frequent contractions and she has previously had premature labor, she should call her obstetrician immediately.

Vaginal discomfort. It is common, especially in the latter part of pregnancy, for a woman to feel "shooting pains" into her vagina, as though the baby were putting its foot through the cervix and out into the vagina. This is not usually a sign that the baby is about to come. These pains, which may vary from a pressure to a sharp, shooting sensation, are not a danger sign and nothing needs to be done. If the pain is quite bothersome, you may need to lie down. This will allow the baby to float up out of the pelvis a little and relieve some of the discomfort.

Both the vagina and the vulva can feel swollen in the second half of the pregnancy. Occasionally this is uncomfortable enough to make intercourse unpleasant. Many women, whether or not they have problems of this type, do not desire intercourse anyway, especially during the latter part of pregnancy. This situation, of course, can put a great deal of pressure on the husband, since his sexual drive is often unabated.

Unfortunately, some men feel that they cannot stand sexual deprivation (or think they can't). There is a greater incidence of infidelity during pregnancy, perhaps in part due to the decreased interest in sexual activity many pregnant women experience. You can alleviate some of his stress— and show your love for him—by meeting his sexual needs. If vaginal sex is too unpleasant for you a great deal of the time, explain this to your husband. Then you might use some lubricating jelly and your hands to bring him to ejaculation occasionally.

Feeling the baby move. Many women actually hurt at times when their babies move. The discomfort may be so bad that the mother thinks something is wrong. When you feel really uncomfortable and are not sure whether it is the baby or your own body, see the doctor and let him or her tell you.

It is normal to have a tender place in the uterus

as a result of the baby poking the uterine wall. This sensation may stay for several hours or several days. It is normal, too, to feel a fairly sharp and uncomfortable pain under the ribs, and this will often happen as early as six months. It can be caused by both the stretching of your ribs and/or the baby's movement. There is nothing you can do about the baby's movement; it is a normal part of a healthy baby's growth.

Some women worry about the baby moving too much. They feel it must be an indication that something is wrong, or that they will have a hyperactive child. In 1983 William F. Rayburn of the University of Michigan studied more than 900 pregnant women who kept charts of fetal movement. Forty-seven of the women recorded more than forty movements of the baby per hour, signs of excessive fetal activity. All of these babies were healthy and normal when they were delivered; none died, and studies on them since that time have shown that none of them had unusual temperaments or delayed development.

Mothers frequently complain that their babies have a repetitive "bumping" activity. This is hiccups, and when I mention this to mothers, they immediately recognize it as such. Studies have shown that all normal babies have hiccups at least once a day from the seventh month on. Don't worry, though, if you don't feel the baby's hiccups; they can occur at night when you are asleep. And it is certainly not worth losing a night's sleep to see whether or not the baby is hiccuping once a day.

On the other end of the scale is the quiet baby. This one is usually normal. You should not worry if you are not constantly aware of your baby moving around. Mothers frequently fail to feel a baby move for several hours at a time and become worried. Normally this fear is unwarranted. If you have any questions about the baby being inactive, you should see your doctor and have the baby's condition checked. You might also try "poking" the baby, eating something sweet, or standing by a loud radio. These things will often awaken a quiet baby.

Leg cramps. Women often get leg cramps during the last half of pregnancy. This is usually due to drinking too much milk. Cow's milk contains excessive phosphorous, which lowers the amount of calcium in your blood. If you experience leg cramps, you should stop drinking cow's milk and start taking calcium pills. These may be obtained without a prescription. If the cramps stop, you can begin to drink milk again, up to the amount that causes the cramps to return.

Insomnia. Many patients have trouble sleeping during the last month of pregnancy. This can make them feel tired and weak. Although most doctors do not like to prescribe sleeping pills during pregnancy, if the woman is really miserable from insomnia—and because this problem is almost exclusively a "last-month" problem—some doctors will offer Benadryl (25–50 mg) to take when a patient wants to sleep.

Nausea late in pregnancy. Nausea during the last month is fairly common. Most women do not need any medication for this late nausea because it is not usually severe. Women often think that they may have a virus or some other illness when late nausea starts. Occasionally this nausea represents preeclampsia, which may pose a danger to you and your baby. Most of the time, however, it is caused by the pregnancy. If you experience nausea, consult your doctor. He or she may want to prescribe Phenergan 25 mg by mouth or by rectal suppository every four to six hours as needed and evaluate you for any serious conditions.

Hemorrhoids. Hemorrhoids are fairly common both during and after pregnancy. It has been thought these are due to the pressure on the veins from the pregnant uterus, and that after pregnancy hemorrhoids are present because of the woman's pushing during labor. This may be partly true. However, in societies where more fiber and less sugar are eaten, women almost never have hemorrhoids, even during pregnancy. It is felt, therefore, that hemorrhoids are related more to the constipating type of diet that we eat in the Western world than to pregnancy.

Hemorrhoids can be treated with cool, moist compresses, Nupercaine ointment, or a cortisone-containing ointment prescribed by your doctor. Because hemorrhoids protrude, it is tempting to push them back inside the anus. Don't do this. Pushing them back will often irritate them and make them more sensitive.

Heartburn or indigestion. This is common in

pregnancy and results from the stomach slowing down its function and passing food through sluggishly. This problem can often be solved by avoiding rich, greasy, or spicy foods. Antacids can help. But, as with any medication, it is probably best to use them only if you cannot make yourself comfortable by other techniques, such as adjusting your diet.

Ill feeling. Some women simply do not feel well when they are pregnant. They feel uncomfortable, full, tired . . . just wretched. There really does not seem to be much you can do to make yourself feel better except to keep in good physical shape through sensible exercise and eating. After your doctor has assured you that nothing is wrong, don't worry if you feel wretched. Keep yourself in good shape and tolerate that miserable feeling until the baby comes. It will be worth it!

Lightening. Some mothers will notice a few weeks before the start of their labor that the baby seems to have dropped lower in their pelvis. They will notice a little extra room at the upper part of their abdomen. Sometimes they may be able to breathe a little easier. After this has occurred, the mother will notice that she has more pressure in the pelvic area. She will often have the feeling that the baby is poking its foot or its hand into her vagina. Occasionally it will be more difficult to walk because of the feeling of pressure in the hips. Increased frequency and urgency of urination as well as increased backache may also occur. Pregnant women normally are not made more uncomfortable by lightening, or dropping, of the baby in the few weeks before the onset of labor. However, it can cause increased pelvic discomfort.

This dropping of the baby occurs most dramatically in mothers who are having their first baby. After the first baby, it seems that the pregnancy starts low, stays low, and does not usually have the lightening that occurs with the first baby.

271 Is it true that a husband may experience symptoms of pregnancy too?

Yes. Not only may you experience nausea in pregnancy but so may your husband. When this occurs, it may include not only nausea but also other symptoms that mimic the discomfort and problems that you may feel, such as abdominal pain, vomiting, diarrhea, and even burning with urination and blood in the urine. These symptoms, called couvade syndrome, are almost always psychogenic and not due to any disease in the father.

Fetal

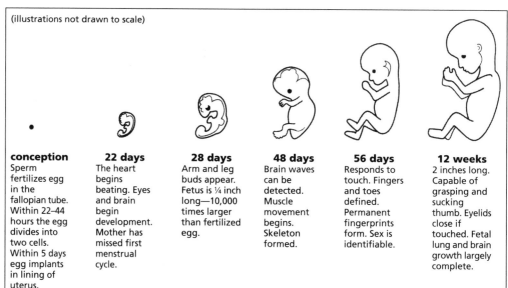

(illustrations not drawn to scale)

conception
Sperm fertilizes egg in the fallopian tube. Within 22–44 hours the egg divides into two cells. Within 5 days egg implants in lining of uterus.

22 days
The heart begins beating. Eyes and brain begin development. Mother has missed first menstrual cycle.

28 days
Arm and leg buds appear. Fetus is ¼ inch long—10,000 times larger than fertilized egg.

48 days
Brain waves can be detected. Muscle movement begins. Skeleton formed.

56 days
Responds to touch. Fingers and toes defined. Permanent fingerprints form. Sex is identifiable.

12 weeks
2 inches long. Capable of grasping and sucking thumb. Eyelids close if touched. Fetal lung and brain growth largely complete.

About 14 percent of expectant fathers are likely to have some symptoms of this type. Most of the time the husband's problems will spontaneously disappear. Men with this problem are not psychiatrically abnormal; they need nothing more than encouragement and a little insight into what is going on.

272 I have heard that women can think that they are pregnant and not be pregnant. Is this true?

What you are talking about is called "false pregnancy." (The medical term for this is pseudocyesis.) This problem of phantom or imaginary pregnancy usually occurs in women who have an intense desire to become pregnant. These women have convinced themselves that they are pregnant even though they have negative pregnancy tests and their sonograms show their uterus to be empty. Some such women often look pregnant and will come to an obstetrician's office wearing maternity clothes. They will actually stop having menstrual periods, develop protrusion of the abdomen, have changes in their breasts, which can include fluid coming from the nipples, and have

morning sickness. They will usually claim that they feel movement in their abdomens.

I remember one woman who came to the labor and delivery unit at Jefferson Davis Hospital in Houston where I was a new student in obstetrics. She was complaining of severe contractions and convinced me she was in labor. When she was examined by physicians, they discovered that she was not even pregnant.

A physician must be very gentle with a woman in this situation. She may need counseling for the intense sadness she will experience when she is finally convinced she is not pregnant.

How Your Baby Develops

273 What is the month-by-month development of my baby inside the uterus?

The growth of your baby is a rapid, miraculous, fascinating process. The chart of fetal development below is only a broad outline of the amazing

Growth

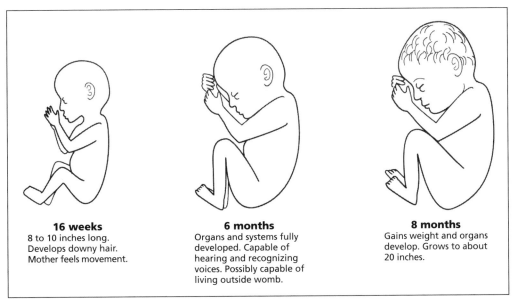

16 weeks
8 to 10 inches long. Develops downy hair. Mother feels movement.

6 months
Organs and systems fully developed. Capable of hearing and recognizing voices. Possibly capable of living outside womb.

8 months
Gains weight and organs develop. Grows to about 20 inches.

pattern of growth in the uterus. It is a process that no human engineering could make happen. There is almost no process in all creation that more clearly demonstrates God's creative genius.

274 How does the placenta function during pregnancy?

The placenta begins forming during the second week after fertilization, and it normally continues to grow until the end of the pregnancy. The placenta stays attached to the uterine wall until after the birth of the baby. Then it separates and is also delivered.

When the baby is able to, it drinks some of the fluid it is floating in. This fluid is absorbed into its bloodstream. Some of the fluid passes through the intestines. The baby urinates some of it. Most of it is carried through the blood vessels into the placenta. The placenta secretes the fluid back into the uterine cavity around the baby. The baby drinks *a gallon of fluid every day* at full term.

By the time of delivery, the placenta normally weighs one to two pounds.

Monitoring Your Health during Pregnancy

275 What are the reasons for routine office visits throughout pregnancy?

Your doctor wants to be sure that your pregnancy is progressing normally. He or she checks for indications that all is well and will watch carefully for signs of any current or potential problems.

Some of the routine procedures involved in this process are:

Blood-pressure check. Your blood pressure throughout pregnancy is an important indicator; it will be checked each visit. Early detection of blood-pressure elevation allows prompt treatment

and a healthier pregnancy. One of the most common causes of poor fetal growth and fetal death is a mother's high blood pressure.

Weight. Checking your weight regularly is important for four reasons:

- Gaining too much weight makes it more difficult for you to deliver the baby, because the birth canal stores fat just as the rest of the body does.
- Gaining too much or too little weight indicates that you may not be eating a healthy diet, which is extremely important for both you and the baby.
- Excessive weight gain can indicate that you are retaining too much fluid in your body. In this event the doctor may suggest decreasing your salt intake if you tend to take in a lot of salt, and increasing your water intake.
- Failure to gain weight, or extreme weight loss, might be an indication of a health problem; if this happens, your doctor will want to determine the cause as soon as possible.

Urinalysis. Your urine will be tested for protein on each visit. If too much protein is present, you may have toxemia of pregnancy, a metabolic disorder characterized by hypertension, edema or swelling, and protein in the urine. This condition can cause several problems. (See Q. 369–378.)

Diabetes can also be detected by routine urine tests. If you are diabetic, your bloodstream is carrying too much sugar; that excess sugar will spill over into the urine and can be detected by the urinalysis. (See Q. 353–356.)

The urine exam will also test for bacteria and pus in your urine. A woman can have a urinary tract infection without having any symptoms. If such an infection is present, it can produce significant problems, such as the onset later in the pregnancy of a kidney infection that can cause premature labor. If your doctor does detect bacteria in your urine, the doctor will discuss the best treatment for this asymptomatic bacteriuria (the medical name for this condition). Normally, you will be treated for five to ten days with antibiotics. After such treatment, the infection can return.

You could need treatment several times during the pregnancy.

Blood count. The doctor will want to check your blood for anemia (the lack of the usual number of red blood cells for carrying oxygen). Many women become mildly anemic during pregnancy, and this is usually not a concern because it is often due to the red blood cells being "diluted." As pregnancy progresses, the volume of fluid in a woman's vascular system increases by 40 percent. Your doctor will usually check your blood count during pregnancy, and, if you are becoming anemic, will let you know if you need treatment or diagnostic procedures. It is because of the possibility of anemia that pregnant women are advised to take iron throughout their pregnancy. The baby does take iron from the mother and that iron needs to be replaced.

Abdominal exam. During each visit the doctor will feel your abdomen to check the location of the top of the uterus. This exam shows the size of the uterus and its monthly growth. The doctor will measure it with a tape measure, with his or her hands, or with a measuring instrument of some type, checking to see whether there is continued growth of the uterus. This tells the doctor not only if the baby is growing at the rate that it should be but also if the uterus is getting larger than it should be, indicating the possibility of twins or triplets, or excess amniotic fluid. Until after the fifth month the doctor cannot tell by an abdominal exam if there is more than one baby.

Fetal heartbeat check. The doctor will listen for the baby's heartbeat. Using a Doppler instrument, the doctor can pick up the heartbeat when the baby is about ten weeks along or he or she can hear it with a fetoscope (a stethoscope-like instrument) about the end of the fifth month. By the way, the heartbeat cannot indicate the baby's sex. If someone tells you the sex of your baby based on its heartbeat, he or she is just guessing.

Check for swelling. The doctor will usually check your legs for swelling. The presence of swelling is not especially significant, as long as your blood pressure is normal and you do not have any protein (albumin) in your urine. Swelling is usually a normal part of pregnancy, but it can be associated with toxemia. (For suggestions on dealing with it, see Q. 266.)

Pelvic exam. Although the doctor probably did a pelvic exam on your initial visit to the office, he or she may want to do another on the next visit or two to make sure that your uterus is growing as it should.

If you are having any bleeding, a pelvic exam will often be done to make sure the cervix is not dilating. Early dilation of the cervix can be a forewarning of miscarriage or premature labor.

During the last month the doctor will usually do a pelvic exam each time (every week) you come to the office. These exams will indicate if the baby is coming headfirst or bottom first (breech), or if the cervix is dilating and effacing (thinning out), a sign that you may begin labor soon. A contraction during a pelvic exam in the last month can also be an indication that you may go into labor soon.

If the baby's head or bottom is not dropping down into the pelvis during that last month, that may be the first indication that your pelvic bones are too small and that you might need a C-section. (See Q. 560–567.) Most of the time, however, when labor actually starts, the baby does drop down.

Ultrasound. (See Q. 398–399.)

Development of a relationship with your doctor. Your obstetrician is interested in developing a good relationship with you, one that will inspire confidence on your part in his or her medical care. If this is your first baby, the doctor knows that you may be somewhat apprehensive. The relationship you build as you see him or her on frequent visits is valuable and in your best interest.

276 Are there any special problems for teenage pregnancies?

Quite definitely. Teenagers are more likely to have medical complications, partly because they often do not have the wisdom, discipline, or money to get good medical care. The children born to teenagers have a statistically greater chance of dying or having serious illnesses during their developmental years. This seems to be due primarily to the fact that teenage mothers deliver more babies prematurely than do older mothers. The low birth weight of these babies can be the cause of neurological defects, retardation, epilepsy, and cerebral palsy.

Although the problems of babies born to teenagers are often blamed on poor prenatal care, a study reported in *Southern Medical Journal* (January 1991, 84:46) by H. L. Brown and his associates, questions that. Their study showed that when a group of teenage mothers were compared to a group of adult mothers, both groups of whom had good prenatal care, there were more babies with problems in the teenage group. The teenagers had more premature deliveries and more low birth weight babies.

There is mounting evidence that premature labor is often caused by bacterial vaginosis and trichomoniasis (common STDs, see Q. 343 and 605). Studies have recently shown that treatment of these infections with antibiotics can decrease the chance of premature labor.

Hopefully, young people will learn that they can abstain from intercourse until marriage. This will not only decrease the number of pregnant single young women but also STDs that can hurt a pregnancy. (See Q. 111–115.)

In the meantime, however, we can help teenagers through pregnancies and deliveries with good obstetrical care. Therefore, to help them avoid serious or fatal consequences for themselves and their babies, these young girls must see a physician regularly during pregnancy and be serious in observing the guidelines that the physician gives them. (See Q. 107–109.)

Multiple Births

277 What is a multiple pregnancy, and how is one detected?

When we use the term *multiple pregnancy*, we are talking about pregnancies with two, three, or more babies. As the doctor follows you in your preg-

nancy, he or she will not automatically assume that you have only one baby, although that is most likely. Twins are much less common than one-baby pregnancies, and pregnancies of more than two babies less common than twins. The natural incidence of twins in pregnancy is about one per hundred and of triplets about one in eight thousand. New treatments for infertility, however, have dramatically increased the number of multiple pregnancies in technically advanced countries around the world.

If you are pregnant with more than one baby, your doctor may notice that your uterus seems larger than it should be for the length of time you have been pregnant. This is almost never obvious during the first three or four months of pregnancy. It is usually during the fifth to sixth months of pregnancy that the doctor might notice that your uterus is larger than it should be. You or your friends may start commenting that you look as though you are ready to deliver any time.

If you are carrying twins, you may feel a great deal of activity in the uterus, with lots of kicking in all directions. This, of course, is not a certain sign of twins; a very active baby can make you think you are carrying half a dozen! Some women feel that kicking in two different places might indicate twins, but this is not necessarily true, either. One baby can kick the lower uterus with its feet and butt its head up against the top of the uterus just as actively as though there were two babies.

Patients often ask their doctor if two heartbeats are audible. Much of the time it is impossible to tell whether there is more than one baby just by listening to the heartbeats. With great care, and with two people listening at the same time, it is possible to tell a difference, but this is a more difficult way to identify a multiple pregnancy. If the listening is done with two different Doppler instruments and the heart rates are distinctly different from each other, the diagnosis of twins can often be made.

The most reliable method for determining a multiple pregnancy is with an ultrasound machine. Because it is important to know if a twin pregnancy exists, some doctors feel that every pregnant woman should be scanned at about the fifth month. I feel that eventually every pregnant woman will have such a scan at least once during her pregnancy. This would detect multiple pregnancy as well as some congenital abnormalities.

An X-ray, too, can detect a multiple pregnancy, but this is not reliable until the fourth to fifth month, when the baby starts depositing calcium in its bones. With the presence of ultrasound scans, however, the use of X-ray for this purpose is not needed, and certainly all unnecessary X-rays are to be avoided. If you are in a community where ultrasound is not available, one or two X-rays to detect a multiple pregnancy will probably not hurt the baby (or babies).

278 Is it more dangerous to be pregnant with two or more babies? If so, how would my pregnancy be handled differently than if I were carrying only one baby?

There is a greater risk to your babies if you are carrying twins, triplets, or more babies in your uterus. There is a greater chance of one or both of your babies dying, and there is a greater chance that they will have an abnormality. In an article in the *Bulletin of the New York Academy of Science* (1990, 66:618), John L. Kiely points out that almost all of the problems of multiple births are caused by low birth weight and premature delivery. This offers some assurance because we know what to do during the pregnancy to increase the chance of the babies being normal.

It is important that you eat more than if you were having only one baby. Your diet needs to be even better balanced. You need to take more iron and probably need at least 1 mg of folic acid a day.

If you have a twin pregnancy, you also need to rest more. The benefit of bed rest is not totally proven, but most physicians feel that if a woman will get more rest, especially during the last half of her pregnancy, she will have a greater chance of having bigger babies and of carrying the pregnancy longer.

Your doctor will probably want to see you more often during your pregnancy if you are carrying two. One reason for this is that toxemia develops more often and more severely in women who have a multiple pregnancy. Your doctor will watch you carefully for high blood pressure, swelling, and protein in your urine. He or she will also want to do pelvic examinations earlier and then more often in your pregnancy to see if your cervix is dilating. If it is, he or she may want you to have even more bed rest.

Your doctor will also watch the growth of your uterus to be sure there are no signs of growth retardation. This will require more frequent office visits during the last half of your pregnancy. Several sonograms may be helpful to observe for adequacy of growth.

Most authorities agree that it is important for you to find out as early as possible in your pregnancy whether or not you are carrying a multiple pregnancy. The sooner you know, the better able you and your doctor are to insure that you get the care required for a healthy pregnancy and delivery. I recommend a transvaginal ultrasound scan if there is any question of whether or not you are carrying more than one baby (see Q. 398–399). A study done by A. Saari-Kemppainen and others (*Lancet*, 336–87, 1990) shows that if twins are diagnosed before the twenty-first week of pregnancy, the chance of one of the babies dying during the pregnancy or at delivery was less than one-half the chance when the twin pregnancy was not discovered earlier.

279 Is a normal vaginal delivery or a cesarean section the best method of delivery for twins?

The answer to that question is determined by so many factors that it is impossible to give a universal answer.

Some physicians feel that if either of the twins is going to be less than three and a half pounds, they should be delivered by cesarean section, but Dr. Kiely's study (see Q. 278) did not show that a cesarean section improved the health of the babies. However, if a woman is pregnant with twins, there is a greater possibility of her needing to have a cesarean section for other reasons. What it comes down to is this: The form of delivery depends on the desires of the mother, the judgment of the doctor, and the available medical facilities.

Occasionally, and rightly, a doctor delivers the first baby through the vagina, discovers at that point that the second baby might have problems, and decides to do a cesarean section for its delivery.

As a matter of interest regarding the vaginal delivery of twins, the first baby (twin A) is born headfirst 75 percent of the time; the second baby (twin B) is born headfirst 53 percent of the time.

280 How are twins produced? How often are they identical?

Twins result from two types of development.

Identical twins. About one-third of the time twins are identical. These twins result from the fertilization of one egg that divides into two different parts early in its development, with each part becoming a child. Though the two babies come from one embryo and often look almost identical, they do not have identical cells in their bodies. Even the earliest cells are different to some extent from each other. Recent studies (Dermon et al.) reported that the number of identical twins is higher among infertility patients who have been given drugs to stimulate ovulation. This means, of course, that both fraternal and identical twins are more common when fertility drugs are taken.

Nonidentical twins (fraternal twins). Twins of this

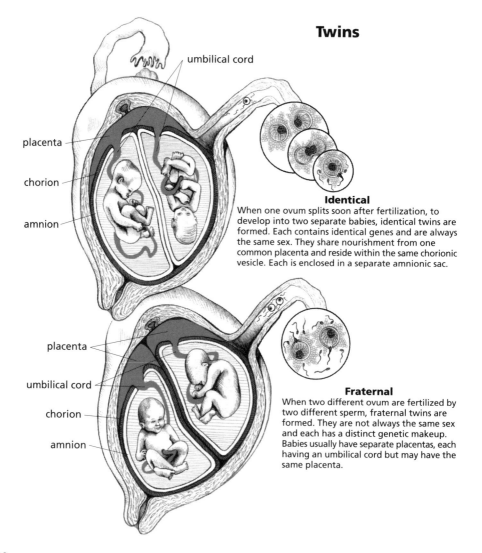

Twins

umbilical cord

placenta

chorion

amnion

Identical
When one ovum splits soon after fertilization, to develop into two separate babies, identical twins are formed. Each contains identical genes and are always the same sex. They share nourishment from one common placenta and reside within the same chorionic vesicle. Each is enclosed in a separate amnionic sac.

placenta

umbilical cord

chorion

amnion

Fraternal
When two different ovum are fertilized by two different sperm, fraternal twins are formed. They are not always the same sex and each has a distinct genetic makeup. Babies usually have separate placentas, each having an umbilical cord but may have the same placenta.

Bearing a Child

type are the result of two separate eggs fertilized by two different sperm. After fertilization, these eggs grow as nonidentical twins. This type of twinning is most common, occurring in about two-thirds of all twins. These babies, of course, can be just as different from each other as any two nontwin children of the same parents can be.

Multiple birth of triplets (or more) may also occur as identical or fraternal babies, or even as a combination of both, but they are usually all fraternal.

281 If there are twins in our family, am I likely to have them? Do twins "skip" generations?

If there are twins in your husband's family, there may be a slightly increased chance of your having twins.

If you are a twin, your chance of having twins is approximately twice that of a woman who is not a twin. One study showed that women who were fraternal twins were likely to give birth to twins at the rate of one in fifty-eight. (Normal is about one in a hundred to a hundred fifty.)

One interesting finding is that the older you are, or the more babies you have had, the more likely you are to have twins. One study in Sweden showed that women having babies were twice as likely to have twins with their fourth pregnancy than with their first.

282 What are the chances of having more than two babies?

The natural occurrence of multiple births more than twins is so uncommon that the subject is barely mentioned in one of the major textbooks of obstetrics commonly used in this country. The chance of a woman having triplets is about one in 8,000 and the chance of quadruplets is about one in 700,000 pregnancies.

For infertility patients using drugs to cause ovulation, however, the statistics are quite different. Women who use clomiphene to ovulate have a 10 percent chance of conceiving twins, rather than the normal 1 percent chance. The chance of their having triplets is 0.5 percent, and there is 0.3 percent chance of conceiving four or more babies.

In my own infertility practice, only one patient taking clomiphene got pregnant with triplets in the past twenty-four years, in spite of my frequent prescription of clomiphene.

Clomiphene is not the fertility drug that causes most of the multiple births you hear about. The drugs that cause three- to six-baby pregnancies are usually Pergonal, Metrodin, or similar drugs. The most recent techniques of administering these drugs are making pregnancies of more than triplets much less common than in the past, however.

Women who conceive by in vitro fertilization (test-tube-baby techniques) also have an increased chance of a multiple pregnancy. (For complete information on fertility drugs and techniques, see chapter 11.)

283 I have heard the term "selective termination." What is that?

See Q. 875.

Miscarriage

284 What is a miscarriage and how often does it occur?

Miscarriage is the term laypeople use to describe the spontaneous ending of a pregnancy before the twentieth week of pregnancy. Medical personnel call this a spontaneous abortion. Abortion actually means the end of a pregnancy, either by an abortionist or by miscarriage, before the twentieth week of pregnancy. (See Q. 169.)

Miscarriages occur in 10–20 percent of pregnancies that are far enough along for a woman to know that she is pregnant. Now that pregnancies can be diagnosed so early by serum pregnancy tests and ultrasound scans, we know that miscarriages actually occur much more often than 20 percent of the time. A study done by Dr. D. Keith Edmonds at South Hampton General Hospital in England showed that 62 percent of all pregnancies were lost within the first twelve weeks of pregnancy! Most of these, of course, occurred before the mother was even aware that she was pregnant. These early pregnancies, and their loss, were detected with serum pregnancy tests. Many other studies confirm this information with the range of pregnancy loss from 50 percent to 70 percent.

What this means is that you may "lose" many fertilized eggs, pregnancies that you will never know about. According to Nathan Kase, M.D., of Mount Sinai Medical Center in New York City, this loss of fertilized eggs is probably due to defects in either the egg or the sperm that would prevent normal development of the baby.

Women often ask me if the heavy periods they are having each month are miscarriages. This is most unlikely. If the pregnancy is in its very early stage at the time you lose it, whether before or at the time of your period, you would probably not notice any unusual bleeding or change in menstrual flow. Even though this could happen, it is highly unlikely it would occur every month.

285 What might cause the miscarriage of an established pregnancy, one the mother is aware of or that is several weeks along?

The cause can be due to abnormal hormones (about 23 percent); an abnormality of the uterus that "squeezes the pregnancy out" (about 15 percent); abnormalities of the baby (25 percent); and unknown reasons (about 37 percent).

Among the reasons for a woman to have a miscarriage are problems that we know cause miscarriages but about which we cannot give precise percentages. These include smoking or alcohol consumption by the mother or father or infections such as from sexually transmitted diseases, toxoplasmosis, and cytomegalic inclusion disease.

286 How will I know if I am having a miscarriage? What should I do if I think I am?

Vaginal bleeding may be the first indication of a miscarriage. Occasionally there will also be cramping. If you begin to bleed, call your doctor. He or she will probably want to examine you. If you are not bleeding heavily and are not cramping, you may be asked to wait until the next morning to come to the office for an exam.

Less than half of the pregnant women who bleed in early pregnancy actually miscarry. Pregnant women will bleed occasionally at the time they would have had a menstrual period, and sometimes each month for several months during the first part of their pregnancy. This bleeding is often implantation bleeding, meaning that as the placenta is "eating its way" into the wall of your uterus to implant itself, it causes bleeding. This invasion of the uterine wall is necessary for a normal pregnancy because the placenta must implant itself to provide food and oxygen for the baby.

Significant bleeding in the early part of pregnancy (the first three months) is often referred to by obstetricians as a threatened abortion. Bleeding as heavy or heavier than a normal period, will often be given this name because it frequently ends as a miscarriage. If you do not miscarry, the bleeding will not have hurt your baby. This bleeding is not from inside the sac where the baby is located. It comes from the area between the placenta and the wall of the uterus. So do not worry about the baby if your pregnancy continues. Just be thankful that your bleeding stopped and that you did not miscarry.

If you should begin bleeding in the middle three months (midtrimester) of your pregnancy, when you have had no bleeding before, let your doctor know immediately. This slight bleeding, with perhaps mild cramping, may be a sign that there is a problem with the pregnancy. (See Q. 294, 384.)

287 What might my doctor advise if he or she thinks I am threatening to miscarry?

First, your doctor will do a pelvic exam to see if you are already miscarrying. He or she would see tissue being squeezed out of your cervix if you are. If you are not miscarrying, your doctor will probably want you to have an ultrasound examination to make sure you have a live baby in your uterus (if you are far enough along for an ultrasound to detect that). Occasionally, a repeat sonogram is necessary about a week later. If the ultrasound indicates that you do not have a good pregnancy, the doctor may recommend that you have a D&C.

If you have a live baby in your uterus, your doctor will probably advise you to stay in bed for two or three days and get up only to use the bathroom. He or she will often suggest that you not have intercourse until about a week after the bleeding has stopped.

Unless it is felt that you have a hormone deficiency, most doctors will not want you to take any hormones. Hormones do not help prevent miscarriage, except where there is a definite hormone inadequacy.

If you continue to bleed after resting for several days, my feeling is that you may as well get up and go on about your business. If the pregnancy is healthy, it will probably "stay" whether or not you get up and return to normal activities. If it is not a healthy pregnancy, losing it is inevitable and bed rest will not prevent your losing it.

If after bed rest you still have slight bleeding (only an occasional change of your pad), and you are not cramping, your doctor will probably allow you to increase your activities, provided your bleeding does not increase when you resume normal activities.

Even if there is increased bleeding and cramping, there is nothing more the doctor can do. If you have increasingly heavy bleeding, especially with significant cramping, you are probably going to miscarry soon. If your water breaks (amniotic fluid surrounds the fetus even in the first few months of pregnancy, and this small bag can break, resulting in a gush of fluid), this means you will definitely miscarry. Call your doctor immediately.

288 What will the doctor do if it is certain I am going to miscarry or have already partially miscarried?

Once it is established that you are miscarrying, your doctor may do a D&C, dilatation of the cervix and curettage (scraping) of the uterus. The material inside your uterus is already degenerating; if it is not removed or spontaneously comes out, it can cause heavy bleeding or infection. An infection in the uterus can cause scarring and damage to the uterus and the fallopian tubes, which could limit your future ability to get pregnant. With new and improved suction apparatus, many doctors now are doing the curettage on an outpatient basis or in their offices.

However, if your miscarriage occurs only a few days past your first missed period, your uterus is very small, you are not bleeding much, and you are not passing too much tissue, you may not need a D&C. Frequently, even if it appears that you have had a "complete" miscarriage, there may be continued spotting and bleeding for many days. If this goes on for more than a few days, it is probably best for you to have a D&C of the uterus to remove any remaining tissue.

You may be surprised by the slow recovery you might have after a miscarriage is over. Although there will not usually be much physical pain, even if you had a D&C, hormonal changes will often make you feel tired and weak for about a month. In addition, the emotional impact of losing a pregnancy will often add to your tiredness.

I generally recommend to patients that they not start exercising until they feel energetic enough to do so.

You may continue to bleed for up to a month. When the bleeding stops, it is okay to start having intercourse again. When you do resume intercourse, I recommend using contraception until normal periods are reestablished (one or two months) before trying to conceive again.

One important thing that is very easy for both you and your physician to forget is administering Rh immune globulin (Rho-GAM) if you are Rh negative and your husband is Rh positive. You need this even if you have a tubal pregnancy. This will keep you from developing Rh antibodies that could affect future pregnancies.

If you have other questions about recovery from miscarriage, be sure to ask your doctor.

289 How is it determined that my miscarriages are chromosomally abnormal, or that I or my husband have abnormal chromosomes? What can we do?

Tissue from a miscarriage can be examined by a laboratory for chromosome abnormalities. This evaluation is not frequently done, as it is expensive and cannot usually determine conclusively that your next pregnancy will have the same problem. If a couple has had more than two miscarriages, however, it may be comforting to have the tissue from the next miscarriage tested for chromosomal abnormality in an attempt to determine the cause of the miscarriage. Occasionally, this testing can give guidance about further pregnancies.

If you or your husband have genetic abnormalities, you could consult a geneticist, who may recommend adoption or donor artificial insemination if the husband has the genetic problem, or egg donation with in vitro fertilization if the wife is genetically abnormal. Whether or not you follow this advice will be determined by your personal choices.

Genetic engineering is still a far-distant development. At the present time there is no way to alter genes to insure a genetically normal baby.

290 How will I know whether I am having a miscarriage or a tubal pregnancy?

This is an extremely important question, especially since the number of ectopic (tubal) pregnancies in our country has increased by about 400 percent in the past twenty years.

Because a ruptured tubal pregnancy is still the second leading cause of death among pregnant women, it is important to identify such a pregnancy very early, when the problem can be resolved safely and easily by laparoscopy. If a tubal pregnancy is not discovered in time, the tube can rupture, causing massive hemorrhage inside a woman's abdomen. (This might necessitate emergency surgery and/or a blood transfusion and could even cause death.)

For a discussion of how a tubal pregnancy is diagnosed and treated see Q. 304–310.

291 What is a "missed abortion"?

A missed abortion is a miscarriage in which the fetus dies but the uterus does not expel the pregnancy tissue immediately. Before ultrasound was available, it was thought this happened only occasionally. Now we know that in many pregnancies the fetus stops growing and dies and a woman will not start bleeding or cramping until much later. Without ultrasound, she would not have known for several weeks that the pregnancy was not still growing in a normal way. She would be unaware of the condition until she finally started the typical bleeding of a miscarriage.

If a woman has a missed abortion, she will often stop being nauseated (if she has been having morning sickness) and, although she may not know it, her uterus will stop growing. She may even lose a little weight. If the woman feels that something is wrong or that the pregnancy is not progressing, or if the doctor determines that the uterus is not growing, an ultrasound (sonogram) will probably be ordered.

If the sonogram shows that the fetus has died, the doctor may want to use a suction machine to withdraw the pregnancy tissue from the uterus unless the pregnancy is very early or little tissue is present. For your health, as in the case of a "regular" miscarriage, the doctor will want to be sure that all the material is removed.

292 If I have had a previous miscarriage, will I ever be able to carry a pregnancy? Should further testing be done?

Usually after one miscarriage you do not need to have any testing to determine why you had a miscarriage. Your next pregnancy will, in all probability, be a normal pregnancy with a normal delivery.

More surprisingly, the same good chance of eventually having a baby still holds after a second miscarriage. Even if you have had four miscarriages in a row, you still have a 60 percent chance of having a live baby in the next pregnancy.

These statistics, though, do not mean that studies and tests on women who are having miscarriages should not be done. They should. If a woman is thirty or older and has one miscarriage, I will usually recommend some tests. When the woman is younger than thirty, I usually do not suggest any testing after one miscarriage. This is because women who are over thirty, and therefore have "less time to waste," need to be sure there is nothing wrong or get the problem treated as quickly as possible if one exists.

Women under thirty generally feel that they have a little bit more time to see how things turn out with the next pregnancy. Although statistically most women who have miscarriages will eventually have a normal pregnancy, some do have abnormalities that cause their miscarriages.

293 What does an evaluation for the problem of miscarriage involve?

Such an evaluation involves several things:

A pelvic examination is done to make sure there are no tumors, cysts, or growths in the pelvis, on the uterus, or on the ovaries.

An X-ray of the uterus (hysterosalpingogram, HSG) is done to make sure that the uterus is formed properly. A uterus with a septum can abort a pregnancy, even though the baby and placenta may be healthy.

A general evaluation for existing or potential medical problems is made. For example, thyroid disease, diabetes, and collagen-vascular diseases such as lupus erythematosus should be looked for because they can cause miscarriage.

A D&C and diagnostic laparoscopy may be done to guarantee the absence of pelvic disease, endometriosis, or severe pelvic adhesions that might cause miscarriage.

The presence of infection must be considered. Spontaneous abortion has been associated with syphilis, toxoplasmosis, cytomegalic inclusion disease, listeriosis, herpes, ureaplasm, and chlamydia. Although tests for these organisms are possible, laboratories frequently will not find them even when they are present. To avoid that possibility, I usually treat a patient who has repeated miscarriages with a tetracycline or erythromycin antibiotic.

Testing for inadequate hormones is done, using a basal body thermometer, or a test to measure the progesterone in the bloodstream, or an endometrial biopsy. If a patient seems to have inadequate hormone production in the last half of her menstrual cycle (the luteal phase), progesterone vaginal suppositories can be used to try to correct the problem and prevent further miscarriages.

Chromosome testing on the mother and the father may be considered, because if either has abnormal chromosomes and cannot produce normal eggs or sperm, this can result in a baby that is abnormal enough to be miscarried. The testing is expensive, but I think it is sometimes important. If it does show an abnormality, the couple then has an answer to their problem and can consult with a genetic counselor.

Abnormal antibodies in your body. If a woman has repeated early spontaneous miscarriages, she may have some forms of abnormal antibodies in her body. These are anticardiolipin antibodies of which lupus anticoagulant antibody is one. Your doctor should test you for these antibodies (a simple blood test) if you have repeat miscarriages and can tell you about the treatments that are available.

Immunologic testing, which is still under research, is a new approach to this problem. It would normally be done only as a last resort. If, after every other type of testing has been done and no cause for repeated miscarriage is found, a couple can check into the problem of histo-compatibility between mother and baby. The mother's body must protect the baby from her own antibodies. Remember that the baby is 50 percent from the father, and the mother's body would ordinarily consider the baby a "foreign substance," like a splinter in her finger, for example. Her body would rally forces against the baby, bring antibodies, white blood cells, and other defenses in an attempt to expel it. This does not normally occur, however, because the mother's body produces "blocking antibodies" that prevent this type of rejection. If a woman does not have enough blocking antibodies, her body will expel her baby—the "foreign" substance—from her body. Research in this area is gradually progressing from the theoretical to the practical. Researchers inject women with their husband's white blood cells to build up enough antibodies in the woman to allow a normal pregnancy to progress. Further information on this subject can be obtained by contacting Dr. Alan E. Beer at the University of Health Sciences, The Chicago Medical School, 3333 Green Bay Road, North Chicago, IL 60064. If you do not live in that area, his office may be able to refer you to someone in your section of the country who is working on this type of immunologic study.

All these tests are usually not necessary for every patient. I would do part of the testing if a woman over thirty miscarries once and wants to undergo the testing. If a woman is under thirty, and has had two miscarriages or more, I would suggest some of the testing.

294 What is a midtrimester loss of pregnancy, and what might cause it?

A midtrimester pregnancy loss is loss of the pregnancy during the middle three months; it is much less likely to happen than loss of pregnancy in the first three months. If a pregnancy loss occurs this far along, a medical evaluation should be done.

Some of the things this evaluation might reveal include an abnormal uterus; a fibroid tumor in the uterus; or an incompetent cervical os (cervix not strong enough to hold the pregnancy). (See Q. 384.)

If an incompetent cervical os exists, it would be wise for you to have a minor operation, a cerclage procedure, either before or during your next pregnancy. In this operation a suture is put around your cervix in purse-string fashion to keep the cervix closed.

If an abnormal uterus (tumor, structural abnormality, scarring inside) is discovered, you should have the problem corrected surgically. This can usually be accomplished by a simple outpatient procedure called hysteroscopic surgery. (See Q. 689, 823.)

Although most pregnancy loss in the middle three months are due to abnormalities of the structure of the uterus, approximately 25 percent of them are due to abnormalities of the baby's chromosomes. In this situation the abnormalities are not severe enough to cause early miscarriage but may cause loss of the pregnancy before it reaches full term.

295 Can chromosome abnormalities cause loss of pregnancy in the last three months also?

Yes. This is much less common, causing only about 5 percent of the pregnancies lost during the last three months. If a baby is chromosomally abnormal, it is common for it to deliver so early that it dies of both its prematurity and its abnormalities. If it is not born too prematurely it will, of course, be born as an abnormal child. Examples of this are babies with Down syndrome or Turner's syndrome.

296 Is it normal for me to feel so emotional about my miscarriage?

Yes, definitely, since you have experienced, in effect, the death of a child you loved and wanted to hold. Your sense of loss may remain for the rest of your life.

A miscarriage is often treated by friends and medical personnel as "just one of those things"; something that is not as major as you feel that it is. Many women, however, have had miscarriages themselves. They know how you feel, whether or not they can express their empathy.

It is especially normal to feel sad on the day your child would have been born if you had not miscarried, especially the first time that date occurs. Knowing this can help you and your husband prepare for it.

There is an especially helpful book that I recommend: *When Pregnancy Fails—Families Coping with Miscarriage, Stillbirth, and Infant Death* by Borg and Lasker (Boston: Beacon Press, 1981).

There are support groups (SHARE) for couples who have suffered miscarriages, stillbirth, or neonatal death (or loss). For more information write:

Pregnancy & Infant Loss Support, Inc.,
National SHARE Headquarters
St. Joseph Health Center
300 First Capitol Drive
St. Charles, MO 63301-2893
Phone: (800) 821-6819
Fax: (314) 947-7486

If you continue to find yourself emotionally torn by your miscarriage, see a counselor. Your intense feelings do not mean that you are abnormal. A counselor can often help you, sometimes with just one or two visits.

297 What can I say to help a friend who has had a miscarriage?

The following excellent suggestions by Leslie Snodgrass were published in *Stepping Stones*, an infertility newsletter (Wichita, Kansas, October 1982).

1. Don't avoid a loved one who is hurting simply because you're afraid you won't know what to say! The Lord gives us grace and wisdom for each moment (see Exod. 4:12), and the feeling of being alone and forgotten during such a difficult time only adds insult to injury.

2. Don't assume your friend doesn't want to talk about it! Chances are, she probably does. I have found that talking about it, reliving the details, helps the person to face the reality of the loss and this is an integral part of the healing process. You can't *assume* she *does* want to talk either, so you must be sensitive to what she says (or doesn't say).

3. If she does want to talk about it, let her! Often, those with the best intentions find themselves filling in an awkward moment by recounting their own personal tragedies, blurting out suggestions or throwing out scriptural reminders without allowing the person in need to get a word in edgewise. *Listening* is the key word; in doing so, you'll be able to learn what your friend's special need is. (What is she having trouble coping with—the loss itself, why God allowed it to happen, whether she did something wrong, whether it is wrong to be angry, etc.?)

4. Don't assume you have all the answers to her questions (or feel inadequate if you don't)! You may not have the answer because the Lord wants your friend to find it in Him. Miscarriage or loss of a child often leads one to feel alone (even with a multitude of family and friends), or abandoned, or even angry. The insatiable need to know the "why" to a myriad of questions will draw her into the arms of the only Person with the answers which give relief to the pain.

5. Do remind her she's loved and being thought of often! You don't have to camp on her doorstep to show her you care. Besides being physically worn-out, she needs time alone, too. Pray for creative ways to show her you care; for example, a ready-to-heat meal is a blessing after a stay in the hospital. A flower stuck in the mailbox with a note attached is a pleasant surprise,

or what about a series of unsigned post-cards with comforting Scriptures?

6. Don't use clichés! They may or may not be true, but more often than not they come out sounding callous and insensitive. For example:

> a. "It's probably for the best." To someone whose hopes and dreams for a child have just been shattered, no matter what the reason, it's hard to believe it could be for the best. (While it may be true, it's a statement that hurts more than helps.)
>
> b. "You're young, you'll be able to have more." Again, it probably is true, but the fact is that even if more children do come along, it doesn't mean the one lost didn't mean as much. Just because it was a life unborn, didn't mean it was any less a life already loved and cherished.
>
> c. "Don't give up, I have a friend who lost two, but then carried a baby full term." This is meant to be hopeful, but what it says is "be glad, it could be worse." It is true, I'm sure, but it also says that the pain they just endured could very possibly happen again. Hurt isn't minimized by comparison. It's a concept that works well in theory but not in practice. Your friend is trying hard to overcome her own grief—she doesn't need to try to work through someone else's!
>
> d. "Time will take care of it." Time may heal the wound, but the memory will probably last forever. I lost my baby three years ago, and have been blest with a beautiful daughter since, but I haven't forgotten.

7. Do continue to be sensitive to your friend's loss in the months that follow. In my own case, it took a while for the initial shock to wear off and when it did, I was left with an incredible emptiness. I needed to be constantly reminded that the Lord loved me, and that He hadn't forgotten me. My loss was more difficult because I knew how long it had taken me to get pregnant, and it took several years to get pregnant again.

Special friends and family continued to pray, and I was sustained by those prayers.

Molar Pregnancy

298 What is a molar pregnancy?

Molar pregnancies, invasive molar pregnancies, and malignant molar pregnancies are growths that result from abnormal pregnancies referred to as trophoblastic diseases. Doctors often use the term *mole* to describe some of these problems; this has nothing whatever to do with a mole on the surface of the skin. The term *trophoblastic disease* is derived from the name of the trophoblast cell, the cell that makes up the placenta.

"Molar pregnancy" is the informal term for what doctors call hydatidiform mole: an abnormal pregnancy in which there is no baby, just an abnormal placenta. As it grows, segments of the placenta (chorionic villi) swell into cloudy, grape-like structures. Often all the chorionic villi change into these cystic structures. When this happens, the uterus becomes literally filled with hundreds of these small, fluid-filled sacs. These little growths are shaped like green seedless grapes and are often about the same size.

About half the time a molar pregnancy results in an apparently normal miscarriage. When this happens, treatment would be the same as with a normal miscarriage. Unless you were told, you would not know that you had had a molar pregnancy instead of the more usual type of miscarriage.

The 50 percent of women who do not miscarry a molar pregnancy may have other problems that indicate an abnormal pregnancy. They may have bleeding; the uterus may get larger faster than it should, indicating development of the molar cysts; or it may not grow as fast as would be expected. When a pregnancy seems to be developing in an abnormal fashion, the doctor will ordinarily order an ultrasound scan. This scan can usually show that a hydatidiform mole is present.

The molar tissue produces large amounts of the pregnancy hormone called HCG (human chorionic gonadotrophin), the hormone that causes a positive pregnancy test. HCG normally stimulates the ovaries, but when it is present in large amounts, it overstimulates them. Because of this, women who have molar pregnancies will often develop cysts on their ovaries. These cysts are not dangerous. They are not growths, and they do not need to be removed.

The cysts will shrink when the molar tissues are removed from the uterus and the HCG returns to the normal low levels.

In addition to this problem, molar tissue tends to make women who have molar pregnancies also have toxemia with its associated high blood pressure, or they may also become hyperthyroid.

Molar pregnancies are not extremely rare. They occur in about one out of every two thousand pregnancies in the United States. Each country, strangely, seems to have its own rate for this problem. Some countries have fewer cases and some have more cases than the United States.

299 How is a molar pregnancy treated?

If your molar pregnancy shows up as a miscarriage, a D&C would be done. If your molar pregnancy was discovered by ultrasound because the pregnancy was not growing properly, the doctor would probably give you general anesthesia and use a suction machine to curette the tissue from your uterus.

After the molar pregnancy has been removed from your uterus, the doctor will want to do blood tests for human chorionic gonadotrophin (HCG). See also the discussion about therapy for malignant moles, Q. 301–303. Immediately after the D&C is done, the doctor will order an HCG test. HCG is produced by the cells of a molar pregnancy. From then on, you will probably have an HCG test every week until you have had three consecutive normal tests. Following that you should have an HCG test every month for six months, and then every other month for six more months to make sure all abnormal tissue is gone from your body.

If your HCG level stops falling and stays the same for three consecutive weeks, or if it starts rising, you need to be treated with chemotherapy, just as does a woman who has a malignant mole. You should have normal HCG levels three to four months after having had the D&C, but it may take several months for the HCG levels to return to normal. Your doctor should follow your HCG levels if you have had a molar pregnancy.

300 What is invasive molar pregnancy?

An invasive mole (*chorioadenoma destruens*) is a condition that is halfway between a molar pregnancy and a true malignant mole. The molar tissue often grows into the muscle of the wall of the uterus, but under the microscope the cells do not look like malignant molar cells.

For the placenta to implant itself in the wall of the uterus to establish a normal pregnancy, it must be able to invade the mother's uterine wall. When trophoblasts start growing abnormally, however, they can become invasive, even highly invasive.

The molar growth that has become mildly invasive requires chemotherapy. Occasionally, but rarely, a hysterectomy might be necessary because the growth may perforate the uterine wall and cause bleeding.

301 What is a malignant molar pregnancy?

A malignant mole is called a choriocarcinoma. This is a condition in which the trophoblastic cells have become cancerous. A malignant mole starts growing (only in women who are or have been pregnant), and can occur after a molar or normal pregnancy. It can also occur after a miscarriage or after a tubal pregnancy. Although this type of growth always starts with a pregnancy, it may not be detected until many months after a pregnancy is over. I realize that this is confusing; it also confuses physicians. One of my patients was found to have a choriocarcinoma growing in her lungs months after a normal pregnancy. She had been admitted to the hospital for tiredness, and a chest X-ray showed the growth.

This malignancy of the trophoblastic cells is the most invasive type of cancer that can occur in humans. If treatment is delayed, or if a woman does not respond to proper treatment, this can be a truly devastating malignancy. Before treatment was available, almost everyone with this cancer died very quickly. On the other hand, because the cells of this tumor grow so fast (much faster than normal cells), they are more responsive to chemotherapy than most other cancer cells; the cure rate with chemotherapy is almost 100 percent, better than with any other solid tumor that can spread in the body.

302 How would I be treated if I had a malignant molar pregnancy?

Treatment is with chemotherapeutic drugs. You would be referred to a specialist in the use of these drugs. He or she would discuss with you which drugs you need and what their side effects are.

Your doctor would want you to have blood tests done frequently to see how much tumor was left in your body during each step of the treatment. Remember that placental cells, even those of malignant molar tissue, produce the hormone human chorionic gonadotrophin (HCG). This is the hormone identified by a pregnancy test. (See Q. 250.) The production of HCG by only a few thousand placental or molar cells can be detected with the test. The doctor would want to keep treating you and testing you until all signs of HCG and the choriocarcinoma were eliminated from your body.

If your doctor does not test for HCG on a regular, organized basis during your treatment, he or she does not understand how to care for this type of tumor. In this situation you should seek further consultation. I suggest that you phone a cancer hospital, such as M. D. Anderson Cancer Hospital in Houston, Texas, and talk with one of the physicians in the department of gynecology.

It is essential that you be treated promptly and properly. If this type of tumor is allowed to grow for very long, it can be irreversible.

303 If I have had a molar pregnancy, should I avoid future pregnancies?

You must not become pregnant until your HCG levels have stayed in the normal range for about one year. It is best that you use birth-control pills to prevent pregnancy until such normal test results have been obtained. Birth-control pills will not affect the test result. Once the tests have become normal and stayed normal, you should consult with your physician about the advisability of pregnancy. Generally, if you have had a hydatidiform mole or invasive molar pregnancy, you may become pregnant once the tests have stayed normal for more than a year. If you have had a choriocarcinoma, a pregnancy may be allowed after an extended length of time. The decision about getting pregnant again must be made after consultation with your physician.

Ectopic Pregnancy

304 What is an ectopic pregnancy and how often does it occur?

An ectopic pregnancy is a pregnancy that develops anywhere outside of the uterus. About 2 percent of pregnancies are ectopic, and the rate is increasing rapidly.

Ectopic pregnancies occur in the fallopian tube 95 percent of the time. The remaining 5 percent may be in an ovary, in the abdominal cavity, or in the cervix.

Ectopic pregnancies are the second most common cause of death among pregnant women; and there is an alarming epidemic of ectopic pregnancy in the United States. The Centers for Disease Control (CDC) *Morbidity and Mortality Weekly Report* (1990, 39:401) outlines the astounding increase in ectopic pregnancies since 1970. In 1970, there were about five ectopic pregnancies per thousand pregnancies. In 1987, there were almost eighteen ectopic pregnancies per thousand pregnancies.

This almost fourfold increase in the rate of ectopic pregnancies is not only causing more deaths, but it also indicates how much infertility women are experiencing. Tubal pregnancies compound the problem of infertility, because they often damage or destroy a woman's fallopian tubes.

305 Why do ectopic pregnancies occur, and why are they increasing?

Ectopic pregnancies can be caused by abnormalities of the tube due to infection, congenital abnormalities, inability of the tube to transport the egg, or tumors. Or they may result from failure of the egg to get into the tube, with the egg being fertilized outside the tube.

The increased rate of ectopic pregnancies seems to be related to societal change. Changed sexual mores have produced more sexually transmitted disease (which includes infections of the uterus, ovaries, and tubes). The use of the IUD (intrauterine contraceptive device) and the number of abortions have increased. In addition, infertility treatment, such as surgery to repair damaged or blocked fallopian tubes, surgery to reverse sterilizations, and the use of fertility pills and drugs is more common. Finally, more women over thirty

are having babies. All of these factors have been shown to increase the rate of tubal pregnancies.

306 What happens with a tubal pregnancy, and is a tubal pregnancy dangerous?

The only place where a baby can safely grow to term size is in the cavity of the uterus. There is no other place in the body where a placenta can properly implant and erode its way into the surrounding tissue to gain adequate nutrition. No other place can allow adequate enlargement to hold a baby at all stages of pregnancy.

When a pregnancy begins in the fallopian tube, bleeding from that tube will soon occur. The tube can stretch only a small amount. When the tube stretches, some of the growing placenta pulls loose and bleeding starts. This damage to the placenta will often kill the fetus, but the placenta itself will often continue to grow until the tube ruptures. When this happens, massive bleeding can occur, and the mother may die before she can get to the hospital. In most cases, however, the pain the woman experiences will be so bad that it will cause her to go to the hospital in time for emergency surgery to be performed. Occasionally, when surgery is done for an ectopic tubal pregnancy, a fetus will be found, but usually none is seen.

Although 10 to 50 percent of ectopic pregnancies, if left alone, would be absorbed back into the body, it would be dangerous to allow the ec-

Ectopic Pregnancy

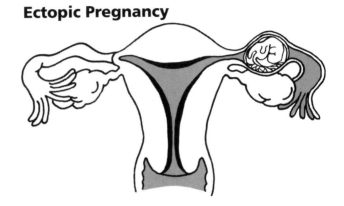

topic pregnancy to continue to see if this occurs. Tubal pregnancies that are not absorbed by the body will grow to the point where the tube ruptures, causing excessive bleeding and even death. In 1978 there were thirty-seven deaths in the United States from ectopic pregnancy, amounting to 11.5 percent of *all* deaths from pregnancy in this country.

It is most important, therefore, that as soon as an ectopic pregnancy is suspected, a definite conclusion be reached as quickly as possible as to the existence and location of the pregnancy.

307 What are the symptoms of an ectopic pregnancy?

You as a patient have a great deal of the responsibility for suspecting an ectopic pregnancy and telling your doctor about your suspicions. If you have the least sign that you might be pregnant, you and your doctor can find your ectopic pregnancy at an early stage.

Remember, you can become pregnant even if you are faithfully using good contraceptives when you have intercourse, have been infertile for years so you don't use contraceptives, or have been less than faithful in using good contraceptives. If you fit into one of these categories and your period is a few days early or late, or it comes on time but is heavier or lighter than usual, call your doctor and insist on a blood (serum) pregnancy test. Have that test even if you have no other symptoms of pregnancy. If a doctor knows you are pregnant, he or she can watch you closely for ectopic pregnancy.

Because ectopic pregnancies are frequent and can be dangerous, it is best that all women know early in pregnancy whether they are pregnant. Pregnancy tests will be positive as early as nine days into the pregnancy, regardless if it is in the uterus or an ectopic pregnancy.

The more traditional and later signs that should make you suspect an ectopic pregnancy are if you miss a menstrual period or seem to have a delayed period, and then have vaginal spotting or bleeding and pain in the lower abdomen. The flow may be heavy and the pain intense, or there may be only spotting and minimal pain. If a menstrual period is missed or was much lighter than normal, and there is a possibility of your being pregnant, contact your doctor immediately when you experience vaginal bleeding and low abdominal pain.

It is important that a diagnosis be made before a tubal rupture, if possible. An early diagnosis can prevent excessive loss of blood, and will involve a simpler operation, but, more importantly, it can prevent loss of the fallopian tube and ovary.

308 How is an ectopic pregnancy diagnosed?

The procedure for diagnosing an ectopic pregnancy has changed dramatically in the past few years. It is now possible to locate a tubal pregnancy in its early stages, which means that an ectopic pregnancy can often be found before it ruptures.

If there is a possibility that you might be pregnant and your period is even a few days late, get a pregnancy test. If your period is "different," such as lighter or heavier, get a pregnancy test. If the test is positive, and you are not having vaginal bleeding or spotting or are not having abdominal pain, you are probably carrying a normal pregnancy.

If the test is positive, and you are having a little vaginal spotting or some pelvic pain, you should see your doctor and get a quantitative HCG test to measure the amount of human chorionic gonadotrophin. About two or three days later, the test for quantitative HCG should be repeated. In a normal pregnancy the level of HCG should double every two or three days. If it does not, you may be having an early miscarriage or a tubal pregnancy.

Once the level of HCG reaches 1500 to 3000 IU/ml, a transvaginal ultrasound scan should show a pregnancy inside your uterus. If it does, the pregnancy is in the uterus, not in your fallopian tube.

If there is no sac in your uterus, you almost certainly are having a miscarriage or you have an ectopic pregnancy. First, your doctor will want to be sure you are not having a miscarriage. He or she may do a D&C and have the pathologist look at the tissue to see if you are miscarrying. If you are not, then the pregnancy must be outside the uterus. If your HCG level is high (greater than about 7000) and the sonogram doesn't show a pregnancy in your uterus, the D&C is usually unnecessary because a pregnancy in the uterus that far along would be visible. If your doctor thinks your pregnancy is in your tube he or she will want to do a laparoscopy to prevent your having a ruptured tube, or treat you with methotrexate.

Studies have shown that progesterone levels are low in miscarriages and in ectopic pregnancies. If your progesterone level is less than 5 mg/ml, you probably do not have a good pregnancy. It is either ectopic or a miscarriage. Testing for progesterone levels has not become standard practice. Other techniques are more precise.

Laparoscopy. By looking through a laparoscope at the inside of your abdomen, the doctor can see whether or not there is a tubal pregnancy. (See Q. 810.)

---

309 What will my doctor do if an ectopic pregnancy is found?

What is done depends on the doctor's training, at what point the ectopic pregnancy is discovered, and on its location.

Early tubal ectopic pregnancy. If you and your doctor have followed the plan outlined in the previous question, you will have discovered your ectopic pregnancy very early. The new standard treatment in the United States for ectopic pregnancy is a laparoscopy. The laparoscope is inserted and, using either cautery or laser, the doctor slits open the side of the fallopian tube and removes the pregnancy. Any bleeding can be stopped by gently cauterizing the edges of the incision in the tube. A patient can normally go home the day of the surgery.

When tubal ectopics are treated with laparoscopic technique, the hole in the tube is not closed with sutures. Normally, the hole will stay in the tube from then on. Such a hole does not seem to interfere with a woman's ability to get pregnant in the future. The original problem that caused the ectopic, though, can still be present and can cause another ectopic in that same tube. Studies, however, show that even after having a tubal ectopic removed with laparoscopic technique, 50 percent of tubes are still open after the laparoscopy and are healthy enough for a pregnancy to occur through that tube.

In laparoscopies done on women with early tubal pregnancies, some of the tissue attached to the tube is almost microscopic. Because of this, it is important that a woman have HCG testing every week following a tubal pregnancy to make sure all cells of pregnancy are gone.

Within two or three weeks, the HCG level should fall to less than 5 IU/ml. If it stays elevated, another laparoscopy may be necessary for removal of the tube, or treatment with methotrexate may be used to get rid of all the pregnancy tissue.

If your doctor does not follow this standard pattern of treatment for you, encourage him or her to call a gynecologist who treats ectopic pregnancy in this way. This is most important. Following this suggestion can save you from a dangerous situation. But if your doctor does not know how to do a laparoscopy, and does not have a consultant who can do one, you should allow surgery through a regular incision if a tubal pregnancy is diagnosed. Delay might endanger your life.

Early tubal ectopic pregnancies can also be treated with the chemotherapy agent methotrexate. This drug, given as an intramuscular injection, is very effective; it is now a common treatment for early tubal pregnancies. A real advantage of this treatment is that it allows the elimination of surgery.

Late tubal ectopic pregnancy. Not all tubal ectopic pregnancies are detected early. Some patients and also doctors can easily miss the significance of the early signs and symptoms of ectopic pregnancy. When these early warnings are missed, the fetus and/or placental tissue will grow until finally the tube ruptures, pouring blood into the woman's abdomen causing severe pain, weakness, fast heartbeat, even shock and death.

The doctor will proceed immediately with a major incision in the woman's abdomen to remove the fetus and/or placental tissue as quickly as possible to save her life. He or she will not even wait to get blood ready for a transfusion. When a tube ruptures, it is usually ruined. Frequently the ovary and surrounding tissues become matted together. Removal of both the tube and the ovary is occasionally necessary. When the portion of the tube affected is the part that goes through the wall of the uterus, a hole may have been blown out of the uterus at that site. This means a hysterectomy is necessary. This is, indeed, a life-or-death situation.

Ovarian ectopic pregnancy. Ovarian pregnancies do not occur very often, but when they do, they closely mimic a tubal pregnancy. The tube is not involved unless scarring and blood clots have affected it. The ovary will usually need to be removed entirely, but it is occasionally possible to save part of it.

Abdominal ectopic pregnancy. An abdominal pregnancy usually results when a tube ruptures but excessive bleeding does not occur. The placenta adheres not only to the ruptured fallopian tube but also to other organs. Surprisingly, women with abdominal pregnancies often have only mild discomfort.

Ultimately, however, the placenta will almost always cause bleeding as it grows on the intestines and other organs in the abdomen. The woman will start having pain, and the doctor will investigate. (Occasionally, a woman may go to term with the pregnancy but will fail to have contractions. This, too, will cause her doctor to investigate.) This is a very dangerous condition and requires the very best of medical care.

310 What are the long-term effects of a tubal pregnancy?

About 50 percent of those who have had ectopic pregnancies experience infertility problems later. It is usually not the ectopic pregnancy that causes the infertility, however, but the abnormality of fal-

lopian tubes that caused the ectopic pregnancy in the first place. In addition to infertility problems, there is a 20 percent chance of another ectopic pregnancy, possibly even in the other fallopian tube.

If a laparoscopy was used to remove the ectopic pregnancy, it is possible later for an egg to travel down that same tube and a pregnancy to develop normally inside the uterus.

If you are Rh negative and your husband is Rh positive, you need to receive Rh Immune Globulin (Rho-GAM).

Deep emotional response to an ectopic pregnancy is not only reasonable but also normal. First, for a pregnancy to end like this is, at the least, a disappointment. Second, you realize that an ectopic pregnancy does affect your future chance of having a normal pregnancy. Finally, you must cope with the depressing effects of anesthetics and pain medications.

If you remain depressed and distressed following a tubal pregnancy, I strongly encourage you to get counsel. Certainly you, your husband, and your doctor need to talk about the way you feel. Help is available.

General Medical Disorders during Pregnancy

311 Are there any specific medical and surgical problems related to being pregnant?

Yes. You may be more susceptible to infections in your urinary tract, but generally any medical or surgical problem that might affect you when you are not pregnant can also affect you while you are pregnant. Some of these problems can have a specific effect on your pregnancy and perhaps on your baby. Pregnancy may also worsen some existing medical problems.

In this series of questions, we will be looking at two groups of problems: those conditions that pregnancy aggravates for the mother, and those problems of the mother that may affect the baby.

312 What is the most common medical problem during pregnancy?

Infection in the urinary tract (including the bladder) is probably the most common problem during pregnancy.

Pregnancy causes the bladder to empty more slowly and drainage of urine from the kidneys is likely to be more lethargic, because of both hormonal changes and pressure of the pregnancy on the organs. Also, the urethra—the tube that empties your bladder—is short, so it is easy for germs to get from the vulva into your bladder and from there into your kidneys.

Because the urine is moving slowly, germs have more time to start growing in the urine and to cause infection. As this is a common occurrence, most doctors routinely use a chemically treated paper strip to check your urine on each office visit. This test also checks for diabetes and albumin.

When infection is found in the urinary tract, it is important that it be treated and then rechecked to be sure it has cleared up. Otherwise a kidney infection may result. A severe kidney infection (pyelonephritis) can cause premature labor.

Your doctor should not treat you with tetracycline in pregnancy (it can stain the baby's teeth and bones). It is also important that you not use sulfa drugs during the last few weeks of pregnancy. If the baby is born while you are taking sulfa, any jaundice the baby might develop in its first few days of life can be more dangerous.

313 What should I know about kidney infections?

A kidney infection (pyelonephritis) is one of the most common serious complications of pregnancy. Your doctor will usually check your urine for bacteria each time you visit the office. If germs are found in your urine, they can usually be treated before they progress to a kidney infection.

Occasionally, however, a woman will develop a kidney infection in spite of this early treatment.

If you start having fever, backache, and shaking chills, you probably have a kidney infection. Call your physician immediately and describe your symptoms. Your doctor will probably want to see you as soon as possible in an emergency room or at his or her office.

This problem is usually easy to diagnose, but it can be confused with other medical problems in pregnancy, such as appendicitis or problems in the uterus. Careful evaluation is important.

Your doctor will probably put you in the hospital and give you fluid through your veins to prevent dehydration. Antibiotics will be given in large doses through your veins to help kill the infection.

A kidney infection can cause premature labor, kidney damage, shock, and problems with blood-clotting mechanisms. If you think you might have a kidney infection, call your doctor immediately.

314 What is anemia? Why is it so frequently a problem during pregnancy?

Anemia merely means that you have a low concentration of hemoglobin, the compound in each of your red blood cells that makes blood red and carries oxygen. Normally, you should have 12 grams (or more) of hemoglobin per 100 ml of blood. A little more than 10 percent of your blood, therefore, is made up of hemoglobin. It is normal for pregnant women to be slightly anemic because the increased amount of fluid in the blood-vessel system dilutes the hemoglobin, making the actual count a little lower than twelve.

Almost all doctors recommend that their patients take iron during pregnancy. Since the baby absorbs iron from the mother's bloodstream, the mother should take supplemental iron to replace that loss.

If a mother is deficient in folic acid, she will not be able to make enough hemoglobin even if she has adequate iron in her system. For this reason, almost all prenatal vitamins contain some folic acid. If you develop a significant anemia in spite of taking adequate iron and folic acid, you need to see a hematologist, a specialist in problems of the blood.

315 What is sickle-cell anemia?

If a woman's hemoglobin is abnormal, the red blood cells break down faster than they should. They can break down so quickly that a woman's bone marrow cannot keep up with production of the hemoglobin and anemia results. The most common form of inherited abnormal hemoglobin is sickle-cell hemoglobin. About one out of every twelve black people in the U.S. has inherited a trait of sickle-cell hemoglobin. This means that there is one gene for the production of sickle-cell hemoglobin and one for the production of normal hemoglobin.

Merely having an inherited trait of sickle-cell disease does not usually affect a woman during pregnancy other than to cause a slightly increased risk of infections of the urinary tract. It doesn't hurt the baby she is carrying, either.

However, if a woman has inherited two genes for sickle-cell hemoglobin, she has "sickle-cell disease." With this disease, a pregnant woman may have attacks of pain, greater anemia, more frequent and more serious infections in the body, and a greater chance of having miscarriages and premature babies.

Currently women with sickle-cell disease tolerate pregnancies better and have healthier babies than before. Expert medical care is necessary; this includes careful treatment of infections and of the anemia, perhaps with transfusions throughout the pregnancy.

In the past, sickle-cell disease was thought severe enough to warrant an abortion, but abortions are done less commonly now because of better prenatal care.

Though modern medical care is helping pregnant women who have sickle-cell disease, it is best for a woman with this disease not to get pregnant. She should discuss this problem very seriously with her doctor. (Preconception counseling is an extremely wise choice for women with sickle-cell disease.)

A woman who has sickle-cell disease should not use birth-control pills or an IUD because she is more prone to infections of the uterus, tubes, and ovaries. She should have a sterilization procedure and until then, without exception, use two contraceptives such as vaginal foam and condoms with every act of intercourse.

316 Is it dangerous to become pregnant if I have heart disease?

I highly recommend that a woman with heart disease talk to both her obstetrician and her cardiologist before becoming pregnant. It is important that she understand the risks involved.

Heart disease is divided into four classifications:

Class I: patients with cardiac disease who have no limitation of physical activity

Class II: patients with cardiac disease who have slight limitation of physical activity

Class III: patients with cardiac disease who have marked limitation of physical activity

Class IV: patients with cardiac disease who are unable to perform any physical activity

Patients who have Class I and Class II cardiac disease can usually deliver normally. Ordinarily they will be admitted to the hospital a few days before their delivery date for stabilization of their heart condition. C-section is necessary only for the usual reasons any woman in labor would need one.

Patients with Class III heart disease must be cared for very carefully. Abortion is usually considered, but if the woman wants to risk pregnancy and delivery, and she has excellent medical care, it may be safe to allow the pregnancy to continue. It is, of course, extremely important that she precisely obey her physician's instructions. She likely will need to spend most of her pregnancy in the hospital. A normal vaginal delivery is best, but a C-section is done, if necessary, for usual obstetric reasons.

Pregnancy for a woman with Class IV heart disease is extremely dangerous and has a high death rate for both mother and baby. In this situation a therapeutic abortion is indicated. Only if surgery can be done to decrease the severity of a woman's

Class IV heart condition should pregnancy be considered. I strongly recommend that a woman who has Class III or Class IV heart disease use careful contraception until after counseling with both her cardiologist and her obstetrician.

Research indicates that if a woman has heart disease, it will not be worse after she has gone through a pregnancy and delivery.

317 What about using nose drops and nose sprays for nasal congestion?

These may be safely used. Afrin, for instance, works locally, on the lining of the nose, and is safe during pregnancy. However, if you use too much Afrin, it can be absorbed into your body and cause you to have a slow pulse, low blood pressure, dizziness, and weakness.

Dependence on Afrin and similar drugs may develop. I suggest that you stop using nose sprays or drops after three days. If you continue using them, your nasal lining may become dependent on them and, from that point on, any time you stop using them you will become congested again, even though the infection is gone. I recommend using these sprays three days on, then three days off.

318 What drugs can I take orally to help with congestion during pregnancy?

There are several. Pseudophedrine hydrochloride (Sudafed) is a good drug to use during pregnancy. For sneezing and runny nose, PBZ (an antihistamine) is useful and quite safe in pregnancy. I prescribe Entex a great deal; my patients find it quite effective.

Remember, though, it is probably best not to use any medication during the first three months of pregnancy because of possible effects on the baby. After the first three months it is unlikely that these relatively safe drugs could cause a problem.

319 Is it advisable for me to have allergy testing or to take allergy shots during pregnancy?

It is probably best not to have allergy testing done during pregnancy. You might have a strong reaction to one of the test substances. This could conceivably affect your pregnancy.

If a woman who is already taking allergy shots when she becomes pregnant is not having fever, rash, or other problems when she takes her shots, she may continue to take them.

If you have not been taking allergy shots, you should not start taking them while you are pregnant. When these shots are given for the first time, a woman does not know whether or not she will have a bad reaction to them. A bad reaction could carry a slight risk of causing a miscarriage.

320 How is asthma best treated during pregnancy?

There is no predictable change in a woman's asthma when she becomes pregnant. There may be no change, or the condition may get better or worse.

The ideal in asthma treatment is to keep you comfortable so that you can sleep well and not become too ill. If your asthma becomes severe during pregnancy, you may need to be admitted to the hospital. Usual reasons for admission include: pulse over 120, respiratory rate greater than 30, evidence of use of accessory muscles of respiration (straining to breathe), severe wheezing, wheezing with decreased breath sounds, severe shortness of breath, EKG abnormalities, and turning blue. In the hospital, the primary concern is to keep the oxygen in your bloodstream high enough to keep both you and your baby healthy. If the oxygen in your bloodstream gets too low, there is a risk of damage to the baby.

Your obstetrician and your allergist will work together to make sure your medications are safe during pregnancy. Steroid (cortisone) treatments, which are often necessary in treating asthma, do not affect the baby. There is no reason to avoid them during pregnancy.

321 Does labor make asthma worse?

No. Asthma during labor is unusual. If a pregnant woman in labor has had a recent asthma attack, though, drugs that she has been taking should be continued. In other words, if she has been using oral theophylline and inhaled cromolyn and dexamethasone, she should usually continue to do so while she is in labor. If a patient has been taking cortisone prior to labor, she should usually continue that drug during and after labor.

322 How does hepatitis affect pregnancy?

Hepatitis can be caused by more than twenty different viruses. The hepatitis that most people develop, however, is caused by either the hepatitis A or hepatitis B virus. If a woman develops hepatitis during her pregnancy, she will normally recover without any major problem. However, if she is malnourished or does not receive good medical care, the hepatitis can damage her liver extensively and could even be fatal.

If the whites of your eyes become yellow, or if you pass urine that is dark brown (cola colored) or stools that are light gray, notify your doctor so you can be tested for hepatitis and properly treated. Care consists primarily of bed rest and good diet.

If you will be traveling to a country where there is a great deal of hepatitis, you should receive a shot of gamma globulin to prevent being infected.

If you are infected with hepatitis A, commonly called infectious hepatitis, the baby is almost never affected and you can breast feed.

If you have hepatitis B, your baby can become infected at the time of delivery, by exposure to you after delivery, or through breast milk. It is not advisable to breast feed if you have hepatitis B unless the baby is vaccinated right after delivery.

You may have hepatitis B and not know it. Because hepatitis B is becoming more common in the United States, almost all physicians now recommend that every pregnant woman be tested to see if she is a carrier of this virus.

If a mother is carrying hepatitis B, it is important that her baby be given gamma globulin against hepatitis B within one hour of delivery and also be started on immunization shots against hepatitis B soon after delivery. Such immunization is quite effective.

It is now recommended by most physicians who take care of children that all babies be vaccinated as newborns for hepatitis B. Hepatitis B is becoming so much more common in our culture that I think this is a good recommendation to consider for your child. Hepatitis B is spread not just by sexual activity, and if a person becomes infected, it can be a devastating infection. And if the baby is a girl, she could give hepatitis B to her own baby. See Q. 1001.

323 What is jaundice of pregnancy (intraheptic cholestasis of pregnancy)? .

Other names for jaundice of pregnancy are icterus gravidarum, idiopathic cholestasis of pregnancy, cholestatic hepatosis, and recurrent jaundice of pregnancy. The problem is caused when the estrogens of pregnancy, which are normally present in high concentration, affect the liver in such a way that it cannot get rid of all the bile salts from the woman's body. The bile salts increase and cause her skin to itch and become yellow (jaundiced).

Treatment for the itching, which can be intense, is cholestyramine (Questran), in varying doses from 1 to 24 grams a day. Often 1 gram taken before breakfast will be very helpful.

A pregnant woman who becomes jaundiced must be tested to be sure she does not have hepatitis or any other abnormality of her liver, gallbladder, or bile-collecting system. After delivery, the itching and the jaundice disappear—until the next pregnancy. The problem usually begins during the last three months of pregnancy.

One difference in the symptoms between hepatitis and jaundice of pregnancy is that jaundice usually does not cause nausea, vomiting, right upper quadrant pain, and other symptoms of hepatitis.

324 What is the effect of pregnancy on ulcerative colitis or on Crohn's disease (regional enteritis)?

Ulcerative colitis is often aggravated by pregnancy. If a woman is having no problem with her ulcerative colitis when she becomes pregnant, she has about a 50 percent chance of its activating during her pregnancy. If she is having trouble with her colitis when she becomes pregnant, the colitis will become worse at least three-fourths of the time. Women with ulcerative colitis who become pregnant will often have more trouble with colitis after the baby is born.

Regional enteritis (Crohn's disease) may activate during pregnancy, but not as frequently as ulcerative colitis.

Ulcerative colitis is associated with a higher risk of premature delivery. One study, reported by H. S. Hum in 1988, showed a 40 percent chance of premature delivery for mothers with ulcerative colitis and a 33 percent chance of premature delivery for mothers with Crohn's disease. In their studies this was compared with a normal rate of prematurity of only 10 percent. Other than prematurity, neither ulcerative colitis nor regional enteritis seemed to damage the baby.

If a colectomy and ileostomy (removal of the colon, with the small intestine made to open and empty to the outside through the abdominal wall) has been done in the past for the treatment of ulcerative colitis, it almost never interferes with pregnancy or delivery.

Infections during Pregnancy

325 What infections are of concern in pregnancy and how are they handled?

Infections in pregnancy may be divided into four groups:

Viral—the multiple viral infections that can infect a pregnant woman including cytomegalovirus.

Protozoan—including toxoplasmosis and malaria.

Bacterial—includes Group B Streptococci infections.

Mixed infections—viral or bacterial, which includes sexually transmitted disease infections.

Information regarding three of the infections—toxoplasmosis, cytomegalovirus disease, and Group B Streptococci infections—will sound rather vague. This is because the knowledge we have concerning them, especially the latter two, is confusing. The symptoms are vague or nonexistent; the treatment is unclear; and opinion on diagnosis, prevention, and incidence is ambiguous.

Fortunately, these diseases are uncommon. I have never had a patient's baby affected by cytomegalovirus disease or by toxoplasmosis. I mention them only because they do exist, and you may read about them in newspapers and magazines.

326 What problems do you include in the "viral infections" category?

Our discussion of viral infections will include the common cold and influenza, German measles, cytomegalovirus, mumps, and chicken pox. Herpes, a common and much-feared viral infection, is discussed in Q. 388.

327 Can my having a cold or the flu affect my baby?

There is no evidence that the common cold or influenza can affect your baby while you are pregnant, but pregnant women do seem to be a little more susceptible to developing pneumonia, bronchitis, long-lasting cough, and other secondary illnesses. To prevent such secondary infections, many physicians give antibiotics more readily to a pregnant woman who has a cold or influenza than to one who is not pregnant. Treatment for a cold or influenza in pregnancy also includes adequate rest and plenty of fluids.

This increased susceptibility to both the cold and to influenza makes preventative health care while pregnant very important. Good food, adequate exercise, vitamins, and plenty of rest are essential for a healthy pregnancy. If a pregnant woman with influenza develops pneumonia, it is important that she get expert medical care.

Since influenza does not affect the fetus, it seems sensible not to expose a pregnant woman to the risk of the influenza vaccine. Although studies have shown that the flu vaccine does not damage either the mother or the baby, any medication can have some side effects.

Most physicians recommend influenza vaccines in pregnancy only for high-risk women, such as those who have heart disease, respiratory disease, asthma, or some other medical problem that would make flu dangerous.

328 What do I need to know about German measles?

German measles (rubella) is the type of measles you need to be concerned about during pregnancy. (This is also called "three-day" measles.)

If you are considering getting pregnant, I encourage you to get a German measles test immediately. If the test shows that you are not immune, you should get the German measles immunization.

Rubella vaccination has been available since 1969, therefore during the last twenty years most people have been immune to German measles. Rubella epidemics became infrequent and complacency resulted. There are now many people who have not been vaccinated. They can, therefore, get the infection and give it to you.

Many people confuse rubella with rubeola, the seven-day or "red measles," which is not a problem for pregnancy but which can make the mother very sick.

Rubella is a mild, short-lived infection; many women do not know whether or not they have ever had it. Women who get a mild rash and a lit-

tle fever during pregnancy are afraid that they have German measles, but often they have some other mild virus infection.

To make sure that you do not get rubella while you are pregnant, be vaccinated when you are not pregnant. If you do not know whether or not you have been vaccinated, have a test at the beginning of your pregnancy to see if you have protection against German measles. If you do, it is highly unlikely that you would develop German measles during your pregnancy.

If you are pregnant, (and do not know whether or not you are immune), and you develop a fever, mild rash, enlarged, sensitive lymph nodes in your neck, and a little sore throat and cough, contact your doctor. You may have German measles.

329 What happens if I get German measles while pregnant?

If you do get German measles while you are pregnant, there is at least a 50 percent chance of your baby having severe abnormalities. These include cataracts, blood-vessel deformities, growth retardation, deafness, jaundice, and glaucoma. The abnormalities are more severe, and the chances for occurrence greater (80 percent), if you have rubella during the first three months of your pregnancy.

If rubella infection occurs after the first three months, the resulting abnormalities are less likely to be severe; it is quite possible the baby will be unaffected.

330 Should I have an abortion if I contract German measles during the first three months of pregnancy?

Because of the serious consequences stated above, many people feel that a woman should have an abortion if she has been infected during the first three months of pregnancy. This means that almost 50 percent of the babies aborted for that reason will have been normal babies, unaffected by the mother's German measles infection. This is a very difficult problem, and I cannot tell you, or anyone else, what to do. I do believe that careful consideration should be given to the course of action.

331 What can I do to be sure I am in no danger from German measles?

Prevent it. I suggest several courses of action:

Before you stop using birth-control methods, be sure that you are either immune or have had the shot for German measles. Wait three months to become pregnant after you receive your vaccination.

If you are infertile and starting a fertility evaluation, be sure the doctor does a German measles test to see if you are immune.

If you become pregnant, insist that you have a German measles test at the start of your pregnancy.

If your children have not been vaccinated, have it done. You are more likely to pick up German measles from your unvaccinated children than from any other source. Even if you are pregnant, there is no danger to you from your child being vaccinated. Apparently the vaccine virus is not transferred from one person to another.

You should not be vaccinated while you are pregnant. However, if you do get vaccinated while unaware of your pregnancy, there is a small chance of this hurting your baby.

332 What is cytomegalovirus disease?

It has been reported that as many as 30,000 babies are born each year in the United States with cytomegalovirus. The virus can be passed from a mother to the baby during pregnancy, or it can be passed in breast milk to the baby while it nurses.

When a mother develops an infection from the cytomegalovirus organism, she is almost never aware of it. There are no specific symptoms that indicate the infection. Fortunately, although the organism can pass to the baby.

It does not hurt the baby if the mother gets a CMV infection during the last half of the pregnancy or if the baby gets CMV from the mother's breast milk. CMV is dangerous only if the baby has become infected from the mother during the first half of pregnancy.

Day-care centers are very high-risk settings for CMV. A pregnant woman who already has a child in a day-care center might consider taking the child out until the first half of her pregnancy is over. This will prevent the possibility of the child's bringing home the infection.

There is no reliable testing to show that a woman has been infected with this organism during her pregnancy, and there is no treatment for the mother or the baby, in spite of the fact that the effect on some babies is catastrophic: microcephaly (small skull), seizures, encephalitis, blindness, changes in the blood vessels, changes in the liver and spleen, and anemia.

Since CMV is transmitted by close contact and from hand-to-mouth, the best way to avoid this infection is to use good hygiene.

333 What if I get mumps while pregnant?

Some studies indicate that the mumps virus can cross the placenta and infect the baby, causing miscarriage or, if late in pregnancy, premature labor. Other reports seem to indicate that mumps does not increase the risk of these things occurring. Most physicians believe that a mother who develops mumps in pregnancy does not need to worry about permanent damage to herself or her baby. Experts do not recommend any treatment.

334 What about chicken pox during pregnancy?

If a pregnant woman develops chicken pox (varicella), she may get pneumonia from that virus that will be serious, and can even result in death. In addition, the chicken-pox virus can pass through the placenta into the baby, causing it to be born weakened and possibly to die after delivery. There is a 3 percent chance of a baby developing varicella syndrome (cutaneous scar, fetal deformation, mental retardation, growth retardation) if the mother has chicken pox in the first trimester.

I urge every mother to expose her little girls to chicken pox while they are young, so they will "get it over with" before they grow up and become pregnant. If a woman has not had chicken pox when she was younger she should consider having herself vaccinated before she becomes pregnant. If she becomes pregnant and has not had chicken pox but has young children already, she should consider having those children vaccinated so they will not bring chicken pox into the home and therefore cause her to become infected while she is pregnant.

If a woman is exposed to chicken pox while she is pregnant, she should notify her physician immediately. There is an immune globulin she can receive that decreases the severity of the chickenpox infection. If your physician is not familiar with this treatment, ask him or her to call the Centers for Disease Control in Atlanta.

335 What is toxoplasmosis?

Toxoplasmosis is a disease caused by a protozoal organism called *Toxoplasma gondii*. This organism is present in raw or undercooked meat, and it can be present in the droppings of cats who are allowed outside where they eat wild rodents or decaying meat.

A human can be infected by cat feces (by touching them or by breathing the air that emanates from them). A woman can also become infected by eating raw or partially raw meat containing the organism.

The *Toxoplasma gondii* organism is killed by dehydration, cooking, or freezing.

If you have had toxoplasmosis in the past, but do not have it now, your baby will not be harmed. If you get your first toxoplasmosis infection while you are pregnant, however, the child you are carrying can get infected. If the baby is infected, there is a 10 percent chance that it can be damaged. The greatest chance of the baby's being damaged is if the infection occurs during the first three months. The baby born with toxoplasmosis can have hypotonia (weak muscles), enlarged liver and spleen, small head (microcephaly), sleepiness, and inflammation of the retina and other parts of the eyes.

In the United States, toxoplasmosis occurs in only about one in 12,000 newborn babies, so routine screening of pregnant women in this country for toxoplasmosis is not ordinarily done. The other problem is that the tests for toxoplasmosis often give false results. They may indicate the presence of the infection when it is not there, or they may show that there has not been an infection when indeed there was.

The signs and symptoms of toxoplasmosis in a pregnant woman are nonspecific and include nothing more than muscle pain, headache, a little tiredness, and weakness. The great majority of women who become infected with toxoplasmosis while pregnant have no symptoms.

Because the blood tests are so inaccurate, if toxoplasmosis is suspected, the only accurate ways to know if the baby is infected is to test the amniotic fluid surrounding the baby in the uterus or to draw blood from the baby's umbilical cord while the baby is still in the uterus. (See the section in this chapter on fetal blood testing.) If the baby is infected, antibiotic treatment is required for the mother during the remaining months of the pregnancy.

336 How can I prevent my being infected by toxoplasmosis?

If before you become pregnant you were infected with toxoplasmosis and have a positive test for toxoplasmosis antibodies, you are almost totally protected against getting the infection in pregnancy and transmitting it to your baby. (About one-third of American women have those antibodies.) You can be tested for the antibodies before you get pregnant and know that you are safe.

If you have not had a toxoplasmosis antibody test or if you have had the test but have no antibodies, you should take precautions against becoming infected. First, pregnant women should not eat raw or undercooked meat. Second, you should not handle cat droppings during your pregnancy. Let someone else clean the litter box. I suggest to my patients that they not even handle the cat! It seems conceivable that some toxoplasmosis germs could be caught in its fur; these could infect you. If you have an "outdoor cat," keep it outdoors during your pregnancy. Don't handle an outdoor cat or its droppings. Don't garden without using gloves—cat droppings and dead animals could have contaminated the soil. And finally, wash fruits and vegetables well before eating. They might have toxoplasmosis on their surface.

More information on toxoplasmosis is contained in "Toxoplasmosis & Pregnancy," a one-page reprint from the *Journal of the American Academy of Family Physicians*, and a six-page fact sheet titled "Toxoplasmosis" available from NIAID Information Office, Building 31, Room 7a50, Bethesda, MD 20892, phone (301) 496-5717.

337 Will my having gonorrhea hurt my baby?

Gonorrhea does not ordinarily affect the baby during pregnancy, but it can cause blindness in newborns if the baby is delivered through the vagina of a woman who has the gonorrhea germ and the baby's eyes are not treated. Though gonorrhea might not damage the unborn baby, it is very important that a woman with gonorrhea be treated while she is pregnant. If a baby is born to a woman who has gonorrhea, the baby should be isolated and treated intensively with antibiotics. The simple application of antibiotics to the eyes may not be adequate, so when doctors know that a mother has gonorrhea at delivery, intensive antibiotics are used to make sure the baby is well.

Because 80 percent of the women who have gonorrhea do not know it, and their doctors may not know it, most states have a law that all babies must have their eyes treated with some type of antibiotic soon after birth to protect the eyes from damage. Generally this is effective. The treatment does not have to be administered immediately after delivery but it should be done in the first few hours of life. See Q. 980–983.

338 Is a chlamydia infection a problem during pregnancy?

Some studies show that a woman with chlamydia has a higher risk of premature delivery or premature rupture of the membranes, or of having an underweight baby. If the woman has chlamydia when she delivers, the baby can get eye infections and pneumonia from the germ. If a pregnant woman is treated for chlamydia with Erythromycin, the possibility of these complications occurring is less.

If you have had past sexual activity (or your husband or partner has) from which you could have become STD infected, be sure to tell your doctor, because doctors often will not ask. It takes a specific test to tell if you have chlamydia.

Remember, if you have chlamydia, your husband or partner will have it, too. Both of you must be treated. (See the section about chlamydia in the STD chapter.) See Q. 984–989.

339 What problems does syphilis cause during pregnancy?

If you have syphilis and do not get it treated, the organism can infect the baby while you are pregnant. About 30 percent of the babies who are infected with syphilis will die before the mother goes into labor; 70 percent of the babies who are born alive will have some signs of infection by the syphilis germ.

Infection that the baby picked up before birth (congenital syphilis) from its syphilitic mother can result in its being anemic, restless, and feverish. The baby can also have a stuffy nose, skin eruptions, and moist sores around the mouth, the anus, and the genitals. The liver, spleen, brain, nerves, eyes, and teeth can all be affected quite severely. (See Q. 994.)

340 What should I do if I think I might have syphilis?

If you might have contracted syphilis during or shortly before your pregnancy, please tell your doctor. It takes about twelve weeks after being infected by syphilis for your blood to produce a positive syphilis test, but it can be positive as early as four weeks. Your doctor will probably wait four weeks before having the test done, but may want to repeat it eight weeks later.

Do not expect the doctor to ask all through

your pregnancy if you have had sex with someone who might have a venereal disease. Tell your doctor if you have such an encounter during your pregnancy.

If you suspect that your husband had intercourse with someone during your pregnancy who might have given him syphilis (which he, in turn, might pass on to you), tell your doctor so that a syphilis test can be ordered twelve weeks after your possible exposure.

341 How is syphilis treated during pregnancy?

Penicillin is the best treatment for it. If you are allergic to penicillin, there are a number of other antibiotics that will kill the germ.

Because syphilis can hurt the baby, most states require a syphilis test early in pregnancy. In some states a syphilis test is also required in late pregnancy. Whether or not it is required, it is probably best that all pregnant women have a syphilis test done in both early and late pregnancy. If there is any possibility that you could be infected with syphilis, tell your doctor so he or she can test you.

If you become infected, your symptoms may be minimal. The initial infection may occur inside your vagina where you cannot see or feel it. This initial infection, called a chancre, heals after two to six weeks. Six or eight weeks later you might have a mild skin rash. When that clears up, you may have absolutely no sign or symptom that you have been infected with syphilis. The only way to know is through a blood test.

At all stages of the disease, however, the baby you are carrying can be severely affected. For this reason, if you have had sexual intercourse with someone who might have syphilis, you may want to be treated even before your blood test has time to turn positive.

342 What is a Group B Streptococci infection?

You may never have heard of a Group B Streptococci infection in a newborn. Phillip B. Mead,

M.D., clinical professor of OB/GYN at the University of Vermont in Burlington, led a symposium on this infection, which was published in *Contemporary OB/GYN* (May 1991). He made these statements:

Early onset Group B Streptococcal neonatal sepsis, the commonest cause of serious perinatal infection [infection that occurs before delivery or just after delivery] represents a difficult challenge for both obstetricians and pediatricians. Protocols [plans] for prevention have been difficult to formulate. The data are frightening. Anywhere from five to forty percent of pregnant women are colonized [carry the germ] in the vagina, vulva, or rectum and 75 percent of colonized mothers will transmit the organism to the fetus during labor or at birth. The attack rate is stated to be approximately one per hundred for colonized women and one to three per thousand births for all women. Mortality [death of the baby] is significant— from nine to twenty percent or higher. About half of the infants who survive Group B Streptococcal meningitis are left with permanent neurologic sequelae.

This obviously is a very serious disease. However, a rate of one to three per thousand live births means that for an individual service [obstetrical unit] it will be a fairly uncommon event. A private obstetrician may practice five or ten years without ever encountering a case. All of these facts make it particularly difficult to design effective protocols to cope with this infection.

Many people ask why doctors do not routinely culture all pregnant women prior to delivery and treat the germ if it is present. Several reasons make the taking of vaginal cultures from all pregnant women not a good idea. First, this organism can come and go during pregnancy. Even if the germ is present at one time during pregnancy, it may be gone later (and therefore will not be a problem at delivery). Culturing and treating throughout pregnancy has not been shown useful or protective to the baby at delivery. Further, vaginal cultures done early in pregnancy may show no Group B Streptococcus, and yet the baby will develop the infection after delivery anyway.

There is no universal agreement about what to do. The Centers for Disease Control recommends that all pregnant women be cultured at thirty-six weeks of pregnancy and if Group B germs are present, be treated in labor. CDC also says it is just as well for your doctor to do what the American College of Obstetricians and Gynecologists recommends: treat for risk factors such as prematurely ruptured membranes, premature labor, etc. regardless of the culture. One suggestion by some physicians who have studied this extensively is that women who go into labor early, whose membranes have ruptured prematurely, or who had a previous baby infected by Group B Streptococcus should be cultured in the last three months of pregnancy and again when they go into the hospital with either labor or ruptured membranes. Women can also be cultured for this organism if they are admitted to the hospital for induction and it is expected that labor is going to be difficult (a long labor can increase the likelihood of infection of the baby).

If the cultures on these patients are positive, treatment is given when the patient is in labor. Ampicillin (a form of penicillin) is usually used. If a woman is in one of the classifications listed above, a doctor may want to start treatment with Ampicillin even before the final result of the culture is back from the lab, especially if a previous child was delivered with Group B Streptococcus.

343 Are there other infections that can cause problems during pregnancy?

Yes, these include:

Lyme disease. This disease may be a cause of premature labor, abnormalities in the baby, and stillbirth. Because of this, a woman who lives in a tick-infested environment should wear protective clothing and shower after possible exposure to ticks. If there is a possibility of having been infected, the antibiotic recommended for treatment is Ceftriaxone.

Listeriosis. Certain foods can contain the listeria organism and if eaten during pregnancy may cause infection that is dangerous for both mother and baby. These include coleslaw made from contaminated cabbage; also, some cheeses can be contaminated with listeriosis. (In 1985, Jalisco brand Mexican-style cheese was associated with an epidemic of listeriosis in California.) If a woman has listeriosis and it passes to her child, the baby can be born early or be stillborn. A woman who is infected with the listeria organism during pregnancy will need to be treated with antibiotics.

Epstein-Barr. These virus infections during pregnancy may or may not cause problems for babies. There have been some reports that if a woman is infected with this virus during pregnancy, the baby can be affected. Researchers merely recommend at this point that a woman with Epstein-Barr virus be monitored very carefully through her pregnancy.

Bacterial vaginosis. This vaginal infection is caused by a group of organisms called anerobes. (In the past, this type of infection was referred to as a hemophilus, or gardnerella infection.) It has only recently been recognized that this infection may increase the chance of premature delivery or a low birth weight infant. Women with this infection are more likely to develop infection in the uterus after delivery. Bacterial vaginosis is usually transmitted sexually. If a woman has a discharge with a fishy or somewhat foul odor, she needs to tell her physician. The treatment for bacterial vaginosis is metronidazole (Flagyl) for her and her partner. (For more information, see the section on vaginal infections, Q. 604.)

Trichomoniasis vaginal infection. This infection can cause premature rupture of the membranes and premature delivery. If trichomoniasis is present, it needs to be treated early in the pregnancy. (For more information, see the section on sexually transmitted disease.)

HIV infection (AIDS). HIV is a serious problem. One percent of pregnant women in Washington, D.C., for instance, are infected with the AIDS virus. About 25 percent of the babies born to women with HIV infection will become infected.

But, if a woman uses AZT during pregnancy, her baby has a two-thirds less chance of becoming HIV infected from its mother than if the mother did not take AZT. This is one of the brightest discoveries of all HIV research—babies are actually being saved from infection. This is a powerful reason for all pregnant women to have an HIV test. Some people advocate abortion for HIV-positive women because of the chance of the baby getting HIV from the mother. This would mean, however, that about 75 percent of babies aborted would be normal. (For more information, see the section on sexually transmitted disease, Q. 1003–1004.)

Chlamydia psittaci. Parrots and sheep (especially in lambing season) can carry this organism. A woman who handles infected animals may become infected herself, which can cause miscarriage.

Thrombophlebitis

344 Are blood clots in the veins a problem during pregnancy?

Blood clots in the veins (thrombophlebitis) occur five and a half times as often in a pregnant woman as in a woman who is not pregnant. These clots are three times as likely to occur during the month after delivery as they are before delivery.

Three things contribute to the development of blood clots in the veins of pregnant or recently pregnant women.

Slower blood flow. In pregnancy, because of the pressure of the enlarged uterus on the veins, blood returns more slowly from the legs to the heart. During the last three months of pregnancy the blood flow in the veins of the legs is only half as fast as the flow in the veins of nonpregnant women.

Damage to blood vessels by infection. There is an increased chance of infection developing in the body during and after delivery. If such infection develops, there is an increased chance of blood clots developing in the pelvis because infection irritates vein walls and this initiates clotting. For example, infection can develop in the uterus, even after a normal delivery. A cesarean section damages uterine tissue and makes it easier for infection to develop in those tissues.

Increased tendency to clotting. The hormones of pregnancy cause blood to clot more easily. This is obviously a God-designed mechanism to protect the woman at a time when she might otherwise bleed excessively. Immediately after delivery the clotting of blood inside the uterus and in any vaginal tears that might be present, keeps a woman from bleeding too much.

345 What is the danger of blood-clot formation in the veins? Can this be treated?

When blood clots form in the large veins of the legs and pelvis, they are very soft. Portions of the clots can break loose, pass through the heart into the lungs, and block blood flow to the lungs, thus causing serious medical problems or even death. This passage of blood clots through the veins into the lungs is called pulmonary embolism. One-fourth of the women who develop these blood clots in their veins have some of that clot break loose and go into the lungs if no treatment is given for the clots.

Even if blood clots in leg veins are detected and treated, 5 percent of such patients will still have the blood clots break loose and go into the lungs; 1 percent will die of this problem.

It is crucial, obviously, that thrombophlebitis be found and treated. Tell your doctor if you see any signs of this problem. A woman can have clots in her veins without knowing it and can have a pulmonary embolism and die suddenly and unexpectedly. An autopsy would reveal she died from such blood clots. (This, of course, happens *rarely*.)

346 What are the signs and symptoms of thrombophlebitis?

There are several signs of blood clotting in the veins:

Pain and tenderness over the veins where the clot is located.
Swelling of the leg that is involved. That leg will often be more than an inch bigger around than the other leg.

Pain on raising the big toe of the leg that is involved.

347 Do these signs always mean that dangerous blood clots are present?

No. Half of the time there will be no blood clot present, even when the above-mentioned signs are present, because other problems such as muscle pain can produce the same signs.

348 What tests are used to determine whether or not I have a blood clot in a vein in my leg?

There is now one standard test for this. It is a totally painless test called a "deep venous Doppler study." A Doppler study uses a machine that emits sound waves like an ultrasound when it does a sonogram. The Doppler study can detect blood flowing through a vein. When a vein is visualized with the Doppler instrument and no blood flow is seen, the Doppler is moved along the vein until the edge of the clot is found and blood is seen flowing in the vein above or below the clot.

The Doppler study does not require injecting dye into a vein and requires no medication. It is a completely safe, simple procedure. It is also very reliable if done by a well-trained physician or technician.

349 How can I know if a blood clot has broken loose and gone into my lungs?

Fast breathing, shortness of breath, anxiety, pain in the chest on breathing, fast heart rate, and coughing blood are symptoms that accompany a pulmonary embolism (the passage of a blood clot through the veins into the lungs).

The problem with these symptoms, though, is that they can also occur in a person who does not have a pulmonary embolus. A woman who has had a cesarean section, for instance, will occasionally have a faster heart rate, shortness of breath, and pain in her chest during the normal recovery from that operation.

Tell the nurse or doctor if you notice unusual or disturbing symptoms of any kind. If a pulmonary embolism is suspected, the doctor will order tests to determine whether or not this is the case.

350 How are blood clots in my legs treated?

Bed rest and anticoagulation drugs are the primary techniques for treatment of thrombophlebitis.

Bed rest. You would be put to bed with your legs elevated so that the blood would drain from your veins more rapidly, decreasing the chance of more clot formation. Elastic stockings would be recommended for the same reason. Application of heat to your legs and pain medication would also be part of your care.

Anticoagulation drugs. The most important treatment is the use of heparin to decrease blood coagulation. This drug prevents the clot from getting larger and allows the body to absorb the blood clot that is already formed. Although the body often absorbs the blood clot, sometimes the blood clot will be walled off, becoming scar tissue. This obstructs the vein, but blood returning from the leg will take an alternate route through other veins going in the same direction.

351 How is heparin given? How long is it used?

Initially the drug is given intravenously (through your veins), but after the problem is under control you would need injections of heparin because it is not available in pill form. You or someone else could administer these shots at home.

The length of treatment has decreased over the years. In the past, heparin was administered for three months. Now we know that the blood clot starts healing after two weeks, so heparin is often used for only three to four weeks. If there is a major complicating factor, such as significant deep vein thrombosis (clotting), you might be treated until the end of your pregnancy and for six weeks after. If your problem develops after delivery and you are started on heparin then, you might be treated with it for as long as six months.

352 Why can't I take a pill to keep my blood from clotting, instead of having injections?

There is a pill—Coumadin—which can be used to anticoagulate blood, but it must not be used in pregnancy. If you are on Coumadin when you get pregnant, there is a great chance (about one in five) that you will miscarry. People who raise cattle know this. They do not let their bred cows into sweet clover, because they miscarry when they eat it. Coumadin comes from sweet clover.

It has been found that Coumadin can cause bleeding into the baby's brain while the baby is still in the mother's uterus. This is like a stroke and can produce abnormalities of the brain in the fetus, resulting in mental retardation, seizures, and a spastic body. If you are taking Coumadin while pregnant, the chance of these abnormalities developing in your baby is about 20 percent.

It is best, obviously, to be anticoagulated with heparin during pregnancy. The explanation for this is that Coumadin crosses through the placenta into the baby, thinning the baby's blood during the pregnancy. Heparin has a much larger molecule and does not pass through the placenta into the baby. Therefore, it does not cause the baby's blood to lose its coagulation ability. If the blood-clotting problem develops following delivery, Coumadin can be used whenever your doctor feels it is indicated.

Diabetes and Pregnancy

353 Is diabetes a special problem in pregnancy? Why do doctors get so concerned about diabetes and pregnancy?

Diabetes is a special problem in pregnancy; doctors are concerned because diabetes can affect the unborn child, the course of the pregnancy, and the woman herself.

If the mother has diabetes, the child can be affected in several ways:

1. Unless the pregnancy is managed very carefully, the risk of losing the baby, either just before or just after delivery, is much higher than if the mother did not have diabetes.
2. Women with diabetes have three times as many babies born with major abnormalities.
3. Diabetic women often have very large babies. This can make delivery traumatic for both mother and baby.
4. Babies of diabetic mothers whose blood sugars are not controlled well may have more breathing difficulties and problems with low blood sugar (hypoglycemia) and low blood calcium levels (hypocalcemia).
5. Babies of diabetic mothers may be born with a predisposition to diabetes.

Diabetes can affect a pregnancy in several ways:

1. The pregnant diabetic has at least a four times greater chance of having preeclampsia or eclampsia. (See Q. 369–378.)
2. Women with diabetes are more likely to have infections.
3. Babies born to diabetic mothers can be large and the delivery difficult.
4. There is a greater chance that a cesarean section will be necessary because of the size of the baby and because of the increased chance that the baby might have a problem.
5. Thirty percent of pregnant diabetic women often develop a much larger volume of fluid around the baby than is normal. This can cause the mother to be short of breath and can also occasionally cause heart problems.
6. Women who are diabetic have heavy bleeding after delivery much more often than women who are not diabetic.

Pregnancy may increase a woman's problems with her diabetes, or may cause diabetes.

1. A diabetic who gets pregnant may have difficulty controlling her diabetes.
2. A woman who is not a diabetic may become diabetic while she is pregnant. Called gestational diabetes, this problem occurs because the pregnant woman's body, because of hormones from the placenta, tends to handle sugar like a diabetic's, thus exposing a tendency to diabetes.

(These complications are explained further in *Williams Obstetrics* by Cunningham, MacDonald, and Gantt [Norwalk, Conn.: Appleton & Lange, 1997].)

354 What can I do to prevent all these complications related to diabetes?

Preconception counseling is one of the most important things you can do to prevent the complications of diabetes. Having counseling before you become pregnant will prepare you for what you will have to do when you are pregnant; if you are in the best possible condition physically and mentally going into the pregnancy, you will go through the pregnancy with less worry.

Recent studies show that if you have your blood sugar under good control at the time you get pregnant, there is less chance of miscarriage and less chance of having a baby with an abnormality.

Getting expert medical care during your pregnancy will increase the chances of a good outcome to your pregnancy, both for yourself and your baby. Good care will require frequent blood tests, seeing your doctor more often, a more carefully controlled diet, and so on. Your reward for all this trouble is a greater chance of having a healthy baby.

Prior to modern insulin therapy for diabetes, very few diabetic women got pregnant. Now, with proper medical care, most diabetic women are able not only to get pregnant but also to have good pregnancies and healthy babies. The following statement, which appeared on the editorial page of the *New England Journal of Medicine* (1988, 319:25), shows the miracle of modern medicine for diabetic women:

The care of women with diabetes who become pregnant represents one of the modern success stories of this century. For decades, stillbirths and neonatal deaths continued to occur in more than one-third of the pregnancies complicated by diabetes, but most major centers now report them in less than three percent of such pregnancies.

Perinatal mortality was prevented initially by the use of new techniques that made it easier to tell when the fetus was about to die in the uterus, so that it could be delivered quickly and sustained in a modern neonatal intensive care unit. Soon thereafter it became clear that fetal compromise could usually be prevented by maintaining the maternal blood glucose concentration at close to normal levels during the third trimester of pregnancy.

Once self-monitoring of glucose became practicable, the intensive management of such pregnancies with the goal of euglycemia (normal blood sugar levels) became the standard approach, creating a much improved prognosis for women with diabetes who desired a family.

355 Should I be tested for diabetes as a routine procedure if I am pregnant?

Most doctors feel that all pregnant women should be tested for diabetes. Studies have shown that half of the women who are pregnant diabetics are not diagnosed during their pregnancy by the now routine practice of watching their urine for sugar. Because of this most physicians recommend that a blood-sugar test be done on every pregnant woman from the twenty-fourth to the twenty-eighth week of pregnancy.

Some women are diabetic when they get pregnant. Other women become diabetic during pregnancy. This is called gestational diabetes. Both groups of women are treated the same way during pregnancy. A woman is a gestational diabetic if her blood sugar level is abnormal two times during a three-hour glucose tolerance test, whether or not she ever needs insulin during her pregnancy. After pregnancy gestational diabetics will usually return to their nondiabetic state, although they often become true diabetics later in life.

Several factors would make it especially important for you to be tested for diabetes during pregnancy. If you have had a very large baby (over nine pounds), prior to this pregnancy, you should be tested for diabetes. Other indications for careful testing would be if you have had diabetes in a previous pregnancy, if you have had an elevated blood-sugar level, or if you have had sugar in your urine with this pregnancy or in the past.

356 When should the test for diabetes be done? How is it performed?

You should be tested during the twenty-fourth to the twenty-eighth week of your pregnancy. This is the time when the production of hormones has become high enough to cause diabetes to reveal itself if a blood-sugar test is done. Testing for diabetes can be done reliably at this stage of your pregnancy.

The test for diabetes is simple. It merely involves drinking a solution, which your doctor will give you, that has 50 grams of glucose. This is followed by a blood test one hour later. This sugary fluid can be taken at any time during the day, and it doesn't matter whether or not you have had anything to eat. If the blood test shows 140 mg/dL, you need to have a glucose tolerance test. This test is done by taking 100 grams of the sugary fluid instead of 50 grams. Blood tests are then done one, two, and three hours after drinking the fluid.

357 What will the doctor do if I am diabetic?

If you are diabetic, you will normally need both an obstetrician and an maternal-fetal medicine specialist. These two doctors will work together to help you have the best possible outcome with your pregnancy. The first goal is to keep your blood sugar as normal as possible throughout the pregnancy. The second goal is to monitor the baby carefully to be sure it is growing properly, is healthy, and does not get too large for a normal delivery. If the baby does get too large, there will be a plan to deliver it in a way that does not harm you or the baby.

There are some principles about the care of diabetes during pregnancy that are important. Your doctors will probably want you to test your own blood-sugar levels at home. They will probably want your fasting blood-sugar level not to exceed 100 mg/dL or your blood-sugar level at two hours after a meal to exceed 120 mg/dL. Your doctors will instruct you as to how often to test yourself.

The primary treatment of diabetes in pregnancy is dietary management. Your doctors will probably have you see a dietitian. The dietitian will stress the importance of eating in such a way that your body does not absorb large amounts of sugar, which would produce high blood-sugar levels and cause the pancreas to be overloaded.

You will probably be told to eat complex carbohydrates; they are absorbed more slowly and do not cause your blood-sugar levels to elevate suddenly. The dietitian may suggest more frequent, lower calorie meals. Since studies have shown that fiber ties up sugar so it is not absorbed as quickly, you may be encouraged to eat a high-fiber diet.

Finally, because studies have shown that people who exercise right after eating do not have such high surges of sugar in their bloodstreams, you may be encouraged to exercise after eating. (Even moving your arms around enough to cause your heart rate to increase seems to have a positive effect.)

If your blood sugars are not maintained with this regimen, you may need to begin taking insulin. If you are already insulin dependent and your blood sugars are higher than they should be, your insulin will need to be adjusted.

Bearing a Child

358 How is my baby cared for during pregnancy if I am a diabetic?

The monitoring of the baby carried by a diabetic mother is highly individualized, but there are some important principles to follow.

It is extremely important that you know exactly how far along you are in your pregnancy so that you will know exactly when to do the tests you will need as your pregnancy progresses. If you are not sure how far along you are, you probably need to have a sonogram in the first few months to date your pregnancy.

Cooperation with your doctors is vitally important. I cannot overemphasize the importance of your doing what your physicians tell you to do to have the healthiest pregnancy possible.

The doctors will be checking you during the last four to six weeks of your pregnancy to see if the baby seems larger than normal. If it does, they will probably order an ultrasound scan. If the baby seems to be under nine pounds, your delivery will probably be handled normally; if it is between nine and ten pounds, the doctors will consider doing a cesarean section; if the baby is larger than ten pounds, they will almost certainly do a cesarean section.

If you have insulin-dependent diabetes, or if you have hypertension or some other complication, your doctors will probably begin nonstress tests as early as the thirty-second to the thirty-fourth week of your pregnancy. If you have no complications and only mild diabetes, doctors may not require the nonstress tests or any other fetal monitoring (such as biophysical profile—see the section in this chapter on that topic) until the thirty-sixth to the fortieth week of pregnancy.

If you are insulin dependent or have some other complication of pregnancy or if tests indicate that the baby seems to be having problems, it may be best to deliver early. If the decision is made that early delivery would be wise, your doctor may want to do a test to see if the baby's lungs are mature enough. (One of the biggest dangers of prematurity is newborn respiratory distress because of immature lungs.) To evaluate this the doctor may want to draw some amniotic fluid from around the baby for a lecithin-spingomyelin ratio. If this test shows that the baby's lungs are mature, your doctor may choose to go ahead with delivery, even if it requires a cesarean. (Cesarean sections are not absolutely necessary for all diabetic mothers; as a matter of fact, if the mother's diabetes is relatively mild, a normal vaginal delivery is probable.)

359 What kinds of abnormalities most commonly occur in babies of diabetic mothers?

These abnormalities are primarily heart defects and neural tube defects. The most common heart defect is a hole between the two major chambers of the heart (ventriculoseptal defect, VSD), occurring in 3 to 5 percent of babies. Neural tube defects occur twenty times as often in these babies as in the general population.

Thyroid Disease and Pregnancy

360 How often is thyroid disease a problem during pregnancy?

Thyroid disease does occur during pregnancy. A woman can have excessive thyroid function (hyperthyroidism) or inadequate thyroid function (hypothyroidism). It is very rare, however, for a woman with significant hypothyroidism to get pregnant. If she does, there is a greater chance of miscarriage, intrauterine growth retardation, preeclampsia, or having a stillborn baby. If a woman has had surgery or radioiodine treatment for thyroid disease, she must be checked for hypothyroidism and treated before she gets pregnant.

Some studies have shown that if thyroid disease is not treated, as many as 45 percent of pregnancies will end as miscarriages, stillbirths, or deaths. It is important, if the expectant mother has abnormal thyroid function, that she be diagnosed and treated.

The diagnosis of hyperthyroidism in pregnancy is somewhat difficult because pregnancy itself produces signs that are typical of increased metabolism, such as excessive warmth, nervousness, and slight tremor. If a pregnant woman develops a fast heartbeat (especially while sleeping), if her eyes become a little protuberant, and if she is failing to gain weight normally, she should be tested for excessive thyroid function. If she is found to have increased thyroid function, this should be treated.

361 How is excessive thyroid function, or hyperthyroidism, treated during pregnancy?

A woman with this problem may be treated in one of the following ways: (1) surgery to remove part of the thyroid after treatment with medicine to "quiet down" the thyroid, (2) antithyroid medicine plus thyroid replacement, or (3) antithyroid medicine alone.

The treatment best for you depends on what your doctors think and on much more specific testing.

The drug usually used in the treatment of hyperthyroidism is propylthiouracil. This drug does cross the placenta and can cause problems for the baby. If the drug is administered properly, however, the chances of its hurting the baby are small. It can, among other things, cause the baby to develop a goiter, and an excessive dose can suppress the baby's own thyroid function and even produce cretinism. Your obstetrician will normally have you see an internal medicine specialist to treat your hyperthyroidism.

There are other medications used for hyperthyroidism. They are:

Tapazole (methimazole), a drug said to cause severe scalp deformities in babies. This has not been confirmed. Your doctor will advise you on whether or not it is safe for you to take Tapazole during pregnancy.

Radioactive iodine, which can cause the baby to have fetal defects including damage to the baby's thyroid gland. It would hardly ever be used during pregnancy.

Breast feeding is generally not recommended for mothers who are taking antithyroid medication.

If there is a question about whether or not you have thyroid disease, I urge you to get it checked before you become pregnant to help insure a healthy pregnancy and baby. If thyroid disease shows up during your pregnancy, however, it can usually be treated successfully.

Arthritis and Pregnancy

362 What about rheumatoid arthritis? Does it get worse or better during pregnancy? Are pregnancy and delivery affected by arthritis? How is arthritis treated during pregnancy?

It gets better! Why this happens no one knows. It may be due to the increase of cortisone in the body during pregnancy, or a change in the immune system.

Unless the hip joints are severely affected, the pregnancy should proceed smoothly, and a woman may have a normal vaginal delivery. If the hip joints are severely affected and stiff, a woman may need a cesarean section for delivery because her legs cannot spread far enough for normal vaginal delivery.

The drug most commonly used for arthritis in pregnancy is aspirin. Since the usual large doses of aspirin that you might take for arthritis can have an adverse effect on the baby, it is important to discuss with your doctor the amount of aspirin—or other medication—you can take.

Cortisone (and prednisone, and other similar drugs) has been used without any sign of abnormalities in babies. (Cortisone has been used in thousands of patients for many years, and most studies indicate that it is quite safe for the baby. Studies on rodents in the past did show development of cleft palates, but the development of the palate in mice is different from its development in humans. There is no correlation between the two.)

Gold is sometimes used for treatment of arthritis, but there have not been enough patients using it to prove whether or not it is safe during pregnancy. It can pass through the placenta and could possibly affect the baby. You and your doctor would need to talk about this.

Lupus Erythematosus and Pregnancy

363 What is systemic lupus erythematosus? I have heard that women with this disease should not get pregnant.

Systemic lupus erythematosus (lupus or SLE) is a disease of the connective tissue (collagen) of a person's body. It can cause tiredness, low-grade fever, anemia, arthritis, kidney disease, neurologic disorders, and other symptoms. It is found primarily in women, but it can occur in men.

For many years women with SLE have been told they should not become pregnant and cautioned that, if they did, they should have an abortion. This advice was given because it was thought that pregnancy caused SLE to become much worse and because there is a high risk of miscarriage, premature birth, and other complications in women with SLE who have not been treated.

New treatment for SLE, and better obstetric care, have changed the outlook for pregnancy for most women with SLE. If a woman with SLE has vascular disease or kidney disease, it is probably best that she not become pregnant. It is unlikely that these women will die from complications

during pregnancy. It is more likely that they will miscarry, have premature babies, or have babies with intrauterine growth retardation. Expert medical care may get them through pregnancy with a healthy baby, but the risk is great.

If a woman with these problems does get pregnant and her SLE worsens while she is pregnant, she would need more intensive medical care during her pregnancy—from both her internal medicine specialist and her obstetrician. The obstetrician would be watching the baby very carefully. If the baby seems to be getting inadequate nutrition with stunted growth, the obstetrician would deliver the baby early.

Women with SLE who also have vascular or renal disease should consider a sterilization; it is best that they not use birth-control pills or an intrauterine device. Birth-control pills can aggravate SLE and IUDs can cause pelvic infections.

364 What is the new treatment that makes pregnancy with SLE acceptable for the health of both baby and mother if the mother does not have vascular or kidney involvement?

If a woman's SLE can be made inactive with drugs, if she does not have blood vessel or kidney disease, and if a blood test for lupus is negative, she has a good chance for a successful pregnancy. The drugs (azathioprine, cyclophosphamide, and methotrexate) used for this purpose are immunosuppressant drugs, the same drugs given to people who have had organ transplants.

Immunosuppressant drugs to inactivate SLE can be given before a woman becomes pregnant. They do not seem to affect a woman's fertility or pregnancy; nor do they harm the baby.

The general medical opinion is that if you have SLE and want to have a baby, you should begin treatment and continue it until your SLE has been inactive for six months. If your lupus blood tests are negative, and your SLE has been inactive for six months, you have a very good chance of an uncomplicated pregnancy and a normal, healthy baby.

An exception to this is that if your SLE has already caused damage to your blood vessels or kidneys, it is best for you not to become pregnant.

365 If the mother has lupus, will her baby get it from her?

No. The antibodies associated with lupus can pass into the baby through the placenta and cause some problems for the baby, but the baby does not get SLE from the mother. The antibodies pass out of the baby's body in a few months.

Problems the baby may have from the mother's lupus may include a transient rash and heart damage. (Occasionally a baby will need a pacemaker to regulate its heartbeat.)

The pediatrician who will care for the baby of a mother with SLE needs to be aware of the problem and needs to know when to expect the delivery. Good communication between the pediatrician and the obstetrician is very important.

366 Is it possible for a woman to have repeated miscarriages caused by SLE and not be aware she has the disease? Can she ever have a baby?

Included in the routine tests we do now for women who have repeated miscarriages are tests for lupus and tests for anticoagulant and anticardiolipin antibodies. These antibodies are found in women who have SLE, but they are also found in women who have no evidence of lupus.

If a woman has these antibodies in her body, she has a greater chance of having miscarriages whether or not she actually has lupus. Yet women with these antibodies have also been able to carry pregnancies to term (even if they have had previous miscarriages).

Some studies have shown that women who have SLE antibodies but do not actually have lupus, and take cortisone (usually given as prednisone) and aspirin, have a greater chance of carrying a pregnancy. Taking these drugs in high doses for several months, however, can cause complications. For example, a woman who uses high doses of cortisone for several months has a chance of developing avascular necrosis of the hip joint, which would then require total hip replacement.

If tests show that you have SLE antibodies, you may need careful consultation with your obstetrician or infertility physician and with an internal medicine specialist if you want to have a baby.

Epilepsy and Pregnancy

367 How does pregnancy affect epilepsy?

Epilepsy is generally not affected by pregnancy. If an epileptic pregnant woman becomes so nauseated or sick from the pregnancy that she cannot take her anticonvulsive medicine, she may have an increased chance of having a convulsion. Otherwise there is not an increased risk of a convulsion while she is pregnant.

An occasional mild convulsion in pregnancy will probably not hurt the baby. It would take a fairly prolonged seizure episode, or multiple seizures, to damage the baby. A woman cannot breathe properly during convulsions and a diminished oxygen supply can adversely affect the baby.

The main problem with epilepsy during pregnancy is the effect of anticonvulsive medications on the baby. It is especially important, therefore, that the diagnosis of epilepsy be confirmed before a woman stays on any drugs during pregnancy. The ideal situation would be that, if a woman expects that she is going to become pregnant, she consult with her neurologist. Together they can pick a drug that is safe in pregnancy and try it before the woman gets pregnant.

It is best, when possible, that an epileptic use only one drug during pregnancy and that this drug be chosen carefully. Drugs women take for epilepsy can hurt the baby. Trimethadione and paramethadione sometimes cause cleft lip and cleft palate, heart abnormalities, growth retardation, and mental deficiency. About 80 percent of babies born to mothers who take these drugs are affected to some extent.

Valproic acid has been found to cause neural tube defects (spina bifida and anencephaly) in 2 percent of newborns. It should not be used in pregnancy.

Carbamazepine seems to have less chance of hurting a baby than Dilantin does. It is probably the best drug to use in pregnancy.

The drug most people are familiar with for the treatment of seizures is Dilantin (diphenylhydrantoin). A past study reported that 10 percent of babies who were exposed to this drug while in the mother's womb developed abnormalities of the face, including cleft lip, and other congenital problems. A more recent study showed no major congenital abnormalities (such as cleft lip), but it did show that 30 percent of babies whose mothers took Dilantin had minor abnormalities of the fingers, skull, or face.

If you have epilepsy, it is very important that you talk to both your neurologist and your obstetrician about medication before you get pregnant.

High Blood Pressure and Toxemia of Pregnancy

368 Why does my doctor check my blood pressure every time I go to the office?

The doctor is checking to see that your blood pressure is not too high. If your blood pressure is elevated it can cause problems for you and your baby during the pregnancy.

Hypertension in pregnancy can cause spasm of the blood vessels of the uterus and therefore a decreased flow of blood through the baby's placenta. This limits the amount of nutrition and oxygen the baby can get from you and can affect the baby's growth, even causing it to die before deliv-

ery. If your blood pressure gets high enough, it can cause a convulsion, which is obviously not good for you or the baby.

High blood pressure during pregnancy is treated with the following goals in mind:

1. Delivery of the baby with the least possible damage to mother and baby.
2. Delivery of a baby who is healthy enough to thrive.
3. Complete restoration of the health of the mother.

369 What is toxemia of pregnancy?

Toxemia, a condition produced by pregnancy, has three components: high blood pressure, preeclampsia, eclampsia.

A woman may have any one of these three conditions when she is pregnant.

1. High blood pressure, discussed in the previous question.
2. High blood pressure with protein in the urine and/or swelling.
3. High blood pressure with protein in the urine and/or swelling of her body, and also convulsions.

370 What causes toxemia of pregnancy to develop?

No one really knows what causes it, but there are some suggestions. One is that the trophoblast cells in the placenta seem capable of causing toxemia. For example, a woman who has a hydatidiform mole (see Q. 298) will sometimes develop toxemia. The presence of the placenta, rather than the presence of the baby, must be the cause of toxemia.

An additional interesting fact is that toxemia will develop if a hydatidiform mole develops in a woman's abdomen, outside her uterus. This is an important consideration, because some theories suggest that toxemia is due to stretching of the uterus in pregnancy. This cannot be true, since toxemia can develop in women whose pregnancy is not in the uterus.

371 Do some women have a high risk for developing toxemia of pregnancy?

Although any pregnant woman can have toxemia of pregnancy, there are individuals in whom this disorder is more likely to occur:

Women who have high blood pressure at the time they become pregnant

Teenagers or older women who become pregnant

Women who are having their first babies

Women who are carrying twins (or more)

Diabetics

Women who have hydatidiform molar pregnancy

Women whose family members (mother, sisters) had toxemia of pregnancy

Women who have had toxemia with a previous pregnancy

372 How will my doctor check for toxemia of pregnancy?

There are three significant indicators.

Hypertension. A blood-pressure reading is written with one number over the other, such as 120/70. The upper number is the systolic pressure and the lower number is the diastolic. If the systolic pressure is 140 millimeters of mercury (mm Hg) or higher, or if, while you are pregnant it rises by 30 points, you have high blood pressure.

If the diastolic pressure is 90 or above, or if during pregnancy it increases by 15 points, you have high blood pressure.

A one-time reading of your blood pressure showing one of these abnormalities is not necessarily anything to worry about. Your doctor would want to check the pressure again, probably the next day, to see if it continues to be elevated.

Protein in the urine. During most office visits your urine will be tested for protein. A trace of protein can merely be the result of vaginal secretions or a temporary, normal spill of protein from the kidneys into your urine. If the urinalysis shows a 3+ or 4+ reaction on the test, you have an abnormal amount of protein in your urine. This is probably due to toxemia.

If you have protein in your urine, but your blood pressure is normal, you might still have toxemia, but your doctor might suggest an evaluation by a kidney specialist to make sure that you do not have a kidney disease. If you have 3+ or 4+ protein in your urine and also have high blood pressure, you almost certainly have toxemia of pregnancy.

Swelling (edema). If you have high blood pressure and either protein in your urine or swelling or both, you have developed toxemia (preeclampsia). Years ago doctors felt that any significant swelling was a sure sign of developing toxemia. If

Toxemia of Pregnancy

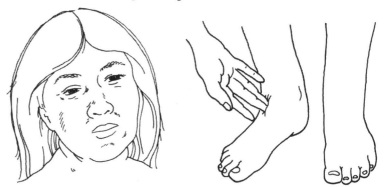

Toxemia of pregnancy. Two signs of worsening toxemia are increasing weight gain and swelling especially of face and ankles.

a woman's blood pressure is normal and she does not have protein in her urine, we usually accept swelling as a normal part of pregnancy.

Diuretics are often given only to women who have so much swelling of their feet that they actually hurt. Some doctors feel that it is unwise to give diuretics even then. (See Q. 266.)

Thiazide diuretics have been found to depress the formation of blood-clotting factors (platelets) in the fetus, causing hemorrhage in the baby when it is born. Diuretics can decrease the blood volume of a pregnant mother enough to lower the flow of blood through the baby's placenta. This can be especially dangerous during the last three months of pregnancy.

Because of these problems with diuretics, and because diuretics do not help in the management of preeclampsia, most doctors feel it is best not to use diuretics in pregnancy. Discuss this with your physician.

373 What if my blood pressure was high before I got pregnant? Will I develop toxemia?

If your blood pressure was high when you became pregnant, you will probably continue to have problems with high blood pressure throughout your pregnancy. You will not necessarily develop toxemia.

The higher your blood pressure is—even if you are not toxemic—the greater chance there is that your baby will be affected. It has been shown that if a woman's blood pressure is 200/120 or greater when she becomes pregnant, she can expect to have her baby die (either before or directly after delivery) 50 percent of the time. Of those babies that don't die, many will be affected by poor growth during the pregnancy.

Most doctors feel that if the high blood pressure is below 150/100, no immediate medical treatment is required. They would watch the growth of the baby carefully to be sure that the baby is growing adequately. If the baby's growth seems inadequate, early delivery may be advised.

If you are taking medication for high blood pressure when you become pregnant, it is prob-ably best that you stay on that medication throughout pregnancy. There are some blood pressure medications, however, that a woman should not take while she is pregnant; your doctor would want to evaluate your medicine to be sure it is proper for you to use it while you are pregnant.

Some women who have hypertension (high blood pressure) when they become pregnant will develop toxemia of pregnancy. Signs of this would usually be swelling, blood pressure getting even higher, and urine having protein. If this happens, both the mother and her baby should be watched very closely. The mother will probably be put on high blood pressure medication; the baby will be watched for intrauterine growth retardation and delivered early if necessary.

374 Why is toxemia a problem? Does it hurt both me and my baby?

Toxemia of pregnancy and its complications are still a leading cause of death of pregnant women in the United States. If you develop severe preeclampsia, you could begin having seizures, which can be dangerous for you and your baby. You could also develop a problem called HELLP syndrome. The "H" refers to hemolysis, the breaking down of your blood cells; the "EL" refers to elevated liver enzymes, which means your liver is being affected by your toxemia; the "LP" refers to low platelets (platelets are required for proper clotting of the blood). If you develop this syndrome, there is an increased risk of bleeding either before or after you deliver—a dangerous situation for both you and your baby.

The treatment of toxemia is especially directed toward your baby since obviously the baby can be affected by toxemia. If your toxemia persists, your baby can have poor growth (intrauterine growth retardation). With significant toxemia, your baby has a greater chance of dying before or after delivery. The seizures that an eclampsia mother has are extremely dangerous for her baby; it is important that they be prevented.

375 What are specific symptoms of worsening toxemia?

Notify your doctor if you experience any of the following symptoms:

Severe, persistent headache. This can be a sign of elevated blood pressure and should be reported to your doctor right away.

Trouble with vision. If your vision is blurred or you have trouble focusing, report it to your doctor.

Pain in the upper abdomen. If you start having really bothersome pain in the upper part of your abdomen, especially on the right side, you should notify your doctor immediately. This can indicate swelling of the liver.

Weight gain and swelling. If you notice a significant weight gain, accompanied by swelling, you may have worsening toxemia.

Convulsions. If your toxemia is bad enough to cause a convulsion, you need to be treated immediately and expertly.

376 How is toxemia treated?

If your toxemia does not seem to be severe (your blood pressure and the albumin level in your urine are not unduly elevated), the doctor will recommend bed rest. Be sure to follow instructions. Stop being the primary caregiver for your other children. Stop cooking, going to the grocery store, and doing car pools. It is important that you actually go to bed and stay in bed except to get up to go to the bathroom, or perhaps to move to the couch to watch television. The doctor will probably want to see you twice a week.

If you will do this and keep your appointments with your doctor, you may be able to avoid having to go to the hospital. In spite of good care at home, though, women will occasionally have worsening toxemia. Hospital admission is then usually mandatory.

If the doctor is fearful that a woman is about to have a convulsion due to the toxemia, she may be treated with magnesium sulfate to prevent the convulsions, and possibly Apresoline (an antihypertensive drug) to keep her blood pressure from getting too high. Doctors will be careful about giving too much medicine to lower the blood pressure, because if blood pressure gets too low, it can limit the amount of blood and, therefore, of oxygen, circulating in the placenta and the baby.

The treatment of toxemia is not only complicated but also somewhat controversial. If you have toxemia, you need to talk with your physician about his or her particular approach to the treatment of this disease. The primary element, though, is bed rest. Not only your life but also the life of your baby may depend on it.

377 Is there a cure for toxemia?

The cure for toxemia is delivery. When your pregnancy is over, your toxemia will soon vanish.

If your toxemia is severe early in pregnancy, the doctor will insist that the baby be delivered so that you will not progress to convulsions. If you have already had convulsions, the baby must be delivered, regardless of the stage of the pregnancy. This must be done, because once severe toxemia develops, and once convulsions start, they do not stop until the baby is delivered. There are few situations in pregnancy in which the lives of both the baby and the mother are endangered, but this is one of them. Even if the baby must be delivered so early that its death is inevitable, this should be done so the life of the mother can be saved.

Fortunately toxemia usually does not get severe until later in pregnancy. Delivery of a premature baby will often require cesarean section. You should certainly give your consent if your doctor recommends delivery of a premature baby by cesarean section. Most babies can be put into a good intensive care nursery where they will be better off than in your uterus if you have toxemia.

Do not be surprised if the doctor wants to monitor your blood pressure, urine output, and urine albumin for the first few days after delivery. During this time there is a chance of your developing very high blood pressure and even of having a convulsion. In some patients, toxemia will persist for days even after delivery.

378 How is my unborn baby cared for if I am toxemic?

Your doctor will be watching the baby's development as your toxemia is treated. He or she will be carefully measuring the baby to be sure that it is growing properly. Failure to grow adequately can indicate intrauterine growth retardation, which could result from inadequate oxygen and nutrients getting to the baby. This seems to occur because toxemia causes spasm of the uterine blood vessels and decreases the amount of blood flow to the baby.

The doctor may want you to have tests done to make sure the baby is developing properly. (See Q. 397–406.) If there are signs that the baby is not developing well, the doctor will want to consider delivering your baby, even if it requires a cesarean section.

Diseases and Abnormalities of the Reproductive Organs

379 Are there diseases and abnormalities of the female organs that might cause problems or complications during pregnancy?

Yes; there may be ovarian cysts, fibroid tumors, cervical irregularities, genital warts, and herpes. These problems are discussed in the following questions. General discussion of these and other disorders will be found in chapters 10 and 13.

380 My doctor says that I have a cyst on the ovary. Does this endanger my pregnancy, and do I need surgery?

The cyst your doctor found may be the corpus luteum cyst of pregnancy, a normal change associated with pregnancy. When your ovary released the egg that was fertilized to become this pregnancy, it immediately formed a corpus luteum cyst. A corpus luteum cyst of pregnancy is responsible for producing progesterone, the hormone that maintains your pregnancy during the first few weeks. Progesterone is absolutely necessary for your pregnancy to continue. You would miscarry if your corpus luteum cyst stopped producing progesterone before the ninth week of pregnancy.

Your doctor can occasionally feel this cyst during the pelvic exam early in pregnancy; if you have an ultrasound scan done early in pregnancy, the cyst will often be seen. Such a cyst may become as large as two to two and a half inches in diameter and may persist for several months into the pregnancy. This cyst is normal and will gradually disappear during the pregnancy.

It is, of course, possible for you to have a growth on your ovary during pregnancy. If an enlargement of your ovary develops during your pregnancy, the doctor may feel that it should be removed. If possible, the doctor would perform the surgery during the middle three months of your pregnancy; this is the time least likely to cause premature labor.

Since a growth on the ovary has a 3 percent chance of being malignant, you and the doctor must make sure that you do not have such a malignancy present. Also, since ovarian growths can obstruct labor, a large one is best removed during the middle part of the pregnancy.

During such surgery the doctor will occasionally find that the enlargement was not a growth but was merely a corpus luteum cyst on the ovary. If this could have been definitely determined beforehand, surgery would not have been necessary. A sonogram of the ovaries can help differentiate between a cyst and a growth. However, whenever an ovarian enlargement continues to be present and seems suspicious to your doctor, there may be no choice but to have surgery. If you have any question about your doctor's recommendation, get a second opinion.

It is possible, although uncommon, for an ovary made heavier by an ovarian growth to twist around on itself and cut off its own blood supply. This will cause a great deal of pain and will necessitate immediate surgery, regardless of the stage of pregnancy. This is called adnexal torsion.

381 How will fibroid tumors in the uterus affect pregnancy?

Fibroid tumors usually do not cause pain or trouble in pregnancy. Occasionally, however, a fibroid will outgrow its blood supply; it will begin degenerating and then cause pain. If you have a fibroid and are having pain in the area of the fibroid, you usually do not need surgery. The fibroid will probably cure itself, gradually turning into scar.

Sometimes a fibroid will be large enough to require a cesarean section because its size or location will interfere with normal labor. This is unusual.

It is, of course, possible for a woman to have fibroids inside her uterus. If so, they can cause a miscarriage. In most cases, though, if a woman had fibroids growing in her uterus, they would have caused bleeding or infertility and she would have had them taken care of before she became pregnant.

Fibroids do not become cancerous. If they are not too large, and you get pregnant without any trouble, and if you can carry the pregnancy without difficulty, the fibroids can be left alone. (See the section on fibroids for more information.)

382 My doctor says that my uterus is retroverted. Is this a cause for alarm during pregnancy?

A retroverted uterus, one that is tipped or turned backward, is not abnormal; one-third of all women have a retroverted uterus. Rarely, however, a woman's uterus will stay in a retroverted position during pregnancy and not "lift up" out of the pelvis. The growth of the uterus can then force the cervix (the mouth of the uterus) up against the bladder, causing the woman to have trouble passing urine.

To correct this the doctor may need to push the uterus up and out of the pelvis. This usually produces immediate relief.

Sometimes a uterus can be so low in a woman's pelvis that the cervix will protrude from the vagina. This is not dangerous, but women who have this problem usually experience a lot of vaginal and pelvic pressure in addition to the discomfort of feeling the cervical protrusion. Most women are able to tolerate this problem once the situation is explained, especially since, as pregnancy progresses, the enlarging uterus will usually draw the cervix back up into the vagina.

383 What are some abnormalities of the cervix that can cause problems with pregnancy or delivery?

There are four conditions of the cervix that can cause problems.

incompetent cervix
cervical stenosis
abnormal Pap smear
cancer of the cervix

These conditions, as they relate to pregnancy, are discussed in the following questions.

384 What is an incompetent cervix?

An incompetent cervix is one that does not have the strength to hold the pregnancy. It relaxes and causes a woman to miscarry or to have a premature delivery. An incompetent cervix can cause loss of the baby during the middle three months of pregnancy.

There is almost no way for the doctor to be absolutely certain that an incompetent cervix caused the pregnancy loss unless a woman had an earlier loss of pregnancy during the middle three months. Most doctors usually suspect an incompetent cervix if everything else is normal and a miscarriage has occurred in the middle three months. (See. Q. 294.)

An incompetent cervical os may occasionally have been caused by previous surgery on the cervix, such as abortions, D&Cs, or conizations. Other causes can be tears at earlier deliveries, or DES exposure. (See section on DES.) Some women, however, have the condition without any previous cervical tearing or surgery. They were probably born with weak cervical tissue.

The woman who has had a previous loss of a pregnancy in the middle three months, and who has no explanation other than incompetent cervix, needs to be treated early in the subsequent pregnancy by having purse-string sutures put around her cervix to hold it closed. These sutures are put in through the vagina, and require that a woman have general, spinal, or epidural anesthesia.

Doctors usually put in sutures that can be removed when labor starts. This is called a McDonald "cerclage" procedure. Occasionally, when cervical damage is extensive, a permanent strip of material is put around the cervix and left in place. Delivery is then by cesarean section. The surgery for strengthening the cervix with sutures or strips of material is called a cerclage procedure.

385 What can be done if I have an abnormal Pap smear while I am pregnant?

Ideally you should have had a Pap smear before you became pregnant and had any abnormality treated. If this was not done, however, and your doctor finds abnormal cervical cells during pregnancy or if your Pap smear becomes abnormal during pregnancy, you will need to be evaluated.

Fortunately with the advent of colposcopy, an examination of the cervix with a magnifying instrument, it is easier to evaluate the cervix than it once was. The doctor will put acetic acid on your cervix. (Acetic acid is the acid in vinegar.) It makes the areas of abnormality stand out more clearly. He or she will then look at your cervix with a colposcope. Frequently the doctor can tell whether or not the cells are malignant just by looking. If there is any question, however, a very small biopsy (pinch of tissue) may be taken and sent to a pathologist for evaluation. This will not harm your pregnancy even though your cervix may bleed more heavily than a nonpregnant woman's would. This is not a dangerous type of bleeding.

If you do not have invasive cancer on your cervix, the doctor will probably do a repeat colposcopy once or twice during the pregnancy just to make sure the growth on your cervix is not progressing, but he or she will not treat the area in any other way. You will usually be allowed to go through normal labor and delivery. You will probably need to return several weeks after your delivery for repeat colposcopy and treatment of the abnormal cells.

If your doctor, after finding abnormal cells in your Pap smear, recommends that surgery be done on your cervix without colposcopic diagnosis, you should ask to be referred to a doctor who does colposcopy. Without colposcopy, the only way that a doctor can make an accurate diagnosis is to put you in the hospital, have you anesthetized, and do a conization of your cervix. This is a bloody operation that can cause you to miscarry or go into premature labor. It is rarely necessary with the availability of colposcopy.

If, however, with colposcopy and biopsies, there is a suspicion that you might have invasive cancer of the cervix, then conization of the cervix would certainly be necessary. (See section on abnormal Pap smears.)

If cancer is found, some difficult decisions will need to be made. (See Q. 394.)

Genital Warts and Herpes during Pregnancy

386 What problems of the vulva or vagina might be present during pregnancy and cause problems?

Two problems of the vulva and/or vagina that might cause trouble are genital warts and herpes. These are discussed in the next two questions.

387 What are genital warts? What should be done if I have them?

Genital warts (condyloma acuminata) are warty growths that can grow in the vagina, on the cervix, on the external genitals, and on the anus. They are virus-caused and are not cancerous. (See Q. 968–972.)

It is a good idea to eliminate genital warts before delivery, not only because they are irritating and bothersome, but also because at delivery they can bleed and tear more easily than normal tissue. Also, pregnancy can cause them to grow extremely fast. As a result, by the time a pregnant woman is at term, she may have such massive genital warts that a cesarean section is necessary.

Podophyllum, a solution that is often used on warts, can cause a pregnant woman to become sick. It usually is not used during pregnancy. Four other methods of treatment are available. In my opinion, the best treatment is the laser, which allows removal of the wart without damaging the tissue from which the wart is growing; warts often seem less likely to grow back after laser treatment than they are with other methods. Laser is safe in pregnancy. It does require some type of anesthesia. A second method of treatment is freezing. A third method is treatment with trichloroacetic acid. Finally, a different method of treatment (with local or general anesthesia) is for the doctor to cut the large warts off and, at the same time, cauterize the smaller warts.

The genital wart virus can be transmitted to babies at delivery and produce small growths called papillomas on their vocal cords. One patient's child has had more than one hundred operations on his vocal cords because of this problem. If you have genital warts at the time of your delivery, tell your baby's pediatrician about them.

388 What if I have herpes and am pregnant?

Even with the large number of people infected with herpes in the United States, herpes-affected babies are not common. It is estimated that only about one child per two thousand to five thousand deliveries will become infected with the herpes virus. Since there are 3.5 million deliveries a year, there are about a thousand babies born with herpes in the United States annually. About 60 to 80 percent of these babies are born to women who had absolutely no symptoms of herpes and no history of ever having had a herpes outbreak.

If you have been diagnosed as having herpes,

the treatment that you and your doctor will want to follow will probably be that which is recommended by the American College of Obstetricians and Gynecologists. In their *Technical Bulletin* (November 1988, no. 122) they offered these recommendations:

During Pregnancy

1. Cultures should be done when a woman has active herpes lesions during pregnancy to confirm the diagnosis. If there is no visible lesion at the onset of labor, vaginal delivery is acceptable.
2. Weekly surveillance cultures of pregnant women with a history of herpes infections, but no visible lesions, are not necessary and vaginal delivery is acceptable.
3. Amniocentesis (withdrawing some amniotic fluid from around the baby) in an attempt to rule out intrauterine infection is not recommended for mothers with herpes infections at any stage of gestation.

During Labor

1. If a woman has a herpes lesion present when she goes into labor, she should have a cesarean section. There is adequate proof now that this lowers the chance of a baby developing herpes, but it does not prevent all cases of herpes in the baby. (Cesarean section should be done even if the bag of waters has been ruptured for many hours.)
2. Scalp electrodes may be used during labor if necessary for protection of the baby.
3. Even though a woman has had recurrent herpes infections, if she does not have a sore or herpes outbreak at the time of delivery, she can be allowed to have normal vaginal delivery.

If the herpes a woman breaks out with right at her delivery time is her very first (primary) herpes infection, her baby has a very high (about 50 percent chance) of becoming infected unless a C-section is done. If the herpes outbreak on the mother is not her first (called a secondary infection), the baby has a much smaller chance of becoming herpes infected (less than 6 percent). Still, a C-section is probably wise.

It is important for the pediatrician who will care for a baby born to a mother with herpes to be aware of her infection. The pediatrician will then make the decision about starting the baby on herpes medication, either vidarabine or acyclovir (Zovirax).

Despite early identification and prompt treatment of herpes in a baby, over half the infants with herpes type II infection still develop severe neurologic disability or die.

Even if you think you could not have herpes, if you have any kind of vulvar outbreak during your pregnancy that might be herpes, you should have a culture done to find out for sure. (See Q. 974–979.)

Surgery during Pregnancy

389 What problems might necessitate abdominal surgery while I am pregnant?

Problems that might require an abdominal incision other than C-section are the same as those that would necessitate surgery on a nonpregnant woman: an acute attack of gallbladder disease, appendicitis, intestinal obstruction, or rupture of a blood vessel inside the abdomen.

Any of these problems that require surgery will give you definite signals that something is wrong. If you begin having unusual abdominal pain, don't delay calling your doctor. This is called an "acute abdomen" by physicians and is a true emergency.

If your abdomen is unusually tender when the doctor examines you, he or she may feel that immediate surgery is necessary.

It is sometimes difficult to diagnose a problem of abdominal pain in a pregnant woman. The obstetrician is the expert in knowing whether a problem is really severe enough to require surgery. A pregnant woman often does not feel discomfort in her abdomen as strongly as a woman who is not pregnant. Because of this, a pregnant woman can have a ruptured appendix, for example, and only

have mild pain. This, of course, can be a very dangerous situation. Your doctor may need to call in a general surgeon for consultation. This expertise will keep your condition from reaching the stage where you become dangerously ill or lose your baby. If an obstetrician feels that a problem is severe enough to warrant surgery, have it done. To delay can result in your dying. It is better to have surgery even if, for instance, an appendix turns out to be normal than to delay and then find out that appendicitis was present and was allowed to rupture and cause generalized infection.

390 Will surgery cause me to miscarry or deliver prematurely?

The surgery itself is not likely to cause you to miscarry or deliver early. The medical problem that makes the surgery necessary can cause your uterus to begin contracting and result in miscarriage or premature delivery. For example, infection of the appendix can cause irritation of the uterus and then premature labor.

There are drugs that can be given to relax the uterus to help prevent contractions. In spite of that, a woman will occasionally lose the pregnancy. Delaying the surgery, however, will not make you less likely to miscarry, since the problem causes the miscarriage, not the surgery itself. The sooner you have the surgery, therefore, the less likely you are to miscarry or to deliver prematurely.

The overriding principle concerning surgery during pregnancy is that if surgery is necessary, have it done.

391 Will anesthetics during surgery hurt my baby?

Studies indicate that all of the commonly used drugs that might be given for anesthesia during pregnancy are safe. This includes Pentothal, nitrous oxide, Halothane, and similar drugs. Also included are the drugs used for relaxation during surgery, such as curare and succinyl choline. In addition, drugs such as lidocaine, bupivacaine, morphine, and Fentanyl used for local injection, for epidurals, and for spinals have not been associated with any abnormality in babies.

If you must have surgery during pregnancy, you can be quite confident that the anesthetic agents will not harm your baby.

Cancer and Pregnancy

392 Does cancer occur during pregnancy?

Cancer in a mother's body during pregnancy is rare, occurring in about one in a thousand pregnancies. The cancers that most often occur in pregnant women are, in order of frequency, cervical cancer, breast cancer, ovarian cancer, lymphomas, leukemia, thyroid cancer, and colon and rectal cancer. Other cancers do occur during pregnancy, but more rarely.

About 15 percent of the cases of breast cancer occur in women who are younger than forty-one years of age. Since more women are delaying childbirth until they are older, doctors are seeing breast cancer in about 3 percent of all pregnant patients.

It was felt in the past that breast cancer grew faster and was harder to cure in pregnant women. The major problem, though, has been the tendency of both patients and doctors to ignore breast lumps during pregnancy because they assumed that the lumps were caused by hormones of pregnancy. This assumption delays treatment, giving the cancer a greater chance to grow and spread.

If you have a mass in your breast that is new and different from anything you have felt before, whether or not you are pregnant, you must bring it to your doctor's attention. Further, you should get a second opinion if you continue to feel uncomfortable about the lump and your doctor does not seem to be paying close attention to it.

Your best chance of cure is to find a breast cancer when it is small, and to get it diagnosed and treated early. With prompt care you are as likely to have as good a prognosis as a woman who is not pregnant when her breast cancer is found. For further information on breast abnormalities, see Q. 756–787.

393 How is breast cancer treated during pregnancy?

Diagnosis and treatment of cancer during pregnancy are essentially the same as if you were not pregnant, though there are some slight risks to your pregnancy from these procedures. It is comforting to know that the chance of your baby being affected by mammograms is essentially zero.

There is a slight chance of miscarriage with any operation during pregnancy. The chance of miscarriage during a breast biopsy is extremely slight, and is still minimal even if a mastectomy is done.

If you have breast cancer, some of the cancer could have already spread to the lymph nodes under the arm, or to other parts of the body by the time you find it. In this case you might need chemotherapeutic drugs. Surprisingly, most chemotherapy drugs given after the first three months do not seem to hurt the baby. There is some increased risk if these drugs are given in the first trimester.

Most experts do not recommend X-ray therapy during any stage of pregnancy.

You do not need to have an abortion done because you have been found to have breast cancer. Terminating the pregnancy will not give you a better chance of cure.

One other concern is whether or not you should ever become pregnant again after having had breast cancer. Formerly, most doctors advised patients not to get pregnant again because of the possibility of hormone stimulation to cancer cells, but statistics now seem to show that if you have gone five years without any recurrence of breast cancer, it is "safe" to get pregnant again.

Statistics show that even those women who get pregnant during the five years after having their breast cancer discovered are not adversely affected as far as survival rates. Further, nursing the baby on the one remaining breast has not been shown to cause the cancer to return sooner nor to have any effect on the cancer or on the baby.

394 Can I develop cancer of the cervix while pregnant? How is it treated?

Cancer of the cervix can occur during pregnancy, as we discussed briefly in Q. 385; as a matter of fact, it is the most common malignancy occurring with pregnancy. If abnormal cervical cells are discovered (from biopsy, colposcopy, or conization) but there are no cancer cells invading your tissues, you can have a normal vaginal delivery. This includes carcinoma *in situ*, a skin-cancer-type growth on your cervix often called CIN III.

If cervical cancer has already begun invading your tissues (true cervical cancer), and you are in the first half of pregnancy, the cancer needs to be treated as though you were not pregnant. This is one of the few medical conditions in a pregnant woman that makes an abortion necessary to save the life of the mother. If a cervical cancer is found when pregnancy has just begun, by the time delivery might occur spontaneously, the cancer would probably have grown so much that it would no longer be curable. For the best chance of a woman's survival, this type of cancer needs to be treated immediately, even if it means an abortion. A hysterectomy may be necessary (which, of course, would involve removal of the uterus with the baby in it) or your cervix may need radiation treatment.

If radiation is used, it will almost always produce a miscarriage. If it does not, the baby, placenta, and membranes must be removed from the uterus either by induction of labor or by the use of abortion techniques. This is because it is necessary for radium to be put up inside the cervix for proper treatment of the cervical cancer.

If you are in the third trimester of pregnancy when the cancer is discovered, the risk in allowing your baby to grow to the point where it can be delivered early and yet be mature enough to live may be an acceptable risk for you. You would need to discuss this with your physicians. The delivery must be by cesarean section, since delivery through a cervix with cancer might cause the cancer to spread. Pregnancy itself does not cause cancer of the cervix to grow any faster or to spread more quickly than it would when one is not pregnant.

395 How are cancers other than those of the breast and cervix treated during pregnancy?

Other cancers, as previously mentioned, occur less frequently in pregnancy. The general rule about treatment is that if the cancer is found in the third trimester of pregnancy, it is acceptable, and usually desirable, to avoid treatment until the baby is mature enough to survive premature delivery. If the pregnancy is not yet into the third trimester when the cancer is found, it is best to treat the cancer as though the pregnancy does not exist.

Since drugs and radiation can affect the baby, a decision about a therapeutic abortion must be reached by the patient and the doctors involved in treatment. This type of problem, of course, produces great emotional conflict. It is a time to have doctors who are very sensitive. It is also a time to have good counsel and comfort from friends, from professional counselors, and from pastor, priest, or rabbi. All these resources are available, and I strongly encourage patients to take advantage of them. This is not a time to try to go it alone. Ultimately, though, it is you and your husband who must make the final decisions.

The Age Factor and Pregnancy

396 Does my being over thirty-five affect my chances for a normal pregnancy and delivery?

I am frequently asked by patients in their thirties if it is "okay" for them to have a baby. These patients are concerned about the ability to conceive, carrying a pregnancy full term, and having a normal and healthy baby. These are legitimate concerns. They are discussed in the following questions and in Q. 792.

One concern is whether or not an older woman can carry a pregnancy to term and if the pregnancy will be dangerous to her. There is an increased chance of miscarriage as a woman grows older. Several studies have shown this. One example is a study that showed that women between the ages of twenty and thirty-five have a 10–15 percent chance of miscarriage; women between thirty-five and thirty-nine have a 17.7 percent chance of miscarriage; and women between forty and forty-four have a 33.8 percent chance of miscarriage. Other studies show the same trend for women as they get older.

Women frequently want to know if it is physically safe to be pregnant after the age of thirty-five. In an article titled "Pregnancy after Thirty-five" in the *Williams Obstetrics Supplement* (no. 2, October–November 1989, Cunningham, Mac-Donald, and Gantt), the summary statement read:

> Although risks are not unequivocally increased, pregnancy in this age group can be concluded to be quite safe, especially in the absence of pre-existing medical disorders. For example, in 1983, maternal mortality for women aged thirty-five to thirty-nine was as low as the rate for women in the ideal reproductive age range (twenty to twenty-four years) during 1960 (Smith, 1987). It is also somewhat ironic that in 1989 we are writing about pregnancy after the age of thirty-five, since, according to Garrett (1988), life expectancy was only thirty-five years in colonial America!

Most studies show that if a woman who is over thirty-five does not have high blood pressure, diabetes, or chronic kidney disease, she has a small chance of having medical problems during her pregnancy. Pregnancy itself does not produce any damage to a woman's body just because she is over thirty-five. The problem is that more women over thirty-five have high blood pressure, diabetes, and kidney disease when they become pregnant.

The third question regarding pregnancy for women who are thirty-five or older is whether or not they will have a healthy baby. They are concerned not only about whether their babies will have a genetic abnormality such as Down syndrome but also about other effects their age might have on a baby's physical and mental health.

Risks do increase as a woman grows older. J. P. Hansen, in an article in *OB/GYN Survey* (1986, 41:726), showed that fetal chromosome abnormalities, such as trisomies 13, 18, 21 and sex chromosome aneuploidy, increase in the middle thirties. At age thirty-five, the fetal chromosome abnormality rate is less than 1 percent; at age forty it is 1.9 percent; and at age forty-five, it is 8.9 percent.

Some studies indicate that women over thirty-five have a significantly higher rate of problems during pregnancy. They have more uterine bleeding, more babies with intrauterine growth retardation and fetal distress, more cesarean sections, and more stillborn babies.

Other studies seem to show that with good obstetric care, these problems are primarily confined to women who have hypertension, diabetes, or some other medical problem when they become pregnant.

Most obstetricians seem to feel that, although there is some increased risk to being pregnant past age thirty-five, the risk is minimal except for the increasing risk of genetic abnormalities. In the majority of cases, a healthy pregnancy for both mother and baby can be anticipated.

Statistics are on the side of the older woman having a healthy, normal baby. For instance, even at age forty-five, taking the highest number of genetic abnormalities that are predicted (10 percent), a woman still has a 90 percent chance of having a healthy, normal baby so far as chromosomal problems are concerned.

To help increase the chance of this happening, Steven G. Gabbe, M.D., a highly respected authority concerning obstetrical issues, reported in *Ob-Gyn Clinical Alert* (December 1995) that

> I have adopted a policy of more intensive antepartum fetal surveillance for women who are 35 or older. I begin all patients on fetal movement counting at 28 weeks' gestation. I also initiate weekly nonstress testing in older women at 32 weeks' gestation and increase the frequency of testing to twice weekly at 36 weeks' gestation. I rarely allow a woman 35 years of age or older to remain undelivered after 40 weeks' gestation.

Monitoring the Fetus

397 What tests can be done to determine whether or not the baby is developing normally?

Every parent and every doctor wants to avoid the agony of delivering a stillborn or defective baby. Modern fetal monitoring makes it possible to avoid, minimize, or at least anticipate problems.

If you or the baby has a problem that might result in a stillbirth, the doctor would want to deliver the baby before that happened. He or she would also want to avoid delivery of a baby so premature that it would have to be on a respirator for weeks or in intensive care for months. Fetal monitoring helps accomplish these goals.

If your physician has any question about your baby's health, he or she will probably do some tests to evaluate the baby's condition. Such evaluation may be quite simple (as in having you count your baby's movements for a time period), or they may be more sophisticated (such as sonogram or amniocentesis).

There are many reasons for doing fetal evaluation tests. It would be impossible to enumerate them all here. They do include problems the mother may have such as diabetes, hypertension, lupus erythematosus, and so on. Fetal testing may be suggested if the pregnancy is going past due or if there is the possibility of intrauterine growth retardation. Evaluation of the fetus may also be done if the mother is a smoker or if there seems to be an inadequate amount of fluid in the amniotic sac.

The entire field of monitoring the baby inside the mother's uterus is constantly changing. There are no absolutes regarding procedure, indications, or time intervals. Your best chance for a healthy baby is to choose a physician who is keeping up-to-date on medical advances and then to do as he or she suggests.

No matter how carefully your physician watches your pregnancy, you do not have a guarantee that you will have a healthy baby. In addition, even if the tests indicate that your baby is having a major problem, the tests could be wrong, and your baby may be in no danger. There is no question, though, that if your doctor is watching you carefully and you are doing the testing that is indicated, you have a better chance of a healthy baby than if you do not do the indicated testing. You may feel that your doctor is asking you to do the tests too often. If the doctor really thinks something might be wrong with your baby, a week between tests can be too long. The baby can seem normal one week, but the next week be dead if there is something seriously wrong. Because of this, your doctor may recommend testing twice a week.

Some of the tests for evaluating the baby's health are:

Sonogram (ultrasound)
Nonstress test (NST)
Contraction stress test (CST)
Fetal movement observation (by the mother at home)
Doppler ultrasound blood flow measurement
Fetal blood sampling (percutaneous umbilical blood sampling, PUBS)
Amniocentesis

An explanation of each of these procedures follows.

398 What is a sonogram (ultrasound) and how is it used to evaluate the health of my baby?

The ultrasound machine has been a revolutionary tool for obstetricians in pregnancy care. The procedure allows a good look at a woman's abdomen, her uterus, her baby, and the related structures without invading those structures. It is not an X-ray nor it is related to X-ray.

There have never been any reports of damage to a baby from ultrasound.

The only preparation for an abdominal ultrasound test is drinking water to fill the bladder. Having an ultrasound is not usually painful. It does not require the use of needles or other "painful" devices. There may be some mild discomfort from the pressure of the transducer on a woman's abdomen or in her vagina, however, and the full bladder can be uncomfortable.

399 How is ultrasound used as a prenatal diagnostic tool?

Diagnostic ultrasonography (ultrasound, scan, or sonogram) involves the use of high-frequency sound waves that are radiated into the body from a handheld transmitter or transducer. The transducer is "connected" to the body by a lubricant through which sound waves can travel. The sound waves bounce off the baby and the organs inside your body and back to the transmitting device. The echoes received are projected on a monitor (TV screen) for evaluation.

In early pregnancy, your physician may want to use a vaginal transducer, which allows a different view of the uterus and the baby. This is very much like a pelvic exam that your physician does but is usually more comfortable. It does not require a full bladder.

The usefulness of the ultrasound scan is in the following areas.

Determination of length of pregnancy. Knowing how far along you are in pregnancy is one of the most important factors in evaluating the health of your baby. If you are not sure when you became pregnant, an early sonogram can accurately determine that. Three weeks after the day your egg was fertilized, the doctor can see a sac in your uterus. Four weeks after the day of fertilization, he or she can see the baby's little body in the sac. Five weeks after fertilization the doctor can see the baby's heartbeat.

Number of babies in the uterus. With ultrasound, the number of babies in your uterus can be determined as soon as you are three to five weeks from the day of fertilization. This is helpful information, because if there is more than one baby, things can be done to help prevent premature delivery.

Evaluation of the baby's growth. An ultrasound can show if the baby's growth rate is too slow. If a baby is not developing quickly enough, it may have intrauterine growth retardation. This can be a sign that the baby is not healthy. If your baby has this problem, further evaluations may be necessary. If poor growth continues, your doctor may want to deliver the baby early, as it may do better in an intensive care nursery than inside your uterus.

Congenital abnormalities. The ultrasound scan can detect certain abnormalities of the baby, such as those of the head, spinal cord, chest, or abdomen.

Amount of fluid surrounding the baby. The ultrasound can show how much fluid is present around the baby. If the amount of fluid around the baby is small, there is a great chance that the baby is experiencing poor growth and needs to be further evaluated or perhaps delivered. Excess fluid is also a clue that something is wrong.

Knowing your due date is very important. A mother may think, for instance, that she became pregnant later than she really did, causing the doctor to believe that something is wrong with the baby because the baby is not as large as it should be. Also, knowing precisely the status of the pregnancy is vital in much of the testing the baby might need later because there are different normal values for different times of the pregnancy.

Knowing your due date also makes it possible for the doctor to know when it is safe to deliver your baby. For instance, if you are going to have your labor induced, or if you are going to have a scheduled cesarean section, your doctor will want you to have an ultrasound between the twentieth and twenty-fifth weeks of pregnancy so the delivery will not be done too early.

Assistance at other procedures done during pregnancy. If your doctor is going to do an amniocentesis, he or she will usually use the ultrasound machine to locate your placenta to avoid inserting the needle into it. (Ultrasound is also necessary for locating the baby's umbilical cord if your doctor needs to draw blood from it for testing or to give the baby a transfusion.)

Biophysical profile. The ultrasound is used to perform a biophysical profile, which is a test to measure various aspects of the health of the fetus. It has changed some from its original design in 1980 by Manning and his associates. It will undoubtedly change more in the future. A biophysical profile as it is practiced by many physicians today includes observation and evaluation of five things: the health of the placenta (placental grade), fetal tone (the tone of the baby's body), fetal breathing, fetal movement, and amniotic fluid volume (whether too little or too much amniotic fluid). Some studies show that if all of these measurements are normal the baby has a minimal chance of being unhealthy and dying before it is born.

400 What is a nonstress test?

A nonstress test (NST) is based on the heartbeat of a baby who is at least twenty-eight to thirty-four weeks along. When the baby moves, that movement should be followed by an increase in its heart rate. If the heart rate does not increase, the baby may not be healthy.

This is quite logical. When you exercise, you expect your heart rate to increase; if it does not, there is probably something wrong.

Studies have shown that about 5 percent of babies whose NSTs are not satisfactory will be sick when they are born.

In addition to watching for an increased heartbeat after the baby moves, the NST checks the heart rate itself. The heart rate of a sick baby may also show other abnormalities. These are:

A too-regular heart rate. The heart rate should vary. When a baby's heartbeat is totally regular, it indicates a loss of the variations in the heart rate that are normal for any baby in the uterus (or for any normal person). When variability is lost, the baby may be in jeopardy.

Decrease in heart rate accompanying false labor pains (or true labor contractions). It is normal for the heart rate to fluctuate, but if the baby's heartbeat drops and stays down for several seconds after the contraction, that baby is probably very sick.

Absence or decrease in fetal movement. Lack of fetal movement for a prolonged time can be a dangerous sign. If this is seen on NST, it demands further evaluation.

401 How is a nonstress test (NST) done?

The nonstress test is usually done in the labor-and-delivery department of the hospital. A nurse will place a fetal monitor on your abdomen to listen to and record your baby's heartbeat. She will then watch for the baby to move and will get a good recording of that heartbeat after the baby's movements. If the baby does not move, the nurse will try to wake up the baby by moving you around, by turning on a television or radio that might be in the room, or by giving you something with sugar in it. She will want to see at least two periods of increased heart rate of at least fifteen beats per minute, lasting for fifteen seconds within a ten-minute period of time.

If the baby does not have such accelerations of the heartbeat—or if there are any factors present that would indicate a sick baby (such as lack of variation in the regular heartbeat or an abnormal dip in the heart rate associated with contractions), the doctor may suggest immediate delivery or a contraction stress test (CST). If the NST is normal, it is called a "reactive NST" and is reassuring evidence that the baby is normal.

402 What is a contraction stress test (CST)?

The contraction stress test (CST) is also called the oxytocin challenge test (OCT) because it usually involves giving the pregnant woman oxytocin (Pitocin). Since it is more accurate than the nonstress test, your doctor may occasionally feel that it would be wise to have an OCT to back up the nonstress test findings. If you are fairly close to your due date and your NST was abnormal, it would probably be easier for you to go ahead with delivery than to have the CST.

The contraction stress test is merely a way of causing the uterus to contract to see if these contractions cause the baby's heartbeat to drop. During a contraction, blood flow through the placenta is decreased. This decreased blood flow will allow less oxygen to get to the baby. This decrease in oxygen will cause an unhealthy baby's heartbeat to drop because of the stress.

If the contraction stress test is negative, it means that the baby's heartbeat reacted normally and the baby is probably healthy. If the test is positive, it means the baby's heart rate dropped abnormally during the contractions and the baby might be having problems and may need to be delivered. If the test is negative, it is very rare for the baby to die within one week of the test. If the test is positive, the baby may be very unhealthy. It is possible that the test could be positive and yet the baby is normal. This is called a "false positive" test. Your doctor will explain the results of the findings and make recommendations as to what should be done.

403 How is an oxytocin challenge test done?

Like the NST, the oxytocin challenge test is done in the labor-and-delivery room of the hospital. After you are put to bed, a nurse will start an IV. (Stimulating your nipples will sometimes cause the uterus to contract. Your doctor may want you to try this method. If it works and causes contractions, the IV may be unnecessary.) Then a heart rate monitor will be put on your abdomen and your baby's heartbeat recorded for twenty minutes. After getting an initial tracing of the baby's heartbeat, Pitocin will be added to the IV bottle and allowed to drip slowly into your vein. The doctor will be trying to produce three contractions in a ten-minute period, with each contraction lasting forty to sixty seconds.

The baby's heart rate will be measured during those three contractions. If it does not drop abnormally during and immediately after the contractions, the baby is probably healthy. If, however, the baby's heartbeat drops after the contractions, and stays down abnormally long, there is a fairly high possibility that the baby is sick.

The problem with the OCT is that at least 25 percent of babies who show a drop in the heartbeat after the contractions, if delivered, will be normal. The physician must evaluate the entire situation, taking into consideration both the NST and the OCT. After discussing the situation with you, a plan of action must be determined: possibly immediate delivery, or maybe a repeat of the tests.

404 How is fetal movement used as a prenatal evaluation method?

Some obstetricians will have their pregnant patients check fetal movement on a daily basis from the twenty-eighth week of pregnancy until delivery. (Others will recommend this only if there is a question about the baby's health.) The most common technique recommended is for the mother to record the fetal movements she feels during three separate hours each day: one hour in the morning, one hour at noon, and one hour in the evening. Most women who are carrying normal babies will feel more than three fetal movements in each one-hour period. If three or fewer fetal movements are felt in one of the hours of observation, the mother should observe fetal activity for six to twelve hours a day until she and her doctor are assured that the baby is healthy, or until delivery. She should normally feel ten significant movements in an eight-hour period if her baby is healthy.

An alternate technique is for a woman to start counting fetal movements at 9:00 A.M. The baby should move ten times by 6:00 P.M. If it doesn't, she should call her doctor.

It is interesting that most fetuses have a peak of activity between 9:00 P.M. and 1:00 A.M. (just what parents have always suspected). Most fetuses do show active periods alternating with quiet periods. If your baby is not too active in the morning, watch for activity late in the day.

A drop in the number of fetal movements over a three- or four-day period can indicate that the baby is having difficulty. If this happens, the doctor would want to do further tests to check the baby.

405 What is the Doppler ultrasound? How is it used for fetal evaluation?

"Doppler ultrasound" measures blood flow through specific blood vessels in the placenta, the baby, and the mother. Its primary use at this time is to measure blood flow through the placenta.

If a baby is not growing well inside the mother's uterus, measuring the blood flow through the placenta can indicate that the placenta is not healthy.

406 What is fetal blood sampling?

Fetal blood sampling is another relatively new technique for fetal evaluation. By inserting a needle through the skin of your abdomen into the baby's umbilical cord, the doctor can retrieve a sample of your baby's blood. This procedure is called percutaneous umbilical cord sampling (PUBS). Another name for it is "cordocentesis." Not only can the baby's blood be tested with this technique, but also a transfusion can be given this way.

New ways of using this procedure are increasing every year. At present, this technique is helpful in determining Rh problems with the baby, infections of the baby with toxoplasmosis, other infections, diagnosis of genetic disease, and so on. This is not a routine test; it requires a physician with a great deal of expertise.

Amniocentesis

407 What is amniocentesis?

Amniocentesis is a very important procedure for evaluating your baby. It is done primarily for two reasons: to make sure that the baby's lungs are mature enough for delivery if it needs to be delivered before term, and to do genetic tests on the baby.

A doctor injects a small amount of local anesthetic in the skin of the abdominal wall. Then a long needle is inserted through the abdominal wall, through the uterine wall, and into the sac of fluid that surrounds your baby. An ultrasound machine is normally used to locate the placenta so that the needle does not go into it. Amniotic fluid is drawn off for testing. The procedure usually does not cause much pain, and most women can tolerate it without complaint.

408 Is amniocentesis dangerous to me?

Risks for the mother from amniocentesis are extremely low. For instance, I know of no maternal deaths from amniocentesis in the United States, and I know of only one maternal death from amniocentesis reported in European literature. I have never seen a mother have any complication from amniocentesis. Occasionally a mother will cramp or bleed after the procedure, but this usually stops after a few hours. The most likely thing that could occur would be a mild infection where the needle is inserted through the abdominal wall. Such an infection might require antibiotics for the mother.

409 Is amniocentesis dangerous to my baby?

Risks to the fetus are greater than the risks to the mother. There is about a 0.5 percent chance of miscarriage as a result of amniocentesis. This means that one out of every two hundred babies will be miscarried. These babies are usually normal and are lost as a result of the procedure.

During the procedure the needle can poke the baby but normally does not damage or hurt it. The baby will merely move to avoid the needle. Before the use of ultrasound during amniocentesis there was a greater possibility of damaging the baby's eyes, puncturing the umbilical cord and causing it to bleed, or perforating the baby's lungs. Such risks have been virtually eliminated today with the use of ultrasound.

Amniocentesis

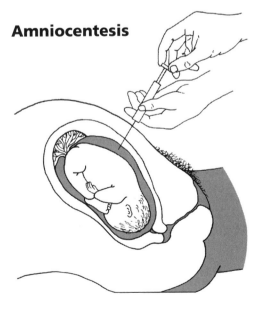

It is possible for the needle to carry germs into the amniotic sac. If this happens, the amniotic fluid can become infected, and this will almost always cause a miscarriage. If a miscarriage occurs after amniocentesis, infection is usually the cause.

410 How is amniocentesis used to determine the maturity of my baby?

If your doctor feels that your baby needs to be delivered before your due date, he or she will usually recommend an amniocentesis to make sure that the baby's lungs are mature enough for delivery. The amniocentesis will allow the measurement of the baby's phospholipids. Phospholipids provide a surfactant effect on the lining of each of the tiny sacs in the lungs. A surfactant is a substance that lines the air sacs in the lungs to allow them to remain open. Without the surface tension-lowering effect of surfactant, the baby's lungs will not stay open for adequate exchange of oxygen. If this happens, the baby will have respiratory distress (major problems with breathing after birth).

The phospholipids measured are lecithin and sphingomyelin. If the L/S ratio is greater than 2, the risk of the baby being born with respiratory distress is very small. Unfortunately, some babies, even with a L/S ratio of 2, will have trouble after delivery. This is more common if the mother has diabetes.

Babies who have an L/S ratio of less than 2 still can survive after delivery, though some of them will have respiratory distress.

411 How is amniocentesis used in genetic testing, and what factors should I consider before having it done?

By studying the baby's cultured cells under the microscope, the doctor can see if they show normal chromosomes. If normal chromosomes are present, the baby does not have Down syndrome (mongolism). Testing for this possibility is the primary reason for doing this type of amniocentesis, but there are other reasons for doing amniocentesis.

I know of an "older" couple who, despite an infertility problem, finally managed to achieve pregnancy. Without adequately considering the consequences, they had genetic amniocentesis performed. It resulted in the miscarriage of a healthy little boy and great heartbreak to these parents. My point is that the consequences of amniocentesis should be carefully considered, and it should not be done routinely or without good reason. For example, if you are fairly certain that if you were carrying a baby with a congenital abnormality you would not have an abortion done, then there is almost no reason to have the genetic amniocentesis.

A woman does not have to have an amniocentesis done. And even if she has an amniocentesis done and learns that her baby has an abnormality, she does not have to have an abortion. Unfortunately some doctors imply that a patient is legally required to have both an amniocentesis and an abortion if certain abnormalities are found. This is untrue! Any patient who has a doctor who would imply this, and she and her husband do not want an amniocentesis and/or abortion, should change doctors.

412 What abnormalities does amniocentesis not detect?

Some of the many problems that amniocentesis would not detect are:

- Isolated body defects not associated with genetic or chromosomal problems, such as absent or shortened fingers and toes, cleft lip, club foot, or absent or shortened arms and legs
- An infant whose growth is affected by its mother's smoking or alcohol intake
- Dwarfism
- Siamese twins
- Abnormalities produced by drugs the mother has taken
- Heart defects

413 Is there a "balanced" approach to amniocentesis?

Even if you and your husband are certain you would consider abortion if the test shows an abnormal baby, you still must be realistic about the fact that one in two hundred times of amniocentesis the pregnancy will be lost anyway. There is a possibility that you would lose a healthy, normal baby. You need thorough moral and medical counseling to help you decide what to do.

If you are so worried about having an abnormal baby that you are having amniocentesis done just to find out if the baby is normal, and you know that you have little risk of having an abnormal child, you need to stop and think about what you are doing. If your doctors tell you that you do not really need an amniocentesis, I suggest that you get some good counseling about handling your anxiety rather than endangering the probably normal baby inside you.

414 What are the problems that justify amniocentesis and abortion if there is a child with an abnormality (in the view of those who favor such abortion)?

There are four major categories to consider. They consist of situations in which there is:

A previous child with chromosomal abnormality

A mother whose age is advanced

A mother or father whose chromosomes are abnormal

The possibility of a metabolic disorder, a neural tube defect, or an X-linked disorder

415 What other tests can be done on the amniotic fluid?

In addition to chromosome studies and fetal lung maturity tests on cells cultured from the amniotic fluid, other tests can also be done. The most common test is having the amniotic fluid screened for alpha-fetoprotein (AFP). If the alpha-fetoprotein level in the amniotic fluid is elevated, the baby may have a neural tube defect such as anencephaly or spina bifida (see Q. 460). Other congenital abnormalities, such as omphalocele, cystic hygroma, and congenital nephrosis, can also produce an elevated alpha-fetoprotein level.

Amniotic fluid can be tested for signs of genetic metabolic disease. (See Q. 461.)

Intrauterine Growth Retardation (IUGR)

416 Tell me about small newborn babies. How are they related to intrauterine growth retardation?

Babies who are in the bottom 10 percent of weight of all babies born at their same stage of pregnancy are termed, "small for gestational age fetuses." If, for example, you delivered an eighth-month baby, it would be considered a small for gestational age fetus if it is in the smallest 10 percent of eighth-month babies. These babies can be divided into two groups.

The first group is made up of babies who are merely small "normally"—their mothers, who may be small, usually have small, healthy babies. Women who weigh less than 100 pounds, for instance, are twice as likely to have babies who are in the bottom 10 percent of weight of all babies born. Babies in this category are healthy and normal and not growth retarded.

The second group of "small for gestational age" fetuses are growth retarded. Some problem has affected their growth in the uterus. A baby who suffers from intrauterine growth retardation may need to be delivered early and put in the more healthy environment of the intensive care nursery.

It is important that the baby not be delivered so early that it will die or have major problems from immature lungs. It is vital that careful evaluation be done of a baby who is growth retarded.

417 Doesn't this just mean my baby is premature?

No, since no matter at what stage your baby is born, if he or she is in the smallest 10 percent of all babies born at that stage, he or she would probably be intrauterine growth retarded. Many babies are born small; one-third of these small babies are growth retarded and two-thirds are small because they were born prematurely.

418 What is the concern about intrauterine growth retardation (IUGR) and its effect on babies?

IUGR babies have a stillbirth or immediately after delivery death rate that is eight times higher than normal. Their deaths frequently occur during labor, delivery, or during the first four weeks of life. They seem increasingly fragile as they get closer to term, unlike normal babies who become stronger, and they are more likely to die during the last month of pregnancy than earlier in pregnancy.

419 What things on the mother's part might cause IUGR?

Medical problems can cause your baby to be growth retarded, but you can also do things that can cause the baby to have poor growth.

Hypertension and toxemia. If you have chronic hypertension or prolonged toxemia, your chance of having a baby with IUGR is greatly increased.

Chronic kidney disease. This can affect the baby's growth.

Sickle-cell anemia. This, or other chronic anemia, causes the baby to be deprived of the normal amount of oxygen and can result in poor growth.

Anorexia nervosa. This problem, manifested by a mother's aversion to food, results in a life-threatening weight loss for the mother and is disastrous for the baby.

Medications. Mothers who take Coumadin (a blood thinner that should not be used during pregnancy), Dilantin (a drug given for seizures that sometimes must be used in pregnancy), and certain other drugs, may have smaller babies.

Smoking. Women who smoke are not able to carry the normal amount of oxygen from their lungs to the baby. This causes the baby to be starved for oxygen and, therefore, not able to develop adequately. This can be illustrated by holding your nose and covering your mouth with your hand so tightly that you can barely get enough oxygen to survive. If you are a smoker, I suggest that you stop smoking. (See Q. 430–433.)

Studies have shown that if a mother stops smoking while she is pregnant, the baby will then start growing in a normal way, as though it is no longer being smothered.

Drinking. Alcohol consumption definitely affects a fetus. Although it is unlikely that a few sips of alcohol during pregnancy will hurt the baby, there is a proven relationship between the amount of alcohol taken in (as little as two drinks a week) and the health of the baby. My suggestion is to drink rarely, or not at all, during pregnancy and to avoid binge drinking completely. (See Q. 434–435.)

420 What problems with the baby can cause IUGR?

Problems with the baby that can cause it to have IUGR include:

Twin (or multiple) pregnancies. The incidence of growth retardation in twins is about one in five.

Abnormalities. Often babies will have abnormalities, including chromosomal abnormalities, which will cause them to grow poorly.

Placental abnormalities. If a blood vessel from the baby to the placenta is missing, the baby can be receiving an inadequate blood supply. If a portion of the placenta pulls loose (and stays loose), it can limit the nutrition of the baby. If there is a large area of the placenta that has been "stopped up" (a large placental infarct), the placenta is less able to provide nutrition to the baby.

Infections. Certain infections, such as German measles (see Q. 328–331), toxoplasmosis (see Q. 335–336), or cytomegaloviral (see Q. 332) infections, will cause a baby to grow poorly. Fortunately these problems occur rarely.

Prematurity. A premature baby is sometimes poorly nourished. Prematurity and IUGR can coexist in a baby.

Naturally small babies. Some babies are small just because their mothers and fathers are small. Such babies must be watched just as carefully as babies that are small for other reasons.

If you have had a baby with IUGR in the past, you have a ten times greater chance of having another baby with this problem.

421 What will my doctor do if he or she suspects that I am carrying a baby with IUGR?

There are several ways the doctor can evaluate the baby; some of them are unreliable. The most reliable ones are:

Measuring the growth of the uterus. Your doctor will measure your uterine growth each time you come in. The actual numbers don't matter; what is important is that there be continued growth. If growth seems to slow down or stop, the doctor will usually have an ultrasound scan done.

Ultrasound (Sonogram). The use of ultrasound has revolutionized the care of women whose babies may have IUGR. Using the scan, a baby can often be diagnosed as being normal or as having retarded growth. This technique involves measuring the baby's head or other body parts, as well as the amount of amniotic fluid around the baby, since the amount of fluid is usually less if the baby has growth retardation. The placenta will also usually be abnormal in pregnancies where the baby suffers from growth retardation. (This can often be identified by ultrasound.)

422 If IUGR is diagnosed, what will the doctor do first?

The doctor will try to determine the cause, and then treat both you and the baby. The treatment will depend on what is causing the problem. For instance, if you smoke or drink, the doctor will encourage you to stop these habits. If you have high blood pressure, it will be treated.

There are some commonsense things you will want to do to help improve your baby's growth. If you are a jogger, it would probably be best for you to walk instead. This would allow more blood to flow through your uterus and less to flow through your muscles. Resting an hour in the morning and an hour in the afternoon during the third trimester of pregnancy has been shown to result in a baby's better growth. If your diet is poor, it should be improved, perhaps with the help of a nutritionist.

423 What else will my doctor do if my baby has IUGR?

Your doctor will try to establish a proper time for delivery. Using the techniques for evaluating the pregnancy that were mentioned in the previous section of this chapter, the doctor will monitor the baby. The goal is to allow the baby to stay in the uterus as long as it is a healthier environment than the intensive care nursery would be.

Making that decision is difficult. You do not want to leave the baby in the uterus too long, nor do you want the baby delivered too prematurely. The nonstress test, stress test, and ultrasound are techniques that can be used to watch the baby until it is getting into trouble, at which point delivery is necessary.

Unfortunately there are times when the baby will be so unhealthy inside your uterus that it will have to be delivered too prematurely to live. Then, too, sometimes the baby will seem to be doing well and yet, when delivered, it will be too sick to live.

On the positive side, though, the techniques now available for evaluating babies before birth are much better than they were several years ago. Even if your baby does start developing IUGR, it has a much better chance of doing well.

Postmature Pregnancy

424 Is there a problem if my pregnancy goes longer than two weeks past my due date?

No one knows why pregnancy sometimes goes past forty-two weeks. Some rare conditions are often associated with prolonged pregnancy.

Among these are anencephaly (the baby with almost no brain), a baby that does not have a normal adrenal gland, a baby that does not have a normal pituitary gland, and a pregnancy in which the baby is not inside the uterus.

A pregnancy that goes over forty-two weeks, or two weeks past the due date, must be watched carefully. This is calculated as forty-two weeks from the first day of the last menstrual period (assuming regular periods and ovulation and fertilization two weeks after that last period).

Only one-tenth of all pregnancies will persist more than two weeks after the expected date of delivery and one-third of those pregnancies will result in a baby who has postmaturity syndrome. (See the next question.) Of those babies with the postmaturity syndrome, 60 percent will have medical problems of some type.

The medical problems of postmature babies can be quite severe; 15–30 percent of these babies can die after delivery because of the effects of the prolonged pregnancy. In fact, the deaths of one half of all stillborn babies are due, at least in part, to postmaturity. This is almost as serious a problem for the baby as prematurity.

425 What might happen to the baby if my pregnancy goes past forty-two weeks?

If your placenta is still functioning well and providing good oxygen and nutrition to the baby, the baby may continue to grow. This extra growth, though, can cause an unusually large baby and problems with labor and delivery.

The life span of the placenta is up to forty-two weeks. After that it gets old and can cause problems. While inside your uterus the baby can lose weight from inadequate nutrition through a placenta that is aging. In this situation, the baby can actually become growth retarded during the last week or two of the pregnancy, causing stress that can result in its death. An aging placenta can cause decreasing amounts of amniotic fluid around the baby. This can result in compression of the umbilical cord and distress in the baby.

Birth Weight and Length of Pregnancy

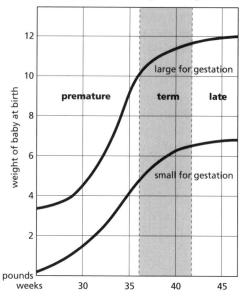

This progression of postmaturity can be categorized by three stages:

Stage 1. In the first stage the baby's skin tends to be dry, cracked, and peeling. The baby looks malnourished—a little skinny, without the robust appearance of a normal newborn—but has an alert, open-eyed appearance.

Stage 2. In this stage the baby also looks malnourished and has an open-eyed look, but he or she is covered with a green film called meconium.

Meconium is bowel movement from the baby, but since he or she has ingested no food, the material has no odor or germs. The baby sometimes passes this material from the colon when under stress. The meconium mixes with the amniotic fluid surrounding the baby and then coats its body.

Meconium staining is especially significant if the baby, the umbilical cord, and the placental lining are all green-stained. The coating itself does not hurt the baby, but a large amount of staining indicates that the baby was under a great deal of stress before birth. Frequently, however, normal babies will pass meconium into the amniotic fluid. When they do, the baby's body is not usually stained green; it is a normal, healthy event and is neither dangerous nor a sign of danger.

Stage 3. In Stage 3 (which includes all of the previously mentioned changes), the meconium is yellow, actually producing yellow staining of the baby's fingernails and toenails. This indicates that the stress was of long duration and the baby is sicker than a Stage 1 or Stage 2 baby.

---

426 What causes a postmature baby to die before it is born (stillbirth) or to become very sick right after delivery?

There are several problems, but two specific ones are:

Inhaling the meconium-stained amniotic fluid. If the postmature baby gets inadequate oxygen and food while inside the mother's uterus, it becomes stressed. This stress is what causes the baby to have a bowel movement inside the uterus. The stress also can cause the baby to gasp and draw the meconium into its lungs. When the baby is born, its lungs cannot expand properly because of the plugs of meconium, causing severe respiratory problems, and even death.

Depletion of fetal sugar. If the baby has been getting inadequate sugar through an "old" placenta, it cannot develop good sugar stores in its own body. Born without these stores of sugar, or glycogen, the baby becomes severely hypoglycemic, characterized by a severely low blood-sugar level. This lack of glucose can cause seizures, brain damage, and death. Because glucose is the one and only fuel that the brain will operate on, the baby must have glucose for healthy brain function.

---

427 If I go over two weeks past my due date, is it not possible that we have just miscalculated the time?

Yes, but please don't let that happen. The due date can be definitely established early in the pregnancy. It is vital that a woman and her doctor determine the date she is actually due while she is still early in pregnancy. If there is any question, a sonogram should be done between the sixteenth and twentieth weeks of pregnancy. When done at this time, the ultrasound study can give a due date that is accurate within about ten days.

---

428 What should be done if my pregnancy is going past my expected date of delivery by more than two weeks?

Most doctors feel that when a pregnancy has progressed two weeks past a definite, well-established, reliable due date, labor should be induced. During the fortieth to the forty-second weeks, if an ultrasound scan shows that the amount of amniotic fluid is decreasing, labor should be induced. Most physicians feel that induction should be done whether or not the cervix seems soft and ready for delivery.

It has been definitely shown that even if the cervix does not seem to be "ripe," labor will usually occur with induction. If it does not, induction can be tried again in two or three days. Most of the time, the induction will be successful the second time.

If labor does not begin with the second induction, your doctor may want to discuss the possibility of your having a cesarean section.

If for some reason your doctor does not feel that induction is best for you when you reach the forty-second week, he or she will almost always start some of the tests described under fetal monitoring in the previous section.

Doctors who have taken the more aggressive approach of induction at the forty-second week have found that surprisingly almost all patients go into labor. This approach has been shown to decrease to very low levels the number of babies dying from postmaturity syndrome.

Even with the best of care, however, some babies will still die because of postmaturity syndrome.

Some postmature pregnancies might be induced by nipple stimulation. The technique is to gently rub the nipple with your fingers for an hour at a time, three times daily, for three days. This exercise sometimes stimulates the release of enough natural oxytocin (from a pregnant woman's pituitary) to produce uterine contractions. Stimulation must be stopped when uterine contractions last as long as one minute. Do not try this technique without checking with your doctor to make sure such stimulation will not cause premature labor and delivery. If you have delivered a premature baby and you and your husband tend to use breast or nipple stimulation a great deal in sex play, it would be wise to discontinue that technique until your pregnancy is full term.

429 Does anything need to be done for my baby immediately after birth if it has developed post-mature problems?

Yes. If there are signs that the baby has inhaled the meconium from the amniotic fluid into its lungs, the doctor would probably use a laryngoscope (lighted viewing instrument) to look in the baby's mouth at the opening to the baby's trachea (main breathing tube). The doctor, while looking into the trachea, can use small suction instruments to remove the meconium. If this thick, jellylike material is not extracted, it can clog the lungs and cause further trouble with the baby's breathing.

If the baby's sugar stores (glycogen) have been depleted because it was not getting enough sugar from its mother, the doctor will probably insert a small plastic tube into a blood vessel in the umbilical cord through which sugar water and drugs may be given, and to provide a way to do frequent testing on the baby to make sure that it is progressing well.

Smoking, Alcohol, and Illegal Drugs during Pregnancy

430 Is smoking harmful during pregnancy?

Your smoking can kill your baby. And, if the baby does not die, your smoking can cause such significant brain and body damage that your child will never be able to function as a normal, healthy person.

The earliest effect of smoking related to pregnancy is infertility. People who smoke are less likely to get pregnant than people who do not smoke. If you do get pregnant, there is a dose-related effect on miscarriage. (The more cigarettes you smoke, the more likely you are to miscarry.)

Women who smoke have a four times greater risk of having a tubal pregnancy. (One study showed that 47 percent of women who had ectopic pregnancies were smokers.) In years past, that may not have been too significant, but since the number of ectopic pregnancies has increased by 400 percent during the past few years, this means that a four times greater risk places a woman who smokes at an enormous risk of having a tubal pregnancy.

It is important to remember, when discussing the effects of tubal pregnancy, that the second most common cause of death among pregnant women is the rupture of a tubal pregnancy.

It has been proven that smoking during pregnancy is not only hazardous to the health of the unborn baby, but it is also a factor affecting its condition during birth, immediately after birth, and also its future mental and physical development. These problems include an increased chance of the baby being very sick or dying before it is born, during birth, or right after delivery. The chance of the baby dying around the time of delivery is increased to about 25 to 30 percent over normal. Because these babies are frail, they often do not tolerate labor as well as normal babies. Because the fetal monitor will show that they are in danger of dying before delivery, this necessitates getting these babies out by C-section more often.

In addition, a smoking mother is more likely to have a premature baby. Studies have shown a considerably higher rate of premature delivery for women who smoke during pregnancy. One report even states that up to 14 percent of all premature deliveries in the United States may be due to the mothers smoking while pregnant.

431 Exactly how does smoking affect the baby?

Cigarette smoking produces a number of abnormalities in a mother's body. First, cyanide (a strong poison) is produced from smoking. This by-product from smoking goes directly to your tissues and to the tissues of your baby, producing hypoxia (lack of oxygen) in the individual cells. In addition to this, nicotine causes constriction of the blood vessels of your body, decreasing the amount of blood flowing through the placenta and adding to the hypoxia produced by the cyanide.

Compounding the action of the cyanide and the nicotine is the fact that when you smoke, your bloodstream absorbs the smoke-caused carbon monoxide from your lungs. When your red blood cells are carrying carbon monoxide, they cannot carry as much oxygen, increasing even more dramatically the hypoxia that is already affecting your baby from the cyanide and nicotine. The lack of oxygen that results from all these effects literally strangles your baby. This oxygen shortage for your child occurs during the most important time of growth in its entire lifetime.

The decreased oxygen supply to the babies of smoking mothers causes such babies, on the average, to weigh about one-half pound less than the babies of nonsmokers. Imagine someone choking you with a rope, limiting the amount of oxygen so much that you lost about one-tenth of your body weight. This is a strong illustration, but what a smoker does to her unborn child is a strong act of selfishness and irresponsibility. I recommend that if you smoke, you either do not get pregnant or you stop smoking before you get pregnant.

432 How does my smoking affect the baby after birth?

In addition to the greater chance of death, there is also a greater chance of having a baby who develops sudden infant death syndrome (SIDS) if you smoked during pregnancy. Dr. Marian Willinger of the National Institute of Child Health and Human Development in Bethesda reported in 1991 that a child's susceptibility to SIDS seems to be established in utero and "the most important thing women can do to prevent sudden infant death among their offspring is to refrain from cigarette smoking and substance abuse during pregnancy."

Also, one study has shown an association between SIDS and smoking after delivery if a mother nurses her baby. If you smoke while nursing, your breast milk will contain nicotine. This may explain why smoking mothers who nurse are more likely to have a SIDS baby. Smoking has also been shown to interfere with the production of milk from the breasts, causing breast-feeding to be less successful.

Smoking during pregnancy has been found to be a cause of hyperactivity in children. In one study of twenty hyperactive children, sixteen had mothers who smoked. The nonsmoking mothers of the other four hyperactive children reported complicated deliveries.

Up until at least the age of five the death rate of children is higher among those born to smokers than among those born to nonsmokers.

Studies have also shown that a child's intelligence can be affected by the mother's smoking during pregnancy. For instance, the attention span of such children has been found to be shorter, causing them to do more poorly in the early years in school.

It appears quite obvious that children of smoking mothers may never "catch up" in certain phases of development with the children of nonsmokers. Your smoking during pregnancy can affect your baby's future for the rest of his or her life.

433 What can I do about my smoking? I want to quit, but it seems almost impossible.

The knowledge that you may be inflicting permanent, irrevocable damage on your helpless baby can help give you the motivation you need to quit. I suggest that you do not try to do it on your own; get every available help that you can.

Do not wait until you want to stop smoking, because that time will never come. You must intellectually realize that you should stop smoking if you are pregnant or plan to be.

Many hospitals, the American Lung Association, and other organizations have programs to help people stop smoking. If you commit yourself to a program to help you break the smoking habit, I urge you to really submit yourself to it. Do what they tell you to do. Don't be ashamed to admit you need help.

It is important to remember that 70 percent of those who stop smoking relapse within three months. Being aware of this should help you to be on guard against it. If you do relapse, don't be discouraged. Return to your support group and try again.

434 What about alcohol and pregnancy?

"Alcohol is now recognized as the leading known teratogen in the Western World. . . . Alcohol ingestion is the most common identifiable cause of mental retardation." (A teratogen is a substance that, if taken by a pregnant woman, can cause damage to her baby.) Drs. Cunningham, MacDonald, and Gantt make these two strong statements in their *Williams Obstetrics* (Norwalk, Conn.: Appleton & Lange, 1997).

Simply stated, when you are drinking, your baby is drinking too. When the alcohol that you drink gets into your baby (and it always does), its development is affected. Problems produced in babies born to mothers who consume a lot of alcohol are so common that these problems are now called the fetal alcohol syndrome.

Fetal alcohol syndrome occurs, to some extent, in every baby born to an alcoholic mother. Following are some of the conditions associated with this syndrome.

Mental retardation. About 44 percent of babies born to alcoholic mothers have IQs of less than eighty.
Growth retardation.
Facial appearance changes. Abnormal growth of the facial bones of babies born with this syndrome results in changes in appearance.
Small head.
Abnormalities in the growth of the joints of the arms and legs.
Muscle abnormalities.

Additional problems. Many of these babies show extreme nervousness and hyperactivity; many have poor attention spans that limit their ability to learn.
Heart and blood-vessel abnormalities.

Fetal alcohol syndrome problems are not just a childhood problem. Many of these disorders continue into adulthood. Adults whose mothers drank too much alcohol during pregnancy show "poor judgment, distractability, and difficulty perceiving social cues." In addition, they tend "to remain short and microcephalic." These problems were quoted in the *Journal of the American Medical Association* (1991, 265:215), in a report by Streissguth and associates in a study of fetal alcohol syndrome.

These abnormalities occur so regularly that it has even been suggested that alcoholic women who become pregnant should have abortions. Compounding an alcoholic's problems with the abortion of her baby does not help her. Rather, an alcoholic mother should use her pregnancy as a reason for doing everything in her power to stop her addiction. This would mean taking advantage of Alcoholics Anonymous or any help that is available.

In the beginning of this section on pregnancy, I spoke of preconception counseling. Such counseling is particularly important if you have a problem with alcohol and cannot limit your consumption. Talk with a counselor or someone in Alcoholics Anonymous before you become pregnant.

435 I am a social, or occasional, drinker. Will this small amount of drinking affect my baby?

Studies suggest that babies of mothers who consume as few as two alcoholic drinks a week may experience neonatal withdrawal syndrome (tension, restlessness, stomach upset, inability to be comforted). Other studies have demonstrated that if a woman drinks two normal-sized drinks a day, her baby will weigh, on the average, six ounces less than the baby of a mother who drinks rarely or not at all. In light of these studies, I would strongly recommend that women abstain from drinking during pregnancy.

436 Do illegal drugs damage the baby if a mother uses them during her pregnancy?

"Our survey shows that the abuse of cocaine, marijuana, heroin, methadone, PCP, and amphetamines in pregnancy often is not recognized until birth. These drugs produce passive addiction in children. These passively addicted children often are born with severe physical or neurological damage, which may contribute to the high rate of infant morbidity and mortality in these infants." These words were spoken by Dr. Ira J. Chasnoff at a recent meeting of the Drugs, Alcohol, Pregnancy, and Parenting Conference. Dr. Chasnoff did a study on this subject that can be obtained from the National Clearing House for Drug and Alcohol Information, P.O. Box 2345, Rockville, MD 20857-2345 or by calling (301) 468-2600.

All of the illegal drugs mentioned cause terrible problems for pregnant women and their babies. (This includes marijuana, which many people thought in the past to be safe in pregnancy.) These drugs increase the chance of miscarriage, cause intrauterine growth retardation, increase the number of congenital malformations, increase the chance of premature labor, and produce babies who have physical and neurological damage.

If you plan to become pregnant, stop using drugs. If you are already pregnant, your baby will have a better chance of being healthy if you stop using drugs immediately. I urge you to go to an alcohol and drug abuse program.

Medications during Pregnancy

437 What do you, as a physician, feel is the proper approach to medications during pregnancy?

My routine advice to a patient is that it is preferable that she take no medications except iron and vitamins, and then only the usual and accepted one prenatal vitamin a day. I always suggest that if she can possibly do so, a woman should get by with no medications during pregnancy. If a woman is taking medications that are medically necessary, she should consult with her obstetrician before she gets pregnant to be sure the medications are safe in pregnancy. If they are not safe, she should change to medications that are safe. This is almost always possible. If it is not, the parents must weigh the risks.

My concern is that, despite the knowledge of the problems caused by thalidomide and DES in the past, the use of drugs by pregnant women has not decreased. The problem is that it cannot be determined conclusively whether or not a drug hurts a baby until that drug has been used for a long time in many human pregnancies.

Thalidomide is an example of the difficulty in knowing whether or not a drug taken during pregnancy affects the baby. No drug given in normal dosages has been proven to have as dramatic an effect on the fetuses as thalidomide, the drug that caused babies to be born with major problems, including no arms or legs. Yet this drug was sold for four years before its terrible consequences were confirmed!

If you want further information on specific drugs, there is an excellent book published by Williams & Wilkins (Baltimore), *Drugs in Pregnancy and Lactation, A Reference of Fetal and Neonatal Risks.* The authors are Griggs, Freeman, and Yaffe. In addition to this book, *The Physician's Desk Reference,* published by Medical Economics (Oradell, N.J.) annually, has information about drugs and their effect in pregnancy with occasional references to drugs during nursing. (See also Q. 543.)

In the next series of questions I will deal with eight classifications of drugs. These are:

sex hormones
pain pills
antibiotics
tranquilizers and antidepressants
cortisone
intestinal drugs
diuretics
acne drugs

438 What effect might sex hormones taken during pregnancy have on the fetus?

Sex hormones, which include estrogen, progesterone (such as Provera), birth-control pills, DES, and androgens may or may not affect the fetus.

Birth-control pills. Women are more concerned about the effect of birth-control pills on a fetus than they are about any other drug. Several years ago physicians thought that these pills might cause abnormalities in babies if women got pregnant while taking them. Further studies, however, have shown that there is no effect on a baby if the mother is taking birth-control pills when she becomes pregnant. This means that it is also safe for a woman to get pregnant immediately after she stops taking birth-control pills, although most doctors recommend that a woman wait until she has regular periods so she will know exactly when she became pregnant.

Provera. A woman should not use Provera while she is pregnant. This drug can cause a female fetus to develop abnormal sex organs, such as a larger than normal clitoris or a vagina that does not quite open up. This is called "masculinization of a female fetus."

Natural progesterone. Natural progesterones do not hurt babies born to mothers who use them during pregnancy. As a matter of fact, if a woman's body does not have enough progesterone, she cannot get pregnant, and if the pregnancy does not have enough progesterone, a woman will always miscarry. Those of us who treat patients for infertility problems often use natural progesterones. (For instance, we always give an in vitro fertilization patient progesterone after we have transferred the embryos into her body.) Almost all gynecologists feel you can take progesterone during pregnancy without worry. It is important, though, that you use a natural progesterone rather than a synthetic one such as Provera.

Pure progesterone suppositories, some progesterone rectal preparations, and some injectable progesterones are semisynthetic progesterone. Most doctors feel that a woman's body cannot tell the difference between semisynthetic and natural progesterone, and their use is not dangerous for

the baby. The use of these preparations is sometimes necessary to avoid miscarriage.

DES. This hormone, diethylstilbestrol, although not prescribed anymore during pregnancy, was used for many years to help prevent miscarriages. We know now that it did not prevent miscarriages, but that it did produce abnormalities of the female organs in some little girls. And some boys born to mothers who took DES also have mild abnormalities of their sex organs. (See Q. 164–168.)

Male hormones (androgens). Drugs such as testosterone and danocrine can cause a female baby to be born with a larger than normal clitoris, or with the labia grown together (fused labia).

439 Can I take pain medication while pregnant?

The discussion of the safety of taking pain pills during pregnancy can be divided into a discussion of the four types of commonly used medications.

Aspirin. It is best not to use aspirin during pregnancy if possible. Aspirin can cause a pregnant mother to become anemic; it can increase her chance of bleeding, both before and after delivery; and because it is an antiprostaglandin (prostaglandins are involved in the labor process), it can stall the start of labor, and then cause it to be abnormally prolonged.

Aspirin does pass through the placenta to the baby, and many physicians think it can cause the baby's ductus arteriosus (located just outside the heart, it connects the aorta and the pulmonary artery) to close before delivery. The ductus arteriosus is an essential part of the baby's circulation prior to birth. It must not close until after the baby has been delivered or the baby will die in the uterus. Aspirin has also been associated with intrauterine growth retardation and a higher incidence of stillborn babies.

In addition, aspirin can keep the baby's blood from clotting properly. This is particularly significant in premature babies. Premature babies whose mothers use large amounts of aspirin during pregnancy have a greater chance of having bleeding into their brain after delivery. Full-term babies of mothers taking aspirin can bruise and bleed after delivery more easily than they would have otherwise.

Very small doses of aspirin probably do not hurt a pregnancy and may be beneficial for a woman who has had repeated miscarriages and has lupus anticoagulant or cardiolipin antibodies. (See the earlier section on miscarriages in this chapter.)

Tylenol. On the other hand, Tylenol does not seem to produce any of these problems if taken for a short time in a normal dose. If it is taken in excessive amounts, it can cause the mother to have severe anemia and the baby to have kidney damage, severe enough to cause death. The usual recommended dose seems permissible in pregnancy.

Narcotics. If taken in large doses shortly before delivery, narcotics can affect a baby's ability to breathe. If a mother is addicted to narcotics, her baby may be born with that same addiction. Narcotics are drugs such as Demerol, morphine, codeine, and "street drugs" such as heroin and cocaine. The baby's withdrawal from narcotics after birth can cause extreme illness and even death.

Nonsteroidal anti-inflammatory agents. These drugs, such as Motrin, Nuprin, Advil, Anaprox, or Naprosyn, are very commonly used for pain and discomfort. Although no conclusive human trials have been conducted, these drugs should probably not be used by pregnant women, especially in the third trimester. They may, as with aspirin, interfere with the onset of labor. They may also cause premature closure of the ductus arteriosus. Studies have shown that one of these drugs, indomethacin, does cause problems in pregnancy. It has been associated with babies having decreased amounts of amniotic fluid, and with having bleeding, edema, and intestinal and kidney problems while in the uterus.

440 Is it permissible to take antibiotics while pregnant?

Obviously, antibiotics are needed at times during pregnancy; unfortunately, there are problems associated with most of them.

Penicillin and cephalosporin-type drugs. No specific pregnancy problems have been associated with these drugs.

Erythromycin. The estolate form of erythromycin increases the risk of cholestatic hepatitis during pregnancy. Because of this, it should not be used. The other forms of erythromycin are probably not dangerous in pregnancy, but they should be used only when specifically indicated. (An example of this is the use of erythromycin to treat chlamydia during pregnancy.)

Tetracyclines. These antibiotics can cause permanent staining of the baby's teeth and bones and should not be used after the third month of pregnancy.

Sulfa. Although sulfa itself does not cause any damage to the baby, if you go into labor immediately after taking a sulfa drug, a baby's jaundice may be complicated by any residual sulfa in its body. If you stop taking sulfa a day or two before delivery, the baby will probably be safe.

Bactrim and Septra. These are sulfa drugs that have trimethoprim in them. Because trimethoprim is a folic acid antagonist and folic acid is necessary for a healthy pregnancy, these drugs are not recommended during pregnancy.

Norfloxacin and ciprofloxacin (Noroxin and Cipro). These drugs have been associated with damage to the bones of animals when they were exposed to these drugs during pregnancy. They are not recommended for use during a woman's pregnancy.

Flagyl. There may be a slightly increased rate of abnormalities in babies born to mothers who take Flagyl in the first three months of pregnancy. This would suggest that it is best not to take Flagyl during that part of pregnancy. Taking it during the last six months of pregnancy probably is not harmful. Since it is the only antibiotic effective against *Trichomonas*, and trichomoniasis can cause premature labor, a mother who has trichomoniasis may actually be protecting her baby if she takes Flagyl.

Aminoglycosides. This includes streptomycin. These drugs can damage a baby's hearing and should be used in pregnancy only with careful dosage calculation. There are several other drugs in this category and the same precaution applies to them.

Clindamycin (Cleocin). This drug seems to be

safe for use during pregnancy, and no abnormalities have been associated with it.

Zovirax (acyclovir). This drug is used to treat herpes. It has not been associated with any fetal abnormality and seems to be safe for use during pregnancy.

AZT (zidovudine). This drug is used in the treatment of AIDS. It has been shown to delay the onset of the clinical disease of AIDS in a person who it is HIV infected. Even more exciting is that if it is taken by a mother during her pregnancy and by the baby after the delivery, it decreases the risk of the baby becoming HIV infected from about 25 percent down to about 8 percent. This is one of the bright spots in the entire AIDS epidemic.

Kwell shampoo. This has been the most common treatment used for lice and scabies infections. When applied to the skin, however, it can cause toxicity to the nervous system of an adult. Because of this, the manufacturer suggests that it not be used by pregnant women as there is some potential for affecting the nervous system of the baby. (Pregnant women who have lice can be treated with a drug such as RID Lice Treatment, which contains pyrethrins.)

Chloramycetin. This antibiotic is not used much anymore because of certain rare, but deadly, effects on both babies and adults. It should not be used in pregnancy.

441 Are tranquilizers and psychiatric drugs safe during pregnancy?

If you are taking tranquilizers, antidepressants, or other psychiatric drugs before you become pregnant, it is important that you talk with your obstetrician about their safety. There are too many of these drugs to discuss here, but I will mention a few of them.

The benzodiazepine drugs, which include Valium and Xanax, have been associated with babies being born with cleft lip, very poor muscle tone, respiratory depression, and with low temperature. Further, these drugs are secreted in breast milk and can cause a baby to be lethargic. A mother who is nursing probably should not use these drugs.

There are conflicting reports, but lithium probably causes congenital abnormalities. The evidence indicates that 15 to 20 percent of children born to women who are on lithium will have some congenital abnormality. Cleft lip, eye and ear abnormalities, and increased miscarriage have been associated with the use of lithium. The primary problem associated with lithium, however, is a heart abnormaltiy called Epstein's anomaly. Because of this, it is probably best that a woman not take lithium unless it is absolutely necessary while she is pregnant.

Many women take Prozac for depression. No congenital abnormalities have been associated with the use of this drug in pregnancy, but, as with all drugs during pregnancy, it would be best not to use it if at all possible.

Phenobarbital should not be used in pregnancy. In a study published in the 1995 edition of the *Journal of the American Medical Association* (274:1518–1525), Reinisch showed that men whose mothers used phenobarbital during their pregnancies had intelligence deficits that were not present in men not so exposed.

442 What about the use of drugs for intestinal problems during pregnancy?

Drugs for nausea were already discussed (see Q. 257). Other drugs used for intestinal disease are:

Laxatives and antidiarrhea medications. None of these have been shown to cause abnormalities in babies.

Antacids. One study, which included a number of different drugs of this type, showed an increase in the number of congenital abnormalities in the babies of mothers who had used these drugs excessively. Most physicians seem to feel that there is little chance of a problem with the moderate use of any antacid preparation, but perhaps cautious use is wise.

Antispasmodics (e.g., Librax, Donnatal). These drugs, given for the irritable bowel syndrome, have been only occasionally associated with a congenital abnormality. It seems that they are probably safe in pregnancy, but they should be used with caution.

Antiulcer medications. No congenital abnormalities have been associated with cimetidine (Tagamet) and other such drugs. They appear to be safe during pregnancy, but no comprehensive studies have been done on them.

443 What about the use of diuretics during pregnancy?

Thiazide diuretics have been found to depress the formation of blood-clotting factors (platelets) in the fetus, increasing the chance of hemorrhage in the baby when born. Diuretics can decrease the blood volume of a pregnant mother enough to lower the flow of blood through the baby's placenta. This can be especially dangerous during the last three months of pregnancy. It seems best, therefore, to use diuretics as little as possible in pregnancy, and unless necessary, not at all in the first three months. (See Q. 266.)

444 Can I safely use acne drugs?

Acutane causes severe congenital abnormalities; a woman must not use it while pregnant. If you are using this drug, you must talk to your dermatologist and to your obstetrician about discontinuing its use before you become pregnant. A similar drug called Retin-A can safely be applied to the skin. No fetal anomalies have been caused by using this skin cream.

Tetracycline should not be used during pregnancy. It can cause staining of the baby's teeth and bones.

445 Can I safely use vaginal fungus or candida medications?

Monistat, GyneLotrimin, Nystatin, and Terazol (and similar drugs) have not been associated with any abnormalities in babies born to mothers who use them. These drugs are absorbed from the vagina into a woman's body, however, so it would probably be best to avoid their use during the first three months of pregnancy. Most obstetricians feel that if it is absolutely necessary for a woman to use

one of these medications to be comfortable, it will probably not cause any harm, even in the first three months of pregnancy.

Caffeine and Pregnancy

446 Is caffeine dangerous during pregnancy?

Some studies show that if a woman takes in more than 150 mg of caffeine per day she has a higher chance of having a miscarriage. Other studies have shown this is not true. The most recent study regarding miscarriages, and a very reassuring one, was reported by Mills et al. in the *Journal of the American Medical Association* (1993) in which they found no evidence that moderate caffeine use increased the rate of miscarriage, intrauterine growth retardation, or small head size.

No association of caffeine with congenital abnormalities has been documented.

Some studies show that women who consume an amount of caffeine equal to more than three cups of coffee per day have a four times greater risk than normal of bearing a low birth weight infant (one that is below five-and-a-half pounds). Other studies have shown that a woman would have to drink as many as six or seven cups of coffee a day before the chances of having a low birth weight baby increased. I am convinced by these studies that decreased birth weight is fairly consistent with the intake of more than 300 to 400 mg of caffeine per day (three or four cups).

I suggest that a woman drink no more than one cup of regular coffee per day. (One cup of regular coffee contains about 100 mg of caffeine.) Decaffeinated coffee seems to be less of a hazard. Brewed decaffeinated coffee has about one-third the amount of caffeine as a regular cup of coffee. Instant decaffeinated coffee has almost no caffeine.

The studies on caffeine and pregnancy are preliminary, but I believe there is enough information to suggest that you should limit caffeine intake during your pregnancy.

Environmental Concerns during Pregnancy

447 Are X-rays harmful during pregnancy?

Diagnostic X-rays, such as X-rays of the chest, intestines, or the pelvic bones, do not produce enough radiation to hurt your baby. Studies have shown that exposures of up to ten rads of X-ray are relatively safe for a fetus. X-rays of the colon (barium enemas) or of the kidneys (IVP) produce only about one and a half rads; chest X-rays and pelvic X-rays produce even less than that.

Unfortunately, a number of unnecessary abortions have been done because of X-ray exposure. Naturally, if a pregnant woman had X-ray studies done before she knew she was pregnant, she would ask the radiologist or her doctor about the effect of the X-ray on the fetus when she learned she was pregnant. Knowing that there is a 2 to 3 percent chance of any baby being born with major abnormalities whether or not it was exposed to X-ray, for self-protection, a doctor might suggest an abortion. The doctor might fear that if this particular mother happened to have a baby with an abnormality, she would blame the X-rays, even though the X-rays had nothing to do with the baby's condition.

An abortion in such a situation might eliminate a potential problem for the doctor, but it would have been an unnecessary abortion for the woman and her baby. It is totally inappropriate to have an abortion done because the mother had been exposed to diagnostic X-rays.

448 Do environmental substances to which I am exposed affect my baby?

This is one of the most common questions asked of obstetricians. Unfortunately, studies are not conclusive about the consequences of exposure to most environmental material. As in all matters related to the pregnant woman, being overly cautious is the safest measure.

Personal and household chemicals.

A. The most recent information is that the following have not been shown to pose any risk to the baby:

> Hair dye
> Permanents
> Video, computer, monitor displays

B. Possibly some effect—though studies have not ever shown any fetal abnormality:

> Hair straightener
> Nail polish (toluene-free polish is okay)
> Most household chemicals

C. Proven problems:

> Paint—long-term, high dose has been associated with abnormal babies. Avoid oil-based paints and solvents. Avoid paints with mildew-killing compounds—they contain mercury. Water-based paints and latex paints are probably okay.

It is probably best for a pregnant woman to let her husband do most of the work with chemicals, paint, and solvents around the house. If she must clean the bathroom and paint, she should have good ventilation not only for the good of the baby but also for herself.

Chemicals at your place of work. The same warning is in effect here. If you are constantly exposed to chemical fumes or agents at your place of employment, it would be best if you changed jobs during the time of your pregnancy.

Anesthetic gases. Female anesthetists and anesthesiologists have been shown to have an increased incidence of miscarriage and of babies with congenital abnormalities. As operating rooms are now more conscientiously watched for gas leaks, I feel it is acceptable for pregnant doctors and nurses to continue working there. In spite of these precautions, time may show that there is still a risk to pregnant mothers who work in operating rooms day after day. This also applies to dental offices that use nitrous oxide regularly.

Genetic Problems and Diseases

diseases that are caused by some of these genes being abnormal. These diseases are passed on as hereditary diseases. An example of a genetic disease is cystic fibrosis.

449 What about genetic problems?

Read Q. 411, 412, 415 for a brief introduction to this subject.

It is estimated that 3 to 5 percent of all newborns have some abnormality. Unfortunately, the causes of these abnormalities are myriad and frequently not identifiable.

Beckham and Brent (1986) suggest the following categories of cause and the estimated contribution of each to fetal damage:

Genetic (chromosomal and single gene defects), 20 to 25 percent

Fetal infections (cytomegalovirus, syphilis, rubella, toxoplasmosis, and others), 3 to 5 percent

Maternal disease (diabetes, alcohol abuse, seizure disorders, and others), < 4 percent

Drugs and medications, < 1 percent

Multifactoral or unknown, 65 to 75 percent

In this section of the book we will discuss the 20 to 25 percent of babies who are abnormal because of an identifiable chromosomal or genetic problem. Remember, though, that 65 to 75 percent of all children born with abnormalities have those abnormalities for no known cause. (Fortunately, the parents of children in this large group are not likely to have the problem repeat itself in later pregnancies.)

An entire chromosome or part of a chromosome or several chromosomes can be abnormal. Some chromosome disorders can be inherited; others can result from a single chromosomal accident in which too much or too little chromosomal material is present in a particular baby's cell makeup. (See Q. 453.) Any of these problems can cause a baby to be abnormal. An example of this is Down syndrome or mongolism.

Each chromosome carries thousands of genes as mentioned in chapter 6. The terms *genetic problem* or *genetic disease* are used in reference to certain

450 Can I know before I become pregnant whether I might produce a baby with a genetic problem? Can I know if the baby I am carrying has a genetic problem?

There are three primary ways to determine the risk of genetic problems.

Genetic counseling. Counseling is available to couples who suspect they might have a problem producing normal offspring. Genetic counseling is usually done when couples already have had a baby that is abnormal, but it is also frequently done when couples know that some family member has a hereditary disease.

Tests before pregnancy. If a couple suspects that they may be carriers of a genetic problem (such as Tay-Sachs disease [see Q. 457] or sickle-cell anemia), tests can be done to determine whether or not one or both of them is carrying such a gene.

Prenatal diagnosis. Your baby can have genetic evaluation while in your uterus by two methods: Amniocentesis, as stated earlier in this chapter, is a prenatal test in which a needle is inserted through the abdominal wall into the fluid that surrounds your baby. This fluid can be tested for hormones or chemicals. Some of the living cells that have sloughed off the baby can also be evaluated.

Chorionic villus sampling (CVS) is a test that has now been used in the United States for several years and is fairly widely available. The only so-called advantage it has over amniocentesis is that it can be done earlier in pregnancy, allowing the couple to have an earlier abortion if that is what they are planning to do with an abnormal baby.

The test involves inserting a tube through the cervix and into the uterus to withdraw some of the placenta for testing. If the baby has a genetic problem, the tissue from the placenta will show the same abnormality.

There are generally problems associated with this test. One is that it can cause about twice as many miscarriages as an amniocentesis. Recent studies also suggest that CVS gives more ambiguous results than amniocentesis. These problems have dampened the enthusiasm of many physicians for this procedure.

451 What does "prenatal diagnosis" mean, and why is it important?

The term *diagnosis* means "to find out what is wrong with," and prenatal diagnosis means "to find out what is wrong with a baby before it is born."

About 3 to 5 percent of babies that are born alive have some major abnormality. Doctors and patients have become interested in trying to find out about the health of the baby before the baby is born. Congenital disease has become the major cause (25 to 35 percent) of infant mortality because other diseases that cause infant mortality have been so well controlled.

452 Why would the doctor or the patient who is pregnant want to know if the baby has an abnormality?

They would want to know for three reasons: to make plans for the care of the baby when it is born; to be able to perform some type of medical care for the baby before birth; or to perform an abortion.

Modern medical technology has made many things possible. We can now find out a lot more about the baby before it is born than we could have in the past. This can help couples be prepared for a child that might not be normal. We can now also do some types of treatment on the baby before birth. Although very new and still experimental, some prenatal surgery is being done for fetuses with certain specific congenital abnormalities.

Some couples may want to know whether or not their baby is going to be normal because they will abort the fetus if it is not. I urge that a couple consider their options carefully before making this

decision. I often point out that none of us is totally normal, and a baby with limitations can often be a great blessing to a family.

Chromosomal Abnormalities

453 What are chromosomal abnormalities?

There are several chromosomal abnormalities. Some involve the 44 chromosomes in each cell that are nonsex chromosomes (autosomes). Down syndrome is an example of this abnormality because it does not involve sex chromosomes.

Down syndrome is the most common chromosomal abnormality. (This was often referred to in the past as "mongolism.") Down syndrome is usually caused by an extra chromosome—usually chromosome 21. (The problem is often referred to as "trisomy 21" because there are three "21" chromosomes instead of the usual two.)

In each cell there are two chromosomes involved with sexual determination, and on each of these chromosomes are a great number of genes. If something is wrong with the genes on one of these sex chromosomes, a person is said to have a sex chromosome or sex-linked abnormality. Three problems of this type are Turner syndrome (see the section of this book where that is discussed), Klinefelter syndrome, and Fragile X syndrome.

Since most children who have a chromosomal abnormality are born with Down syndrome, we will discuss that here. In addition, since most Down syndrome babies are born to mothers who are older, we will discuss that in some detail.

A mother who is over thirty-five will often be advised to have amniocentesis to test her baby for Down syndrome. Many people have the mistaken idea that at age thirty-five suddenly there is higher risk of having a baby with abnormalities. This is not true. What the geneticists are saying is that thirty-five is the earliest age at which it is reasonable statistically to do chromosome testing with amniocentesis. Before the age of thirty-five such abnormalities do not occur often enough to warrant testing; the occurrence rates at age thirty-five merely make such testing reasonable (except possibly when an earlier baby had Down).

Starting at about age thirty, there is a gradual increase in the chance of conceiving a baby with Down syndrome. The risk figures I usually quote are:

Mother's age, thirty: 1-in-1,000 chance of a Down baby

Mother's age, thirty-five: 1-in-400 chance

Mother's age, forty: 1-in-100 chance

A woman is twice as likely to give birth to a defective child at age forty than she was at age twenty-five; she is five times as likely to have an abnormal baby when she is forty-five than when she was twenty-five. Almost all of these age-related abnormal babies have Down syndrome.

The father's age may have something to do with the baby's being born with Down syndrome. It has been shown that approximately 30 percent of Down syndrome births resulted from the father's sperm rather than the mother's egg. The statistical rate of risk with the father's age has not been determined as it has with the mother's age.

Most geneticists at this point do not consider the father's age that much of an issue. One significant point is that fathers should not blame the mother of a baby with Down syndrome; the abnormality could have come from either parent.

drome than the woman who has not had a previous child with the abnormality. If the woman is below the age of twenty-four, there is only a 0.7 to 1 percent increased chance of this happening a second time.

The facts from these studies mean that a woman who has had one baby with Down syndrome does not need to have amniocentesis to evaluate future pregnancies unless she is younger than twenty-four, and even then there is not as much chance of it happening a second time as had previously been thought. The exception to this is if the mother has had a baby with Down syndrome caused by chromosomal translocation. There is then a greater chance of having another baby with Down syndrome. If the translocation came from the father, there is a 5 percent chance of the couple having another baby with Down syndrome. If the translocation came from the mother, there is a 15 to 20 percent chance of having a baby with Down syndrome with a subsequent pregnancy. This means that if a person below the age of thirty has had a baby with chromosome abnormalities, both the mother and the father should have their chromosomes checked to see if they are carriers.

Other chromosomal abnormalities, such as Turner syndrome (a baby girl born without ovaries because of having only one X chromosome), have no known risk for recurrence and are much less common than Down. There is no reason for amniocentesis in future pregnancies even if this problem was present in a previous child.

454 If I have had a previous child with a chromosomal abnormality, what are the chances of this happening again?

In the past, a mother whose previous miscarriage or live baby showed abnormal chromosomes of Down syndrome (mongolism or trisomy) has been counseled that there is a 1 to 2 percent chance of having another baby with the same disorder. Newer studies reveal that if a woman is over twenty-four years of age, she does not have a greater chance of having a baby with Down syn-

Single Gene Genetic Abnormalities

455 What are single gene abnormalities of babies?

A person can carry a single abnormal gene that can have devastating effects if it is a dominant gene. If a woman is carrying a defective dominant gene, she will pass this to 50 percent of the children she has. This type genetic defect includes Marfan syndrome, achondroplastic dwarfism, and many others.

A single gene defect can also be devastating if it is recessive and a person with the recessive gene marries a person with the same abnormal recessive gene. When this happens, one out of four children born to these parents will usually have the disease the abnormal genes produce. Included in single gene defects are about four thousand different diseases.

Many of the diseases produced by recessive gene abnormalities cause metabolic disease. These are diseases that exist because abnormal "metabolism" is caused by the absence of certain enzymes and the lack of enzymes is caused by the abnormal gene. When the metabolism is interrupted in this way, it is as though a dam has blocked the normal pathway of metabolism, allowing toxic products that can cause diseases and death to build up in the baby's body. These diseases include Tay-Sachs disease, sickle-cell anemia, phenylketonuria, and many others.

The tests are time-consuming, and testing for metabolic disorders must usually be started in the early months of pregnancy.

If there is a question about the possibility of there being a metabolic disorder in any child you bear, you should make plans before you get pregnant or at the beginning of your pregnancy, so you will know who will do your studies, where they will be done, and what the testing will require.

456 How do we know if either my husband or I have abnormal genes and should undergo genetic testing?

A couple cannot really know that they carry and could pass on a genetic abnormality unless they are tested for it. They would not ordinarily have such testing unless they have had several miscarriages or have produced a baby with some abnormality. It is usually during an evaluation of a couple who has a problem in producing a normal baby that a genetic abnormality is detected. When this type of abnormality is found, consultation with a geneticist is very helpful. A geneticist can give a couple some idea of their chance of producing a normal baby in the future.

When a parent has a genetic abnormality, the chance of producing an abnormal baby is theoretically high. In actual practice, however, far fewer abnormal babies are born to parents with genetic abnormalities than would be expected. When the father is the one with the abnormal genes, the risk of producing a baby with a genetic abnormality is far less than if the mother is the one who has a genetic abnormality.

457 I have heard of Tay-Sachs disease. What is it?

Tay-Sachs is a metabolic disease (a deficiency in the enzyme necessary to metabolize fatty substances for proper functioning of the nervous system) that occurs with high frequency in one particular population group. Tay-Sachs is carried by one in thirty Ashkenazic Jews, the Jews of eastern Europe who are the ancestors of most of the Jewish population of the United States. If two Ashkenazic Jews marry and both carry the genes for Tay-Sachs disease, they have a 25 percent chance of having a baby with that disease. Such babies seem to be normal at birth but soon show signs of slow development, paralysis, blindness, and other disorders of the nervous system. Tay-Sachs is usually fatal by age three or four.

Since the gene is also carried by both Sephardic Jews and by Gentiles, or non-Jews, at the rate of one in three hundred, it is possible for a baby to have the Tay-Sachs gene and have a gentile or Sephardic parent who is carrying the gene. This does not happen very often, but it is possible.

When only one partner is an Ashkenazic Jew, the chance of that couple producing a baby with Tay-Sachs is very small. Scientifically, it is probably unwise for them to have amniocentesis and testing done, because there is a much greater chance of damaging a normal baby by amniocentesis than of identifying Tay-Sachs in their unborn baby.

The best approach to this problem is for any

Jewish husband and/or wife to delay pregnancy until chromosome studies are conducted to see if either or both carry the gene for Tay-Sachs disease. The reason for this approach is that there is such a mixture of genes in the world's population that Jewish people cannot know for certain that they are not part Ashkenazic, and gentile people cannot know for sure that they are not part Jewish. When such a Jewish or Jewish/gentile couple later achieve pregnancy, they do not need to worry about their baby having Tay-Sachs disease unless both were found to be carriers of the disease.

Abnormalities Caused by Several Abnormal Genes Working Together

458 What is an example of a problem produced by several abnormal genes?

There are some abnormalities that are the result of several genes "working together" in an abnormal way to produce a child with abnormalities. Some diseases that are produced in this way are neural tube defects, congenital heart defects, cleft lip, and so on. One of the most common and most devastating examples of this type of genetic problem is neural tube defects.

Neural tube defects are problems in which the baby can be born with most of its brain absent (anencephaly, which is incompatible with life) or with spina bifida, in which the spine has a defect that exposes the spinal nerves (these babies are often paralyzed from that part of the spine down).

One or two babies per thousand are born with such problems. If you have previously had a baby with anencephaly or spina bifida, your chance of a future baby having this same problem is about two per hundred. For some reason, if you have had the same abnormality and you live in England,

the chance of this happening to a future baby is about five per hundred.

If you would like to know more about spina bifida, contact:

Spina Bifida Association of America
Suite 317, 343 S. Dearborn St.
Chicago, IL 60604
(800) 621-3141

459 What causes a neural tube defect?

This can be caused by one of two things: the abnormal function of several genes working together or by the baby being born with a whole group of abnormalities, one of which happens to be spina bifida or anencephaly.

Although one of those two factors can cause neural tube defect, it is important to know for future reference which one caused the problem. If your previous baby had only spina bifida or only anencephaly, then the chance of recurrence is only 2 percent. If the baby had several different problems, and one of those happened to be spina bifida or anencephaly, then there may be as high as a 25 percent chance of another baby having a neural tube defect.

In calculating your chances for a normal birth the next time, you should make sure that your medical records are clear; you should also keep a set of them to show to any future doctor to intelligently discuss further pregnancies.

460 Which tests are available to determine whether or not my baby has a neural tube defect?

Two tests are available: amniocentesis and ultrasound (sonogram).

Amniocentesis involves testing the amniotic fluid around the baby for increased levels of alpha-fetoprotein. Although this is a normal protein, if there is a neural tube defect this protein can leak from the baby's blood vessels into the amniotic fluid. If a baby's amniotic fluid has elevated amounts of alpha-fetoprotein, it can be a sign of a neural tube defect.

When amniocentesis is done to check for elevated alpha-fetoprotein levels in the amniotic fluid, almost 100 percent of the babies with anencephaly can be detected and 90 percent of babies with spina bifida can be detected.

The second test for neural tube defect is a sonogram. A sonogram can detect almost all cases of anencephaly and most cases of spina bifida. The procedure is painless but not totally accurate. (See Q. 399.)

It is possible that neither the sonogram nor amniocentesis would show the baby as being abnormal when it does indeed have an abnormality. The sonogram does not reliably indicate when the baby has spina bifida low in the spine near the tailbone; when the baby has that lesion and the skin is completely covering it, the alpha-fetoprotein level in the fluid might not be elevated and would not show the defect.

461 How is blood testing done on the mother's blood for elevated alpha-fetoprotein (AFP) used to find babies with neural tube defects?

When the amount of alpha-fetoprotein is abnormally high in the amniotic fluid around the baby who has a neural tube defect, some of this protein seeps into the mother's bloodstream and can be detected. An elevated level of alpha-fetoprotein in the mother's blood may mean that the baby is abnormal.

Most doctors now offer maternal serum alpha-fetoprotein (MSAFP) screening to all pregnant women. As a matter of fact, the test is now mandatory in some states. The sequence in the screening program for the woman who chooses to have the following testing done is explained in the next few paragraphs.

By the time the baby with a neural tube defect is fourteen to eighteen weeks along, the level of AFP in the mother's blood is high enough to be detected as abnormal. The best time for the test is between the fourteenth and twentieth week of pregnancy. All pregnant women who choose to have this test should have their blood tested during that time. It is absolutely imperative that the length of the mother's pregnancy be very well established. The amount of AFP in the mother's blood changes as the pregnancy progresses, and misleading results can occur if the dates of the pregnancy are wrong.

If the MSAFP test on the mother's blood is normal, no other testing is done. This does not prove that the baby is normal in all respects, but it does mean the baby probably does not have a neural tube defect.

About 2.5 to 5 percent of pregnant women will have a higher AFP level than is normal; 4 to 5 percent will have a lower AFP level than is normal. This does not mean that the baby is definitely abnormal, but it might indicate a potential problem. If the level is low (about one in eighty-five to ninety pregnancies have a low MSAFP), the baby is twelve times as likely to have abnormal chromosomes and three times more likely to die fetally than those with normal MSAFP levels. Further testing may be suggested. A couple can have that done if they desire. (Because the abnormality is often Down syndrome, see Q. 453–454.)

If the first MSAFP level is elevated, your doctor may recommend that you have the test repeated. About half of the women who have an elevated MSAFP the first time will have it again the second time. If the second test is normal, however, the woman is probably carrying a healthy baby.

Sonogram studies are done on women who have a second elevated MSAFP. Recent studies have shown that if an ultrasound is done very carefully by a physician who is an expert in using it for this purpose, almost all (80 to 90 percent) babies with neural tube defects can be identified. About half of the time, the problem will not be a neural tube defect but something else, such as a dead fetus, twins, or inaccurate pregnancy dates.

Generally, if the sonogram does not show the problem and the second MSAFP was abnormal, your doctor may recommend that you have an amniocentesis. The amniocentesis is done to detect elevated AFP in the fluid surrounding the baby, which would mean that the baby almost definitely is abnormal. Fortunately, 90 to 95 percent of women with high levels of alpha-fetoprotein in their blood will have normal levels in their amniotic fluid, indicating that the baby does not have a chromosome problem. However, although the babies of these pregnancies are structurally normal, the pregnancies should be handled as high-risk pregnancies because there is a higher than normal possibility of premature delivery, intrauterine growth retardation, and intrauterine death of the baby.

Following the above sequence would allow the doctors to find 90 percent of the women who are carrying a baby with anencephaly and 80 percent of the women who are carrying a baby with spina bifida. Some studies even show that almost 100 percent of these babies can be found this way. Overall, 34 percent of major congenital abnormalities, 11 percent of all fetal losses, and 19 percent of all pregnancy complications are associated with abnormal MSAFP results. This test, therefore, can warn a pregnant couple and their doctor of problems and allow them to do things to protect the baby.

There are several problems with screening all pregnant women for MSAFP.

First, 4 to 7 percent of all pregnant women in the group being tested will be told that they have an abnormal level of AFP in their blood, yet only 0.2 percent of the entire group will actually have an abnormal baby. This results in alarming an extremely large number of pregnant women about a major complication their baby might have, when only a very few of those women will actually be carrying an abnormal baby.

In addition, this testing is demanding. It requires that physicians and laboratory personnel be well trained and careful as they do these tests. Otherwise abnormalities would be missed, or women would be told they had babies with abnormalities when they did not.

Finally, the initial testing cannot be done until after the fourteenth week. By the time all the tests are performed, several weeks will have passed. An abortion—if that is the decision—this late in pregnancy carries increased risk for the mother.

If you are sure that you would want to abort an abnormal baby or if you want to know if something might be wrong with your baby and your physician suggests that you have MSAFP screening done, I would encourage you to follow that advice. Be aware, though, of the problems associated with this type of screening.

462 What are the advantages of genetic testing for neural tube defects?

There are two major reasons for the testing. First, the testing will find babies who have an abnormality that is incompatible with life, so the mother, if she desires, may go ahead and have an abortion for that complication. A baby with anencephaly, for instance, is totally incapable of living more than a few hours. Some women prefer to have the baby aborted when they know this is the problem. Others prefer to carry the pregnancy to term. Induction of labor will usually be necessary since labor does not usually begin on its own with an anencephalic baby.

Second, the testing can reveal abnormalities that need to be handled immediately after delivery. When spina bifida is found to be present in the fetus, the mother can be transferred to a hospital that will have a team of neurosurgeons standing by in the next room, ready to repair the baby's defect as soon as it is born. This will decrease the danger of infection and paralysis that could develop in the baby from this problem.

463 I keep reading about gene therapy for genetic problems. Is this type of therapy a reality? Where can I get more information about genetic abnormality testing and treatment?

From reading the newspapers, you might have the impression that genetic engineering is on the verge of curing genetic disease. As yet, however, there have been no diseases cured by gene therapy. This science is still in the research stage.

You may have read that the cystic fibrosis (CF) gene has been cloned. This is exciting, because cystic fibrosis is the most common, potentially lethal, autosomal recessive disease affecting white people. There is no cure yet for CF, but being able to identify the gene, and thus screen carriers, is an important milestone in the search for a cure.

However, even if both the husband and wife are carriers of the gene, not all of their children will have the disease, and even if the test does not show them to be carriers, they can still have a baby with CF.

The idea behind genetic testing for cystic fibrosis at this point is to identify couples with a high possibility of having a baby with CF so they can use contraceptives and not get pregnant, or choose to abort if they do get pregnant. There is no way at the present time to use the testing to effect a cure.

Genetic screening, even with the astounding ability to identify the cystic fibrosis gene, is still a very complex and difficult problem. In April 1990, the American Society of Human Genetics said that they do not recommend routine carrier testing for cystic fibrosis.

Another possible use for genetic testing is the in vitro fertilization process. An early embryo, which consists of only a few cells, can "give up" one of its cells and still grow into a normal child. It is possible, therefore, to take one of the cells of an embryo and test it for genetic abnormalities. If an abnormality is found, the embryo could be destroyed. Again, the technology for identifying the defective gene is only useful for destroying an embryo, not for effecting genetic or chromosomal healing. I do not mention this to approve of it. This is the type of ethical dilemma we will be facing in the future.

This is a complex subject and one that is approached with a great deal of concern and emotion by both patients and doctors. The American College of Obstetricians and Gynecologists has an excellent booklet titled *Causes and Treatments for Genetic Disorders*. You can order it from:

The American College of Obstetricians and
  Gynecologists
409 12th Street NW
Washington, D.C. 20024
(202) 638–5577

The United States Department of Health, Education and Welfare also has an excellent booklet containing pictures of the amniocentesis technique and a short discussion about this subject. You can obtain this booklet by writing to:

Centers for Disease Control
Attention: Chronic Disease Division
Bureau of Epidemiology
Atlanta, GA 30333

464 All of this discussion on genetic problems is frightening and sad. Is there any other perspective one can take?

Just because children are born with limitations does not mean that they are "nonpersons" or worthless. These children do have limitations, but then so do you and I.

I have frequently referred my patients with babies who were not normal to the book *Angel Unaware* by Dale Evans Rogers. Dale and Roy had a child with Down syndrome and Dale wrote this book as a result of that experience. I believe her perspective is helpful.

No matter how much testing we do on pregnancies or how many abortions are done, we will never be totally able to prevent the birth of babies with some of these problems. I believe it is important to point out that with the development of infant-stimulation and early-intervention techniques, retarded babies are able to function more normally as they grow up than was previously thought possible.

In addition, these babies are greeted with more opportunity in our society than they have been in the past. They are no longer shut up in state schools where they cannot develop to their fullest potential, but are being treated as persons who do have worth.

If you desire to learn more about Down syndrome, you can write:

National Down Syndrome Congress
1605 Chantilly Dr., Suite 250
Atlanta, GA 30324

This group has a twenty-four-hour hotline for information, (312) 226-0416. They also publish *The Down Syndrome News*.

For information about Turner's syndrome, I encourage you to write:

Turner's Syndrome Society of the U.S.
15500 Wayzata Boulevard
Wayzata, MN 55391
(612) 475-9944

Down babies, although limited in their ability to function in various areas, are persons. It is important that we approach them—before birth and after—with the dignity, compassion, and thoughtfulness that we ourselves would want. I realize that there are tremendous problems and expenses involved when parents are faced with the care of one of these individuals, but I believe our entire society is elevated a notch when we care properly for less fortunate individuals.

In thinking of this subject, my mind always turns to the autobiography of a Dutch woman named Corrie ten Boom. During World War II, this fifty-two-year-old watchmaker was arrested by the Nazis in Holland and held in the German concentration camp at Scheveningen. In *The Hiding Place* (Lincoln, Va.: Chosen Books, 1971), written by John and Elizabeth Sherrill, Corrie gives an account of an interrogation by a German lieutenant:

> "Your other activities, Miss ten Boom. What would you like to tell me about them?"
>
> "Other activities? Oh, you mean—you want to know about my church for mentally retarded people?" And I plunged into an eager account of my efforts at preaching to the feeble-minded.
>
> The lieutenant's eyebrows rose higher and higher. "What a waste of time and energy!" he exploded at last. "If you want converts, surely one normal person is worth all the half-wits in the world!"
>
> I stared into the man's intelligent blue-gray eyes: true National-Socialist philosophy I thought, tulip bed or no. And then to my astonishment I heard my own voice saying boldly, "May I tell you the truth, Lieutenant Rahms?"
>
> "This hearing, Miss ten Boom, is predicated on the assumption that you will do me that honor."
>
> "The truth, Sir," I said, swallowing, "is that God's viewpoint is sometimes different from ours—so different that we could not even guess at it unless He had given us a Book which tells us such things."
>
> I knew it was madness to talk this way to a Nazi officer. But he said nothing so I plunged ahead. "In the Bible I learn that God values us not for our strength or our brains but simply because He has made us. Who knows, in His eyes a half-wit may be worth more than a watchmaker. Or—a lieutenant."
>
> Lieutenant Rahms stood up abruptly. "That will be all for today." He walked swiftly to the door. "Guard!"
>
> I heard footsteps on the gravel path.
>
> "The prisoner will return to her cell" (p. 166).

The Rh Factor and Pregnancy

465 What is all the talk about "Rh negative" and "Rh positive" in pregnancy? How does it concern my baby and me?

Before I tell you exactly what Rh factor is, let me explain some facts about it.

The term *Rh positive* means that a person's red blood cells have particles of a specific type of protein on their surface. About 85 percent of all people have that blood type. The people with Rh-negative blood do not have these particles of protein on the surface of the red blood cells and are therefore called Rh negative. They make up 15

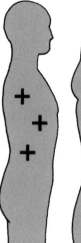

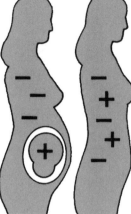
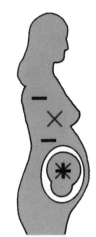

Father, Rh positive

You, Rh negative

Your baby, Rh positive (possibly)

If your baby is Rh positive, near or during delivery some Rh-positive cells from the baby may enter your bloodstream and mix with your Rh-negative cells.

Then your blood system produces antibodies that attack "foreign" Rh positive cells.

These antibodies become a permanent part of your bloodstream and your next baby will receive them into its blood system.

If your next baby is Rh positive, these antibodies will fight to destroy the baby's Rh-positive cells. Rh hemolytic disease results.

The Rh Factor

percent of the general population. If you lack these particles on your blood cells but your body is exposed to them through a transfusion or through an Rh positive baby in your uterus, your body can develop antibodies against those particles.

If you are Rh positive (a blood test that is ordered at the beginning of pregnancy determines this), you do not need to worry about the Rh problem.

If you are Rh negative, your husband needs to be tested.

If both you and your husband are Rh negative, you do not need to worry about the Rh factor.

If, however, you are Rh negative and your husband is Rh positive, you could be carrying a baby that is Rh positive and this is the situation that can cause problems.

About 16 percent of the women with Rh-negative blood who are carrying an Rh-positive child will develop antibodies to Rh-positive blood. They will usually have a baby with some degree of jaundice from the Rh problem in their next pregnancy.

The process that occurs, if you are Rh negative, carry an Rh-positive baby, and are one of the 16 percent who develops Rh antibodies, is this:

During the later months of your pregnancy, or at the time of delivery, some of your baby's Rh-positive red blood cells leak from the placenta into your bloodstream.

Your Rh-negative blood system reacts against these Rh-positive blood cells by producing antibodies. Your body considers these cells as "foreign objects" that it must react against.

The antibodies that you form are then a permanent part of your blood system.

The next time you become pregnant with an Rh-positive baby, during the pregnancy your anti-Rh antibodies gradually pass through the placenta into the baby's bloodstream, where they can destroy a number of the baby's Rh-positive red blood cells.

When a small number of the baby's red blood cells are destroyed, the baby may be born jaundiced (the yellow color results from the breakdown of blood cells just as the yellow color of a bruise does) or develop jaundice after birth. When a large number of the baby's red blood cells are destroyed, the baby can die inside your uterus because of heart failure from severe anemia and an inadequate amount of blood in its bloodstream.

If you are found to have reacted against Rh-positive blood in the past and you are pregnant again, your doctor will want to watch you carefully so that he or she will know if your baby is being affected. If the baby is affected, the doctor may need to give it a blood transfusion while still in the uterus or deliver it early so it will not be affected so severely. The shorter the time that the baby is exposed to your antibodies, the less severely affected the baby will be.

The scenario I just described happens rarely. This is because we can now administer an immunization to prevent your body from reacting to Rh-positive red blood cells.

If you are Rh negative and your husband is Rh positive, you need to get a shot of Rh immune globulin (RhoGAM) within seventy-two hours after delivery. You must do this whether you have an abortion, a miscarriage, an ectopic pregnancy, or a normal delivery. If you have delivered a child, the baby's blood can be tested. If it is Rh negative, you do not need Rh immune globulin. It is easy for your doctor to forget that you need this injection. Immediately after your delivery ask for your Rh immune globulin.

Even if you have a sterilization done after delivery, you should get your injection of the Rh immune globulin if your baby is Rh positive. A fairly large number of women return to their gynecologist to have their tubes repaired in later years to try to get pregnant again. You might do the same thing. Have the shot even if you plan never to become pregnant again.

Additional protection for Rh-negative mothers with Rh-positive husbands is afforded if the pregnant mother gets an Rh immune globulin shot at twenty-eight weeks of pregnancy and also right after delivery. I feel that this is a wise procedure because 1 to 2 percent of women will become sensitized during the last months of pregnancy instead of after pregnancy. An Rh immune globulin shot at twenty-eight weeks prevents this, and this is now a routine recommendation for Rh-negative women with Rh-positive husbands.

The Rh immune globulin is a wonderful medical breakthrough! There is essentially no risk to receiving the Rh immune globulin and it almost totally prevents the possibility of the Rh problem affecting your future babies. There was some concern at first about the possibility of the HIV virus being passed to mothers through immune globulin. This has never happened, however; apparently the manufacturing process destroys any HIV virus present.

During my training program I did exchange transfusions on babies after delivery who had the Rh problem. We always worried that the babies would die during the transfusions. We also worried about the possibility of brain damage if the babies became too jaundiced. These worries are almost a thing of the past.

An Afterword

We have discussed a great number of things in this chapter, and many of them seem frightening. I think it is important at this point to come back to reality about pregnancy and newborns.

Most pregnancies and most babies are normal. If you walk by the nursery of a hospital, you will see that almost all of the babies there are normal. In some fantastic way God has made us so that, in spite of the myriads of things that can go wrong, we and the babies we produce are usually normal.

We have discussed alarming things in this chapter primarily as a warning. Knowing these factors exist, and knowing what *can* go wrong, should help women be on the lookout for indications of a problem with their pregnancy or with their baby and help insure that they deliver a normal child.

If you suspect that any of the things that have been discussed in this chapter might apply to you, please tell your doctor. Today more and more mothers are able to participate in their medical care. Increased knowledge and better care can increase the probability that their babies will be healthy and normal.

I think it is important to mention that much of what we have discussed in this chapter could not have even been written thirty years ago. Many of these facts were not known. The techniques for following the baby in pregnancy were not available. Although knowing all these facts makes pregnancy seem a great deal more complicated, it certainly has added to a couple's ability to deliver a healthier baby.

It is my firm belief that God has given us the insight and the information that we now possess to help us in this whole process. He loves us more than we love ourselves and even more than we love our own children. He wants the best for us in everything.

8

Preparation for Childbirth

Childbirth classes are exciting. When it is time to sign up for them it means this business of having a baby is "real." Most obstetricians encourage patients and their husbands to go to classes, whether or not they are interested in "natural childbirth."

Husbands who attend childbirth classes usually find to their surprise that they not only learn a lot, but they actually enjoy the learning. These husbands are a great physical and emotional help to their wives during labor and delivery. With training, expectant mothers know more about the growth of the child in the uterus and are more aware of the danger signs that might indicate problems with their pregnancy. In addition, they are taught effective pain-control techniques that really do help during labor.

The team effort involved in producing a baby from conception to delivery helps a couple see the pleasure they can have in continuing as a team to rear the child they, and God, have produced.

I encourage patients who might need a C-section to attend cesarean section classes; these classes help both a woman and her husband to relax during the last few weeks of pregnancy. Also, even though a cesarean is anticipated, a woman may go into labor and deliver so quickly that there is no time for a cesarean. Classes will help a couple know what to do in that situation.

Training for Childbirth

466 How can we prepare for childbirth?

I suggest two things. First, enroll in childbirth classes. Some information about childbirth can be learned from books, but you will probably learn it more effectively in a series of classes. Second, read some of the books listed below. (If you attend childbirth classes, you will probably be referred to other books by your instructor.)

> *Six Practical Lessons for an Easier Childbirth* by Elizabeth Bing (Bantam, 1980)
> *Thank You, Dr. Lamaze* by Marjorie Karmel (Harper & Row, 1981)
> *A Lamaze Guide—Preparation for Childbirth* by Donna and Rodger Ewy (Formur, 1982)
> *Husband-Coached Childbirth* by Robert A. Bradley (Harper & Row, 1965)
> *Commonsense Childbirth* by Lester D. Hazell (Berkley, 1981)
> *Awake and Aware* by Irvin Chabon (Delacorte Press, 1969)
> *Moving through Pregnancy* by Elizabeth Bing (Bobbs Merrill, 1975)
> *Childbirth without Fear* by Grantly Dick-Read (Harper & Row, 1981)
> *Painless Childbirth* by Fernand Lamaze (Regnery, 1970)

Most of these books represent the materials that popularized "natural childbirth." Most childbirth-preparation classes now have their own individual syllabuses. Many are excellent, and some quite complete. The advantage of such individualized booklets is that they can be custom-fitted to the hospital where you deliver your baby.

467 Aren't preparation-for-childbirth classes the same as "natural childbirth" classes?

To most people, *natural childbirth* implies the birth of a baby without any pain medication, or at most a local anesthetic for repairing a small episiotomy. But preparation-for-childbirth classes are not offered to convince mothers that "natural childbirth" is the best way to have a baby.

Some teachers do stress "natural childbirth," but they do not necessarily represent the mainstream philosophy. If you are in a class in which the teacher seems to be trying to push everyone toward having labor without pain medication and you disagree with this, you may be in the wrong class.

The goal of childbirth classes is to produce an expectant mother/father team who will approach labor and delivery with the attitude that they can handle whatever comes. The parents will have studied the anatomy and physiology of childbirth and learned techniques to cope with both the emotional and physical aspects of having a baby. The mother will have learned that if the pain becomes too uncomfortable, there are medications that can ease her discomfort without affecting her baby or interfering with normal labor.

The mother and father also learn that if there is a medical problem, a cesarean section can be done. This procedure enables them to complete the childbirth process with the ultimate goal attained: the delivery of a healthy child.

468 What are the advantages in going to preparation-for-childbirth classes?

The advantages agreed on by physicians, nurses, and patients are the following.

Reduction of anxiety for the father and mother. Most women who have not experienced childbirth are at best uneasy about it, and at worst scared to death. Many women find that knowing what is going on during labor and delivery, and using learned techniques for dealing with pain, keeps them from being as anxious as they expected to be. The same is true for fathers: Increased knowledge usually results in lessened anxiety.

Parents have an active role. With training the father can be involved in the process. Without training he is just a bystander. With training the mother and father can become a team and actively participate in one of the most exciting events of their lives: the birth of their baby.

Prepared parents work better with the medical staff. Prepared parents are better able to do the things suggested by the doctors and nurses that will help ease distress. Most medical personnel enjoy working with patients who have some knowledge of what is going on and who want to be involved in the birth process.

Prepared patients are ready for emergencies. Simple things, such as knowing whom to call if you start heavy bleeding, can save a baby's or mother's life. In the hospital, a patient's cooperation in the event of an emergency cesarean section can make delivery easier for the baby and thereby allow the birth of a healthier child.

Prepared mothers use pain medications intelligently. Although recent studies have shown that prepared mothers do not use less pain medication, I believe that prepared mothers are more knowledgeable in their requests for pain medication.

Prepared parents are more alert at the time of delivery. Patients who have not had any preparation for childbirth often seem so frightened during the entire birthing process that when delivery is accomplished, they are too agitated to appreciate the deliciousness of the moment of birth. Prepared mothers are often more alert and thus better able to enjoy the thrill of having given birth.

Prepared mothers seem to have a better outcome. This is controversial, but some studies show that prepared mothers have fewer episiotomies, fewer cesarean sections, fewer episodes of fetal distress, fewer episodes of infection after delivery, and less toxemia. The reasons for this are neither proven nor clear. It may be that mothers who take preparation-for-childbirth classes are also more likely to take good care of themselves and to choose doctors who are more sensitive, conservative, and careful.

Doula. This is the name for a professional labor-support person who remains by the side of the couple throughout labor. This is a new concept, and it will be interesting to see if it becomes popular. A doula is trained in the physiology of birth and the emotional needs of a couple having a baby. A doula does not take the place of a doctor or a nurse, but is present to aid them in the care of the patient. They are not available in most locations now, but it is quite possible they will become more prevalent as time goes by. If you have no one who can be with you or if you feel that your husband would appreciate having someone more highly trained with him during labor, you might inquire at your hospital about a doula.

---

469 How can childbirth education help relieve pain?

Most women who have not experienced labor and delivery (and many who have) are afraid of the pain that labor will cause them. If this were not true, it is unlikely that Dr. Lamaze would have caused such a stir when he wrote *Painless Childbirth*. Without question, labor contractions are uncomfortable. It is also without question that pain can increase or decrease according to the way a woman perceives these contractions.

When a woman enters labor frightened, tense, and unaware of what is happening, she perceives her contractions as being much more painful than they really are. The beginning of a contraction signals to her that she should feel pain, even if the contraction itself is not very uncomfortable. Since she perceives contractions as very painful, as they become closer and stronger she envisions that they must hurt even more. She can become disoriented and exhausted as she perceives herself to be wracked with pain.

A woman in this condition is totally out of control and unable to cooperate as labor progresses. For her, the entire process of labor and delivery is such a wrenching experience that instead of enjoying the birth of the baby, all she can think of is getting relief from pain.

Although the situation just described is extreme, untrained women will often have this experience with labor. We have all been conditioned to recognize pain as an indication that something is wrong. In labor, however, pain usually is a sign that things are right. Understanding that contraction pain is natural and good helps a woman relax and "go with the flow" of the contraction.

470 **Will preparation-for-childbirth classes insure a pain-free delivery?**

Not necessarily. Although many women who have their baby "naturally" receive no pain medication, experience very little pain during labor, and are up walking around the day of delivery, there are many who have a great deal of discomfort with their "natural childbirth." Even women who are well trained, unafraid, and enthusiastic about childbirth without medication can become so uncomfortable during labor that they require medication for pain relief and an epidural for the last part of labor and for delivery. Others enter labor without any preparation, progress through labor quietly and without any significant discomfort, and deliver with only a local.

Each of us is made with different thresholds of pain tolerance. No woman who has had a fairly painless "natural childbirth" should push this technique on another woman. The other woman may have nerves that are "hooked up" to be much more sensitive. Likewise, someone who has had a great deal of discomfort while trying to deliver without pain medication should not tell another woman how "terrible" it was. That other woman may have nerves connected in such a way that labor for her will not be so painful.

471 **Do women who have had preparation-for-childbirth classes require less medication?**

Several recent studies of medication and anesthesia given during labor have shown that medication rates have not been affected by childbirth preparation. This surprised many of the strong advocates of such training, but I doubt that it was a surprise to most obstetricians.

My experience with women who have had childbirth classes is that most of the time they are able to go without Demerol through the early part of labor (from one or two centimeters to five centimeters of cervical dilatation). At this point the contractions become stronger and more fre-

quent. Those patients unable to tolerate labor comfortably or who do not want to feel the pain of contractions will then request drugs or, if available, an epidural. (See next three questions.)

Whether or not less medication is used, however, childbirth classes make for an easier, healthier, and more enjoyable labor and delivery.

Medication for Pain

472 **Is it better not to use drugs during labor and delivery?**

I believe that the less medication, the better—within reason. It is good if a woman can go through the early stages of labor without drugs such as Demerol, but I do not see any medical reason why she should not have medication, even in early labor, if she needs it to help her relax. A woman would do well to attend childbirth classes and be as prepared as she can. Then, if she needs medication, she should go ahead and use it.

In my opinion there has been too much hysteria about the effects of drugs like Demerol and techniques like epidurals on full-term babies. Since physicians stopped using large doses of Demerol (common prior to the mid-sixties), I have never seen a full-term baby affected in any significant way by Demerol, nor have I ever seen one affected in a negative way by an epidural.

473 **What anesthesia options are available for labor and delivery?**

There are seven anesthetics that we will discuss in the following questions:

epidural	pudendal block
spinal block	local anesthesia
general anesthesia	twilight sleep
paracervical block	

474 What is an epidural?

An epidural is an anesthetic given in the lower part of the back. It stops pain by numbing a woman from the waist down. The plastic catheter through which the drug is administered is left in place for subsequent injections. This catheter does not interfere with a woman's movement.

An epidural seems to be ideal for a woman who decides during labor that she needs an anesthetic. It can be started when she is about five centimeters dilated, if the baby's head is far enough down in the birth canal.

In administering an epidural, a needle is inserted in the lower middle part of the back between the vertebrae. Since it does not penetrate the sac surrounding the nerves, the drug does not go into the spinal fluid. It is injected, rather, into the cavity between the bones and the sac that contains the nerves, anesthetizing the nerves as they come out of the sac from the spinal cord.

Because the nerves that control the muscles of the abdomen and legs are surrounded by a covering and are thus partially protected from the anesthetic agents, these muscles are not totally anesthetized. This allows some movement on the part of the woman. The nerves that carry the pain sensation, however, do not have a covering over them, and they are totally anesthetized.

A woman does not feel much pain when the epidural is working properly. Occasionally, however, accumulations of fat or connective tissue may result in uneven distribution of the anesthesia, or problems encountered in placing the tubes may prevent an epidural from working properly.

An epidural may be used for many hours. Since the plastic tube is left in place in the back, the anesthesiologist can merely inject another dose of the anesthetic as the previous injection begins wearing off.

It is possible for labor to be slowed down by an epidural but, conversely, as some women relax with an epidural the cervix dilates faster and delivery is quicker than it might have been otherwise.

Even with an epidural in place, a woman can still push, although she will not feel the need for pushing. By following the techniques she learned in childbirth class and the instructions of the coach and the nurse who are helping her, she can be effective in pushing the baby down.

Forceps must be used more often with women who have epidurals than with those who do not. This, however, is not a bad thing, since forceps use in this situation is done when the baby's head is low in the birth canal and merely assists the baby's head out.

An epidural wears off within one to two hours after delivery, depending on the drug used.

One advantage of an epidural is that a woman who wants to undergo a sterilization procedure immediately after delivery can have it done with the epidural eliminating a second anesthetic. Another advantage is that in the event of a sudden need for a cesarean section, it can be done with the epidural in place without any further anesthetic.

The epidural does not hurt the baby if the mother's blood pressure is not allowed to drop, a problem that can usually be prevented. Complications for the mother from the use of the epidural are extremely rare and unusual.

475 What is a "spinal"?

Spinal anesthesia is administered much like an epidural. Instead of stopping outside the sac containing the spinal nerves, however, the needle is pushed into that sac and the drug is injected into the spinal fluid in which the spinal nerves float. Because both the muscle and pain fibers are uncovered while inside this sac, both pain and muscle activity are totally stopped by a spinal. A woman is numb from her waist down and cannot move her legs.

476 What is general anesthesia?

With general anesthesia a woman is normally first given pentothal in the veins to make her unconscious. Then a mask is put over her face or a tube is put in her trachea for administration of an anesthetic gas and she is "put to sleep" completely.

Except for special situations, this type of anesthesia should not be used for a delivery. When a woman begins labor, her stomach stops working and any fluid or food in her stomach will still be there when she delivers the baby. If a woman vomits while under general anesthesia, the vomited material can get into her lungs. This is dangerous and can cause pneumonia and even death. An epidural anesthetic is much safer for a routine delivery.

A general anesthetic can be used with reasonable safety for a planned cesarean section. Ordinarily the anesthesiologist will put a tube into the woman's windpipe (trachea) and inflate a small balloon around the tube. With this in place, even if the woman vomits, that material cannot get into her lungs.

A baby can be delivered without any significant effect from general anesthesia if the woman is being cared for by a competent anesthesiologist and obstetrician. The baby may be slightly sleepy, but it usually wakes within moments with a lusty cry.

477 What is a paracervical block?

This technique involves the injection of an anesthetic drug beside the cervix, at the top of the vagina to deaden the nerves coming from the woman's body into her uterus. It fairly effectively stops the pain of contractions and cervical dilatation. If the drug is injected into the blood vessels that flow into the uterus, the absorption of the drug into the baby's blood supply causes its heartbeat to slow and can, in rare cases, result in death. Because of this problem paracervicals are almost never used today.

478 What is a pudendal block?

Pudendal blocks are used extensively for women who do not want or need epidural or spinal anesthesia, but who need some type of anesthesia for an episiotomy or repair of a tear. The nerves to the lower vagina and the area around the opening of the vagina come up near the surface of the vagina, about halfway up the vagina. The pudendal is given by injecting an anesthetic agent first on one side and then on the other into the tissue around the nerves. A doctor competent in giving a pudendal can completely numb this area 75 to 80 percent of the time. When a pudendal is given, the doctor can use forceps, if necessary, with little discomfort for the mother, and the mother can have tears or an episiotomy sewn up without much discomfort. (See Q. 523.)

This type of anesthetic is usually given only after the cervix is completely dilated and when the baby's head is low enough in the birth canal that the mother's pushing will soon deliver it.

479 What is local anesthesia for delivery?

A local anesthetic is given in the tissues around the opening of the vagina or in the vagina. It can be given immediately before delivery, allowing an episiotomy to be cut, or it can be given after delivery so that tears can be repaired.

Because of the large number of blood vessels in the area around the opening of the vagina late in pregnancy, local anesthetic agents are often "carried away" quickly. Although a woman may be numb in that area when the doctor begins sewing, feeling may return before the stitching is completed. If this happens, the doctor will sometimes inject more local anesthetic agents. This in itself can, at times, be so uncomfortable, however, that the doctor may just finish the repairs without it. The woman would probably be as uncomfortable from more injections of the drugs as she would be from completion of the sewing.

The only side effects from a local or a pudendal would be a mother's adverse reaction to the drug. It is possible for a woman to react to any medication, even the medication used for local and pudendal anesthesia.

When a patient tells me she wants a "local" for her delivery, I give either a local or a pudendal, depending on which seems best at the time of the delivery. The same amount of drug is injected, and the results are much the same.

Birthing Rooms

480 What is a birthing room? What is an LDR (labor, delivery, recovery) room?

A variety of labor-and-delivery room options are now part of most modern obstetric units in the United States. They offer an alternative to the usual labor in one room and delivery in another, providing a more casual, homelike setting.

There are advantages and disadvantages to different situations. There are certain things that patients and their families may do in birthing centers that they cannot do in the regular labor-and-delivery unit. There are also certain things that patients may do in the regular labor-and-delivery unit that they may not do in the birthing room.

LDR rooms. These rooms are equipped so that all obstetric care can be given in one place. Women are allowed to labor, deliver, and recover in the same bed. In contrast to birthing rooms, LDR rooms are usually set up for any obstetric care except for cesarean sections. Women who develop some problem in their pregnancy can be cared for, drugs or anesthesia may be given, and forceps delivery can be done. More people than just the father or a coach may be present during the labor and delivery. In most birthing rooms, family or friends may also be present.

If a woman has a significant medical problem or high risk pregnancy, or develops a problem during labor, she may need to labor in a regular labor room and will probably need to deliver in a regular delivery room.

If there is a breech presentation, the woman will probably need to labor in the regular labor room and deliver in the cesarean section room so that surgery could be done quickly, if necessary.

Regular labor rooms. These rooms are set up for more intensive medical care, and the equipment is geared for care of high risk, complicated pregnancies.

LDRP rooms. These rooms are for labor, delivery, recovery, and postpartum care. A woman can go through all these stages and stay in an LDRP room until she goes home. These rooms are also commonly called birthing center rooms.

LDR and LDRP rooms are good options. These rooms were developed by physicians, nurses, and laypeople who have felt that labor and delivery in the United States had been "dehumanized." They believed that if there were a "special room," where the mother and father could be in a homelike, casual situation, they could have a more pleasant hospital experience.

This type of pressure has caused most hospital labor-and-delivery units to respond to the expressed needs of mothers and fathers during labor and delivery. Although the improved sensitivity on the part of the regular childbirth units has not made regular labor rooms and delivery rooms extinct, it has made them less necessary.

We are achieving a balanced approach to the use of the hospital for delivery. A woman with no problems can deliver in a homelike environment with family and, if she desires, friends present. A woman with a high risk pregnancy can deliver in a more intensive medical atmosphere. And, of course, a woman who needs a cesarean section can have that done, all within the same obstetric unit.

Home Births

481 Is a delivery outside a hospital a good alternative to a hospital delivery?

I feel that this is a dangerous option. There have been incredible advances in the care of women in labor and delivery in the past twenty years. Not only have the sensitivity and humaneness provided by health care professionals improved, but the ability of doctors and nurses also has improved because of training and technical advances. If you choose to deliver outside the hospital, you cannot take advantage of these advances in the event that you or your baby have problems.

Although a mother could suffer medical complications during labor and delivery because she is not delivering in a hospital, it is likely that the baby would suffer the more severe complications. For example, something as simple as a plug of meconium getting sucked into the baby's lungs can damage the baby severely. In that event a suction machine with a laryngoscope, commonly available in delivery rooms, could have been used to remove the meconium in a matter of seconds, avoiding such a catastrophe.

There are other problems that women and their babies can suffer during labor and delivery. One in ten babies has some problem during the delivery process that requires expert medical attention. Midwives may say that you or the baby can be taken to the hospital by ambulance if an emergency does develop, but if a baby's brain is deprived of adequate oxygen for more than four minutes, it will be either severely brain damaged or dead. No emergency service in the United States could get your baby to the hospital fast enough to make any difference in that case.

Certainly there is a statistical chance of getting by without having anything happen, but it is like playing Russian roulette. Once the unforeseen occurs, it cannot be changed. If you make the choice to have a home birth, and your baby is brain damaged or dies because of that decision, you will regret your choice for the rest of your life.

482 Would a home delivery be safe with a qualified nurse-midwife in attendance?

Certainly a home birth would be safer with a nurse-midwife than with a lay midwife or no midwife. Nurse-midwives generally have excellent training, whereas lay midwives typically have no medical background except for a couple of years of apprenticeship. In my opinion there is no place for lay midwives in the care of a pregnant woman unless there is no other medical care available. Even a qualified and competent nurse-midwife taking care of patients in labor outside the hospital cannot provide safety for the mother and baby.

If you want to have a nurse-midwife care for your labor and delivery, and she can do that in a hospital where there is a doctor to help if a problem develops, then I believe a nurse-midwife may safely be used. In the United States in the past few years, nurse-midwives are being allowed to work in concert with obstetricians in more and more hospitals.

Since they usually work in home situations, midwives will point out the "bright side" of delivering at home. They will assure you that it is uncommon for problems with labor to develop and they will point out the pleasure of being in a home environment for delivery. They might also point out the economic advantage of delivering at home.

There are reasons that midwives rarely see problems during home deliveries. First, they usually will not take care of a mother who has a complicated or high risk pregnancy. With this policy, they have eliminated from their practice most of the mothers who are likely to have problems with pregnancy, labor, and delivery.

Second, there are about fourteen deaths per thousand babies born, most of whom die from premature birth. If a woman goes into premature labor, the midwife will send her to a hospital, eliminating those babies from home delivery statistics.

Because midwives care for only those women who are carrying healthy pregnancies and who have no complications, they eliminate essentially all potentially dangerous situations. This is, of course, what they should do. Even with these guidelines, it is still possible for the baby or mother to develop a problem.

If you choose to have a delivery outside of a hospital, I encourage you to use a certified nurse-midwife. These midwives have very strict standards. They are certified by the American College of Nurse Midwives and must have an affiliation with an obstetrician.

Further, if you choose to use a midwife, I urge the following guidelines:

Don't choose this route for a first baby. In a study on outcomes of care in birthing centers published by Rooks and associates in the *New England Journal of Medicine* (1989, 321:1804), it was reported that 29 percent of women having their first babies had to be transferred to hospitals for delivery.

Only 7 percent who had already had one pregnancy and delivery needed to be transferred to the hospital.

Don't try to deliver outside the hospital if you have a high risk pregnancy or a medical complication.

Don't try to deliver outside the hospital if you have a breech baby.

If you will abide by these fairly strict guidelines, you have almost as good a chance of having a successful outcome for both you and your baby outside the hospital as you would in the hospital. You are taking a risk, however, and I advise against it.

Preparing for the Hospital's Routine

483 **The labor-and-delivery units of the hospitals I have seen recently seem much more attractive and thoughtful than in the past. Is this a trend?**

When you walk into the labor-and-delivery unit of a hospital or onto the floor where mothers stay after they have delivered, or when you peer into the nursery, you will sense a totally different atmosphere than exists anywhere else in the hospital.

There is a flexibility existing in most labor-and-delivery areas that is pleasant for both the patient and her family. When patients ask about the possibility of doing things a little differently, their physicians will usually now tell them that they can do anything they want to while they are in labor and delivery, unless a medical problem develops to prevent their carrying through with their plans, or unless there is something they want to do that would be medically unwise. This type of attitude prevails among most obstetricians today.

The nurses on most labor-and-delivery units are flexible enough to work with people who have had childbirth classes and with those who have not. Nurses at our hospital care for many totally untrained patients in such a way that, by the time these people had finished their labor and delivery, they had had an amazingly complete course on how to breathe, how to relax, and how to push to have a baby with a minimum amount of analgesia or anesthesia.

Patients often ask if the hospital "requires" that they have an enema or some other medical treatment. The "hospital" doesn't ordinarily require anything that has to do with your routine care. All medications, treatments, and food are ordered by your physician. While hospitals have superbly trained staffs prepared to meet the needs of the patient, the attending physician is the one who orders the medication and treatments.

Do-It-Yourself Emergency Deliveries

484 **What should I do if I start delivering on the way to the hospital?**

Prior knowledge in the "basics" of delivering a baby will be extremely helpful in an emergency birth. There are some clear "dos" and "don'ts" in this situation. For clarity of discussion, the husband will be addressed, but the advice is applicable to anyone who might need to help you deliver.

Don't panic. Even if you do absolutely nothing, your wife will almost certainly deliver with no problems. Deliveries have been taking place for thousands of years, and your wife's will occur whether or not you do anything.

Don't start driving faster. This merely endangers you, your wife, and your baby.

Don't stop the car and try to get the doctor on the phone. At this point there is nothing he or she can do.

Do listen to your wife. If she says the baby is coming NOW, it probably is. Stop the car in a safe place and help her!

Do help your wife remove her clothing from the waist down and assist her in lying back on the car seat.

Do tell your wife to gradually push while you gently hold your hand against the top of the baby's head. The head will look like a grapefruit pushing its way out of the vagina. The primary thing you can do at this time is to keep the baby's head from "popping" out of the birth canal. If it pops out without control, there is a possibility that some blood vessels inside the skull around the brain can tear, causing damage to the baby.

Do help ease the baby's head out. If your wife is pushing too hard, and you can see that it is likely that the baby's head will pop out, tell her to stop pushing. Keep gentle, but firm pressure against the top of the baby's head, letting it ease out over a few seconds' time.

Do "catch" the baby gently, then hold it face down to allow any mucus to drain from the mouth and nose. The baby will normally cough, gasp, and gag a little.

Do lay the baby on your wife's tummy, once it is breathing freely.

Don't take off your shoestring and tie the umbilical cord. Leave the cord alone and let the doctor or hospital personnel cut it later.

Don't worry about the placenta (afterbirth). It may deliver on its own while you are driving to the hospital or it may not. Either is fine.

Do wrap the baby gently in a blanket, or in anything you have handy, to keep it from being chilled.

Do assist your wife in lying back comfortably in the car, with the baby snuggled up on her abdomen. You can proceed to the hospital with this beautiful addition to your family.

Do drive carefully to the hospital.

Do congratulate yourself and enjoy the accolades of your friends! You are one of the select few husbands in the United States who has delivered his own child.

An Afterword

There is probably no stronger anticipation in any couple's life than that which starts the day they know they are pregnant, especially with their first child. I encourage you to take time to savor the excitement and joy of that anticipation. You have never done anything like it in your life. Prepare well! Not only is it fun, but the reward is enormous—a precious, beautiful child of your own.

9

Labor and Delivery

When labor starts, the waiting is almost over. Soon that individual who has so completely filled your womb will fill your arms and your heart.

Your baby is a separate and unique individual. Although we know approximately when the birth will take place, unless we do something artificial, the sex of the child and the exact time of its birth are beyond our control. It matters not that we want the baby to come on December thirty-first nor that we already have two boys and want a girl. The baby almost shouts aloud at birth, "See me! I am a separate creation of God. I came when God wanted me to. I am a boy or a girl as God wanted me to be. I am an individual, not an object to be manipulated."

So labor begins as the unborn baby issues the first of his or her thousands of untimely, unexpected, and usually selfish demands: "I want out!" Your bills may be piled up, your other children may have the chicken pox, your hair may be dirty, but the baby couldn't care less. Those first contractions herald the entrance of a brand-new person onto the stage of this world.

Ready or not, here that baby comes!

Before Labor Starts

485 What if my bag of waters breaks before I am at term in my pregnancy?

The rupture of the bag of waters before term is serious because no matter what a physician decides to do, there is danger to the baby. If the pregnancy is allowed to continue, there is a risk of infection. Germs can ascend from the vagina and cervix up into the uterus where they can infect the baby, causing damage or death. If labor is induced and the baby delivered prematurely, there is also danger of permanent damage or death. If labor is induced and your uterus is not ready for labor, you might need to have a C-section that would have been unnecessary if your bag of waters had not ruptured.

No matter how far along in your pregnancy you are, if your bag of waters breaks, it is common for you to start labor. (About 50 percent of the time, you will go into labor within twenty-four hours; 85 percent of the time you will begin labor within a week.)

Sometimes it is difficult for you to know if your bag of waters has broken or if you are leaking urine. Your doctor will use various techniques to determine which has happened. One technique is to test the acidity of the fluid. Amniotic fluid is alkaline; vaginal secretions are acid, but this test can be inaccurate.

If your bag of waters has ruptured prematurely, you will probably be hospitalized by your physician unless you have not yet reached twenty weeks of pregnancy. If you are under twenty weeks, your doctor may just let you start your miscarriage on your own at home because you may not miscarry for a day or two and hospitalization during that time would be unnecessary.

If your bag of waters ruptures between twenty and thirty-six weeks of pregnancy, your doctor may choose to keep you in bed and check for signs of infection. At this point, premature delivery and infections are major problems. If you stay in bed and do not develop infection, your labor might

not start, and your baby may mature enough to survive delivery without problems.

If your bag of waters ruptures after thirty-six weeks of pregnancy, most physicians will want to induce labor. At this stage, the chance of the baby's being premature is low. Because of the risk of infection, your doctor may feel that it is best to go ahead and deliver the baby.

Giving antibiotics to prevent infection is not effective if your bag of waters ruptures. While antibiotics can keep the mother from developing any sign of infection, they cannot keep the baby from being infected. Antibiotics therefore can keep the doctor from knowing whether or not the baby is infected until it is too late.

Occasionally, a woman will stop leaking fluid. If this happens, she may be released from the hospital. Sometimes, even if a woman is still leaking fluid, a doctor will allow her to go home if she can stay in bed there and call if any problem arises. If a patient is at home, she still must not have intercourse, douche, or put anything into her vagina. If rupture of the membranes has occurred and signs of infection develop, the baby must be delivered so that it can be put on antibiotics in the nursery. A woman will usually have a normal vaginal delivery unless there is a medical reason for a cesarean section.

486 What if I have light bleeding or spotting?

One of the most likely causes of this type of bleeding during the last month of pregnancy is your doctor's pelvic examination. As the doctor examines your cervix, he or she will gently place a finger against the cervical opening to see how dilated it is. This can tear some of the delicate blood vessels of the cervix, causing light bleeding, which may be bright red and actually run out of your vagina. If it is not as heavy as a menstrual period, you need not worry about it. Such bleeding may occur the night after an exam rather than immediately following it.

Bleeding late in pregnancy not associated with a pelvic examination is called a "bloody show" and merely indicates that your cervix is beginning to dilate. The material that is passing is the mucus that has been plugging the cervix during pregnancy. In the later months of pregnancy the cervix will often stretch open a little, tearing small blood vessels and causing spotting and passage of some of the cervical mucus. This can happen at least two or three weeks before you actually go into labor. You do not need to call your doctor because of this bloody show, unless you are also having contractions and think you may be in labor.

If you have a bloody show at any time other than the last month, though, you need to call your doctor immediately. It could be an indication of premature labor or a miscarriage.

487 What is false labor?

Most women seem concerned about the "embarrassment" of being in false labor. You should not be embarrassed if you go to the doctor or to the hospital with some contractions and are told that they are not true labor contractions. Not even your doctor can tell whether or not you are in true labor without feeling your cervix. If the contractions you are having are not causing your cervix to thin out and to dilate, you are not in labor, no matter how strong they are. It is better to go to the doctor several times in false labor than it is to ignore significant contractions and risk having your baby at home because you thought you were in false labor.

We have all heard stories of women who were "in labor" for a week. These stories are almost never true. These women have usually had strong false labor contractions for the six days that preceded the onset of true labor on the seventh day! A woman should not take any aspirin or prostaglandin inhibitors, such as Advil, Nuprin, or Motrin, near the end of her pregnancy because they can interfere with labor.

488 Should labor be induced if false labor continues to occur?

After a patient has been examined several times and found to be in false labor, the question will

arise as to why she cannot be "induced." Induction should usually not be done unless the cervix is adequately dilated (about two centimeters), soft, and the baby's head in good position. (See Q. 551.)

It can be unsafe to do an induction of labor, even if you are having numerous Braxton-Hicks contractions (false labor pains), if your body is not ready for induction.

The How, When, and Why of Labor

489 When should I call the doctor if I think I might be in labor?

There are three primary indications of the onset of labor. You should call your physician if any of the following occur:

Broken bag of waters. When your bag of waters ruptures, you may have a slow leak, a moderate flow, or an embarrassing gush of fluid from your vagina. When that happens, call your doctor immediately. After your membranes rupture, germs are likely to get up into the fluid around the baby and cause infection.

It is possible, however, that the fluid you are leaking is urine. The baby can "poke" your bladder, causing a squirt of urine that you may mistake for amniotic fluid. This happens to many pregnant women.

It is important for you to understand that your bag of waters can break at any time during your pregnancy. When it occurs very early in pregnancy (third or fourth month), the pregnancy will almost inevitably end as a late miscarriage. If the bag of waters breaks from the twentieth to the twenty-eighth week of pregnancy, you and your physician have a very difficult situation to deal with. (See the question about prematurely ruptured membranes.)

Contractions that are becoming hard and regular. Most physicians will want first-time mothers to call when their contractions are about three to five minutes apart, unless they are more than an hour away from the hospital. Even if they wait until contractions are this close together, there are usually still several hours until delivery.

Most physicians will want patients who are having their second baby to call when their contractions are eight or ten minutes apart, are coming regularly, and are getting harder.

Mothers with a third baby (or more) should call when they think they are in labor. By the third baby most women know what labor feels like. Also, labor can progress faster than with previous births. It is best, therefore, for a woman to call as soon as she thinks labor has begun, even if contractions are fairly far apart.

Heavy bleeding. If you begin to bleed heavily any time during pregnancy, call your doctor. (Most physicians would consider heavy bleeding to be soaking a pad every three or four hours.) If you cannot reach your doctor, go straight to the hospital and have someone continue trying to notify the doctor that you are on your way to the hospital so that he or she can meet you there.

test may be inaccurate, if the pH paper seems to indicate leaking amniotic fluid, the doctor will have you go to the hospital. Occasionally the doctor and you can tell without an exam that your bag of waters has broken because you are losing so much fluid.

The first sign of the onset of labor may be the breaking of the bag of waters, but the bag of waters can break without labor starting. If this happens, your doctor may need to use Pitocin to start your labor.

Patients frequently ask me if their bag of waters will break with a second pregnancy if it broke with the first one. The answer is, "Not necessarily." One labor may be ushered in by breaking of the bag of waters and another with contractions.

If you are bleeding heavily. If this occurs the doctor will probably have you go immediately to the hospital. Once you have arrived at the labor-and-delivery unit, your doctor and the nurses will evaluate you to see if you can have a normal delivery or will need a cesarean section.

490 What will the doctor do when I call?

If you have called because of the reasons discussed in the previous two questions, your doctor will probably want to see you immediately either at his or her office or in the hospital.

If you are having contractions. The doctor will examine you to see if you have dilated since your last examination. If your cervix is thinning out (effacing) and opening (dilating), it means that you are probably in labor and should go to the hospital.

If your water has broken. If this has happened, the doctor will usually do a pelvic examination with a speculum. If you are definitely leaking fluid from the cervix, you will be sent to the hospital. If the doctor cannot tell if there is a definite leak of fluid, he or she will probably test some fluid from the opening of your cervix with pH paper. Since amniotic fluid is alkaline and vaginal secretions are acid, pH paper will turn blue if there is a leakage of amniotic fluid through the cervix. While the

491 May I eat a meal before going to the hospital?

If the doctor has asked you to go to the hospital, do not eat or drink anything from that point until you are told specifically that you may have something to eat or drink. Any food or drink that you take in once labor has started will stay in your stomach for hours, because when the uterus starts working, the stomach seems to stop working. If you should suddenly need general anesthesia for a cesarean section, you could vomit while receiving your anesthesia, and such vomiting can cause breathing of the food into your lungs, an extremely grave complication.

During labor your doctor may allow you to sip water or eat ice chips. If your labor is not progressing well, however, and a C-section may be necessary, he or she may require that you ingest absolutely nothing through your mouth.

Many obstetricians allow their patients to eat hard candy and to use glycerin swabs, which are available in most labor-and-delivery departments, because these items do not add much to the contents of the stomach.

492 What is labor? When does it start?

A basic definition of labor would be "contractions that produce progressive dilatation and effacement of the cervix." Incidentally, if the cervix does not dilate and thin out, the contractions are not true labor contractions. Labor, then, is the natural process which produces the birth of a baby.

No one knows why labor starts. In the practical sense, about all we can say is what was said of the virgin Mary in Luke 2:6 (NASB): "And it came about that while they were there, the days were completed for her to give birth." In other words, when it is time, you will go into labor.

493 How do uterine contractions—labor pains—bring about the birth of a baby?

Uterine contractions are unique. If the entire uterus were to contract in exactly the same way, producing exactly the same pressure in all parts of the uterus, nothing would happen except that the baby would be squeezed. This is not what happens, however.

The uterus basically has two segments—the upper and the lower. As the muscle of the upper segment contracts, it does not relax back to its original length, but gets thicker and thicker as labor progresses. The muscle of the lower part of the uterus thins out and is actually pulled into the upper segment and up around the baby's head. This explains why the cervix dilates. The whole process is an extraordinary example of a functional design created by God.

494 How frequent are labor contractions?

Labor contractions can occasionally be frequent even at the beginning of labor. I have had many patients whose contractions began three to four minutes apart. Generally, however, contractions will start ten to fifteen minutes apart, and gradually get closer and closer together.

During the active part of labor, contractions usually last about sixty seconds, with about one to three minutes between each contraction. After the cervix is completely dilated, contractions may last sixty seconds, with only sixty seconds between each contraction. At this point the mother's uterus is working hard to get the baby out.

495 Why are there periods of time between contractions?

Women in labor welcome the respite between labor contractions, but this "breathing space" is primarily for the baby's benefit, not theirs. During a contraction, there is almost no blood flow through the uterus. Periods of relaxation between contractions are essential for the baby's well-being, because the mother's blood can then flow into the uterus to provide the oxygen and nutrients necessary for keeping the baby healthy. This oxygen is transferred from the mother's blood, across the placental membrane, into the baby's blood. This allows the baby to tolerate the process of labor in a healthy way. Contractions that come too frequently could cause an inadequate oxygen supply for the baby and could be a reason for an immediate cesarean section.

496 What happens at the hospital if I am sent there in labor or with ruptured membranes?

Normal, routine procedures include:

Admission to the hospital. If you earlier completed procedures for preadmission to the hospital, you will merely pass through the admission office. They will lift the information from their computer or records and take you immediately by wheelchair to the labor-and-delivery section.

Admission to labor and delivery. The nurses will make you comfortable in your labor room. Your history will be taken, including a record of past health problems, past pregnancies and labors, and of this particular pregnancy. Your blood pressure, pulse, and temperature will also be taken and recorded.

Change of clothes. You will be asked to undress completely and put on a hospital gown.

Examination. After you have changed clothes and gotten into bed, a labor-and-delivery nurse will examine you. Even if the doctor examined you in the office, the nurse may want to examine you, too, to compare her findings with the earlier ones. Since labor can progress quickly, it is important that the nurse know how fast you are progressing and how far along in labor you are when you are admitted to labor and delivery. The nurse will check your uterus for contractions and examine you to see if your bag of waters has broken.

A primary reason for this initial exam is to determine the position of the baby. If the baby is coming headfirst, then the nurse knows that it is safe for you to progress in labor. If she finds that the baby is not coming headfirst, she will call your obstetrician immediately.

A call to your obstetrician. After the nurse has completed the exam, she will call your obstetrician. If, as they discuss your situation, they feel that you are in labor, the doctor will ask the nurse to do the procedures he or she thinks are right for you: blood tests, enema, IV, and the application of a monitor, as described below.

If the nurse and the doctor are quite certain that you are not in labor, the doctor will ask the nurse to discharge you from labor and delivery. You will go home and probably go to the doctor's office within a few days.

If it seems to them that you may be in false labor, but they are not sure, you may have to stay in the hospital for a couple of hours to be observed.

Once it has been determined that you are truly in labor, nurses will monitor your progress. Most physicians will have the nurses call them when their patients are dilated five centimeters. At that point, if it is during the night, your physician may come to the hospital and stay; if it is during the day, he or she may continue working in the office if it is near the hospital.

Prior to five centimeters of dilatation there may still be many hours of labor, and it is extremely

rare for any unexpected problems to develop in that time. If, however, a patient has had a previous fast labor, or if she has already had several babies, your physician will usually come to the hospital sooner and then stay close by once active labor has begun.

Blood and urine tests. When your doctor admits you to labor and delivery, he or she will usually want you to have a blood count, a test for syphilis, and blood typing done. (The latter is so that your type blood will be available should you need an emergency transfusion.) If you have not had prenatal care, the doctor caring for you now will want to know if you are Rh negative or Rh positive and will test for this. You will also be asked to collect a urine specimen to check for urinary-tract infection or other kidney problems.

Enema and prep. During the pushing phase of labor, anything not attached in the lower part of your body is pushed out, including not only the baby but also urine and stool. To avoid having both baby and stool passed at the same time, most patients and doctors prefer that an enema be given. I feel that having an enema is wise. In addition to preventing a messy birth, it also decreases contamination of vaginal tears and episiotomies and thus reduces the chance of infection. One additional advantage of an enema is that it can actually stimulate labor contractions to be more effective. Occasionally a patient will have her bag of waters rupture and yet have no contractions. Such a patient usually needs Pitocin to start her labor, but occasionally an enema will have that effect before the Pitocin is started.

It is not absolutely necessary that you have an enema. Some patients do not want one. If you do not, discuss it with your doctor. If he or she agrees, you may be able to avoid having the enema.

Most doctors prefer some cleansing of the perineal area and having some of the hair around the lower part of the vulva and around the anus shaved or clipped. Sometimes this is done soon after admittance to the hospital, and at other times it is done after you are moved to the delivery table. The purpose of shaving is to avoid any vulvar hair being caught in the sutures as the episiotomy or vaginal tears are sewn. If that happens, the incision can become infected and break open.

Intravenous fluid. Most physicians like their patients to have an IV going in the event it is needed quickly later. To avoid the tubing, a needle can be inserted into the vein and a "heplock" attached to it. The heparin in this device keeps the tube open and an IV or blood transfusion can be attached immediately if it becomes necessary to treat sudden bleeding or an unplanned C-section. A patient's sudden collapse into shock because of heavy uterine bleeding or a ruptured uterus or some other problem is dangerous enough by itself—but it could cause an even more serious problem if an IV were not already going, as it could be difficult to get one started under those conditions.

It is better to plan ahead, even though such complications do not occur very often. Your doctor wants both you and your baby to survive this whole process in a healthy fashion and thus may take certain precautions to insure that.

Some women worry about dislodging their intravenous needle. This fear is unwarranted because most IVs are started with plastic needles that will not come out of the vein, even if the arm moves around wildly.

If you feel strongly that you do not want an IV, talk to your doctor. He or she may agree that it is okay to do without it.

Fetal monitoring. Many obstetricians feel that continuous fetal monitoring is wise during every labor. If fetal monitoring is not done by a machine, someone should listen to your baby's heartbeat frequently with a doppler device or a fetoscope during labor. (See Q. 502.)

The Stages of Labor

497 What are the stages of labor?

The stages of labor are Stage One, Stage Two, and Stage Three. These will be discussed in the following questions. (Childbirth classes label the stages differently. See Q. 501.)

498 What does the first stage of labor include?

This stage of labor includes the time from the start of true labor until the cervix is completely dilated. It is characterized by the following events:

Gradually increasing strength and frequency of labor contractions. Once the cervix is dilated five centimeters, the effectiveness of the contractions often increases. This is called the "phase of acceleration." Some women progress fairly rapidly from one or two centimeters up to five; others will take many hours to reach five centimeters of dilation.

Once the "phase of acceleration" is reached, the cervix often dilates much more quickly. Obstetricians expect the cervix to dilate at the rate of one centimeter an hour from five centimeters on; if progression is not that fast, the doctor will be watching carefully for a problem.

Most obstetricians rupture the bag of waters (when they know a woman is in active labor) if the baby is coming down headfirst. This seems to make contractions more effective and, therefore, makes labor a little shorter.

Descent of the baby's head in the birth canal. During the first stage of labor, not only is the cervix dilating up to ten centimeters (complete dilation), but the baby's head is progressing down into the birth canal.

A woman's pelvic bones have some prominent projections called ischial spines, which are easily felt by the doctor on vaginal exam. When the top of the baby's head progresses down the birth canal to the level of the ischial spines, it means that the largest part of the baby's head has come through the ring of bone at the top of the birth canal and is probably going to deliver without a cesarean section, though many C-sections are still necessary even then. When the top of the baby's head is at the ischial spines, the baby is said to be at "station zero." For each centimeter above the ischial spines that the top of the baby's head is, you are said to be at "minus one, minus two," and so on. For each centimeter that the top of the baby's head is past the ischial spines, you are said to be "plus one" or "plus two," as the case may be.

Cervical dilatation. The pregnant woman's cervix can be almost totally closed just before labor starts or it can be as much as three or four

Cervical Dilatation

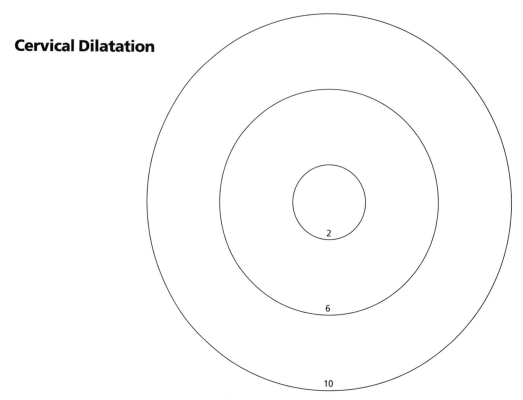

2

6

10

Cervical dilatation in centimeters, shown actual size

10 cm = 3.9 inches

Fetal Head Stations

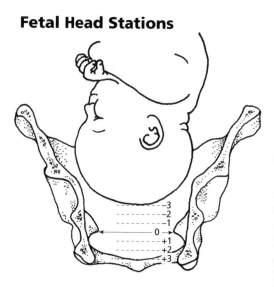

−3
−2
−1
0
+1
+2
+3

centimeters dilated before labor starts. The amount of dilatation of the cervix before labor starts does not cause the onset of labor. The changes in the woman's body that cause the start of labor are much more complicated than that. When labor starts, the cervix starts dilating (opening up). (See Q. 492.) The dilatation of the cervix enlarges the small round opening present at the start of labor to an opening big enough for the baby to deliver through. For normal-size babies a dilatation of ten centimeters is required for delivery.

Effacement. Effacement of the cervix means the shortening of the cervix. The normal cervix is about one inch long, and during effacement the cervix gets shorter. This can happen during the last few weeks of pregnancy without any labor contractions occurring. A woman may go into labor with her cervix 100 percent effaced but dilated only a small amount. If the cervix is not to-

Effacement

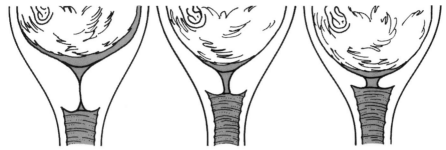

tally effaced when a woman starts labor, the contractions of labor will result in the cervix being totally effaced by the time the cervix is completely dilated.

If a woman's cervix is about one inch long, it is not effaced (0 percent effacement) since the normal cervix is that long. If the cervix is about one-half inch long, it is said to be 50 percent effaced. If the cervix is totally flattened out and amounts to no more than a circular opening with a paper-thin edge, it is said to be 100 percent effaced.

499 What does the second stage of labor include?

The second stage starts when the mother's cervix is completely dilated—ten centimeters—and ends with the delivery of the baby. This stage may be brief, because as soon as the mother reaches ten centimeters of cervical dilatation, the baby may progress immediately out of the birth canal and be delivered.

During this stage of labor the lower part of the vagina is dilated and the perineum (the area be-

tween the lower vagina and the anus) is stretched out. An episiotomy may be done to keep the tissue of the perineum from tearing. Especially with the first baby the choice is almost always either tearing or episiotomy. After the first baby, episiotomies are sometimes necessary, sometimes not.

I am frequently asked by patients if I routinely recommend episiotomies. Few doctors "routinely" do episiotomies, but most agree that it is better for your tissues to have a clean straight cut as in an episiotomy, than ragged, bloody tears. Both of these, of course, must be sewn, but it seems that tissues heal more normally if they have been carefully cut than if they have torn. (See Q. 510.)

500 What does the third stage of labor include?

This stage begins with delivery of the baby and concludes with delivery of the placenta. As soon as the baby is born, the uterus continues to contract, eventually squeezing out the placenta. As

Dilatation

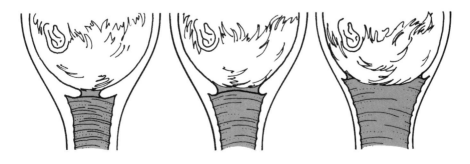

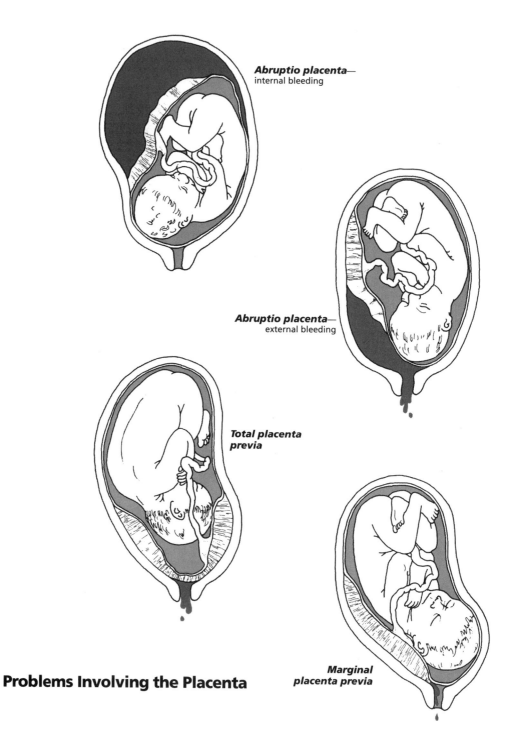

Abruptio placenta—
internal bleeding

Abruptio placenta—
external bleeding

**Total placenta
previa**

**Marginal
placenta previa**

Problems Involving the Placenta

the placenta is extruded from the vagina, a gush of blood occurs. This happens because, as the placenta separates from the uterus, blood collects behind it, helping to make the separation complete.

This loss of blood is not dangerous, and as the placenta leaves the uterine cavity, the uterus continues to "contract down," pinching off its blood vessels so that little further bleeding occurs.

The placenta may not deliver for hours if left alone. Usually if the placenta does not fairly soon come out spontaneously, the doctor will put his or her hand up into the uterus, grasp the placenta, and pull it out.

Patients occasionally tell doctors that they want the placenta to deliver on its own. This is fine, except that it sometimes takes two or three hours and can heighten the chance of bleeding and infection. Most doctors believe that it is best to get the placenta delivered within ten or fifteen minutes after delivery of the baby.

Most doctors today carefully examine the inside of the uterus with their hand if the placenta did not seem to come out intact. They want to make certain that all the membranes and placental tissue have been removed. In spite of this exam, however, it is fairly common for even large pieces of placental tissue to pass from the uterus a few hours or a few days later. The lining of the uterus and the placental tissue feel similar (soft and mushy), and it is impossible to know for sure that all placental tissue is out.

Before the episiotomy or vulvar tears are sutured, most doctors will visually check the cervix and the vagina to make sure there are no tears of these tissues. If there are, these are sewn prior to the repair of the episiotomy or of the tears around the opening of the vagina.

501 How does this account of the stages of labor correlate with the phases taught in childbirth classes?

Patients can be confused by the differing terminology used by their physicians and their childbirth-class teachers. Obstetricians talk in terms of first stage, second stage, and third stage. Childbirth classes teach that the first stage of labor (the time during which the cervix dilates from one or two centimeters to ten centimeters) is made up of three different phases:

The first phase equals dilatation from zero to four centimeters; the second phase equals dilatation from four to eight centimeters (essentially the first part of the "phase of acceleration" that was

discussed in Q. 498); the third phase, "transition," equals dilatation from eight to ten centimeters (the last part of the phase of acceleration).

The reason the teachers of childbirth classes divide labor into these three phases is that progressively increasing amounts of effort and concentration are required for the mother and father with each successive phase. It is easier for the mother to anticipate what to expect if she considers labor divided into these segments.

Practicalities in the Labor Room

502 How is monitoring done during labor? Why is it so important?

Monitoring your baby during labor merely means observing how it is doing. This is done by watching both the baby's heartbeat and your contractions. In most hospital labor-and-delivery units, mothers wear electronic fetal monitors that not only observe the baby's heartbeat but also record the "character" of the uterine contractions the mother is having. The straps of these monitors are fairly comfortable and do not interfere with the mother's movement or activity during labor.

Fetal monitors are usually kept in place throughout labor, allowing the doctors and nurses to compare the baby's current heartbeat with earlier records to check for a pattern that might indicate a problem.

Monitoring of the fetus can also be done with a fetoscope (a stethoscope designed specifically to hear the baby's heartbeat), or with an electronic monitor. The baby's heartbeat will normally be between 120 and 160 beats per minute, though it is normal for the rate to drop or to rise a little from those norms.

If the heartbeat develops an abnormal pattern of slow or fast rates, immediate delivery may be indicated, even if it involves a cesarean section. This is a situation in which the doctor's judgment is important. If you are in the second stage of labor, it may be possible for the baby to be delivered vaginally before it is damaged.

Observation of your contractions is also important. This may be done by the nurse's or the doctor's hand on your abdomen or with the electronic monitor. Either way, both the intensity of the contractions and their frequency are evaluated. If the intensity suddenly becomes abnormally strong, or if the uterus is not relaxing between contractions, the baby might need to be delivered immediately, even if it requires a cesarean section. Occasionally a woman's uterine contractions will slow down and even stop. It is important that the nurses and your doctor be aware of this because you will need medication to make the uterus continue contracting. (See Q. 507.)

Some labor-and-delivery units have telemetry systems. This means that you can wear the equipment to monitor your baby and your contractions. The information is "telegraphed" wirelessly to an external recording unit at the nurses' station. This leaves the woman in labor without wires or tubes to tie her down. If, therefore, her doctor feels it is okay, she can be up walking around and still be safely monitored while she is in labor.

503 What examinations will take place during labor?

The nurse and doctor will be performing vaginal exams throughout your labor. Only occasional examinations are necessary when you are less than five centimeters dilated, but more frequent exams are necessary when contractions increase in frequency and intensity.

These examinations are done for two reasons. First, they show the progress of dilatation; second, they show the progression of the baby's head through the birth canal. If the baby's head is staying high, even with good contractions, you may have an obstructed labor and need a cesarean section.

The doctor will want your blood pressure, temperature, and pulse checked intermittently. Normally these are checked about every one to two hours.

The doctor and nurses will be watching your abdomen to make sure that your bladder is not too full. If your bladder is filling up, and you cannot urinate on your own, you will need to be catheterized. This involves the insertion of a hollow rubber tube through your urethra into your bladder for the drainage of urine.

504 How much will labor hurt?

The terms used to refer to the process of having a baby, *labor* and *pains,* should offer some clues to the woman who has never had a child as to how it feels.

The term *labor* indicates that the process is a lot of work. For this reason women should be in good physical condition as they approach the end of their pregnancy.

The term *pains* has been applied to the process of labor for thousands of years. Labor does hurt, but the amount of pain that women have with labor varies from individual to individual. A patient of mine described it as "like a gas pain that you cannot get rid of, which makes you feel like doubling over and bearing down." This is a good description of the pain of labor.

As labor starts, the pain is like a menstrual cramp. This cramping becomes increasingly more intense and more frequent, and about the time that a woman in labor is five centimeters dilated, the pain begins changing to a type of pain that she has never had before, similar to a severe gas pain that does not go away and that causes a great deal of discomfort.

Because each woman's nerves are "hooked up" differently, some women feel labor pains a great deal and others very little. I read a newspaper article several years ago about a pregnant woman who took a nap and awakened to find that she had delivered her baby! It would be wonderful if all women were like that, but few are.

One problem with "natural childbirth" classes is that they can sometimes play down the pain aspect of labor. Many teachers tend to imply that if a woman prepares herself adequately, she will not hurt during labor. This is untrue. Most women will have a great deal of discomfort during their labor, although often it is a discomfort that they can tolerate. Women tend to "forget" about the severity of the pain after the delivery is over. The fact that most women get pregnant again shows that labor pains are not intolerably severe for most women.

505 What about pain relief during labor?

Many women in early labor, whether or not they plan to have anesthesia for delivery (see Q. 472–479), will want something in addition to their breathing techniques to help relieve pain. Most obstetricians normally give some type of narcotic in the vein through the IV tubing if the patient requests it.

The drugs usually given are 25 mg of Demerol with a mild tranquilizer. This is not enough to put a mother to sleep, nor can it hurt the baby. If the mother is still uncomfortable, that dosage can be repeated two or three times almost immediately without harming either mother or baby. The 25 mg dose of Demerol can be repeated at intervals, and giving it every thirty to forty minutes is not excessive.

Some mothers feel that they "lose control" when they have been given Demerol, or they don't like its effect. Those women should not receive a repeated dose of it. Many mothers, however, feel better with Demerol, and I encourage its use. Pain medication used this way does not hurt the baby. Very little of it gets through the placenta—certainly not enough to depress the baby or cause problems. Years ago, women received 100 mg of Demerol several times during labor without significant problems to the babies.

During the earlier part of labor whirlpools or at least showers can provide a surprising amount of distraction and relief from labor "pains." Of course, if you have had pain medications, you may be too groggy to be up for these things.

506 Can regional anesthetics, such as an epidural, be given during the first stage of labor?

Epidural anesthesia is the most widely used form of anesthesia for labor and delivery in the United States. It allows a woman freedom from pain and yet she still has some awareness of the position of her legs and some movement of her legs. (See Q. 474 for more on "epidurals.")

In the first stage of labor, the only type of anesthesia that can be given is epidural. A spinal stops labor and therefore can be given only during the second stage of labor. An epidural is usually given when a woman having her first baby is dilated to five centimeters and the baby's head is at "plus one" (engaged). If the baby's head is higher than that, the doctor may not feel comfortable with the first-time mother's receiving an epidural even if she is six or seven centimeters dilated. (See Q. 498.)

If a woman has had a previous baby, she may be able to have an epidural when she is only three or four centimeters dilated. Most doctors feel that it is important, in an ordinary situation, that a good labor pattern be established before the epidural is given.

507 When and why is Pitocin given?

Pitocin (oxytocin) is normally given in the IV fluid when a woman is not having good contractions. The contractions in the first stage should gradually increase in intensity and frequency; if they are irregular and ineffective and the woman is dilating very slowly, it is probably best that she have Pitocin added slowly to the intravenous fluid. This is not given in an attempt to make contractions harder than normal contractions; it is given only to bring the quality of contractions and their frequency up to what is expected of normal labor.

The advantage of Pitocin is that it keeps a patient from staying in labor for longer than normal and prevents the woman and her uterus from getting weak, dehydrated, and tired. If labor is prolonged, infection can develop in the amniotic fluid and in the baby. Keeping good contractions going can prevent this. If a mother's contractions are monitored carefully by the medical attendants, there is almost no chance of any damage to her or her baby from Pitocin. (See Q. 563.)

Pitocin may also be given to start labor. If a woman's bag of waters has broken, she needs to deliver the baby before germs from the vagina get into the uterus and infect the baby. Occasionally a woman and her doctor will want to induce labor because of convenience or because a pregnancy has gone more than two weeks past the due date. In these situations the doctor will usually break the bag of waters and start Pitocin.

The Basics of Delivery

508 Does monitoring continue through delivery?

It is helpful if the baby can be monitored, either with the electric fetal monitor or with the fetoscope, all through the second stage of labor, which concludes with delivery. During this time the baby's head is being pressed by the birth canal. Contractions can become so forceful and prolonged that oxygen to the baby is compromised. If there is any indication that the baby is being affected, delivery can be quickly accomplished by the use of forceps. The problem is that at this stage of labor the mother is usually pushing hard with contractions, and the baby is so low in the uterus that its heartbeat can be hard to find. However, if monitoring can be done with a scalp electrode attached to the baby's scalp (or even intermittently with the abdominal electronic monitor or with the fetoscope), it can be reassuring during this very active period of the labor.

509 When does it help for me to "push"?

Up to the point when you are completely dilated, you have probably been told that pushing would do no good. This is true. Finally, though, with your cervix completely dilated, pushing does help the progress of the baby through the birth canal. Many women find pushing to be a great relief; others find pushing uncomfortable and want to avoid it.

It is important, though, that you do push dur-

ing this stage of labor. If you have an epidural, you will not feel the urge to push, but because of your childbirth-class training, your pushing will be effective in helping the baby come down anyway.

The urge to push, when you do not have an epidural, feels like the need to have a bowel movement. This is because the baby's head is putting a great deal of pressure on the rectum.

Patients these days have learned to push so effectively that they can put a great deal of pressure on the baby's head. I have seen babies born "depressed" (low Apgar score) after the mother had been allowed to push too long and too hard during this second stage. If you have been pushing for a length of time that the doctor feels is adequate, and the baby is still not ready to deliver, it would be safer to let your doctor go ahead with a forceps delivery than for you to continue pushing longer. Forceps almost never hurt a baby and their use can save many minutes of pushing. (See the next two questions.)

510 What happens next if my delivery proceeds normally?

As you push and the contractions continue to be effective, the baby's head will cause your perineum (the area between your vagina and your rectum) and vulvar areas to bulge. The skin of this area will become tense, and a portion of the baby's scalp will show between your labia. If it is your first baby, you will almost certainly need an episiotomy at this point. If you do not have an epi-

Episiotomy

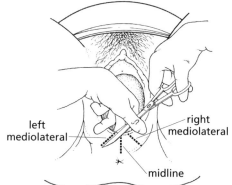

left mediolateral

right mediolateral

midline

Cardinal Movements of Delivery

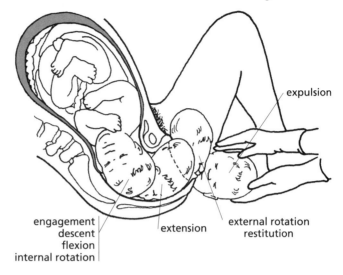

expulsion

engagement
descent
flexion
internal rotation

extension

external rotation
restitution

siotomy, the tissues all around the vaginal opening will usually tear in a jagged, irregular way. Some physicians feel that without an episiotomy, there is great stretching of the underlying ligaments of the vagina, making it more likely that you will need surgery to repair your vagina later in life after you have had all your children.

If this is your second child, an episiotomy is less likely, and for each child thereafter there is a decreasing chance of your needing an episiotomy.

An episiotomy is a small incision cut into the back of the vagina toward the rectum (midline episiotomy) or cut to the right or the left of the lower vagina (mediolateral episiotomy). It is not uncommon for an episiotomy to tear on into the muscular ring that is around your anus or even into the anus and rectum. This is not dangerous unless the physician doing the delivery is unaware that such a tear occurred. This type of tear must be sewn so that you do not end up involuntarily leaking stool in the future.

As the baby's head progresses down through the birth canal, it will gradually bulge through the labia. At this point, progression is normally very rapid. The baby's head suddenly appears totally outside the vagina and the baby's body quickly follows.

It is important that the baby's head not "pop" out of the vagina. While still in the vagina, there is pres-

sure on the baby's head. The pressure decreases as the head emerges, and if this happens very rapidly, this decreased pressure and the expansion of the baby's skull bones can tear blood vessels inside the skull, causing the baby to have brain damage.

When the doctor tells you to stop pushing, it is important that you not push. If you are delivering the baby at home, in a car, or at someplace other than a hospital, the one helpful thing that a person can do is to hold the baby's head gently as it is coming out so that it does not pop out of your vagina.

---

511 How do you feel about the use of forceps?

Forceps have received an unwarranted bad reputation, one that resulted from the way they were previously used.

Forceps were invented in the early 1600s, making it possible for doctors to complete some difficult deliveries and save the mother's life. Until then the cesarean sections that were necessary for difficult births would almost always result in the mother's death. Prior to 1882 almost every woman who had a cesarean section died.

With the use of forceps, many babies were killed during difficult vaginal deliveries, or they were already dead at the time the forceps were used. Of the babies who survived, many were terribly brain-damaged because of either the long, difficult labor that had preceded the use of forceps or because of the forceps themselves. In these situations, however, without the use of forceps both mother and baby would have died.

The big difference now is that forceps are no longer used for difficult deliveries. Cesarean sections are done instead—safely. When forceps are used, it is merely to assist the baby's head in its completion of the passage through the birth canal.

Forceps tend to hold the walls of the vagina away from the baby's head, and they pull only on the strongest part of the baby's skull, the facial bones of the baby that are rarely damaged by the forceps' pressure. The forceps, therefore, actually protect the baby's brain to some degree from the pressure of the birth canal.

It is true that forceps can sometimes scrape or bruise the baby's skin, but any significant damage is unusual. For instance, in my years of practice I know of only one child in which my use of forceps produced a significant scraping of the facial skin, and this skin healed with very little scarring.

In my opinion, the use of forceps by a competent physician is extremely safe and almost never causes any problems. I encourage you to let your doctor use forceps if there is any indication that they would help your labor.

512 What might indicate the need for forceps?

As stated previously, contractions may become so forceful and prolonged that the baby's oxygen supply is threatened. In that situation a speedy delivery is important, and if you are ten centimeters dilated, forceps can help get the baby out quickly.

In addition, a baby delivers most easily face downward, looking toward your rectum. If the baby's head is in any other position, the doctor will probably want to rotate the baby. If this can be done with his or her hand, the doctor will do so; if not, forceps may be tried, because the head will sometimes fail to deliver unless it is turned. Normally the head is not stuck but has just been inadequately turned by the labor process.

If the doctor cannot rotate the baby's head, it may be possible to deliver it with the baby facing up. If not, the only other choice is to have a cesarean section.

513 What is a vacuum extractor and how is it used to deliver a baby?

A vacuum extractor is a simple device that is put on top of the baby's head while it is still in the mother's birth canal to pull it out. It consists of a "traction cup," a tube, and a chain. The cup is small enough to fit into the vagina of a woman whose cervix is completely dilated; it is placed over the top of the baby's head and, through a tube attached to it, vacuum is applied to the cup.

After the cup is sealed to the baby's scalp with a moderately strong vacuum, the physician gently pulls on a small chain attached to the cup. It is usually recommended that only three or four pulls be applied and that the device not be left in place for more than fifteen minutes.

Vacuum extractors are not used extensively in the United States, but most labor-and-delivery units have one for the situations where it can be helpful. It is not used when the head is truly stuck in the birth canal, but only when it seems the mother is unable to push hard enough to get the baby out and the doctor thinks the head will come down easily with the vacuum extractor.

514 Can the baby become stuck even after the head is delivered?

After delivery of the baby's head, the remainder of the body normally comes through easily. Occasionally, however, a shoulder will get stuck in the birth canal behind the mother's pubic bone.

If the doctor indicates to you that the head is out but the shoulders are stuck and then asks you to push, it is important that you push with all your might. The nurses will normally be pushing up above on your uterus, and the doctor will be doing his or her best to turn the shoulders to a position where they will deliver. If that is not working, the doctor may put a hand up into your uterus, grasping one of the baby's arms to pull it out of the birth canal. This allows the "stuck" shoulder to fall away from the pubic bone, allowing delivery of the baby. Occasionally these maneuvers will result in some tearing of the nerves of one of the baby's arms, causing temporary or permanent paralysis of that arm; occasionally a collar bone (clavicle) or an arm can be broken in this process; and occasionally a baby will be so badly stuck that the doctor cannot get it out and the baby will die.

To avoid this frightening situation, your physician might recommend a cesarean section if your baby seems to be growing very large during the last few weeks of your pregnancy.

515 When is the umbilical cord clamped?

The cord is clamped after the baby is delivered, suctioned, and placed on the mother's abdomen. There have been long-standing arguments about the best time to clamp the cord. Most doctors today do not adhere to a specific timetable.

Clamping the cord after some delay allows about three ounces of extra blood to get to the baby, but babies are almost always born with an excess of blood that must "break down." This breaking down of the excessive blood is what causes the mild degree of jaundice that almost all newborn babies have. Perhaps it is just as well that they don't also have the extra blood from the placenta to break down unless they are anemic at birth. If they are anemic at delivery, a rare occurrence, the extra blood can be of benefit.

It is unhealthy for some babies to get the extra blood because it might overload their blood-vessel volume. These include premature babies, growth-retarded babies, and babies of diabetic mothers.

516 Why does a newborn need to be "suctioned"?

As soon as the baby is delivered, whether by C-section or by vaginal delivery, a bulb syringe is used to suction the baby's throat, mouth, and nose. This is important, not because the baby must breathe immediately, but because when the baby does take its first gasping breath, it could suck the material in its throat down into its lungs, causing breathing difficulties later.

517 What is done if the baby does not begin breathing immediately after birth?

Physicians and nurses are carefully trained in resuscitation of the baby, and this is done quickly and gently.

First, the baby will be suctioned again to make sure there is no material blocking its breathing tubes. If there is not, the baby will be stimulated often by gently rubbing its back. These things often make the baby take a breath and become active.

If the baby is still not breathing after a few seconds of stimulation, the doctor or nurse will listen to its heartbeat. At this point the doctor may use the laryngoscope, a lighted instrument for looking at the baby's vocal cords. This allows direct suctioning of the area of the vocal cords and of the trachea for removal of meconium and mucus. It may be necessary to put a small endotracheal tube into the trachea to give the baby oxygen directly. During this time the medical personnel would have already had pure oxygen flowing over the baby's mouth and nose.

The baby is in the delivery-room bassinet while these techniques are being performed. Most modern delivery rooms have an open bassinet, with an overhead heater that provides radiant heat to keep the baby warm. Being open, it allows medical personnel to work with the baby more easily.

With this care the baby usually begins breathing and crying spontaneously. If it does not, it would require continued close observation and care.

518 What is the Apgar score?

There was no standard way to evaluate the birth status of newborn babies until a few years ago. It was then that the late Dr. Virginia Apgar, former professor of anesthesiology at Columbia College of Physicians and Surgeons, devised her scoring system. Using her system, based on five different signs, she began evaluating newborns, and the Apgar score soon came into routine use.

Most hospitals now give the baby an Apgar score when it is one minute old and another when it is five minutes old. Although the one-minute Apgar was the initial recommendation of Dr. Apgar, most physicians believe that the five-minute Apgar score tells more about the baby's true health. The Apgar score evaluates heart rate, respiratory effort, muscle tone, reflex irritability (no response, grimace, or vigorous cry), and color. (See diagram on the Apgar scoring system.)

The Placenta and Other Considerations after Delivery

519 When is the placenta delivered?

Most doctors feel it is best to facilitate delivery of the placenta; this may be done by applying moderate pressure on the uterus or by massaging the uterus while pulling on the umbilical cord. Normally, the doctor will ask the mother to bear down as when she was trying to push out the baby.

The placenta will come out fairly quickly about 75 percent of the time. In the 25 percent of situations where it does not, the doctor will ordinarily put a hand inside the uterus, grasp the placenta, and pull it out. The cord occasionally breaks off as the doctor is pulling on it, but that does not matter since the placenta will usually come out easily without using the cord for a handle anyway. After the placenta and membranes have been removed, if there is any question that some of the tissue may

remain in the uterus, the doctor will put his or her hand up into the uterus to check. It is, however, very easy for a piece of placenta to be missed on that type of examination because the placenta can feel exactly like the wall of the uterus. It would not be good for the doctor to dig into the wall of the uterus to make sure that all of the placenta was out. The most that he or she would do is to feel for it, and if it is felt, take it out. (See Q. 500.)

520 After the placenta is delivered, what happens next?

The doctor will probably ask the nurse to give you some Pitocin (oxytocin) and/or a shot of Methergine to make your uterus contract down. These drugs cause the uterus to contract better than it would on its own, and the uterus is firmer than without them. This decreases the amount of blood loss that you will have immediately after your delivery.

Nursing the baby immediately after birth also helps the uterus contract. Nursing causes the mother's pituitary gland to release natural oxytocin, which makes the uterus contract. Injections of the drugs work more quickly and effectively than nursing the baby, however, and do not in any way interfere with the natural contractions produced by nursing. The drugs just add to the effect of nursing.

521 Are there any problems that can develop soon after delivery of the placenta?

Bleeding is a fairly common problem immediately after delivery of a baby. This bleeding is usually

Apgar Scoring System

Sign	Score of 0	Score of 1	Score of 2
Heart rate	Absent	Slow (below 100)	Over 100
Respiratory effort	Absent	Slow, irregualr	Good, crying
Muscle tone	Flaccid	Some flexion (bending) of extremeties	Active motion
Reflex irritability	No response	Grimace	Vigorous cry
Color	Blue & pale	Body, pink; extremities, blue	Completely pink

Bearing a Child

caused by the uterus being so relaxed that the blood vessels are not pinched off by the normal firm uterine contractions after delivery and remain open and continue bleeding. This is most likely to occur during the first hour or two after the placenta is delivered.

As mentioned previously, Pitocin or Methergine is given to make the uterine muscle contract down and pinch off the blood vessels so they will stop bleeding. Since you should be carefully observed at this time, you are usually brought to a recovery area instead of to your room. In past years patients occasionally died because they were sent to their rooms, not carefully watched, and bled heavily while no one was there.

If you have heavy bleeding, the doctor would give you more oxytocic drugs. If these drugs did not work, other techniques might include packing the uterus, making an incision into the abdomen to tie off some of the arteries of the uterus, or even an abdominal hysterectomy.

This situation is frightening. The doctor never likes the thought of causing sterility in someone who might want to have more children. However, you would want to have a doctor whose primary concern is saving your life, one who would expeditiously do whatever lifesaving procedures are necessary.

522 Can the uterus turn "inside out"?

Yes, an inverted uterus can occur and almost always surprises the doctor and the nurses. The patient will often not even know what has happened.

It is important that the doctor push the uterus back into place before the mouth of the uterus can constrict down and keep its body from going back up inside the abdomen. If the uterus will not go back into position, an abdominal incision may be necessary to pull it back. An inverted uterus can cause hemorrhage and shock. It can require blood transfusions. Therefore, no matter what is required, the uterus must be put back quickly into its normal position.

523 What happens after delivery of the placenta and membranes?

There are several things that normally take place.

Repairing cervical tears. The doctor will examine the cervix. If large tears are found, the doctor will use absorbable stitches to sew the cervix back together. It is hoped, of course, that this will allow the cervix to heal in such a way that it will be as strong as it was before delivery. In so doing, the doctor can help prevent premature delivery of the next pregnancy due to a cervix so damaged from a tear that it cannot hold the baby inside the uterus for the entire pregnancy. (See Q. 294, 384 for information on incompetent cervix cerclage procedures.)

Repairing vaginal tears. As the doctor explores the vagina, tears may also be found there. These too would be sewn with absorbable sutures to prevent bleeding and to prevent the vagina from being excessively scarred.

Episiotomy repair. Before sewing an episiotomy the doctor will first see if there are any tears into the muscle around the anus or into the anus or rectum, since episiotomies will occasionally tear all the way into the rectum.

Once the doctor makes sure of the extent of the episiotomy, it will be repaired properly so that you will be able to have normal bowel movements after proper healing. Occasionally episiotomy repairs will break open later. If this happens and it involves the rectal wall or the muscle ring around the anus, a future surgical procedure would be necessary to keep a woman from losing stool involuntarily.

524 What happens to the baby and me after the delivery is complete and episiotomy and tears have been repaired?

The nurse will put an arm band on your baby and take its footprints. She will also fingerprint you. This is for identification purposes in case of any confusion in the nursery. If you have delivered in a regular delivery room and the baby is not too chilled and is breathing well, you will usually be able to hold your baby until the doctor finishes examining you and doing any necessary repairs.

The baby will usually go to the nursery to be evaluated while you go to the recovery room. You can usually have the baby with you in the recovery room for a while before you go to your room on the postpartum floor. If you delivered in an LDR room (labor, delivery, recovery), you will probably be given the choice of keeping your baby with you or having the baby go into the nursery until you get to the postpartum floor.

If you delivered in an LDRP room (labor, delivery, recovery, and postpartum care), you will usually stay in that room until you go home. If you delivered in an LDR room, about two hours later you will leave this room for a room on the maternity floor. If you labor in a regular labor room and deliver in a delivery room, you will go to a recovery room for one or two hours before going to your room on the postpartum floor.

Parent/Baby Bonding

525 What does the term bonding mean?

In this context, bonding usually refers to the attachment that develops between a mother and her baby, but it also refers to the attachment that occurs between the father and the newborn. Studies have shown that close contact between the new parents and the baby during the first few hours and days after delivery is very important.

The best pattern seems to be for the mother, father, and healthy baby to be together for thirty to sixty minutes after delivery. Skin to skin contact between mother and baby seems to produce healthy emotional feelings in many mothers and may be important for the baby. Nursing the baby, of course, fits into this pattern. Nursing the baby on the delivery table or in the LDR room before the doctor is through is a clumsy affair. It is probably best to try nursing after the physician has

completed repairs and everything is cleaned up. Waiting for this brief time before starting the nursing process will help insure a pleasant, successful "first feeding" for mother and child. This short delay will not interfere with bonding.

526 Is "rooming in" a good idea?

I think it is best for mother and baby to be together almost constantly during the first few days of life. Some experts maintain that "rooming in"—having the baby stay in the mother's room rather than in the hospital nursery—is the best thing. With adequate help in the hospital, most new mothers can handle this. Being with the baby during her hospital stay can teach the new mother how to meet the needs of the baby.

Studies have indicated that spending this time together does appear to cement the bond between mother and baby. Mothers will want to hold their babies more and will often kiss and look at them more than mothers who have not had a bonding time. These things indicate a good, healthy relationship and attachment between the mother and the baby. Babies who have had such close contact with the mother early in their lives seem to smile and laugh more, according to some studies.

Postdelivery Details in the Hospital

527 Are "the blues" normal after delivery?

Postpartum depression, or postpartum blues, has been reported in more than 80 percent of mothers. The problem, usually indicated by depression and crying during the hospital stay or soon after going home, is generally limited to a few days and goes away spontaneously. This response may be partly produced by the habit many hospitals still have of separating the mother and the baby immediately after delivery, allowing them only short visits every four hours or so during the hospital time. However, I doubt that this is usually the cause today, since most hospitals no longer have those restrictions. Yet most mothers still experience some postpartum depression.

Most obstetricians feel that postpartum blues are caused by hormonal changes. Just before delivery there are amazingly high levels of estrogen, progesterone, and other hormones in the mother's body. Immediately after delivery these levels fall dramatically, and the mother's hormones do not return to normal for about two to three months. It seems reasonable to assume that these dramatic hormone changes contribute to a mother's feeling of depression.

In addition, the changes in a mother's life must be considered. She may not be confident about her ability to care for the baby; financial concerns may be present; family problems may surface when a new family member arrives. All these things (and many more!) can certainly contribute to depression at a time when the mother is already physically "below par."

The depression usually lifts in just a few days. If it does not and you find yourself becoming more and more depressed, mention this to your physician. If it seems to be a serious problem, your doctor will help you find a psychiatrist or counselor to help you with therapy so the depression does not ruin this special time in your life.

528 Is infection of the uterus a common problem after delivery?

Uterine infections may occur after delivery. Most fevers that women develop after delivery are due to some degree of infection in the uterus.

Often this infection is due to the fact that a woman's waters ruptured several hours before delivery. The longer the bag of waters was ruptured prior to delivery, the greater the chance of uterine infection after delivery.

Also, the wall of the uterus is raw after delivery, and this entire surface is open to infection. The area of the uterine wall where the placenta was attached is especially raw, making this the area in which bacteria generally will grow after a delivery has occurred.

Infection in the uterus can become quite severe and can spread to the ovaries and tubes. It can extend into the large veins of the pelvis, producing clots in those veins. These clots can break loose and travel to the lungs. Death can result from this. Infection of the female organs can also cause infection of the abdominal tissues, or peritonitis.

Although infections of the uterus do not often develop after vaginal deliveries, even with the best of care they do occur. Such infections, especially the more severe forms, are much more common after C-sections.

529 Is circumcision advisable for baby boys?

If you find yourself having difficulty in making this decision, you are in good company. The American Academy of Pediatrics, which is the primary organization of American pediatricians, had a task force study this question. They reported in 1988 that they could not reach a concensus on whether or not a newborn should be circumcised.

The task force did find, however, that in the studies they reviewed, newborn boys who had circumcisions had far fewer urinary tract infections than boys who were not circumcised. The task force also reviewed evidence that showed that circumcision almost completely prevented cancer of the penis in the future.

The chairman of the committee, Edgar J. Schoen, M.D., reported in the *New England Journal of Medicine* (1990, 322:18), "The benefits of routine circumcision of newborns as a preventive health measure far exceed the risks of the procedure, although some may question its cost effectiveness and priority in the delivery of health care." Others, however, do not share his views that the health benefits are so dramatic.

If a male is not circumcised as a baby, he has a 10 percent chance of needing to be circumcised in later life for some medical problem. This might be an infection under the foreskin. It could be a foreskin that is too tight to let the head of the penis out with an erection. Circumcision done when a man is older is not only painful but requires hospitalization, anesthesia, and significant expense. For these reasons many parents choose to have their baby boy circumcised.

The baby can have some pain when the circumcision is done. Some physicians will inject local anesthetic into the skin before the procedure, but babies often cry as much from the injection as they do from the circumcision itself. Also there may be a slight risk to the baby of having a reaction to the anesthetic. I recommend that you allow your doctor to do the procedure in the way (with or without anesthesia) that he or she is most comfortable.

Traditionally, the obstetrician rather than the pediatrician does the circumcision. However, some pediatricians do circumcisions. If you have a family practitioner or a general practitioner caring for both you and your baby, he or she would do the circumcision.

Bris or *brit* (the modern spelling) is a Jewish ceremonial circumcision often performed by a *mohel*, a person who does such circumcisions as a profession but is usually not a physician. Conservative, Reform, and Reconstructionist Jews allow a Jewish doctor to perform the circumcision, provided a rabbi is in attendance. The ceremony is normally scheduled the eighth day after birth. The date may be changed if there are valid medical reasons. Usually held in the parents' home, the ceremony is a joyous occasion and includes the naming of the child.

delivery. If the tip of their spinal column (coccyx) curves forward toward the front of the body as the baby's head delivers, the coccyx pops back (it actually does not break) at one of the joints between the different segments of the coccyx. This can cause significant pain that can continue to be moderately severe for many weeks. There is no treatment, except for pain medications and sitz baths; the condition usually clears spontaneously. If coccyx pain persists, check with your doctor. He may suggest that you see an orthopedist.

Most hospitals these days have liberal visiting hours and will allow your husband and your children to visit frequently. Statistics show no increased infection in newborns because of family visitation, and the benefits from such visitation far outweigh any potential risks.

Almost all hospitals allow "feeding on demand." Years ago this was felt to be an imposition on the hospital staff, but now hospital staff members encourage mothers to feed their babies when they are hungry. This, of course, fits right in with "rooming in."

It is common for a woman to go home one or two days after a normal vaginal delivery and two or three days after a C-section. If you do not feel well enough to go home either physically or emotionally, tell your doctor you would like an extra day in the hospital. Perhaps he can arrange it with the hospital and the insurance company.

530 What can I expect during my stay in the hospital?

If you have had a cesarean section, or if you have had an episiotomy or torn tissues, you will have some pain. You should take the pain medication that your doctor prescribes. Taking it will keep you from hurting, will allow you to sleep better at night, and will keep you from becoming tense. The less pain and discomfort you feel and the less tense you are now, the better you will feel later. If you are nursing, the pain medications you take will not hurt your baby.

Some women will "break their tailbone" with

Health Care Once You Are Home

531 What instructions do you give your patients when they go home from the hospital?

Most physicians give these very simple instructions:

Housework. Have somebody else do the cooking, housekeeping, and other work around the house for two weeks. You can take care of the baby as long as you feel up to it, but if you get tired, let someone else do that too! Most obstetricians have found that patients who follow this advice feel better a month or two later. Women who get too busy right after leaving the hospital will often feel tired for several months after having a baby. Don't fall into this trap. If people want to take care of you, let them!

Constipation. It is important that you not become constipated. I encourage my patients to use a tablespoon of Metamucil or similar product three times a day. Metamucil is basically just fiber; it is not a laxative. If your stools are not soft, increase the amount of Metamucil until they are. Be sure to drink plenty of fluids, or the Metamucil can cause constipation.

Bleeding. Bleeding can last as long as two months. It may come and go, and may be bright red or with clots, all of which is normal. You do not need to call your doctor unless the bleeding is heavier than a normal menstrual period and is causing you concern. You should not use tampons during the first three weeks following delivery. Their use could conceivably be uncomfortable or cause infection of the uterus.

Intercourse. Do not have intercourse until your physician permits it. This is normally about three weeks, allowing any tears or the episiotomy or the C-section scar to heal before you begin having sexual relations again. Your doctor will discuss techniques for contraception, giving you information and/or a prescription for pills. (See also chapter 12.)

Douching. Do not douche until your physician allows it. The time interval is usually three weeks from delivery. (Actually, I do not believe women should douche unless specified by their physician.)

Exercise. Women should not begin aerobic and muscle-strengthening exercises until six weeks from the time of delivery because such exercise can cause muscle strain. The abdominal muscles have been stretched out of shape, but even without exercise they will shrink back to near-normal length. I feel it is best to let those muscles shrink on their own and then, six weeks after delivery, to begin exercising those now-shortened muscles. I certainly feel that it is normal and desirable for a new mother to go outside and stroll around and climb stairs as soon as she gets home.

Personal care. It is fine to take a bath or shower and to wash your hair immediately. Being well-groomed and attractive is important at this time. The better you look, the better you will feel!

Episiotomy care. The episiotomy or tear repair requires no special care; normal cleansing and gentle towel-drying are all that is necessary. While heat lamps and spray medication are soothing to the area, neither speed healing. Care should be taken, however, in using heat lamps. The bulbs can cause leg burns if your legs touch them. These burns can be very painful.

Occasionally the episiotomy will come open. This is not due to your doctor's negligence. In fact, it is amazing that this does not happen more often. When it does open, the wound cannot be resewn. It will heal by itself. After healing, most women cannot tell it ever happened. Occasionally, an episiotomy will break down completely. When this happens, a surgical repair is necessary if it affects the anus and causes leakage of stool.

Driving. It is fine for you to ride in a car when you are comfortable doing so. I suggest that you refrain from driving, however, until you are confident that you can apply the brake quickly in an emergency situation.

Iron and vitamins. If you are nursing, continue taking your prenatal vitamins as long as you nurse. If you are not nursing, finish taking all your prenatal vitamins, then start taking an iron pill a day. Do this for six months. Most women need to make up for the iron they lost to the pregnancy. You do not need an expensive or prescription iron preparation. Ask your pharmacist for a reliable, cheap iron preparation that you can take once a day.

532 When will my doctor want to examine me again in the office?

Most obstetricians see patients back in the office about three weeks after delivery, or within one or two weeks following a cesarean section.

Most obstetricians will want to see their patients again when the baby is about three months old. At that time they will usually do a Pap smear, a pelvic examination, and answer any further questions about contraception. After this three-month visit, the next visit is usually one year later unless there is a special problem that needs to be checked sooner.

533 When do menstrual periods begin again?

Women who are not breast-feeding will normally ovulate four weeks after they deliver a baby (or after a miscarriage or ectopic pregnancy, or after stopping birth-control pills). A period will normally start two weeks after that. Most women, then, will have a period approximately six weeks after they are no longer pregnant. It is just as normal though for a woman not to have an ovulation or a period for up to six months after delivery, although 90 percent of women will have started their periods within three months after delivery.

Many nursing mothers will not ovulate or have periods while they are nursing, but it is also quite normal to have menstrual periods while nursing, especially after a mother begins to supplement her baby's diet with other foods. Many women will have menstrual periods on a regular monthly basis even though they are not supplementing the breast feedings.

It is important to understand that you can become pregnant even if you have not yet had a period. When ovulation occurs, which can happen even when you have not had a period, you can become pregnant. Therefore you cannot wait for a period to come and use that as a sign that you are fertile from that point on. You are fertile when you ovulate, whether or not you have had a period. (See Q. 546.)

534 How long should I wait to become pregnant again?

Most obstetricians recommend that a woman wait three months before trying to get pregnant again. Though most of the hormone changes from a delivery, miscarriage, or even from birth-control pills are gone after about a month, a woman's ovulation may not become regular for another two or three months. If pregnancy occurs during this time of unpredictable ovulation, a woman would not know when she actually got pregnant. She could be confused if she has spotting, bleeding, or needs to know the exact date she became pregnant.

If a woman does get pregnant immediately after having a baby or a miscarriage (or stopping birth-control pills), the new pregnancy will not be damaged as a result of getting pregnant so soon.

A woman who becomes pregnant almost immediately after a previous baby needs to exercise more vigorously during that subsequent pregnancy to keep her body in good shape. Other than this, a pregnancy that closely follows a previous delivery can, in general, be considered and treated as a normal pregnancy.

Breast-Feeding

535 Is breast-feeding my baby a good idea?

Yes! Without any question, breast-feeding is superior to bottle feeding a newborn baby. Studies show that babies who are breast fed tend to be healthier, have a lower mortality rate, seem to develop better physically and mentally, and have fewer problems with allergies in later life. In addition, other studies show that babies who nurse have greater immunity to respiratory and digestive tract disease than babies who do not. Also, babies who nurse seem to have straighter teeth and better mother/child bonding. A recently conducted study showed an amazing thing that God has done to help premature infants grow. Mothers of infants born one to three months prematurely produce milk especially adapted to the needs of such preterm infants. It is much different from the milk of a mother who delivers at term. The milk of the mother of the "preemie" is easily digested and contains a higher proportion of the nutrients that promote neurological maturation. I strongly encourage my patients to breast-feed their infants or to collect their milk if the baby is too sick or premature to nurse.

Millions of babies, however, have been bottle fed, and if there is a difference in babies who are breast-fed and those who are not, it is not an enormous difference. A baby who is bottle fed can be healthy and happy.

Many things can prevent a mother from breast-feeding; a mother should not feel guilty because she cannot breast-feed her baby. She may be physically unable, she may have to return to work, or she may become ill.

I believe that breast-feeding is the best of two choices but that either choice is acceptable.

536 I have heard that breasts do not produce milk for several days after delivery. Is this true?

Yes. Breast milk does not "let down" for several days, but your breasts begin immediately to produce colostrum, a very important fluid for the baby. Some women produce colostrum for weeks before delivery. This is normal.

Because babies are born with excessive fluid in their bodies, just as your body had excessive fluid right up until the time that you delivered, they do not need fluid other than colostrum for the first two or three days. This thin, bluish fluid seems to have important antibodies and helps protect the baby from developing diarrhea and other intestinal illnesses. Although babies probably do not need anything but colostrum at first, most pediatricians will give babies water or formula by bottle until the mother's milk comes in.

537 My nipples are inverted— sunken back into the areola. Can I still nurse my baby?

Yes. It may take a little work, but inverted or flat nipples will not keep you from nursing, and some women with nipples that are flat or "sunken in" have absolutely no trouble nursing. The lips and gums of babies encircle the areola (the dark area surrounding the nipple), and the sucking is concentrated on this area.

Some babies, though, seem to have trouble nursing when the mother's nipples are inverted or flat. There is a solution to this. If a woman uses a "breast-feeding shell" for a week or two before delivery, the nipples may become more everted (protuberant) and perhaps help the baby nurse more easily. A "shell" is simply a dome-shaped plastic device with a hole in the middle to allow the nipple to protrude. The device is put inside the bra. The pressure of the shell around the nipple encourages it to protrude. While this device can be used for the first time after you have had your baby, it seems to work better if it is used for a week or two beforehand.

If the breast-feeding shell does not work adequately, you can use a nipple shield while you are nursing to help the baby.

538 My breasts are small. Can I nurse my baby?

Yes. The old wives' tale that suggests that small breasts cannot produce enough milk is unfounded and untrue. Women with small breasts have adequate enlargement of the gland tissue of their breasts after delivery and can usually provide an ample supply of milk for their babies.

539 If I were to have breast implants, could I still nurse?

In a study reported by Hurst in the journal *Obstetrics and Gynecology* (January 1996, 87.1:30–34), women who had breast implants were much more likely to be unable to provide adequate breast milk for their babies.

You might want to know that the silicone that was used in breast implants for so many years is not a reason to avoid trying to nurse. There have been a small number of children with a variety of problems of their muscles, their skin, and their esophaguses who were breast-fed by mothers with silicone implants. The number, however, is so small that it is not likely that the implants were the problem. Remember that the benefits of breast-feeding are substantial and it is best to not deny it to a child unless necessary.

540 Do I need to eat differently while nursing?

Certain foods that you eat may cause your baby to be irritable. Many women find that chocolate and some spicy foods will cause their babies to become a little cranky. This seems to be an individual issue, but is almost never a health problem. If you notice your baby is consistently irritable after you eat a certain food, common sense tells you to stop eating that food, not only for your baby's comfort but also for your own personal peace.

While you are nursing you need more calories and more protein. The Food and Nutrition Board of the National Research Council recommends 2,600 calories a day, 64 grams of protein, and vitamin supplementation while nursing. So, stay on those prenatal vitamins while you nurse, and eat heartily.

541 Will I gain weight while nursing?

Most patients stay a few pounds overweight while they nurse because of the increased calories we just mentioned. When they stop nursing, those pounds go away. It is desirable to limit sugar, soft drinks, and desserts for health reasons. This will help with weight control during the period of nursing. A healthy, well-balanced diet is important during pregnancy and while nursing.

542 Is it normal to have cramping of the uterus during nursing?

Most women have some degree of cramping when they first begin to nurse, and some will continue to have cramping every time they nurse their baby. Most of the time, however, women do not feel significant cramping after the first few days.

It is normal to have even severe cramps with nursing at first. One of the benefits of nursing is that it helps the uterus "contract down" and return to normal size. A woman who has this type of cramping can take a pain pill thirty minutes before she nurses. The small amount of medication that the mother would pass to her baby in her breast milk will not hurt the baby and will help relieve the uterine cramps caused by the nursing. Cramps are usually worse in women with their second and third children.

543 May I take medications and smoke and drink while I am nursing?

Almost everything you eat, drink, or take by mouth or injection will be excreted into your milk to some extent. It makes sense, therefore, that a nursing mother exercise caution in this regard.

A modest amount of alcohol may not affect your baby adversely, other than perhaps to make it a little sleepy, but no one knows that for sure. Consistent and more-than-modest alcohol intake is certainly not good for you or your baby.

For instance, a study reported in the *New England Journal of Medicine* (August 1989, 321:425) reported that if a mother had one drink of alcohol daily while she nursed, her child showed some slight retardation in motor development at one year of age compared with the children of mothers who did not drink while breast-feeding.

Aside from its detrimental effects on you, cigarette smoking is dangerous for your baby and may increase the chance of the child getting cancer later. Smoking can also decrease your milk production.

The same cautions about smoking and drinking pertain to drugs. It seems best for a nursing mother not to take any drugs unless necessary as suggested or prescribed by her doctor.

An excellent book on this subject that your doctor may have is *Drugs in Pregnancy and Lactation, A Reference Guide to Fetal and Neonatal Risk* by Griggs, Bodendorfer, Freeman, and Yaffe (Baltimore: Williams & Wilkins).

544 What medical complications can occur during nursing?

In the first few weeks you may develop nipple soreness. This usually occurs because you let the baby use your nipples as a "pacifier" before your nipples have become toughened by the infant's sucking.

A baby gets most of the milk from the breast in four or five minutes. If the baby continues to nurse, that can cause your nipples to become sore. The key, then, if your nipples are sore or cracked, is to let the baby nurse only long enough to get most of the milk but no longer. After nursing, put nipple cream (Masse or A&D ointment or some other brand) on your nipples to help them heal. Later, when your nipples are healed, you can let the baby nurse as long as you and the baby want to.

Nursing mothers will sometimes develop mastitis—sore, red places on their breasts. (Mastitis means breast infection.) Fever often accompanies these infections. It is common for nursing mothers to have several episodes of these infections during the time they nurse a baby. Most women, though, can continue to breast-feed even with this type of infection. Call your physician immediately if you develop mastitis; he or she will probably start you on antibiotics. You may also find that warm, moist heat helps healing. The best way to apply this heat is to put a towel soaked in warm water on your breast, cover that with plastic wrap, and put a hot water bottle on top of that. Keep this heat on your breast as much as you can night and day. Do not use a heating pad; it could burn you.

545 If I nurse my baby, will my breasts become smaller, and will they sag more?

Many women will notice that their breasts are smaller and sag more if they have nursed a baby. This does not always occur, but you should be aware that it can happen and not be disappointed if you find a significant difference in your breasts after you nurse your first baby.

546 I have heard that nursing mothers cannot become pregnant. Is this true?

Absolutely not! It has been shown that it is the baby's hard sucking on the breasts that makes a woman less likely to ovulate and thus unlikely to become pregnant. After nursing for several weeks the baby and breasts usually form a pattern so that the baby does not need to suck as hard to get milk flow established at each nursing. The less hard a baby sucks, the more likely you are to begin ovulation.

Since you will not know when ovulation has occurred, you can become pregnant if you have unprotected intercourse. This can happen even though you have not had any menstrual bleeding during the time you are nursing.

Studies presented at the Bellagio, Italy conference on lactational infertility in August 1988 did show that if a woman is providing all or most of her baby's food by nursing, and is not having periods because of that, she has 98 percent protection from pregnancy in the first six months of her baby's life. If a woman doesn't like even this small chance of pregnancy, she can take a progesterone-only birth-control pill without affecting her milk supply. Of course, you can also use a barrier method, such as foam, condoms, or a diaphragm, or have an IUD inserted. Most physicians feel that a nursing mother should not use birth-control pills. No serious side effects have been found in babies whose mothers used birth-control pills while they nursed, but taking regular birth-control pills may cause a decline in milk production and nutritional value. There are no known side effects from the progesterone-only birth-control pill. (See Q. 902.)

547 After weaning a baby, is it common for the breasts to continue to secrete milk?

It is common for a mother to have milk coming from her nipples for many months (or even years) after she has weaned her baby. As long as the mother's menstrual periods are regular, this does not indicate a medical problem.

If there continues to be fluid from the nipples after nursing has been stopped and the menstrual periods do not return to normal for several months, a prolactin test (a simple blood test) should be performed. Fluid from the nipples with a failure to have periods may indicate a tumor in the pituitary. The prolactin test can show whether such a tumor is present.

548 I have many questions about nursing and my doctor doesn't seem to know the answers. What should I do?

Many hospitals have lactation specialists or know lactation specialists to whom they can refer you. If that is not available to you at your hospital, then the LaLeche League will be of inestimable value to you. I encourage you to contact them. Also, before delivery, you could obtain a copy of their excellent book, *The Womanly Art of Breast-feeding*, rev. ed. 1981 (LaLeche League, Intl., 9616 Minneapolis Ave., Franklin Park, IL 60131).

The LaLeche League also has members to contact in large cities. They are often listed in the phone book under LaLeche League.

Another excellent book on breast-feeding is *The Nursing Mother's Companion* by Kathleen Huggins, R.N., M.S. (Boston: Harvard Common Press, 1990).

549 What do I do if I choose not to or cannot nurse my baby?

Physicians used to prescribe Parlodel for their patients. This drug suppresses the production of prolactin from the pituitary gland and therefore stops production of breast milk. (Prolactin is the hormone the pituitary secretes to cause milk pro-

duction.) When there is less prolactin in the woman's body, there is less milk production. Most women who use Parlodel 2.5 mg twice a day for fourteen days stop milk production and will not have breast engorgement.

However, physicians are not currently prescribing this drug as much. They don't like the fact that about 25 percent of women will have rebound engorgement after they finish taking Parlodel. Even worse is that some medical problems have been associated with this drug, including hypertension, seizures, and stroke. These complications are rare but can be severe.

If your doctor is one who feels that it is best for you to not use drugs to stop milk letdown, there are several things you can do. You can try binding your breasts with a breast binder. (Be sure it is not too tight.) You can put cold packs on your breasts. You can use pain medication for breast discomfort. At first the breasts will become hard, but after a few days of not nursing, they will usually start softening. Milk production will cease, and the breast engorgement will go down. It is best not to pump your breasts. This merely encourages the breasts to continue milk production.

Special Labor-and-Delivery Situations

550 What are some of the special problems that need to be considered in relation to labor and delivery?

Some special situations will be discussed in the next few questions.

Labor induction
Breech deliveries
Multiple-birth deliveries
Premature labor
Premature deliveries
Cesarean sections

551 What is your opinion on inducing labor?

Inducing labor for convenience is called elective induction of labor. I feel that the induction of labor in a woman who is certain of her due date and is "ripe" for labor is a safe process; it is unlikely to increase the necessity for cesarean section or to endanger the baby. It should not, however, be done flippantly.

Before an induction is done, certain elements must be considered.

Due date. If a patient has any question about her due date, and her doctor has not been able to determine a reliable date for her, I would not recommend that she be induced unless there is a medical reason for doing so. If a woman who is unsure of her due date sees her doctor by the twenty-fifth week of her pregnancy, the doctor can do ultrasound measurements of her baby's size and thus determine a reliable due date most of the time. If a woman and her physician have not established an accurate due date by the twenty-fifth week of pregnancy, they will not be able to be as certain of the true due date as they would like to be. This is one reason it is important to see a physician early in pregnancy.

"Ripe" cervix. Even if a woman is at term, she should usually not be induced for convenience purposes unless the cervix is ripe. Most physicians feel that a woman must be at least two centimeters dilated, with a cervix that has effaced (see Q. 498) at least 50 percent before she should be induced. The cervix must be soft and the baby's head down against it. The baby's head must be down because, if the doctor breaks the bag of waters and the head is not down against the cervix, the umbilical cord could be washed down through the cervical opening. This would precipitate the need for an immediate cesarean section.

To summarize my position, inducing labor should not be done as a matter of course or without appropriate medical evaluation. It should not be done unless there is an accurate due date established. The cervix should be "ripe" and the baby in proper position. If these criteria are followed, I feel that induction of labor is quite safe—even when there are no medical problems and it is done merely for convenience.

Though I would not necessarily advocate that all women be induced for convenience, there is an advantage in having labor start in the morning so that delivery takes place during the day while a full labor-and-delivery staff is present. Another advantage to planning the time for your delivery is that you would most likely have your own physician doing the delivery. Still another advantage of induced labor is that when it is planned, a woman can arrive at the hospital with an empty stomach, which is always a safer situation for the mother.

552 Why would labor need to be induced other than for convenience?

There are many reasons that labor might need to be induced that have nothing to do with convenience. A few of these are:

Toxemia that is becoming dangerous for the mother or the baby

Premature rupture of the membranes

Fetal jeopardy, which can include fetal growth retardation and post-term pregnancy

Maternal medical problems such as diabetes or kidney disease

A baby that has died inside the mother's uterus

A mother who has had rapid labor in the past or who lives a long way from the hospital

These indications for induction are listed in the *American College of Obstetricians and Gynecologists Technical Bulletin* (July 1991, no. 157).

If a woman needs to have labor induced and her cervix is not ripe, she is not yet at term, and/or the baby's head is not in the ideal position, the doctor will need to make a judgment call. If he or she feels it is possible to induce labor successfully, that will be suggested. If not, a cesarean section may be recommended.

The physician may try to "ripen" the cervix by putting prostaglandin medication in a woman's vagina (either suppository or vaginal gel). When this medication is absorbed into the cervix, it softens and ripens it, making the induction process more successful. The drug seems to be very safe for the baby and the mother.

Once the cervix is ready, the physician will start Pitocin. When good contractions have developed, he or she will rupture the membranes (or rupture the membranes first and then start Pitocin).

If induction does not develop into normal labor that progresses to normal delivery, the obstetrician will need to do a cesarean section for the health of both mother and baby.

553 Is there anything I can do to start my own labor?

Unless it is time for labor to start anyway, physical activity, such as washing walls or riding over railroad tracks, will not induce labor. Taking castor oil or an enema may produce contractions, but those contractions could be either intestinal or uterine. If you do try the castor oil or enema routine (or some other activity), you may have such strong intestinal cramping that your doctor will want to put you in the hospital to see whether or not you are in labor. If you are not, he will send you back home. Trying to stimulate labor in this way is usually futile and can result in unnecessary expense, inconvenience, and frustration.

There is one activity that can cause such strong contractions that labor can start—this is nipple stimulation. If you or your husband massage your nipples (be sure not to do this even in sex play if you are not at term because it can start premature labor), or if you even put a warm washcloth on your nipples, your pregnant uterus will contract. The danger of nipple stimulation is very strong contractions. Don't do nipple stimulation even when you are at term pregnancy without consultation with your doctor. The stronger the nipple stimulation, the stronger your uterine contractions will be.

There is one thing your doctor might try: "stripping the membranes." When you are definitely at term, and you and your physician feel it would be good to do something to make labor

start soon, he can strip your membranes. This is a simple procedure in which the doctor, while doing a pelvic exam, can insert a finger into your cervix and separate the membranes from the cervix.

This procedure has been done for at least 175 years. A study in *Obstetrics and Gynecology* (October 1990, 76:4), showed that it is safe and it works.

It is possible that the bag of waters can be ruptured during this procedure, but if a woman is ready for delivery, that will not make any difference. She would simply go in to the hospital as though she had ruptured her membranes on her own.

Some bleeding may occur after the membranes are stripped. If the bleeding is heavy, the woman should call her doctor. (This is rarely ever significant. It is usually equal to the amount of bleeding that occurs in early labor for most women.)

Breech Deliveries

554 What about breech deliveries?

Breech babies (babies who come bottom first) occur in only 3 to 4 percent of all deliveries. Mothers frequently react with some degree of fear when their physicians tell them that their baby is coming breech. This fear is based on tales they have heard about the dangers and difficulties of breech labor and delivery. Let me reassure you that the risks of a breech presentation have mostly been eliminated today because physicians almost always perform a cesarean section for a breech birth.

The reason for a C-section with a breech presentation is that your baby can be damaged if it is born bottom first in a vaginal delivery. The umbilical cord can be pinched off, preventing adequate blood supply from getting to the baby's brain during the delivery. The baby's head can also be caught in the birth canal, causing damage or death. This can happen because the baby's head is larger in diameter than the rest of its body. This is especially true if the baby is premature. The birth canal may not be sufficiently dilated to allow passage of the baby's head without damage.

To avoid such damage, most doctors agree that it is "legitimate" (not mandatory) for all breech babies to be delivered by cesarean section. It is more important that they be delivered by cesarean section if the following conditions exist (see also Q. 560):

It is a woman's first pregnancy

The baby is very large

The baby is premature

The mother's pelvic bones are small

The mother desires to have a sterilization procedure. Since she is going to have an incision in her abdomen anyway, this incision can be enlarged and accommodate both the delivery and the sterilization.

If your doctor is going to do a vaginal delivery of your breech baby, he or she would evaluate your pelvis to be sure that there are no deformities or constrictions of the bones and soft tissues of the pelvis that might hinder delivery. If a problem developed during labor, a C-section would immediately be performed.

555 Can the baby be turned, either before or during labor, so that it will come headfirst?

Some women who have a breech baby can have the baby's position changed from breech to vertex by a technique called "external version." If your baby is breech, and you and your doctor want to try this technique, you would be admitted to the labor-and-delivery unit. You would be given medication intravenously to make your uterus relax (tocolytic agent). When the uterus is relaxed, the doctor would do an "external cephalic version." This means that with his or her hands on your abdomen, the doctor would try to push the baby around until the head rotates down into the pelvis. This procedure often works, and usually the baby stays down in the headfirst position.

There are some dangers to this procedure. In pushing the baby around, the placenta can come loose from the wall of the uterus—a dangerous thing for the baby. Even if this does not happen, manipulating the baby in this fashion can cause its heartbeat to drop, causing death. This is extremely rare. These possible complications scare some doctors and some patients out of trying this useful procedure.

To avoid this happening, doctors who do this procedure carefully observe the baby with the ultrasound machine and fetal monitor as they rotate the baby. They do the manipulation very gently, with the woman's abdomen well-coated with oil.

There are some conditions that make an external version unsafe. Even if you have had a successful external version, the baby can move back to a breech position before you go into labor. A repeat external version can be done, but the closer you get to term, the more difficult it is to turn the baby. An example of this is if the baby does not have an adequate amount of amniotic fluid, or if the baby has intrauterine growth retardation.

Although your doctor may find your baby to be in the breech position during the last few weeks of pregnancy, and you are not going to have it rotated, the baby can still switch around on its own and be headfirst by the time you go to the hospital.

Multiple-Birth Deliveries

556 Are the deliveries of twins, triplets, and so on, managed in the same way as single babies?

No. Careful consideration must be given to the management of multiple-birth labor. For one thing, one of the two babies in a twin pregnancy will often come as a breech. Statistics show that the first baby is born headfirst 75 percent of the time, and the second baby is born headfirst 53 percent of the time.

Whether the delivery should be by normal vaginal delivery or by cesarean section depends on several factors. Since studies of delivery of twins do not show any significant difference in the health of the babies born vaginally or by C-section, you and your obstetrician must make the decision based on your individual situation.

Most obstetricians prefer that twin babies be born vaginally unless they are premature. If your babies are more than four weeks early, it is probably best for them to be delivered by cesarean section. The reason for this is to avoid damaging the babies' heads or having to deliver the second baby by breech in case it gets "stuck" in a difficult position after the first baby is born.

If you are in the last month of pregnancy, it is probably best to do the delivery vaginally unless some complication develops during the labor and delivery. It is sometimes necessary for the doctor to deliver one baby through the vagina and then, because of some problem, do a cesarean section for delivery of the second baby. Most doctors will do cesarean sections on all triplets or more-than-triplet deliveries. See Q. 277–282.

Premature Labor

557 What is premature labor and what causes it?

Premature labor is labor that starts before the thirty-seventh week of the pregnancy. It can be caused by premature rupture of membranes, infection in the amniotic fluid, abnormalities of the uterus, death of the baby, and many other problems. A large percentage of premature labor is caused by unknown reasons.

Every woman has contractions of the uterus throughout pregnancy. These are not dangerous and do not lead to premature labor. If, however, a woman starts having strong contractions that become increasingly regular and frequent, they may be caused by an "irritable uterus." She may be in premature labor and should call her physician. If it is labor and it continues, the baby will be born prematurely, a condition that carries significant risks for the baby.

Occasionally a woman thinks she is going into labor prematurely when actually she is not; experts estimate that 15 percent of due dates are miscalculated. You may be starting labor on time and just think you are early. This is another reason that it is so important early in pregnancy to accurately establish your due date.

If you are having contractions that you think might be labor, call your physician. He or she will check to see if your cervix is dilating, run tests to see if you have a bladder or uterine infection, and order a sonogram to check for abruptio placenta (see Q. 564).

If you are having contractions that are worrisome but are not labor, your doctor may want you to use a home contractions monitor to record the contraction activity of your uterus. The information is transmitted once a day by telephone from your recorder to a center that evaluates the information. If significant contractions are found, the center will notify your physician. Although this system is somewhat expensive, it is less expensive than a hospital stay to accomplish the same objective.

If you are having increased contractions, your physician will probably want you to stay in bed most of the time and abstain from intercourse and stimulation of your nipples (which can cause uterine contractions).

Occasionally, early in a pregnancy a doctor will find a woman's cervix to be "incompetent." This means it is so weak that it will not hold the baby in the uterus. If you are having some contractions and your cervix seems to be dilating, your doctor may want to put a "purse string" suture (cerclage) in your cervix. This procedure will often help prevent premature labor though it does not guarantee that there will be no further dilation. (A woman's bag of waters could break as the stitches are put in or even later, after they are in.)

558 What about medications that are used to stop labor?

There are drugs that appear to decrease the frequency and intensity of uterine contractions of an irritable uterus if you are not actually in labor. If you are in labor, the drugs may stop it for about forty-eight to seventy-two hours. Even though these drugs don't stop true labor most of the time, physicians may use one of them to try to extend your baby's stay in your uterus for a few extra days or to keep you from delivering until cortisone-type drugs can help your baby's lungs mature.

The drugs usually used to inhibit labor are either magnesium sulfate or Beta-adrenergic receptor agonist (Ritodrine, Terbutaline). These drugs can have dangerous side effects and must be used with great care.

A pump device that provides medication to stop labor continuously through a small needle placed just under the skin has not been proven to work long-term in preventing a baby from being born prematurely. The FDA has recently advised not to use this device and the medicine in it because of this failure.

Premature Deliveries

559 How dangerous is it for a baby to be born prematurely?

A baby born before the twenty-fifth week has only a slight chance of survival. From twenty-five to twenty-eight weeks the chance of its living increases. Babies born at or after twenty-eight weeks of pregnancy will usually survive. However, they may have a difficult time for several weeks.

One of the frightening things about having a premature baby is the possibility that it may die or have a handicap that results from its prematurity. One recent study from Vanderbilt University (the *Journal of Pediatrics*, 1990, 117:139) by Jens B. Grogaard et al., reported that of the babies who weighed three and a half pounds or less at birth, 12.5 percent had a handicap that seemed to result from their early delivery.

At least two things have improved the chances of healthy survival for a premature baby. The first is a revolution in intensive care nurseries. In recent years technology in these nurseries has improved dramatically. For example, there is a new treatment—surfactant replacement—that your physician might use for your premature baby in the newborn intensive care nursery. Surfactants coat the inside air sacs of a premature baby's lungs to help them stay open and can prevent the development of respiratory distress. It does not always work, but recent studies are very encouraging.

A second development has been the use of a cortisone-like drug given to the mother if she is expected to have a premature baby. If the mother is given a drug such as betamethasone before delivery, and delivery can be delayed for twenty-four hours, some premature babies' lungs will be more mature and better able to maintain life. Many obstetricians routinely use these drugs now if a mother is going to have a baby when she is less than thirty-four weeks along. Occasionally they are used when the mother is from thirty-four to thirty-six weeks along, but they may not be of any advantage for such babies. There is some evidence that these drugs are not helpful if a woman is carrying more than one baby.

If you have a "preemie" this book may help you: *Premature Baby Book: A Parents' Guide to Coping and Caring in the First Years,* by Helen Harrison with Ann Kositsky, R.N. (New York: St. Martin's Press).

560 Are premature deliveries handled differently from normal deliveries?

Because a premature baby is more fragile than a full-term baby, it is normally delivered with gentleness and care. Special consideration is given to making the episiotomy generously large (to give the baby's head plenty of room), limiting the amount of pain medication the mother gets (to avoid depressing the baby), avoiding inductions unless necessary, and doing C-sections more freely (to provide a gentle delivery).

Although one would think that an episiotomy to deliver a premature baby would be unnecessary or quite small, most obstetricians do a liberal episiotomy so that as the baby comes through the birth canal it is not unduly pressed, or hurt, by the mother's pelvic muscles.

Forceps can help protect the baby. If you will read the section in this chapter on forceps, you will see that forceps actually protect a baby's head most of the time. This is especially true of a premature baby. The forceps can hold the vaginal walls open for the passage of the baby's head. Your physician, of course, will decide what is best for you, but don't be afraid of forceps use for your premature delivery.

As for pain medication for the mother during

Cesarean Skin and Uterus Incisions

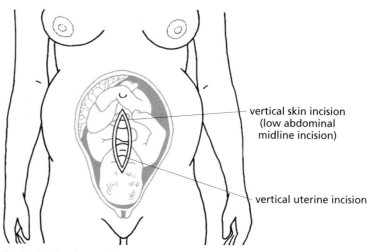

vertical skin incision (low abdominal midline incision)

vertical uterine incision

The skin incision does not have a bearing on whether or not a woman may labor with her next pregnancy; either uterine incision can be used, regardless which skin incision is used.

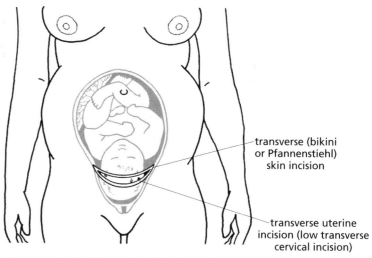

transverse (bikini or Pfannenstiehl) skin incision

transverse uterine incision (low transverse cervical incision)

If a woman has had this uterine incision she may be a candidate for labor with her next pregnancy.

labor, the use of Demerol is extremely limited. Most obstetricians prefer not to use it during premature labor, as premature babies are more susceptible to the effects of drugs, which can cause the low Apgar score at birth. In a premature delivery it is probably best that a mother use an epidural for her labor unless she has a medical problem that makes that unwise (for example, high blood pressure or uterine bleeding).

If a medical problem has made it necessary for you to deliver before full term, the doctor will most likely do a cesarean section rather than an induction before the cervix is ready, because an early induction can be dangerous for the baby. If you are not at the end of your full nine months, it is best that your baby be delivered by cesarean section.

A premature breech baby should be delivered

320

by cesarean section because of its small body and proportionately large head, which can cause the head to become trapped after the delivery of the body.

Cesarean Sections

561 Why are cesarean sections necessary?

Some of the most common reasons for cesarean sections include:

failure to progress in labor
fetal distress
breech baby
prolapse of the umbilical cord
placental problems
problems of the mother
repeat cesareans

A baby too weak to tolerate labor can be delivered safely by cesarean section. If the placenta comes loose, a baby can be delivered before it detaches completely, thus saving the baby. Likewise, if the placenta obstructs the uterine outlet, a C-section preserves the lives of both the mother and the child.

In addition to cesarean sections saving the lives of many women and babies, C-sections have also decreased the number of babies born with cerebral palsy and physical damage from difficult deliveries.

There is a great debate currently raging in our country about the "high cesarean section rate." Your primary concern as an individual is to choose a physician you trust and with whom you can communicate. Should a cesarean section become necessary for you, you can then feel confident with your doctor's advice.

562 If cesarean sections are so beneficial, why are they not used routinely?

Although there is not a great deal of risk to cesarean sections, there is always some potential danger in any surgery. Studies do indicate that a mother has a slightly greater chance of dying from delivery with a cesarean section than if she has a vaginal delivery. Infections of the wound in the uterus, the abdomen, or the urinary tract are more likely with a cesarean section. The rate of such infections varies from as low as 12 percent to as high as 50 percent, the higher numbers usually occurring in indigent populations in large, public hospitals.

It is important that neither the doctor nor the mother feel that a cesarean section is an option to be taken lightly. The doctor must not use it as an easy out from working with the patient in labor toward a vaginal delivery—and the patient must not feel that a cesarean section is a simple way to avoid painful labor or some other aspect of delivery she finds distasteful.

563 What causes labor to "fail to progress"?

There are two primary reasons for a failure to progress in labor, and they are the most common indications for a cesarean section to be done on a mother who has not had a previous C-section. (The first cesarean a woman has is called a primary cesarean section.)

Cephalopelvic disproportion (CPD). Some babies are too large to get through their mother's birth canal, and some women have pelvic bones too small to allow even a normal-sized baby through.

A good obstetrician knows that labor usually follows a fairly normal pattern. It is normal, for instance, for it to take many hours to go from one to four centimeters of dilatation. Once a woman has dilated four centimeters, her labor should progress at about one centimeter an hour. If it does not, her doctor will watch carefully to see if she has cephalopelvic disproportion. If a woman progresses normally in her labor and dilates to ten centimeters, she should not need to spend more than two to four hours pushing to bring the baby's head down far enough for delivery. If she cannot get the baby's head down in that time, she may have cephalopelvic disproportion.

A woman who is completely dilated may get the baby's head down far enough for a forceps delivery. However, since "aggressive" forceps deliveries are rarely done anymore, if there is any question about the baby's inability to get through the birth canal, a cesarean section is usually done.

Abnormal position of the baby's head. If the baby's head is coming into the birth canal "cockeyed," with the brow or chin coming first, a cesarean section may be necessary.

Ineffective contractions (uterine inertia). Although the uterus is a big muscle whose contractions usually push the baby out, there are times when it does not contract effectively. Some women begin labor with ineffective contractions (primary inertia); other women will begin labor with good contractions, only to have the uterus stop contracting effectively at a later point (secondary inertia). If the baby's position seems to be affecting the ability of the uterus to contract well, a cesarean section may be necessary. From 2 to 4 percent of mothers in labor will need a cesarean section for this reason. Normally, however, the baby's position is not a problem and Pitocin can be used to stimulate ineffective contractions. Many C-sections have been prevented by the use of Pitocin.

Pitocin is one of the most useful drugs for a woman in labor. Pitocin is like the hormone produced by a woman's body that makes the uterus contract. It is given through the veins in gradually increasing amounts, causing the uterus to contract increasingly longer and more often, until the contractions are occurring about every three minutes and lasting about sixty seconds, thus duplicating normal labor. When the uterus is made to contract effectively in this manner, labor will often progress normally, concluding with a healthy vaginal delivery. (See Q. 507.)

Doctors do not use Pitocin to cause stronger-than-normal contractions. When Pitocin is used, it is used to duplicate normal labor. Pitocin-stimulated contractions are no more painful than normal strong contractions.

Pitocin is a safe drug when used properly. For labor and delivery Pitocin must always be given in an IV. If a woman's uterus contracts too hard, the IV (intravenous solution) containing the Pitocin can be stopped. The Pitocin in the bloodstream is dissipated in just a few seconds and will not cause any more contractions. After delivery a woman may be given Pitocin in the form of an injection.

564 What other circumstances might indicate the need for a C-section?

During the first stage of labor, some problems may develop that make a cesarean section necessary.

Placenta previa. If the placenta is growing over the inside opening (the cervix) of the uterus, the baby cannot be delivered vaginally. You would probably know about this condition before you actually went into labor.

A woman with a placenta previa will normally have some bleeding from the vagina during the last few weeks of pregnancy. If she did not have bleeding before, she will probably start having heavy bleeding as labor starts.

If a woman starts bleeding during the last few weeks of pregnancy, her doctor will probably order a sonogram to locate the placenta. With the sonogram, the doctor can tell if the placenta is over or near the cervix. If the woman has placenta previa and is within three weeks of a definite and accurate due date, the doctor may want to admit her to the hospital and do a direct examination of the cervix in the operating room by introducing a finger through the cervix to feel the placenta. If the placenta is definitely present, the doctor will do an immediate cesarean. (This exam is done in the operating room with a C-section setup ready because of the possibility that a blood vessel in the placenta could tear and cause heavy bleeding, making an immediate C-section absolutely mandatory.)

Abruptio placenta. Occasionally, either before labor starts or during labor, a placenta will pull loose partially or completely from the wall of the uterus. When this happens the uterus becomes tense and does not relax properly. Sometimes a pregnant woman in this situation will bleed from her vagina.

When abruptio placenta occurs, the whole placenta can pull loose and cause the baby to die immediately. More commonly the placenta pulls loose only partially, causing irritability of the uterus. When this happens an immediate cesarean section is often necessary. If only a very small part of the placenta has pulled loose, the uterus may not develop a great deal of irritability, the baby's heartbeat may remain stable, and a C-section may not be necessary. Normally, however, if abruptio placenta develops, a C-section must be done.

Fetal distress. Fetal monitoring (observation of the baby's heartbeat) detects any distress the baby might be having. If your baby develops significant distress during the first stage of labor, you will probably need to have a cesarean section. Your doctor will usually be able to determine whether or not the fetal distress is a significant emergency or whether the baby can be watched further.

If the distress is seen on the monitor, and your bag of waters has broken and your cervix has dilated a couple of centimeters, your doctor can attach the scalp electrode. This allows monitoring of your baby's heartbeat without interference from the abdominal wall, from your movements, and from other variables that a nondirect observation of the heartbeat produces. With the scalp electrode, the baby's heartbeat is transmitted directly to the monitoring machine. (See Q. 496 for more about fetal monitoring.)

Obstruction to the progress of labor. The term *cephalopelvic disproportion (CPD)* is normally used to describe a disproportion between the size of the baby's head and the size of your pelvis.

If you have dilated to five centimeters and do not progress a centimeter an hour, your labor is going slowly. If your labor continues to be relatively slow but is progressing, the doctor will probably allow labor to continue to a vaginal delivery. If the labor is too slow, however, the doctor may feel that the baby's head is being compressed too hard by your contractions and that a cesarean section would be best. In this way you can avoid damage to the baby. (See Q. 560.)

The physician's recommendation in this situation will depend on his or her own judgment. There is no absolute criterion, other than those mentioned. If you have trusted your doctor this far in your pregnancy, then I recommend that you trust your doctor's judgment now about the need for a cesarean section. You will be more likely to have a healthy baby than if you allowed your labor

to progress too slowly and possibly cause damage to the baby.

565 What causes prolapse of the umbilical cord? Why is a C-section necessary in this situation?

When a baby's head is down into the pelvis, either before or during labor, it is unlikely that the umbilical cord will slip past it down into the vagina (prolapsed umbilical cord) and be a problem. This situation occurs more often when the baby is in a breech position, when the baby's head is not positioned correctly in the pelvis, when the baby is premature, and in a few other unusual conditions. If the cord has prolapsed, contractions could push the baby's head or bottom against the umbilical cord, pinch off the flow of blood from the mother to the baby, and kill the baby before delivery could be accomplished. Your physician is trained to be aware of the possibility of this problem and knows how to treat it. Labor is dangerous when the umbilical cord has slipped past the baby's head and an emergency cesarean section is usually necessary.

566 What problems might the mother have that would make a cesarean section necessary?

Problems the mother might have can be separated into three groups. Many conditions of this type were discussed in the chapter on pregnancy, and most of these problems are not commonly found to be causes of C-sections.

Problems of the mother that could cause the baby to die before birth if delivery is not accomplished. A good example of this is diabetes. Review the discussion of diabetes in Q. 353–359. You will recall that when a mother is diabetic and pregnant, her baby can seem healthy one day and be dead inside her uterus the next. A well-timed C-section can often prevent this.

Problems of the mother that could cause her to die if the baby is not delivered. One example of this would be an expectant mother who is critically ill with heart disease. Another would be a woman with cervical cancer that was found during the pregnancy.

Problems of the mother that could cause the death of both mother and child. Eclampsia is a classic example of this situation. Review the discussion of toxemia in the chapter on pregnancy, especially Q. 369–371.

567 If a woman has a C-section, do all future pregnancies have to be delivered this way? Is it risky for me to have a vaginal delivery with my next pregnancy?

Few obstetricians still feel that the standard dictum, "Once a cesarean section, always a cesarean section," still holds. Still, however, more cesareans are done for that reason than for any other. This feeling is because, years ago, cesarean sections were done by making vertical incisions in the uterus, thereby cutting through the uterus in its thickest part. When the healing occurred, it left a thin scar where there should have been strong, thick muscle tissue. When the patient became pregnant again and was allowed to labor, instead of the presence of strong muscle in the upper part of the uterus, there was strong muscle—but with a weak place in it. Occasionally this weak place ruptured. When that occurred, 50 percent of the babies and 5 percent of the mothers died.

Most C-sections in the past thirty years were done with a horizontal (transverse) incision low in the uterus. Recent studies have shown that there is very little chance of a uterus rupturing if a woman's previous cesarean was done this way. This portion of the uterus provides very little of its contracting power; it is a more passive area that thins out gradually during labor. Because of this passive nature it is much less likely to rupture during labor.

If a patient who has had a previous cesarean section does not go through labor, but simply has a repeat C-section, any risk of the uterus rupturing through the previous scar is eliminated. A cesarean section, however, carries with it risks that

are greater than the very slight possibility of rupture of a previous cesarean section scar.

Another consideration is that cesarean section is much more expensive than a normal delivery. Because of these reasons most obstetricians now discuss VBAC (vaginal birth after cesarean) with their patients who have had previous cesarean sections. Many studies done during the 1980s proved conclusively that VBAC is a safe procedure. In *Clinical Obstetrics and Gynecology* (1985, 28:735), V. L. Flamm reviewed this topic. He reported that out of 6,258 women who tried VBAC, 5,356 (or 86 percent) delivered vaginally. There was not a single death among the mothers in this group, and the number of babies lost was not higher than would be expected for normal vaginal deliveries.

The advantages of having a vaginal delivery are numerous. Studies have conclusively proven that risk for the mother and child is no greater with a VBAC than with having another cesarean section.

No medical procedure is 100 percent safe. It is possible for a mother's uterus to rupture with VBAC. In the review by Flamm (mentioned above), one of the 6,258 women had a uterus tear. But the previous incision in her uterus was vertical, considered a reason not to do VBAC. (A woman whose incision in the uterus goes from one side to the other instead of up and down has only a minimal risk of her uterus tearing.)

Not all women should try to have a vaginal delivery after a previous cesarean section. If a woman is carrying twins or has excessive amniotic fluid, this increased distention of the uterus might cause a rupture. Additionally, women who have had more than two previous cesarean sections should, perhaps, not try VBAC.

These guidelines were established in 1988 by the American College of Obstetricians and Gynecologists for attempting vaginal delivery after a previous cesarean section:

1. The concept of routine repeat cesarean birth should be replaced by a specific indication for a subsequent abdominal delivery (C-section), and in the absence of a contraindication, a woman with one previous cesarean delivery with a low transverse in-

cision should be counseled and encouraged to attempt labor in her current pregnancy.

2. A woman with two or more previous cesarean deliveries with low transverse incisions who wishes to attempt vaginal birth should not be discouraged from doing so in the absence of contraindications.

3. In circumstances where specific data on risks is lacking, the question of whether or not to allow a trial of labor must be assessed on an individual basis.

4. A previous classical (vertical) uterine incision is a contraindication to labor.

5. Professional and institutional resources must have the capacity to respond to acute intrapartum obstetric emergencies, such as performing cesarean delivery within thirty minutes from the time the decision is made until the surgical procedure is begun.

6. Normal activity should be encouraged during the latent phase of labor; there is no need for restriction to a labor bed before actual labor has begun.

7. A physician who is capable of evaluating labor and performing a cesarean delivery should be readily available.

Studies have shown that it is safe to use Pitocin carefully to stimulate labor if a woman is attempting to have labor and delivery after a previous cesarean section.

Epidural anesthesia is usually safe for pain relief during such a labor.

No woman should be forced to go through labor and vaginal delivery after having had a previous cesarean section if she does not want to. Obstetricians often find that many of their patients prefer having another cesarean section rather than trying to go through labor. This is a reasonable request and few obstetricians will argue with it.

Vaginal delivery for previous C-section patients marks a major and dramatic change in the method of care for patients all over the United States. Many patients and doctors are still uncomfortable with the idea, but this procedure will undoubtedly be more and more accepted with the passage of time.

568 What does recovery from a cesarean section involve?

Recovery following a C-section takes about a week longer than after a vaginal birth. Patients are about a week slower in resuming normal activities at home and in "feeling good" again.

After a cesarean section is performed, the mother will go to the recovery room for a one- or two-hour stay. She is then taken to her room, where she is carefully watched. Fluids will probably be given intravenously for a day or two, and she may have a catheter in place for a day. A catheter is simply a hollow rubber tube that is usually inserted into the bladder just before a cesarean section is done. Urine drains through this catheter into a bag that is tied to the side of the bed. This is used for two reasons. First, with a C-section the obstetrician is cutting so near the bladder that it must be empty so the doctor can see where to cut and does not cut the bladder itself. Second, immediately after surgery a woman is often in too much discomfort to empty her bladder properly.

After a C-section, over a period of about two days, the woman's diet will progress from a few sips of water to clear liquids, and then, by a gradually increasing schedule, to regular food.

Most women can go home by the second or third day after the surgery.

A cesarean section does not interfere with nursing, but a woman will not want to be alone in the hospital room with her baby as long as she is taking strong pain medication because she might go to sleep. Pain medicine following a C-section is normally given by injection every three or four hours. I strongly encourage patients to ask for pain medicine any time they hurt. As soon as a patient eagerly begins a liquid diet, she can usually start taking a pain pill. By this time a pain pill will usually be adequate to relieve pain.

When the patient goes home, I think it is best for her not to cook or keep house for two weeks; I give the same recommendation to patients who have had normal vaginal deliveries. Though a woman may not feel quite as well as if she had delivered vaginally, at the end of three weeks from the day of surgery she will usually be ready to resume most normal activity.

Most physicians feel that it is fine for a woman

to climb stairs slowly as soon as she feels comfortable doing so. She can ride in a car when she wants to. She can drive a car when she knows she can jerk her foot up to brake in a hurry. She can go outside and stroll. The primary recommendation is that for two weeks after she goes home from the hospital she has someone else do all the work so she can allow her body time to recover.

Doctors generally allow patients to have intercourse about three weeks from the day of delivery, whether the baby was born vaginally or by cesarean section.

569 What if my C-section incision comes open?

Infections in the wound can occur, causing it to come open. Usually this opening is only in the skin itself. The strong sutures that hold the fascia (material surrounding your abdominal cavity that keeps everything inside) are generally unaffected by such superficial openings in the wound. If the fascia does break loose, it must be sewn back together. This problem might be developing if your wound is becoming tender, red, and swollen. You might even notice some bloody fluid draining out of a small hole in the wound. If you see these things, call your doctor.

Patients who have been in labor and had their bag of waters rupture always have some germs inside the uterus. With a cesarean section, these germs can implant on the walls of the wound, start growing, and cause the wound to become infected and then to break open. If your wound comes apart superficially, it is inconvenient but not dangerous. You may have an irregular scar. After about a year, there is not much difference in the scar's appearance from one that did not come open.

570 Is a hysterectomy ever done following either a cesarean or vaginal delivery?

A hysterectomy may be necessary after delivery if a mother has bleeding that will not respond to any other procedure, such as receiving Pitocin through her veins or having her uterus packed with gauze.

Hysterectomy after delivery may also be necessary if there are tears in large blood vessels in the uterus, or if the placenta has so imbedded itself in the wall of the uterus that it cannot be removed.

Occasionally hysterectomies are done at the time of a cesarean section if the mother has developed precancerous cells on the cervix or wants to be sterilized or has something wrong with her uterus.

Although the woman will be sterile after such surgery, the ovaries are normally left in so that she will neither go through menopause nor have to take hormones.

A hysterectomy done immediately after delivery involves the loss of a moderately large amount of blood and will occasionally require transfusions. Additional problems can occur if either the bladder or the ureters (the tubes that lead from the kidneys down to the bladder) are damaged at the time of a cesarean-hysterectomy; such damage is much more likely to occur than after either a C-section or hysterectomy done separately.

Recovery is similar to the recovery after any hysterectomy or a normal cesarean section. A cesarean-hysterectomy is major surgery and should not be undertaken lightly by a patient or her doctor.

An Afterword

Having a baby is one of life's most interesting, exciting, and mysterious events. For nine months your body has been building toward the climactic event of delivering its precious burden. During this time, changes have taken place in your body and in your baby's body, and while the most visible changes took place in your body before birth, your baby will steal the stage from now on with an amazing display of constant change and growth.

Your mind has been cleared of some questions: Will the baby be all right? What will we name the baby? Should I have natural childbirth? Now it is cluttered with new ones: Cloth or disposable diapers? Breast or bottle? Why is the baby crying? Why am I sad? You long for form-fitting clothes. You can't wait to put on makeup and wash your hair. You wonder how soon you can play tennis!

Caring for your new child will be a series of constant contradictions—thrilling and trying, sweet and sad, fulfilling and emptying—yet you know that rearing this child will be one of the most satisfying, rewarding, and challenging tasks of your life.

Pregnancy, labor, and delivery are in the past. The result is a truly miraculous "harvest."

Now the *real* labor begins!

Part Three

Special Concerns

10

Disorders of Sexual and Reproductive Organs

The female organs, like the women who have them, are a study in contrast. On the one hand these organs are intricate, sensitive, and delicate; on the other they are functional, sturdy, and hardworking. Remarkably, they are usually normal, performing efficiently and capably their vital roles.

Sometimes things go wrong, resulting in a variety of problems for the female. Disorders of the female organs—vulva, vagina, cervix, uterus, fallopian tubes, ovaries, and breasts—are discussed in this chapter.

As background information, a review of chapter 1, "Basic Anatomical Facts," will be helpful. That chapter includes a description of how the various female organs were formed during uterine life, the anatomy of these structures, and a broad overview of how they change from birth through the postmenopause period.

Chapters 2, 3, 4, and 5 continue a survey of the anatomical and functional changes of the female body, highlighting in turn four somewhat arbitrarily chosen age groups: childhood, adolescence, the reproductive years, and middle age and beyond. The items in this chapter cross over all age limits, and are discussed according to the specific body organ involved.

Cross-referencing the material in this chapter to the discussion on intrauterine development in chapter 1 should help you understand disease processes. The same will hold true as you cross-reference this material to the chapters on conception, pregnancy, and delivery. Studying these problems from different perspectives will make them easier to understand. Consult the glossary and index for help finding information about particular subjects and problems.

Problems of the Vulva

A woman's vulva—a term referring to the external part of the female genital organs—is an extremely important area of her body. It serves as guardian of the much more sensitive areas of her female organs, provides an outlet for the urine and stool, and is a source of a great deal of pleasure during sexual intercourse. In fact, the clitoris is the only organ of either male or female that is provided for no other purpose than sexual pleasure. Because of its location and functions, the vulva is subject to certain medical problems.

571 Does my vulva need any special daily care?

If you are having no problems with vulvar irritation or vaginal infection, you can continue the basic hygienic measures that you are now using because you are probably employing a very good program of care. However, if you have episodes of vulvar irritation or infection, it will be helpful to consider the following recommendations:

Bathe daily with a mild soap. Some soaps marketed today are very strong and may contain perfumes and other chemicals that can cause irritation. Don't use these; choose a milder nondetergent soap such as Ivory.

Cleanse the vulva frequently if there is vaginal discharge. At ovulation time and just before a period there may be increased vaginal secretions. During menstruation, blood that is not washed away may cause irritation. Merely cleansing the vulva with a moist washcloth as often as necessary during the day is usually adequate.

Use tampons instead of pads. Tampons absorb menstrual flow internally and do not hold moisture against the vulva as sanitary napkins do. If you do use pads, change as frequently as necessary to avoid the irritation a moist pad can cause. Do not use tampons or pads that have any deodorant or perfume; these chemicals can be extremely irritating. (See Q. 87, 630–631.)

Wear cotton panties. If you do not have vulvar irritation, there is no need to change your clothing habits. If you do, however, cotton panties are a big help. They absorb secretions and allow air flow, thus reducing moisture in the vulvar area.

Don't wear panty hose or panty girdles. Panty hose and panty girdles hold moisture against your vulva, greatly increasing the possibility of vulvar irritation, especially if you already have an infection. Panty hose with a cotton crotch are better, but these are not entirely satisfactory because they still inhibit good air circulation in the area. Women who feel that they cannot do without panty hose may have to pay the price by suffering the irritation that often accompanies their use.

Use no drugs, medications, or feminine-hygiene sprays on the vulva. Unless your physician prescribes these things for a specific problem, do not use them. You can become sensitive to various drugs, chemicals, and medications; the best practice is not to use any of them except for a specific problem.

Practice good toilet habits. When you cleanse yourself after urinating or having a bowel movement, wipe from front to back. This avoids contamination of the vulvar area by urine or feces.

Choose toilet tissue carefully. Use tissue that does not contain deodorants or coloring. The chemicals in the dyes and perfumes can be quite irritating to your vulva.

Wash your underwear with mild soap. Avoid using detergents for your underwear. Detergents are likely to be more irritating than soap.

If you have an infection, these measures will not cure it, but they will keep irritation or infection from being quite so severe and will encourage faster healing when you do start specific treatment.

572 For what reasons should I see a doctor about a vulvar problem?

I encourage you to have an annual physical examination or, at the least, an exam every eighteen months. In addition to a routine Pap smear, the doctor can check your vulvar area for any growths or tumors that may have developed. The doctor can record any changes and, by seeing you regularly, he or she can more easily detect any important change. He or she will probably also examine your vagina. Infections of the vulva and vagina are so often connected that an infection of one usually indicates an infection of the other. Most of the time, for instance, a vulvar irritation is caused by a vaginal infection. (See Q. 601–611.) Vulvar problems caused by sexually transmitted diseases are discussed in chapter 13. Other than the routine physical, the following problems should prompt a visit to the doctor's office.

Discharge. If secretions cause you to wear a pad all the time, or if your secretions have an odor or cause itching, you should see your doctor. He or she can probably prescribe something that will solve this problem. Some women, however, have normal discharge that is heavy enough to require the constant use of small pads for protection. If the discharge is odorless and does not cause itching, there is usually no infection present and there is no medical reason for a woman to try to get rid of such discharge. This type of normal discharge at most may cause a mild "body-type" odor. Increased secretions at the time of ovulation, just before a period, and during pregnancy are normal. If you have discharge other than this, it may or may not be normal.

Itching. If you have vulvar itching, see your doctor so that he or she can determine the cause of the problem and treat you for it. If you have one spot on your vulva that always itches and there is no sign of infection, it may be a precancerous growth starting in that area. Such a precancerous growth can cause itching before it is visible. If you have itching that is persistent, continue to go back to your doctor until it is determined exactly why you have that uncomfortable spot of skin on your vulva. (See Q. 578–580.)

Nodules or growths on your vulva. Bumps in the tissues of the vulva are not usually malignant, but they can be. If you have a knot or a growth on your vulva, be sure to see your physician about it as soon as possible. (See Q. 584–585.)

Trauma. See your physician if you have damaged your vulva in some way, unless you know for sure that it is no more than a mere bruise or slight tear.

Other problems. Other problems can develop in the vulvar area, such as pain, tightness or dryness with intercourse, and varicose veins. If you have any question about this area of your body, see your doctor. If the doctor is not sure what is going on or is not successful with treatment, or if you have a spot that continues to itch, you may need to see a gynecologist for consultation. (See Q. 578, 582.)

573 What might cause a lump or bump on my vulvar area?

A lump or bump is the second most common vulvar problem that prompts women to see their doctor. The most common is irritation. A patient usually thinks of cancer when she discovers such a lump. Usually, however, the growth is not malignant. It can be one of a number of things, including epidermal inclusion cysts, genital warts, or molluscum contagiosum. These and other vulvar growths are discussed in the next questions.

574 What are epidermal inclusion cysts?

These cysts prove to be the most common cause of a vulvar bump. They are rarely larger than a small pea and are located on the outer side of the labia majora.

The cause of epidermal inclusion cysts is undetermined, but it is most likely that some of the ducts in the skin become stopped up because of irritation or infection. When the duct is obstructed, a cheesy or gritty material builds up behind the blockage.

No treatment is necessary unless a woman wants it removed, it becomes infected, or it gets bothersomely large. A doctor can use local anesthesia, slit the cyst open, and squeeze out the material.

575 What are genital warts?

Genital warts, or condylomata acuminata, can occur anywhere on the vulvar area, including the anus. These warts look like ordinary warts and can grow to a very large size. For more information on this subject, see the discussion of human papillomavirus infection (HPV) in Q. 968–973.

576 What is molluscum contagiosum?

Molluscum contagiosum is an infection that causes dome-shaped bumps to grow on the inside of the thighs and on the vulva, in the groin area, and at times in the low abdomen. These bumps are small; the largest ones are rarely more than an eighth of an inch across. They contain a pearly white core and do not hurt, although occasionally one of these bumps may become irritated and tender.

Molluscum contagiosum is caused by a virus that is spread primarily by sexual contact. Treatment is simple: Scraping the core out of each bump causes it to go away. If all are removed, these little growths normally do not come back. As this area is a little sensitive and difficult to reach, you will probably need to let your doctor scrape away the growths. This is not a dangerous problem and these growths do not become malignant or cause other problems.

577 Are there other nonmalignant growths and cysts of the vulva?

There are a large number of different types of growths and cysts of the vulva. It is important to realize that the doctor may not know exactly which one of these you have even after he or she examines you. A biopsy of the growth may be necessary to make a definite diagnosis. The doctor will inject a local anesthetic and take a small piece of the growth for biopsy, or, if the growth is not very large, snip it off entirely. Either way, tissue from the growth is sent to a laboratory for examination and diagnosis under a microscope.

If you have several of the same type of growths, the doctor may feel it is unnecessary to biopsy or remove all of them if they are not bothersome. Some of these growths may be so large, so extensive, or so numerous, however, that your doctor may recommend hospitalization and general anesthesia to have them removed after a diagnosis has been made.

Some of these growths may hang from your body on a thin, narrow stalk. Their removal is simple and can be done in the office. The doctor will merely inject some Xylocaine (a deadening agent) into the base of the growth, tie a suture around it, and cut it off.

A woman in her late teens came to see me once because of a five-inch-long growth of tissue hanging from her vulva. At its tip, the growth was about three inches across. Most of her life this woman had had to keep this growth tucked into her panties to keep it from hanging between her legs. Embarrassment and fear had kept her from seeing a doctor. It took less than five minutes to remove the growth. When I saw her four weeks later, she was completely healed and totally free of what for years had been a bothersome and embarrassing problem.

578 I have a persistent itching of my vulva. What should I do?

As stated previously, if your vulva itches persistently and is not relieved by the usual treatment for vulvar infection, you must continue to see your doctor until the cause is discovered. This warning does not include women who have recurrent fungus infections that require intermittent treatment, nor women who have recurrent *Trichomonas* infection, but rather those whose itching is unexplained and unrelieved.

If your doctor has not been able to give you a specific diagnosis and an organized approach for treatment, you probably need to see a gynecologist.

If you have seen one gynecologist and are still not free of your itching problem, get a second opinion from another gynecologist. Occasionally, seeing a dermatologist for a problem of this type is helpful.

The problem of vulvar itching is a most frustrating problem for a patient and for her physician. It can be difficult to find the cause, and even the best treatment does not always give relief. I will merely give some general guidelines to help you understand what might be done if you have this problem.

579 What procedure will a doctor follow to find the cause of itching?

There are several basic steps that a doctor may take.

History of the problem. The doctor will want to know how long the problem has been present and whether or not you have been treated for infections of the vulvar area. He or she will also want to know if you have been using medications on the vulvar area and whether you have been using toilet tissue containing perfumes or dyes or tampons or pads that contain chemicals.

Treatment of infection. The doctor will want to treat you for any infection found, to see if that will eliminate the problem.

Biopsy. The doctor will look for any areas of abnormal tissue. In some women there may be thickened vulvar tissue present, and in other women there may be areas that have become thin and sensitive. The doctor may want to take several biopsies if there are several areas that look abnormal. Occasionally a cancer of the vulva will first show up as itching.

Further treatment. If you do have premalignant or malignant tissue, the doctor will obviously treat that. (See Q. 584–588.)

If changes of the vulvar skin persist, you may need to continue seeing your doctor intermittently. He or she may want to do repeat biopsies of the tissue. If your doctor suggests this, I urge you to follow the suggestions. Such conscientiousness may help you find abnormal cells on your vulva before they become malignant.

580 How will a doctor treat itching caused by thickened skin?

This is known as hyperplastic dystrophy. Cotton dressings soaked with cool Burrow's solution can be applied repeatedly to the areas of thickened skin. This helps clear up the irritation and oozing. In fact, Burrow's solution, a preparation available without prescription from a drugstore, is helpful for many skin problems. In addition, an antibiotic cream can be applied to the area if it seems infected, and cortisone-type ointments can be applied when the oozing and irritation have resolved. These cortisone preparations can be applied two or three times a day and may need to be continued intermittently for many years. Women tend to use them when they are itching and stop when the itching is better. See your doctor if the problem persists.

The thickened skin usually becomes much more normal looking, but sometimes it does not. Occasionally the itching will not clear up either. Further medical consultation may be necessary.

581 My doctor did a biopsy of my vulva and said that I have lichen sclerosis. What is that? How is it treated?

Lichen sclerosis is a condition of the skin of the vulva of unknown cause. With this condition, part or all of the skin of the vulva gets thin, shrunken, white, and itchy. It is not an infection or a malignancy.

Your doctor will take a biopsy to confirm his or her impression of your problem and to make sure you do not have a malignancy. Once certain of the diagnosis, your physician can prescribe medication. An application of 2 percent testosterone propionate in petrolatum, used two or three times a day for at least four weeks, has been found to be the best treatment. If the itching is intense, application of the testosterone ointment can be alternated with cortisone cream, or the two may be mixed together. It may be helpful to wrap a sanitary pad in plastic wrap and wear it to hold the ointment against the skin of the vulvar area more effectively.

After about a month most women will have much less itching and will be able to use the testosterone ointment less frequently. This less-frequent use is desirable because continued use of this male hormone can produce masculine changes in a woman such as increased hair growth, decreased breast size, oily skin with acne, and increased sexual desire. But don't run to the pharmacy to get this drug just to increase your sexual interest! For most women, the amount of this medication required to significantly increase libido will also be enough to give them a beard!

Lichen sclerosis can cause shrinking of the vulvar tissues. Women who have shrinking of these tissues may find intercourse painful or impossible. In this situation, Premarin vaginal cream should be used in the vagina in addition to the testosterone on the vulva. One-half an applicator full of the Premarin cream in the vagina three times a week is the usual dose. It can take up to nine months for this medication to have its maximum effect. If intercourse remains difficult, the doctor may be able to make a "relaxing incision" to open the vagina more widely. This would, of course, need to be done under anesthesia.

An exciting new treatment has recently shown marked improvement in patients with this problem. The use of clobetasol propionate (Tenovate cream) applied twice daily to the uncomfortable area not only made most women much more comfortable but made their vulvar tissues appear more healthy (Dalzeil and Wojnarowska, *Journal of Reproductive Medicine*, 1993, 38:25).

582 What if my vulvar itching does not respond to treatment?

If itching continues, injections of a cortisone-type drug (10 mg of triamcinalone diluted 2:1 with saline) directly into the itching skin may be given. If the cortisone injections do not work, an injection of an alcohol solution into the tissues to kill the nerves can be tried (under general anesthesia). This is effective only for itching. It will not usually eliminate any burning in the vulva.

583 My doctor says I have leukoplakia on my vulva. What is this?

The term *leukoplakia* means "a white patch." Until recently, doctors were afraid that any time such a white patch was present it heralded the possible development of cancer. It has now been shown that this is not true and that leukoplakia is usually due only to thickening of the tissues.

If your doctor says that you have leukoplakia and suggests that a large part of your vulva be removed (a vulvectomy), you should generally refuse to have that done without expert consultation, unless you know that your doctor is a specialist in problems of this kind.

584 There is a growth on my vulva that itches. My doctor biopsied it and the report says it is premalignant. What does this mean and how should it be treated?

A premalignant growth contains cells whose chromosomes have changed in such a way that they no longer respond to normal growth controls. At this stage your growth is somewhat like an early skin cancer. It is not dangerous in its present form. However, if such a growth is neglected, it can become dangerous by growing down into the deeper tissues of the body. A premalignant growth, therefore, is at the stage doctors like to find a growth— before it is dangerous.

Premalignant growths of the vulva are of different types and have been given many names in the past: Bowen's disease, erythroplasia of Queyrat, squamous cell carcinoma in situ, and Paget's disease. Presently specialists recognize only two different groups of this type of problem: squamous cell carcinoma in situ and Paget's disease. The symptoms and treatments for both are the same.

Once a biopsy has determined premalignancy, the doctor will suggest further treatment. It will be one of the following.

Excision of the growth. To insure getting all the growth, a doctor normally must cut wide of the outside edge of the growth by at least one-third inch. If the pathologist determines that the growth has actually extended to the edges of the tissue that the doctor has removed, the doctor will need to make a wider circle of incision around the area. You must continue treatment until all abnormal tissue is gone.

Laser treatment. The laser is now being used to vaporize these growths. The initial procedure is easier and there is less scarring. If the laser is used, it is usually easier to tell when a growth is coming back because there is less distortion of the vulva after healing.

Chemotherapy treatment. A 5 percent 5-fluorouracil cream (a chemotherapy drug) applied to a premalignant growth on the surface of the vulva will frequently make the growth go away. The problem with this treatment is that it can cause a great deal of irritation to the tissue. Many women are unable to continue the use of this drug long enough for it to be effective. However, if a woman can tolerate it, it is often good therapy.

Vulvectomy. See the next question.

585 Is a vulvectomy ever necessary for premalignant growths?

Doctors in the past have felt that a woman with precancerous growths needed to have her vulva removed, a procedure involving the removal of both the labia majora and minora and often the clitoris and surrounding skin. Very few doctors feel this is necessary today, unless the premalignant growths are extensive or severe, or unless these growths continue to recur.

A vulvectomy is not particularly dangerous, but it does occasionally require skin grafting to cover the raw areas. It changes the way a woman's vulva looks and also causes a problem with urination. Urine is normally guided by the labia into forming a stream; after a vulvectomy urine tends to splatter in a bothersome fashion.

Another problem with treating this type of growth with a vulvectomy is that the same type of growth for which the vulvectomy was done can regrow along the edges of the healed surgical incision. This requires further surgery.

586 What about cancer of the vulva?

Cancer of the vulva is usually squamous cell carcinoma of the labia majora. In other words, cancer of the "skin" of the labia majora is the most common cancer of the vulva, although vulvar cancer can originate in any of the other parts of the vulvar tissues: sweat glands, Bartholin's glands, clitoris, and urethra.

There has been a dramatic increase in the number of cases of both premalignant and malignant growths of the vulva in the past few years, many of these occurring in young, premenopausal women. Cancer of the vulva had always been considered to be a cancer of women of the postmenopausal age until this trend started a few years ago. During this same period of time, there has been a marked increase in the number of precancerous and cancerous growths on women's cervixes and vaginas. Most researchers feel that the increase in all of these problems is related to infection by the same virus that causes genital warts, the HPV organism. (See Q. 968–973.) The increased presence of the genital wart virus seems to be due to the increased number of infected sexual partners to whom so many single women are exposing themselves today.

It is important that both patients and doctors understand that if a growth is present on the vulva, or if there is an itching or uncomfortable area that persists, a biopsy should be done to make sure that no cancer is developing.

A cancer of the vulva is normally slow-growing, but after it has been present for a while, it will finally grow into the deeper tissues of the labial skin and from there spread inside the body to lymph nodes of the groin and the pelvis. Often, even then, this type of cancer will remain confined to these lymph nodes for a long time before it spreads on to other parts of the body.

587 How is vulvar cancer treated?

Treatment for this type of cancer has traditionally been an operation that removes the labia, the mons pubis, and the lymph nodes of the groin and inner thigh. Skin grafting of the vulva, of the pubic bone, and of the groin is often necessary. This operation is called a radical vulvectomy.

If a pathologist studies all of the tissue removed at surgery and finds no lymph node involvement, which means that the cancer is growing only on the vulva, the patient has up to an 80 percent chance of being completely cured by the operation. If some of the lymph nodes are involved, however, the chance of complete cure drops to as low as 30 to 40 percent.

Because this type of cancer is occurring more often in younger women, and because the operation is so disfiguring to the external genital appearance, doctors are trying to determine ways to do a less radical operation. For instance, some of these cancers can be removed by laser or wide local excision. If a cancer can be treated this way, it is much less disfiguring and debilitating. If you have a cancer of this type, be sure you are in the hands of doctors who are specialists in the care of female-organ cancer. Then you will be able to get surgery and treatment that is custom-made to your particular needs, avoiding surgery that might be unnecessarily extensive.

If, after surgery for vulvar cancer, the cancer begins growing again, it is absolutely necessary that you be treated by a female-organ cancer specialist. There is still a chance for a cure, but only if it is handled with great expertise and care.

588 What does a biopsy of my vulva involve? How important is it for me to have such a biopsy?

Having read this chapter, you will have seen the common thread winding through all our discussions about vulvar lumps, bumps, growths, and irritations. That common thread is the vulvar biopsy—an absolutely mandatory part of the care of vulvar disease in women. A report on cancer of the vulva indicated that diagnosis of cancer of the vulva is delayed, on the average, by sixteen months. In other words, the patient went to the doctor with a complaint (usually itching), but the doctor did not make the diagnosis for another sixteen months! During that time the patient's can-

cer was enlarging and getting worse. All it takes to diagnose a cancer of the vulva is a simple biopsy.

If you have a small growth on your vulva, or an area that continues to itch and be uncomfortable, you should insist that your doctor do a careful examination of your vulva and consider doing a vulvar biopsy. I am talking about itching or pain that persists in a particular spot on the vulva, not the "all over" vulvar irritation of chronic vulvitis that so many women have.

The vulvar biopsy is not extremely uncomfortable. It is done in three simple steps:

The doctor injects anesthetic into the area to be biopsied.

The doctor twirls a small, round "punch" biopsy onto the numbed area of your vulva and snips away a small, round piece of tissue.

The doctor uses silver nitrate sticks to cauterize the bleeding from the walls of the small hole. This procedure eliminates the need for sutures.

The biopsied tissue is sent to a pathologist for diagnosis. If the report shows a malignancy, proper treatment can be started immediately.

589 What problems can affect the urethra?

A red, tumorlike growth can occur at the opening of the urethra, usually in women who have gone through menopause. The problem is usually a urethral caruncle, a condition in which the lining just inside the urethral opening protrudes from the urethra and is exposed to the irritation of underwear, intercourse, and other irritants. This delicate tissue, which is normally inside the urethra, cannot stand this type of trauma and becomes reddened and swollen.

Most of the time this problem, if not too bothersome, can be left alone. If the caruncle bleeds or is sensitive, an application of a vaginal estrogen cream or estrogen by mouth will normally clear it up. If it does not, the doctor may give a woman general anesthesia and cut out the irritated tissue. If a caruncle does not seem to be clearing up as quickly as it should, the doctor should certainly take a biopsy of it and send it to a pathologist. Carcinoma (cancer) of the urethra does occur.

Occasionally a reddish, bleeding urethra is caused by the inner lining of the urethra actually falling out. This problem, called urethral prolapse, can occur in young girls before they begin their menses and in women after the menopause. It rarely occurs in women of reproductive age. Urethral prolapse is uncommon. Treatment for the problem is done with freezing (cryocautery), using the laser to evaporate the tissue, or with use of a catheter and sutures. In the latter method a catheter is put in the urethra and the suture tied down on the catheter, over the prolapsed tissue. After a few days the tissue falls off.

590 What causes a cyst of the urethral opening?

There are glands at the entrance to the urethra (Skene's glands) that produce mucus that moistens the opening. When the outlet to these little glands gets blocked, they fill up with mucus and form small cysts. This may happen following an infection with gonorrhea, but it may also occur in women who have not had such an infection.

These urethral-opening cysts may cause discomfort during intercourse, or they may become infected and cause a great deal of pain. Occasionally they can block the opening of the urethra, making it difficult to empty the bladder.

When these glands are infected, they can be opened and drained. If the glands have become cystic and are problematic, a urologist can cut them out in a simple but effective procedure.

591 My doctor said I have a Bartholin's duct cyst. What does that mean?

Every woman has two Bartholin's glands, one on either side of the entrance to the lower vagina. These glands produce secretions that lubricate the vaginal entrance and are especially active during intercourse. They empty their secretions just inside the labia through two small tubes, or ducts.

Even if the ducts become obstructed, the glands will continue to secrete mucus. This will cause the ducts to begin "ballooning up" from the pressure and presence of mucus.

Bartholin's gland ducts may become blocked for several reasons: infection from germs around the vaginal entrance (including sexually transmitted disease such as gonorrhea or chlamydia), underdeveloped ducts, and occasionally, stitches from episiotomies.

It is fairly easy for a doctor to tell if the swelling at the lower part of the vagina is a Bartholin's duct cyst or an infection. Once he or she has diagnosed the problem, treatment will be suggested.

592 How is a Bartholin's duct cyst treated?

If the cyst is not bothersome, it may be left alone. If it is bothersome, however, one of three treatments may be suggested. The doctor may want to open the cyst in an operating room and sew around the edges so that it stays open. This requires general anesthesia and is called "marsupialization." Second, the doctor may suggest the use of local anesthesia in the office so he or she can make a small nick into the cyst to insert a small rubber catheter called a Word catheter. The balloon on the tip of the catheter would then be inflated to keep it in place. A third alternative treatment is to cut out the entire Bartholin's gland.

I have been using the Word catheter for years and prefer it to sewing the gland open. The catheter can be inserted in the office and does not require general anesthesia. Patients tolerate it well and are less likely to develop a subsequent Bartholin's gland cyst after use of a Word catheter than after marsupialization. Occasionally a woman finds the catheter too uncomfortable and must have it removed after only a few days.

Intercourse may be difficult but is permitted with a Word catheter in place. The catheter hangs out of the Bartholin's gland about an inch.

When the Word catheter is removed after about four to six weeks, a sufficient opening is left to permit outflow of mucus allowing the duct to remain collapsed.

It is rarely necessary to cut out an entire Bartholin's gland. If, however, you have had a great deal of trouble with your Bartholin's gland and a competent doctor suggests that you have the gland removed, it is probably best to follow that advice. By "a great deal of trouble," I mean many episodes of the recurrence of the cyst, with its presence causing persistent pain and problems. If a doctor suggests—on first seeing you for a cyst that has not been too troublesome—that you have the cyst cut out, it would be best to get another opinion.

593 How is a Bartholin's duct abscess, or infection, treated?

Occasionally a Bartholin's duct cyst will become infected. When this occurs, your lower vagina, either on the right side or on the left, will be inflamed and extremely tender. The doctor will usually cut open the abscess in the office under local anesthesia to allow drainage of the pus and relief of the painful pressure that has developed. Sometimes a Word catheter can be inserted at this time. I have been able to use the Word catheter with a number of patients at the time an abscess was opened. This saved their having to come back later to have a second procedure done. However, many times the infection will prevent any treatment beyond opening the abscess.

594 The blood vessels of my labia seem swollen and distended. What does this mean?

Swollen, distended blood vessels of the labia are probably varicose veins. Most women are surprised when this situation develops. Although varicose veins of the vulva occur most often during pregnancy, they can occur any time. If the veins are not too bothersome, they can and should be left alone. If they do cause trouble, they may be treated.

If vulvar varicose veins develop during pregnancy, a woman may be able to make it through the pregnancy by lying down whenever the vulvar area becomes engorged and uncomfortable. A vulvar support (produced by Ortho-Vascular Products Company in Yonkers, New York) may help.

Vulvar varicose veins can bleed during pregnancy. If repeated bleeding occurs, surgery may be necessary. If so, it is probably best to have it done before the end of the seventh month of pregnancy.

Surgical treatment for varicose veins is to have them ligated (tied off), just as if they were present in a woman's legs.

595 How should injuries to the vulva be treated?

Most injuries to the vulva occur in children: falling on a bicycle seat, a fence, a toy, and so on. However, they do occur in adults too, usually as a result of waterskiing, motorcycle or bicycle accidents, or because of some similar type trauma. (See Q. 43–45, 632.)

Injuries from intercourse also occur, but they are unusual except in rape cases. (See Q. 189–191.)

If an injury to the vulva produces only a bruise, there is no need for treatment other than an ice pack during the first twenty-four hours, followed by sitting in a bathtub filled with warm water (sitz bath) several times a day until pain and swelling have subsided.

Although most of the time it is best not to open a hematoma, if the bruise includes a very large accumulation of blood, the area may need to be opened surgically. This may be best done under general anesthesia in an operating room because, when the wound is opened, there may be bleeding from the raw area inside that requires suturing.

If there are tears of the vulva, these may require suturing. This would usually require anesthesia and treatment in an operating room. Tears of this type need to be washed thoroughly. Careful examination of the tissues is necessary to make sure that no foreign material is left embedded in the tissues.

If a vulvar injury occurs it will not normally interfere with future sexual activity. If this area can tolerate delivery of a baby, which includes tears, bruising, and even hematomas, it can obviously tolerate other injuries. The vulva was designed to heal well and to allow normal sexual function after trauma.

Problems of the Vagina

As you well know, your vagina is an important part of your body. Though you cannot see it, and you probably do not think of it often, the vagina performs several vitally important functions.

It serves as a passage for the menstrual flow.
It receives your husband's penis during sexual intercourse.
It serves as a receptacle for semen.
It serves as the walls of the birth canal for delivery of a baby.
It allows a doctor easy access to your cervix for Pap smears and permits easy examination of your uterus and other internal organs.

Most of the time a woman is as unaware of her vagina as she is of other internal body organs. Even when the vagina is diseased, she is primarily concerned with the blood or discharge or odor that comes from the vagina rather than with the vagina itself. If there is a problem of the vagina, the symptoms may include:

abnormal discharge
abnormal bleeding
unusual odor
pain with intercourse
itching
tissue protruding from the vagina

If it takes your doctor a while to help you get rid of a vaginal problem, be patient. The solution may not be simple. It may be reassuring to learn that the vagina rarely has a malignancy, a tumor, or a problem that is dangerous to your health.

596 Do I need to provide any special care for my vagina?

If you are not having trouble with your vagina now, and have had no problems in the past, you are probably doing things right.

There are several topics I am frequently asked about by patients concerning the vagina and its care:

the use of tampons
lubrication with intercourse
avoiding sexually transmitted diseases
douching
intercourse after hysterectomy
first intercourse

597 Should I use tampons?

I recommend that girls begin using tampons as soon as they begin having a menstrual flow. (See Q. 87.)

The advantage of internal protection is that it keeps the vulva drier, making it less likely to become irritated by moisture. However, although this is true for menstruation, using tampons throughout the month for vaginal discharge is not advisable because of the possibility of developing toxic shock. (See the question in this section on toxic shock.)

Another advantage of a young person's using tampons is that it helps her become familiar with her hymen and with her vaginal structure. The tampons stretch the hymen a little, making a girl's first pelvic exam and first intercourse easier. It is my impression that my young patients who use tampons are more relaxed about and comfortable with their bodies.

It is true that toxic shock syndrome has been

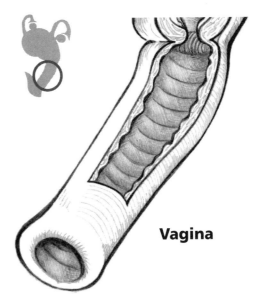

Vagina

associated with tampon use, but this was primarily in the past when high-absorbency tampons were on the market. Toxic shock syndrome has also been found in non-tampon users and even in men and small children. (See Q. 630–631.)

598 Should I use a lubricant during intercourse?

I advise my patients to purchase a vaginal lubricant and keep it at their bedsides from the first night of marriage on. When women have times of poor sexual lubrication, a little vaginal lubricant could help.

Vaginal dryness occurs under numerous circumstances in all women. For instance, lubricants are helpful for intercourse immediately after a menstrual period, or soon after a bath, or in cases of limited sexual excitement. Lubricants are especially important if you have gone through menopause and find that you have less-than-satisfactory sexual lubrication. Because lubricants tend to kill sperm, you should not use one if you are trying to become pregnant.

Several vaginal lubricants can be purchased without a prescription. For example, the Ortho Company has one called Ortho's Personal Lubricant. Maxilube ointment is pleasant to use because it is nongreasy and is quickly absorbed by bedsheets or by your skin. Lubrin and Replens are two other good lubricants. I advise you to try several kinds until you find one that feels most like your own normal vaginal moisture.

599 Should I douche?

Douching (cleaning the vagina by directing a stream of water or a prepared solution into it) is quite common, and many women consider it to be a necessary—although unpleasant—part of good hygiene. I do not recommend the practice, however. Douching is not necessary and can, in fact, be quite harmful. There is no reason for a woman to douche unless a physician recommends it as part of treatment for infection.

Many women douche because they feel the vagina needs cleaning after their menstrual period

or following intercourse, but that is not the case. The normal, healthy vagina is "self-cleaning." Neither semen nor blood leave it "dirty," and external cleaning is all that is necessary for good hygiene and freshness. (When I examine a woman the day after her period ends, I rarely find any evidence of blood and her vagina almost always looks clean and healthy.)

The natural secretions of the vagina make some women uncomfortable, and these women may douche to feel clean and dry. The moisture from the vagina is normal, however, and serves an important function. It provides lubrication to keep the vaginal entrance from becoming raw and sore, thus preventing cracks and tears.

Until fairly recently, most doctors considered douching to be a harmless practice. Recent studies have shown that this is not always true. Women who douche have a greater risk of tubal pregnancies, and women who have STD (sexually transmitted disease) germs appear to be more likely to suffer PID (pelvic inflammatory disease) if they douche.

Some general guidelines concerning douching are:

1. Do not douche if you are pregnant.
2. Do not use douching as a contraceptive. Sperm are in the uterus within seconds of intercourse.
3. Do not douche before seeing a physician for a vaginal infection. You could temporarily wash away germs needed to identify the cause of the problem.
4. Do not douche if you think you have a vaginal infection or if there is a possibility that you may have STD germs. This could cause PID. See a doctor instead.
5. Do not use douche equipment more than once. Always use disposable bags and nozzles, even if you use water or diluted vinegar (one or two tablespoons per quart of water).

Finally, let me urge you to reconsider your practice of douching. I assure you that you will be just as clean with only external cleansing, and I am certain that within a few weeks you will not even notice the slight increase of moisture.

600 Should I prepare my vagina in any way before I have intercourse for the first time?

The best preparation of the vagina for first intercourse is to have a doctor examine it. He or she can warn you of any existing problem, detect a hymen that is too tight and firm, and tell you if you have any kind of vaginal abnormality.

Even if you have been examined and found normal, you may still have some discomfort with your first intercourse. You are unlikely to have severe pain, but if you do, that pain is more likely a result of your tightening up your body out of fear of intercourse than it is of your hymen actually being resistant to intercourse.

If you have significant pain with your first intercourse, there are a couple of things you might do to make it more comfortable the next time.

First, try to relax! If you are tensing up during entry of his penis, ask your husband to stop pushing in. Then consciously relax your "bottom." You will be amazed at the amount of control you have over the entrance to your vagina. When you have relaxed some, you can then push down on your husband's penis, as though you are trying to have a bowel movement. This tends to open up your vagina a little, allowing further penetration. In addition, use lots of vaginal lubricant. If your pain persists, see your doctor.

It is normal to have soreness of the hymen after having intercourse the first few times. If this occurs, refrain from intercourse for a few days to allow the irritation caused by the normal tears in your hymen to clear up.

It is also normal for you as a virgin to have a little bleeding with the first intercourse, but it is just as normal not to.

601 Is it normal to have some vaginal discharge?

It certainly is. As a matter of fact, it is remarkable that women do not have more discharge than they do. Secretions come from the sweat and oil glands of the vulva, and from the Bartholin's and Skene's glands; fluid oozes through the vaginal walls; cells slough off the vaginal walls continually; and the cervix, uterine lining, and fallopian tubes contribute fluids to the vagina that are either absorbed by it or passed to the outside.

In spite of the secretion of all these fluids, most women do not require external protection for the vaginal secretions. Some women, however, have enough normal secretions to make them feel wet all the time; they will often be uncomfortable without some type of external protection.

Most women have increased secretions at the time of ovulation (fourteen days before the next period is going to start) and just before a menstrual period begins. Some women may notice it only as slight moisture at the opening of the vagina. Other women do not have any increased secretions at this time (also a normal situation).

Secretions produced by normal body function will usually be white or off-white in color. Their consistency will be "curdy or mucouslike." If vaginal secretions are milky or runny, they are usually not normal. The normal, curdy secretions cause some women to think they have a fungus infection even though they have no itching. If a woman has enough fungus infection to produce the typical "cottage cheese" discharge of such an infection, she will also have irritation.

If you are not sure that your secretions are normal, have your doctor check their acidity. The acidity of normal secretions should be in the range of a pH of 3.8 to 4.2. If your secretions have this acidity, no odor, cause no itching, and have the normal off-white, curdy appearance, they are normal secretions.

Normal vaginal secretions do not have a foul odor. A woman with or without vaginal secretions can, of course, have some "body odor" from the vulvar area. (This is especially common if a woman is a little overweight.) If the vaginal secretions have a foul odor, there is probably an infection present.

602 What should I do if I have an abnormal vaginal discharge or odor or itch?

You need to see a physician for abnormal vaginal discharge, itch, odor, and so on. Your doctor will question you about your symptoms. Since problems of this sort almost always indicate a vaginal infection, he or she will ask you if the discharge causes itching or has a bad odor and will determine how heavy the discharge is and what color it is. Since the irritation might be caused by some medication or drug that comes in contact with your vulvar skin, you will be asked about materials or medications that have come in contact with that area. If you have had a vulvar irritation for a long time, for instance, you may have been using some medication to which you have become sensitive. Your symptoms may now be due to the medication and not to the original irritant.

The doctor will examine you, checking the vulvar area to see if it is red, scratched, or has sores, and will look inside your vagina to see what the discharge looks like. Your physician will often take some of the secretions on a Q-tip, daub them onto a drop of saline (salt water) on a slide, and look at the suspension under a microscope. On a wet mount of this type, gardnerella germs can sometimes be seen, indicating a bacterial vaginosis infection. (See Q. 604.) The gardnerella germs are small and stick to the normal vaginal cells seen under the microscope. A doctor can often identify gardnerella infection just by looking in the microscope for these normal cells with bacteria clinging to them ("clue" cells).

Trichomonas organisms can usually be seen quite easily in a saline (salt water) preparation.

The doctor might do a KOH prep with your secretions: a drop of your secretions is placed on a slide and a drop of potassium hydroxide (KOH) placed on that. The potassium hydroxide will dissolve all the vaginal cells, leaving only fungus organisms, if there are any present.

The doctor may check the acidity of your vaginal secretions to help determine what type of infection you have. If the test shows a pH of 4.7 or higher, and you have an odorous discharge, you almost certainly have bacterial vaginosis, formerly called gardnerella vaginitis or hemophilus vaginitis. (See Q. 604, 1002.) If you have an infection causing itching, and the pH of the secretions is 6.0 or above, you probably have trichomoniasis.

Since trichomoniasis and bacterial vaginosis are treated the same way—with Flagyl, a med-

ication taken in pill form by mouth—the decision as to which drug you need can sometimes be made simply by testing the acidity of your vaginal secretions.

The doctor may feel it necessary, however, to take some of the secretions from your vagina for a culture. The culture can show whether or not you have fungus organisms in your vagina, even when you have such a minimal amount of infection that it cannot be directly seen on a microscope. Vaginal cultures can also identify gonorrhea, chlamydia, or herpes, but each germ must be tested for separately.

Occasionally, poorly informed doctors will worry a patient about normal but unusual vaginal germs that they find on a vaginal culture. For example, it is normal to have an *E. coli* organism or a streptococcus organism in the vagina; if a doctor begins treatment for these organisms, you are being treated for a normal germ that is not usually the source of a vaginal infection. You should get further consultation if your doctor insists on continuing treatment for such organisms. Of course, if you have gonorrhea, chlamydia, herpes, fungus, trichomoniasis, or gardnerella, treatment is usually necessary.

603 What is trichomoniasis? How is it treated?

This is an infection caused by a protozoan organism called *Trichomonas vaginalis* and occurs only in the genital organs of men and women. Although it does not usually damage the people it infects, trichomoniasis can be extremely irritating, especially in women. If a woman is having a discharge that is irritating, she should be checked for "trich," as was described in the previous question.

Flagyl is effective in clearing up 99 percent of trichomoniasis. It is normally as effective for a person to take two grams of Flagyl at one time as it is to take one-half gram twice a day for five days.

More important than which dosage schedule a woman follows is the fact that her sexual partner also be treated. Trichomoniasis is primarily a sexually transmitted disease. If a woman has it, her partner will also have it in his internal genital organs, even though he has no symptoms. If a woman is treated and her sexual partner is not, he will give the infection back to her as soon as they have intercourse again. Physicians call this a "ping-pong" infection.

There is no doubt that this infection can be transmitted sexually. As a matter of fact, if both partners are being treated, but infection recurs, it may be that one of the two has an involvement with another sexual partner that is causing the reinfection. There are, however, some exceptions to sexual transmission. Trichomoniasis does occasionally occur in people who have not had extramarital intercourse. Also, 1 percent of trich patients do not respond to Flagyl because their *Trichomonas* germ is a resistant organism.

If an infection seems to be resistant to the usual doses of Flagyl, larger doses may work. Some women, however, will develop nausea, light-headedness, and a metallic taste in their mouths with larger doses. These symptoms are not dangerous, however, and if a woman can tolerate them, the medication should be continued. If she can continue the medication she will usually be cured. At the same time, of course, her partner must be treated with the same high doses as he undoubtedly has the same resistant organism. Women who cannot tolerate higher doses of Flagyl can be treated through the veins. (There are vaginal suppositories of Flagyl, but they probably offer no advantage over the use of Flagyl by mouth.)

For control of irritation, a woman can use Vagisec suppositories or douches or similar medications, which do not cure trichomoniasis but may help her be more comfortable. It is important that a woman not use such medication in her vagina for several days before she sees her physician. The medication can kill some of the germs and make her appear free of infection when she is not.

A woman who is considering becoming pregnant should be treated until she is free of *Trichomonas*, since pregnant women with trichomoniasis have a higher chance of going into labor early. In addition, the germ can be passed to a baby, although it does not seem to damage the baby in any way.

Recently (1995) researchers reported evidence that *Trichomonas* can cause or be a part of the cause of infection of women's fallopian tubes (PID). If this research is true, it can make a woman infertile (see PID Q. 827). This is why it is so important to get treatment for trichomoniasis quickly.

Recent studies have indicated that if a woman with trichomoniasis has intercourse with a man who is infected with HIV, she will be more susceptible to becoming infected with AIDS. Some studies suggest a three times greater risk.

604 What is bacterial vaginosis (BV)? How is it treated?

Bacterial vaginosis (BV) is a vaginal infection that is the most common cause of abnormal vaginal discharge in women who are in their reproductive years. It accounts for at least 30 percent of the abnormal discharge that women have. The usual symptom of this infection is an increased amount of vaginal secretions with a strong, fishy odor. However, more than half of those who have this infection may have absolutely no symptoms.

Bacterial vaginosis infection is usually, but not always, considered a sexually transmitted disease. This infection seems to be caused by a mixture of organisms, called anaerobic organisms, which grow without oxygen. This type of infection has a discharge that is "fishy," foul-smelling, watery, and often heavy. It does not cause burning or itching. If itching is associated with the above symptoms, a mixed infection—vaginosis and fungus, or vaginosis and *Trichomonas*—is probably present.

The doctor can make the diagnosis (as stated earlier in Q. 602), by putting a drop of the vaginal secretions in a drop of saline and looking at this under a microscope. The "clue" cells are the normal vaginal cells to which the offending germs have adhered. The doctor may check the acidity of the secretions. If the pH is between 4.7 and 6.0, the infection is probably vaginosis.

The best treatment is with Flagyl, 500 mg taken twice a day for seven days. If you are also being treated for trichomoniasis, it might be wise to have the 500 mg-twice-a-day-for-seven-days regimen instead of the one-time dose often given for trichomoniasis alone. This would insure that you will get rid of both bacterial vaginosis and *Trichomonas*.

Because bacterial vaginosis is often a sexually transmitted disease, for a woman to be free of it, her sexual partner must also be free of it. It is necessary, therefore, that both partners be treated. If the infection keeps recurring, it is possible that one of the couple has another sexual partner. But no treatment is perfect, and failure to eliminate the infection may not necessarily be due to outside exposure.

Also, as with *Trichomonas*, a man may not have any symptoms of the infection, but if a woman has it, her partner also does, and he must be treated too.

Bacterial vaginosis can occur in women who have not (and whose husbands have not) had extramarital intercourse. If you have developed a bacterial vaginosis infection, therefore, don't assume that your husband has been unfaithful.

If a woman is planning to get pregnant, she should get rid of this infection before she gets pregnant. Recent studies have shown that women with bacterial vaginosis have a four or five times greater chance of having complications with their pregnancy. The primary complication has been premature labor with delivery of a premature infant. It has also been shown that a woman with bacterial vaginosis is more likely to have uterine and tubal infection after delivery (pelvic inflammatory disease).

Since the discharge from this infection does not cause itching or irritation, many women will tolerate being infected for years. If you have a heavy discharge with an odor, especially if the odor is slightly "fishy," it is important to get this evaluated and treated.

As with trichomoniasis and other STDs, if a woman is infected with BV she is more susceptible to becoming infected with the AIDS virus (HIV) if a man she has intercourse with is infected with HIV. Some studies suggest a three times greater risk.

605 What are monilia vaginitis, candidal, yeast, or fungus infections? How are they treated?

Monilia vaginitis, also called fungus or yeast or candidal infection, is a very common vaginal infection. A woman who has a fungus infection will usually have itching, ranging from mild to severe. The vulvar area may be red and often thickened from the woman's scratching. Though this infection can be very irritating, it does no permanent damage to a woman's body, nor is it dangerous during pregnancy.

Examination by the physician shows a cheesy, white discharge, which can be identified as fungus by putting a fleck of the white secretions on a slide, applying a drop of potassium hydroxide and looking at that under a microscope. What the doctor sees is an organism that looks like a tree branch with no leaves; he or she may also see small, round spores that look a little bit like holly berries stuck to the branches.

Occasionally a patient will have enough infection to cause her to have itching without the fungus showing up on a smear. In this case the doctor may want to do a culture to prove that monilia is the culprit. A culture is fairly reliable for detecting the presence of the fungus organism, but even then there are women who are bothered by a fungus infection when a culture is negative. This situation may require several cultures to find the infection. Sometimes it is best for a woman to just try vaginal candidal medication. If this clears the infection, it was probably *Candida*. If the infection comes back, she may need to go back to her physician for reevaluation.

Treatment for fungus infection is with drugs such as Monistat or Gyne-Lotrimin. (These are now available without prescription.) Normally a seven-day course of nightly vaginal applications takes care of the infection. A woman can also apply some of this medicine over her vulva. This not only soothes the area but also helps kill any infection that might be developing on the vulvar skin. A pill taken by mouth called Diflucan (fluconazole) can have as much benefit as one week of the vaginal creams. The cost for the one pill is about the same as a tube of cream. Since the effectiveness is about the same, it probably doesn't matter which you use. Diflucan does require a prescription.

Some women have persistent fungus infections. Occasionally these recur because a woman is predisposed to the development of fungus infections. For example, pregnancy is a situation in which infections will often return soon after treatment has been completed. Diabetics and those who have poor immunity because of being on immunosuppressive agents (such as a kidney recipient) or those who have some other condition that affects their immunity will have problems getting rid of a fungus infection. Markedly debilitated women, weakened because of cancer or old age, will also have trouble getting rid of fungus infections.

Persistent vaginal candidal infection can be the first sign in an otherwise unsuspecting woman that she has AIDS. If you are having a continual problem with vaginal candidal infections, and you (or your husband) have been involved in activity that might make you at high risk for AIDS, contact your doctor so you can be tested for HIV.

For many years physicians thought that a woman on oral contraceptives was more likely to develop vaginal fungus infections. Recent studies have shown that this is probably not true. In spite of those studies, if I have a patient who takes oral contraceptives and cannot get rid of her vaginal monilia, I suggest that she try stopping her oral contraceptives for a few months to see if she gets better; occasionally this seems to help.

Some women will continue having fungus infections, even though they have none of the above problems. Apparently their bodies just grow fungus easily. Chronic fungus infections can be one of the most frustrating problems women can have. Some suggestions in the next answer may help if you have this problem.

A man may occasionally have penile or skin irritation (a form of "jock itch") from fungus infection. If he has such an irritation, he can use some of his wife's medication on himself once or twice a day.

Candida vaginitis is not a classic sexually transmitted disease, but a person with a candidal infection can infect his or her sexual partner.

606 What is the treatment for persistent candidal infection?

A study in 1992 showed that if women consumed yogurt daily, it markedly decreased the amount of monilia in their vaginas and markedly decreased the number of vaginal infections they suffered. If a candidal infection does not clear up with this and other treatments (see previous question), other techniques may be helpful. Before trying them, ask your physician about giving you a prescription for terconazole (Terazol), a new antibiotic for candidal infections. It is used in the same way that Monistat, Gyne-Lotrimin, or similar medications are used. One technique for a woman with a persistent infection to follow is to use the antibiotic cream every day for four to six weeks, followed by the use of one of the medications for two or three days at the beginning of the menstrual period for six months, or even indefinitely.

In addition, medication should be used for an entire week whenever there is any discomfort or itching.

If the irritation persists in spite of the above-mentioned treatment, the woman can usually keep it under control by inserting fungus medication into the vagina every two or three days indefinitely.

If the woman is having external irritation, the medicine should be put not only in the vagina but also on the vulvar tissues. The fungus medicine that the woman uses should be applied to the man's penis every few days also. He needs to get it under the foreskin if he is not circumcised. One good technique is to have intercourse within a few hours of a vaginal application of fungus medication.

Another form of treatment, an inexpensive one, is the use of boric acid capsules vaginally. You can use 600 mg of boric acid in capsules twice daily for two weeks. (Your pharmacist can make the capsules for you.) If you are still uncomfortable, repeat the treatment. If the fungus persists, use 600 mg of boric acid in capsule form in your vagina once daily during your period only for four months, or a capsule high in the vagina every third night for 12 months or longer. Recent test results indicate that this procedure has helped 98 percent of women with yeast infections to eliminate them.

Any time antibiotics are taken, the same vaginal fungus medication should be used during the entire time the antibiotics are taken. As far as is known, these medications are safe for indefinite use, even during pregnancy.

Finally, since it is felt that fungus organisms are harbored in the rectums of some people, drugs should be taken by mouth to clear up such organisms. There are two medications for this: Mycostatin and Nizoral. Your doctor would need to give you a prescription for one of these if this seems to be a factor.

For persistent vaginal monilia some experts advocate Ketoconazole (Nizoral) 400 mg by mouth daily for two weeks, followed by a half tablet (100 mg) daily for twelve months or longer. This treatment is expensive and can cause hepatitis. It should be used, therefore, only if nothing else works and then only with close medical supervision.

607 How is vaginitis treated if it is caused by a sexually transmitted disease such as gonorrhea, herpes, or chlamydia?

The most important thing concerning such infections is that you tell the doctor if you think there is any possibility that you have a sexually transmitted disease. If you think there is a possibility that your husband may have had intercourse with someone else, tell your doctor so that you can be checked for infection. Don't let embarrassment keep you from being truthful with your doctor so that you can receive good medical care; delay could cause your body unnecessary damage.

I often have patients who say that it is impossible for them to have a sexually transmitted disease because their sexual partner has not had intercourse with anybody else for at least two or three months. Such a statement indicates ignorance of sexually transmitted disease. If you have intercourse with anyone who has had relations with anyone else, even several years ago, he can still give you the germs that can cause you to contract a sexually transmitted disease. If you have questions about this, read chapter 13.

608 My doctor says that my IUD is causing my discharge. Is this possible?

Yes, an IUD (intrauterine contraceptive device) can cause vaginal discharge. Some women can use an IUD for several years without any problems and then suddenly begin having a discharge. In this case it is best to remove the IUD. In some women, IUDs can set up an irritation of the lining of the uterus that causes discharge. This may actually be a low-grade infection.

If you develop this type of discharge and do not want your IUD removed, your doctor may want to take secretions for a culture and treat you with antibiotics. Be sure and tell the doctor if there is a possibility of STD. If this does not stop the discharge, it may be best for you to have your IUD removed. If such a discharge is caused by infection, getting rid of the IUD would be best, since it would allow the uterus to clear itself of such infection.

609 Is there anything other than infection or disease that might cause an abnormal vaginal discharge?

There are two other causes of vaginal discharge that should be mentioned, although both are relatively rare in the United States. These are discharges caused by a hole from the vagina into the rectum (rectovaginal fistula) or by a hole from the vagina into the bladder (vesicovaginal fistula). The discharge associated with these fistulas is irritating, bothersome, and offensive because of the continual drainage of urine or feces into the vagina.

610 What are the causes of vesicovaginal fistula? How is this treated?

In undeveloped countries the most common cause, and unfortunately, a very common problem, is erosion of the wall between the vagina and the bladder, caused by the pressure of the baby's head on these tissues in extremely prolonged labor. In the United States a vesicovaginal fistula (hole from the vagina into the bladder) is usually a result of a hysterectomy or of surgery to repair a loose, relaxed vaginal wall.

If your gynecologist suspects a vesicovaginal fistula, he or she might suggest that you see a urologist. This specialist would look into your bladder to detect a hole and would probably order X-rays of the urinary tract for the same reason. In addition, your doctor might have you insert a tampon, drink colored water, and check the tampon later to see if the color has come through a hole into your vagina. This is all done to detect a vesicovaginal fistula.

The treatment for a vesicovaginal fistula is surgery. It is important that the doctor who does this performs it carefully and with great expertise. Since this problem occurs rarely in this country, few doctors have extensive experience in repairing such fistulas. Good gynecologists can do a competent job, however, if they will study the available literature to determine the best surgery for your particular problem.

611 What causes a rectovaginal fistula? How is this treated?

The most common cause of a rectovaginal fistula (hole from the vagina into the rectum) is an episiotomy. No matter how well an obstetrician sews up an episiotomy, occasionally it will break open, either partially or completely. The opening can be through a part of the episiotomy, or the entire episiotomy can tear open into your rectum so that you have no control of your stool.

Other causes of rectovaginal fistulas can be from treatment with radiation for cancer of the cervix (this can occur up to ten years after the radiation treatment has been used) and from a diverticulum (an outpouching of the colon) eroding into the vagina.

If there is any suspicion of a leak of stool into the vagina, your gynecologist will probably consult with a proctologist, a specialist in colon and rec-

tal disease. This specialist will look into your rectum to see if an opening can be seen, and X-rays might be ordered in an effort to detect a hole. The gynecologist, of course, would have already looked into your vagina to check for a hole, but sometimes an opening is so small that it cannot be easily detected.

The treatment for a rectovaginal fistula is the same as for a vesicovaginal fistula: surgery. It is important that careful, competent technique be used for repair of a rectovaginal fistula. The best chance of cure is for the surgical operation to be done correctly the first time. In spite of great care and skill, however, a fistula can break down after an operation and would then require further surgery.

612 Can my vagina be "too loose"? What causes this?

Yes, a woman can have vaginal looseness. Physicians call this pelvic relaxation or, if a woman has had a hysterectomy, vaginal relaxation. Pelvic relaxation has multiple causes. It is commonly present in women who have had children, since childbirth stretches the vaginal tissues. Some women have had many children with no pelvic or vaginal relaxation, however, so childbirth is not always the cause. Some women seem to have inherited weak tissues. Some women seem to have vaginal relaxation because their tissues are weak from poor nutrition. A good example of this is that women who smoke have a greater chance of having vaginal relaxation. Women who are overweight have more problems with pelvic relaxation. Excess weight seems to push the vaginal tissues down.

An overweight woman with vaginal relaxation can sometimes avoid surgery if she will lose weight. The loss of weight can release some of the pressure that tends to push the vagina down and out.

Vaginal relaxation seems to worsen with age. As a woman's vaginal tissues get thinner, they get weaker and tend to prolapse more. Using estrogen after menopause can help keep those tissues from weakening. Exercise also seems to help keep the tissues healthier and stronger, decreasing the chance of pelvic relaxation.

There are several symptoms of this problem. (See the symptoms listed in the next question.) Occasionally the symptoms of pelvic relaxation are much worse than those listed. The uterus may lose its support and fall down far enough in the vagina so that the cervix will actually protrude. In some situations the entire uterus will hang out of the vagina. At times the vaginal walls will bulge out of the vagina, causing a woman to actually sit on her prolapsed vaginal tissues when she sits down. When problems of this sort develop, it is best to have surgery. Women with this condition are almost always uncomfortable enough to ask for surgery. In fact, when uterine prolapse is this severe, if it is not corrected, much more major surgery may be necessary later, as it gets even more severe.

Physicians will often irresponsibly recommend a hysterectomy with vaginal repairs for women who feel perfectly fine. The doctor recommends this merely because the patient's uterus has dropped down some and her vagina appears loose on examination. Surgery for looseness that is not bothering you is absolutely unnecessary. It does not matter how many children you have had nor how relaxed your vagina may appear to a physician nor that your uterus has fallen—you do not need surgery to repair it unless it bothers you. You do not have to have surgery just because it might get worse later.

613 What problems might result from vaginal looseness?

There are several symptoms or problems with vaginal looseness.

Looseness with intercourse. A relaxed vagina may seem to be very "open," resulting in decreased friction with intercourse. This lack of friction can result in less stimulation with intercourse, both for you and for your husband. The looseness may also cause an embarrassing gush of air in and out of the vagina during intercourse. This is a bothersome but not a dangerous problem.

Pelvic pressure. Vaginal looseness, with its associated protrusion of the bladder and rectal walls into the vagina and prolapse of the uterus, can cause a feeling of pelvic pressure. This may be especially noticed when a woman has been on her feet for several hours.

Loss of urine with coughing, sneezing, or laughing. It is normal for a woman to lose some urine occasionally with a hard sneeze or laugh. If this happens often, however, and is a real problem for a woman, she should consider having vaginal repairs. I have had patients stop exercising because of loss of urine while walking, jogging, or doing aerobics. It is much better to have the tissues repaired than to stop living a healthy, normal life.

Inability to have a bowel movement without finger pressure ("splinting"). If you are unable to have a bowel movement without using your fingers to put pressure on the rectal wall, you probably have looseness of the back wall of the vagina (rectocele). If you have this problem, the first thing to do is to start eating more fiber—either unprocessed wheat bran, Metamucil, or a similar product. If you still need rectal splinting with looser and softer stools, you may need rectal wall repair.

Pain with intercourse. When the vaginal walls are very relaxed and the uterus has lost its support, it can tend to fall down or even "fall out" of the vagina. When the uterus is this low in the vagina, there may be discomfort with intercourse when the penis pushes against the uterus.

614 What do the terms cystocele, rectocele, and enterocele mean?

A cystocele is a relaxation of the front wall of the vagina. This wall is actually made up of the lining of the vagina plus the lining of the bladder. When they become loose and bulge down into the vagina, a woman is said to have a cystocele. This bulge can actually protrude outside the vagina. A woman can occasionally feel this protruding tissue if she touches her vulvar area when she stands or pushes down. When the problem becomes severe, a cystocele may constantly protrude outside the vagina.

Surgery to repair a cystocele is called anterior vaginal colporrhaphy. (Anterior means toward the front of the body; colporrhaphy is the name used for repair of the vaginal wall.)

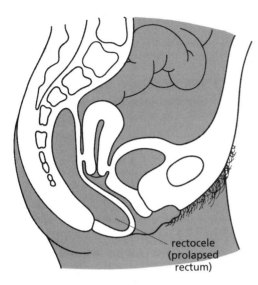

rectocele
(prolapsed
rectum)

A rectocele is a weakness of the back wall of the vagina. The back wall is made up of the vaginal lining plus the rectal wall lining. When there is a weakness of these tissues, the vaginal wall bulges forward and is said to be rectocele. The repair for this condition is called a rectocele repair, or a posterior vaginal colporrhaphy.

An enterocele is a hernia inside the pelvis. It occurs behind the uterus and in front of the rectum. Pressure of the intestines in that area can push down between the uterus and the rectum and on down between the vagina and the rectum so that a sac exists there. The primary problem with an enterocele is pressure. The pressure from an enterocele can cause a lot of discomfort. (It is not a dangerous hernia, like an inguinal hernia can be.) Often a physician is not aware that an enterocele is present until it is discovered during pelvic surgery for vaginal reconstructive repair. A physician can usually tell by physical examination before surgery that there is some possibility that an enterocele is present.

615 I have heard of Kegel's exercises for vaginal looseness. What are they?

If a woman has pelvic relaxation she will rarely have just one problem. Usually she will have two or three problems. She may have a feeling of pelvic

pressure and also have stress incontinence. She may have a uterus that descends so that she can feel her cervix protruding slightly out of her vagina and also have a rectocele. If she has pelvic relaxation, unless her tissues are actually protruding outside of her vagina, I suggest that she try Kegel's (pronounced Kay´-gulls) exercises.

The late Arnold Kegel, M.D., clinical professor of gynecology at the University of Southern California School of Medicine, developed strengthening exercises for the pubococcygeus muscles. These muscles are shaped like a sling that goes from the front to the back of the pelvis and holds the abdominal and pelvic contents up in place. The urethra, vagina, and rectum are like tubes poking down through this sling of muscle to get to the outside. When these muscles become weak, the vagina, rectum, and urethra lose their support. Strengthening these muscles can give better support to those tissues.

The exercise consists of doing the same tightening movement (and holding it for a second or two) that you would make if you would purposely stop your urine flow. One does not need to be urinating to tighten these muscles. To learn which muscles need to be contracted for Kegel's exercise, it is helpful for a woman to begin urinating and then shut off the flow by tightening her muscles. Once she has discovered which muscles are

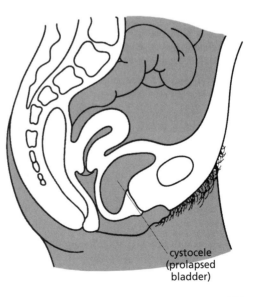

cystocele
(prolapsed
bladder)

tightened to stop urine flow, she has discovered how to do a Kegel's exercise! I encourage a patient to think in terms of tightening the muscles all the way around to her anus also, so that, in essence, she is tightening her whole "bottom" when she does the exercise.

616 Are Kegel's exercises effective?

If a woman will do these exercises for twelve weeks, she may gain the vaginal tightness she wants and can stop doing the exercises. If the same symptoms return, a woman can do the Kegel's exercises again for just a week or two, or she may need to do the full twelve weeks again. It takes real commitment, however, to do the exercises effectively and consistently, and some women may need to do them on a regular basis indefinitely to benefit from them.

A woman needs to do three hundred contractions a day. I suggest to my patients that they do them in six groups of fifty each. These exercises can be done while riding in a car, watching TV, or even while having intercourse. Kegel's contractions during intercourse can be quite stimulating to a man but can be a distraction for the woman.

In all honesty, I find that most women will not do these exercises adequately. Many who have done them do not get much improvement in pubococcygeal muscle strength. Others, however, do find them a great deal of help, and I continue to recommend these exercises to patients.

Women who do Kegel's exercises often have an unexpected pleasure in store: better sexual responsiveness. Dr. Kegel became interested in this aspect of his exercises when some patients returned to him to say that although they had never had an orgasm before, after doing his exercises they became orgasmic. Therefore, books dealing with sexual problems will often suggest Kegel's exercises as a partial solution to failure to achieve orgasm.

A woman may purchase a device (inserted into the vagina) for electrical stimulation of her pubococcygeus muscles. It is about twice the size of a tampon and is called the Intimate Trainer. It may be ordered by calling (888) 303-0123. It can make

development of strong pubococcygeus muscles easier.

617 If vaginal exercise does not stop the vaginal relaxation, is there anything else besides surgery that might help?

There is a device called a pessary that can be put into a woman's vagina. One type of pessary fills the vagina so completely that it pushes the rectal and bladder walls back into position and holds up the uterus; another type pushes the uterus up but does not hold the vaginal walls in place. (Occasionally a large tampon will hold the tissues in better position, but the continual use of a large tampon can cause an ulcer of the vagina to develop or perhaps cause toxic shock.)

If a pessary is used, the entrance of the vagina must be tight enough to hold it in place. If it is not, the pessary will fall out. Pessaries come in different sizes and must be fitted by a physician.

My experience is that pessaries are not acceptable to most women. They irritate the vaginal walls and almost always cause a discharge that becomes foul smelling and almost intolerable. If a woman is so debilitated that she cannot tolerate surgery for vaginal prolapse, a pessary might be helpful, but this device is almost never the answer for women who are healthy and active.

618 Is the problem of vaginal relaxation treated by surgery?

Most women who have pelvic relaxation and the symptoms listed in Q. 613 will finally decide to have surgical repair. This type of surgery is not generally done until a woman has had all the children she wants because ordinarily it is best to have a hysterectomy done with the repairs. The procedure in this case then is usually a vaginal hysterectomy with repairs of either the front wall of the vagina if there is bladder prolapse (cystocele), or the back wall of the vagina if there is a bulge of the rectal wall (rectocele), or of both front and back walls of the vagina. For some women, removal of a prolapsed uterus is all that is necessary.

If a woman chooses to have corrective surgery for vaginal looseness, she should have it done by a physician who will do it carefully and properly. Some doctors are so proud of their ability to do surgery quickly that they do not take the time to carefully sew the bladder and urethra back in place or to meticulously rebuild the back wall of the vagina in such a way that the vagina has appropriate size for intercourse. Occasionally, even if the surgery is done properly, the tissues can quickly lose their support again and all the symptoms a woman had previously will recur.

If your tissues are healthy and you have a good surgeon you will probably experience excellent results from this type of operation. Although there is some discomfort for a few days after surgery, most patients do not find it a terribly uncomfortable procedure.

The surgical technique and recovery from this problem is partially described in Q. 135–137.

When the operation is done to repair a cystocele (the front wall of the vagina that is under the bladder) or a rectocele (the back wall of the vagina, over the rectum), the vagina can become tighter. This tightness can cause pain with intercourse. It may take many months for intercourse to be comfortable again, because the scar must soften and become elastic after the vaginal surgery. I always tell my patients that they can expect to have some pain with intercourse for about a year.

The discomfort of intercourse following vaginal surgery is not usually severe, but it can be bothersome, especially if a woman does not expect it. It may seem that the vagina has been made too tight, but time and patience will solve the problem. Actually the end result is for the woman's vagina to dilate to the size that she and her husband need for tighter but comfortable and more pleasurable intercourse.

After a cystocele repair, a woman may be unable to void for several days or even weeks. Either case is normal. To empty the bladder, a woman will need to wear a catheter until she is able to void on her own. Some physicians put in a suprapubic tube that goes through the skin, above the pubic bone, and into the bladder. This procedure is not painful, because it is done while the woman is still under anesthesia. It is generally painless to have

the suprapubic catheter in place, and its removal is also painless. A suprapubic catheter does not damage a woman's bladder and allows drainage of urine without a woman having to wear a urethral (Foley) catheter, which is more uncomfortable. A woman must wear some type of catheter till she can adequately empty her bladder when she urinates. Getting rid of the tube or catheter will be under the physician's direction.

619 I have heard that there are new surgical procedures for the problem of loss of urine. What are they?

Many conditions cause the problem of leaking urine, and we cannot discuss all of them in this book. The condition we are concerned with is stress incontinence—leaking urine with coughing, sneezing, laughing, or exercise. This condition can generally be corrected surgically.

There are many other bladder problems that cause women to leak urine that often can be easily corrected nonsurgically by a urologist. For instance, many women leak urine just because they have a full bladder. Some women have such urgency to urinate that even a small amount of urine in their bladder will leak if they don't rush to the bathroom. Some women have a problem called interstitial cystitis. If you leak urine, see a urologist and determine what the problem is. If it is stress incontinence, surgery will probably be necessary.

The objective of the surgeries designed for urine control is to elevate the urethra where it enters the bladder so that it is higher than the lowest part of the base of the bladder as seen when a woman is lying down and also to compress the urethra with surrounding tissue. When a woman leaks urine, she has usually lost the support of this portion of her bladder and urethra. Stress incontinence can be treated by one of several types of surgery. If a woman has a cystocele, a bladder repair done through the vagina (anterior vaginal repair) is usually the recommended procedure and has the best chance for stopping the loss of urine.

If an anterior repair does not seem to be the best procedure, a woman may need a retropubic suspension of the urethra (and sometimes the bladder also). This means an operation is done with an incision in the abdomen just above the pubic bone with the urethral and bladder surgery being done behind that bone. This type of operation can sometimes be done with the laparascope to make it a more minor operation.

The standard operation (still done more than any other) is called the Marshall-Marchetti-Krantz procedure. Newer procedures that accomplish much the same things are also done. These include the Burch and paravaginal operations. Needle operations such as the Stamey, the Stamey-Martins, the Pereyra, or the Raz are also done.

Another new procedure for this problem is the injection of collagen into the vaginal tissues under the urethra. The bulky collagen under the urethra elevates it, producing the same effect as surgery. You need to be aware that the decision to use this procedure may not be a simple one. However, it is a useful technique in certain special situations.

Your physician will probably have an approach that he or she feels is best. If you know your physician is a good surgeon, is careful, and has had good results with similar surgery with other women, you are probably better off having your gynecologist do the surgery than trying to chase down the very latest and most up-to-date operation. At a conference on urogynecology and pelvic surgery presented at the Medical College of Virginia, in Richmond in 1991, R. Peter Beck, professor of obstetrics and gynecology at that college said that if a physician does an operation that elevates the urethra and compresses it, good results are obtained no matter which technique is used. A gynecologist should use the technique he or she is most familiar and most comfortable with.

620 I've heard that women who have had bladder repairs usually start leaking urine again. Is this true?

It is possible for a woman who has had one bladder repair to start leaking urine again. This may happen for a couple of reasons.

First, if a woman has had bladder repair that did not stop her loss of urine, her problem may

have been something other than stress incontinence. She should see a urologist for evaluation.

Second, some surgeons do seem to have better results than others. If you have had an operation to stop your loss of urine and you have started having leakage of urine again, perhaps it would be good to get a second opinion about the problem. A urologist would be a good choice.

It is important to remember, though, that all surgeons who do this type of surgery will have some patients who start leaking urine again even when they have done the operation correctly. If you trust your gynecologist and you know that he or she usually has good results, perhaps you should stay with that physician if he or she feels that a solution can be found.

If urologic examination shows that your bladder is functioning normally and your loss of urine seems to be caused by problems that surgery can correct, you may need to have another operation. Careful consultation and planning with your physician is important before another operation is done.

621 I had a vaginal hysterectomy with repairs, but now my vaginal tissues are beginning to protrude from my vagina again. Is there anything that can be done?

Some women will have vaginal repair that is successful in stopping their loss of urine, but they will later notice that they are having vaginal tissue protrude from their vagina again. The bladder (or the rectum) might start bulging slightly out of the vagina. Occasionally, however, a great deal of tissue will start protruding again. At times the entire top of the vagina will come down as though the vagina is turning inside out and is protruding far outside of the vagina.

If you have prolapse of the vagina, be sure you are seeing a good gynecologist who can give you a very thorough evaluation of your problem before you allow him or her to operate on you again.

Occasionally, all a woman with this problem needs to do is have a repeat repair of the front or back vaginal wall, but some women have a more complicated problem than this. There are several procedures for correcting these more complicated situations. These repairs are done vaginally or abdominally, or as a combination of these two types of operations. Your doctor will usually have a procedure that he or she prefers, is most comfortable with, and one which gives good results for your particular problem. For example, in an operation done through the vagina, the upper vagina can be sutured to some ligaments inside the body (a sacro-spinous ligament fixation of the vagina). Another operation that seems to work well uses a synthetic, plastic mesh to tie the top of the vagina to the sacrum. This operation requires an incision but is usually more reliably permanent than the vaginal operation.

One factor for deciding on which type of vaginal or abdominal repair to select is that of sexual activity. If you are sexually active, your physician must choose a surgical procedure that will not only give support to the vagina but will also allow you to continue to have normal intercourse. This will often involve an abdominal incision to suspend the vagina from above in some way.

If a woman is not sexually active and knows she never will be again because of age and/or marital status, her physician may plan to do the operation through the vagina by doing extensive repairs to the front and back walls of the vagina. These procedures are usually simpler than those done with an abdominal incision but will usually leave the vagina too tight for intercourse. Be frank with your doctor about this.

Another matter to consider concerns estrogen. If you were not using estrogen before your first surgical operation for vaginal relaxation problems, I urge you to start using vaginal estrogen cream. This cream can make your vaginal tissues healthier and less likely to prolapse again.

It is a great disappointment to have surgical repair of the vagina be unsuccessful. Unfortunately, the human body is not a totally perfect machine; this is true especially in older women whose tissues have begun getting thinner. I encourage you, however, to have surgery again if that is what it takes for you to feel well and be active. You need to feel comfortable and healthy so that you can exercise, have normal intercourse if desired, and be free from discomfort.

622 What types of growths can occur in the vagina?

There are a number of different types of growths that occur on the vaginal walls. Premalignant and malignant growths can develop (see Q. 627–629) as can nonmalignant growths and cysts. These do not occur often, but when they do, they are usually easily diagnosed and treated. The most common growths that occur in the vagina are: cysts and polyps, endometriosis, adenosis, and condyloma.

A growth that is uncomfortable, protrudes from the vagina, or causes any problems can be surgically removed. Such surgery usually requires general anesthesia. After surgery the patient ordinarily has minimal discomfort and no long-term pain with intercourse. For further information on the above growths and treatment, see the next five questions.

623 What is a Gartner's duct cyst?

Of the cysts and polyps that can occur in the vagina (fibro-epithelial polyp, leiomyoma, dermoid cysts, and Gartner's duct cysts), the most common is the Gartner's duct cyst.

A Gartner's duct cyst seems to arise from tissue "left over" from fetal life that would have been part of the sperm-carrying tubes if the fetus had developed into a male. It has recently been found that many of these cysts come from remnants of female-type fetal tissue that lines the vagina rather than male-type tissue. These tissues generally lie dormant as mere fragments of tissue resting in the vaginal walls. Occasionally, though, enough of this tissue may be present to collect fluid and form a cyst. This type of cyst is known as a Gartner's duct cyst.

Gartner's duct cysts are not painful, but they can be quite large and there can be more than one of them. They do not become malignant, and if they do not bother a woman, surgery is not indicated.

Your doctor can usually tell the difference between a polyp and a cyst by looking. If you are told that you have a polyp or growth in your vagina, you should have it removed even if you cannot feel it. However, if the doctor tells you that you have a "cyst" that needs to be removed, and it is not causing you any pain or discomfort, you should ask if it is a Gartner's duct cyst. If it is, you can feel quite confident in telling your doctor that you do not want it removed. If he or she insists, it would probably be best to get a second opinion.

624 What is endometriosis of the vagina?

The most common cause of this condition is endometriosis inside the pelvic structures that has grown down through the vaginal wall behind the uterus into the vagina. This would mean that a woman has fairly severe endometriosis. Such endometriosis can cause pain with intercourse, and a woman will often have vaginal bleeding from it. She would ordinarily not know this, however, because she would usually bleed only during her period, at which time she could not differentiate between endometriosis bleeding and the menstrual blood from her uterus. A woman with vaginal endometriosis may have more symptoms, such as pain with intercourse or pain with menstrual periods, than a woman whose endometriosis is contained inside her pelvic structures.

Occasionally a woman may have vaginal endometriosis because the endometrial tissue that comes out with her menstrual flow can "seed" onto the vagina or into the episiotomy at delivery and start growing there. Such endometriosis would usually be treated with the laser, a freezing instrument, or by excision with scissors or knife.

If the endometriosis is perforating through the upper vagina from inside the pelvis, treatment is much different. The doctor may want you to try Danocrine or Lupron, hormones that can cause the endometriosis to stop growing. These drugs, however, can be taken for only six months; then the endometriosis usually starts growing again.

Treatment may be a combination of these drugs and surgery. Occasionally the endometriosis can be so extensive that a hysterectomy, with removal of the area of vaginal endometriosis, is necessary. (The tubes and ovaries are usually removed also as with any complete endometriosis operation.) Such endometriosis can often be removed without a hysterectomy. For further information about endometriosis, see Q. 138–140 and Q. 849–856.

625 What is adenosis?

Adenosis is a condition in which small areas of the normal vaginal lining are replaced by a lining similar to that of the cervical canal. Most of the time adenosis occurs in women who were exposed to DES in their mother's womb, but occasionally women who have not had such exposure can have small patches of adenosis in their upper vaginas. (See Q. 166.)

Most women who have adenosis are not even aware of its presence. The first indication they have of the problem is usually during a checkup when a doctor sees a patch of pink or red tissue on the vaginal wall.

Most physicians feel that treatment is unnecessary for these small areas of adenosis. However, just as a doctor watches your cervix for the development of cancer, so will he or she watch your adenosis. You do not have your cervix removed just because there is a possibility of developing cancer of the cervix. Likewise you do not need to have adenosis taken out just because it is structurally similar to the lining of the cervical canal and thus capable of cancer.

Occasionally, however, adenosis can cause a discharge just as the cervix can cause mucous discharge. If this does not bother a woman, she can leave it alone. If it does become a problem to her, she can have it treated. The laser can "wipe away" this adenosis much like a pencil eraser erases pencil marks. This is by far the best treatment. If your doctor does not have access to a laser, he or she can cut out the area or use a freezing machine to get rid of it. However, this is not nearly as successful and as free of complications.

Your doctor will probably suggest that you

have a general anesthetic for the procedure. The laser (a machine that emits an extremely hot ray) vaporizes away the abnormal tissue and yet leaves the tissue immediately under that abnormal tissue undisturbed and undamaged. As healing takes place the normal vaginal lining covers the area where the adenosis was treated. Healing is faster after laser treatment than after either freezing or surgical excision.

My principal warning concerning adenosis is that if you have it and are having no trouble with it, you can afford to be a little skeptical about any suggestion to have it removed. If a doctor insists on its removal, you should probably get a second opinion.

626 Are precancerous or cancerous growths in the vagina common?

Both precancerous and cancerous growths can occur in the vagina, but they do so rarely. Their frequency has increased during the past thirty years, however, just as the frequency of cancers of the vulva and cervix has increased, apparently due to the rising incidence of sexually transmitted HPV infections. (See the section on HPV.)

Precancerous changes of the lining of the vagina are called vaginal intraepithelial neoplasia (VAIN). In the past, these abnormalities were more likely to occur after menopause. However, they are now occurring at younger and younger ages apparently because of the sexual spread of HPV.

627 How is a precancerous or cancerous growth of the vagina discovered?

Precancerous (see Q. 584) or cancerous growths of the vagina might show up as abnormal vaginal bleeding—bleeding after intercourse, between periods, or after menopause—or as red or brown vaginal discharge. Most of the time, however, precancerous growths are found on routine Pap smears, with no symptoms having occurred.

Cells that cause an abnormal Pap smear can come from the cervix but they can also be from the vaginal walls. If a Pap smear is abnormal, the physician will do a colposcopy (see Q. 659) to magnify the cervix. As the cervix is viewed, the doctor will usually look carefully at the vagina with the colposcope. The physician is usually surprised to see an abnormal area in the vagina because abnormal cells on a Pap smear are so much more likely to come from the cervix. When it is discovered, it is biopsied, just as would be done with abnormalities of the cervix. Because the area is magnified, only a very small piece of tissue is necessary for an adequate biopsy; therefore such a biopsy is not very painful.

628 How is a precancerous vaginal growth treated?

If the doctor finds a precancerous growth of the vagina, treatment is necessary to keep the growth from becoming cancerous. The treatment that seems best at this time is laser therapy (see Q. 584), which can be used to wipe away this type of growth on the vaginal wall without penetrating the important underlying structures of the body. Other treatments are available. If the area is small, the doctor might want to cut it out. Or a doctor might suggest the use of a cream containing an agent (5-fluorouracil) that will kill cells. This cream can be quite irritating. If you use it you should also use a lot of Vaseline on the vulva to avoid irritation.

629 How are cancerous growths of the vagina treated?

If your doctor is not an expert in the treatment of vaginal cancer, he or she should refer you to an experienced physician in that field. Such a specialist is called a gynecologic oncologist.

The main reason for great care in this treatment is that radiation is usually used, and if not given properly, it can cause holes between the vagina and the bladder or between the vagina and the rectum. (See Q. 609–611.) Also, surgery is occasionally indicated for this type of cancer. It is major surgery and the decision as to whether or not to do surgery or use radiation is a critical one. This decision should be made by doctors who have had a great deal of experience with this type of cancer.

Vaginal cancer has been found in women who were exposed to DES in their mother's uterus. Because DES affects several parts of the female organs, it is discussed in Q. 164–168.

Most vaginal cancers occur in women who have (or had) precancerous or cancerous cells on the cervix or vulva. It is important, therefore, that careful vaginal examination be done during each annual checkup, especially if a woman has previously had cancer of the cervix or vulva.

Also, if a woman has had a hysterectomy for precancerous cells of the cervix—but her doctor did not do a colposcopy before surgery to find out exactly where the abnormal cells were—she should be even more meticulous about having follow-up Pap smears, because before the surgery some precancerous cells could have already spread out onto the vaginal wall and have been left behind to continue growing even though a hysterectomy was done.

630 What is toxic shock?

Toxic shock is a condition caused by a bacterium called *Staphylococcus aureus*. The most commonly held theory concerning toxic shock is that when this germ grows in the body of a male or female who does not have natural immunity (antibodies) against the germ, it produces a chemical called a toxin that spreads through the body and causes severe illness.

Toxic shock occurred more often when women used high-absorbency tampons. When these tampons were taken off the market the risk of tampons causing toxic shock decreased dramatically. With the tampons available today, the risk of toxic shock is extremely small. To help decrease even that small risk, change tampons at least every six to eight hours.

Foreign objects such as a vaginal sponge, diaphragm, and tampon are all associated with toxic shock. It seems best that those objects not be left in the vagina any longer than necessary.

Although 5 percent of reproductive-age women have *Staphylococcus aureus* germs in their vaginas, the large majority of these women are immune to the toxin that these staphylococci can produce. Though the toxic shock syndrome can occur, it certainly does not occur very often. The chance of a reproductive-age woman developing toxic shock syndrome is about 10 out of 10,000 per year.

It is important to understand that the *Staphylococcus aureus* germs occur in both men and women, and that their growth and release of toxin can affect them both. Toxic shock syndrome has been reported in both men and nonmenstruating women. Toxic shock has been identified in patients who have staph infections in burns and abrasions, lacerations, abscesses, insect bites, surgical wounds, vaginal deliveries, and abortions.

631 What symptoms might indicate toxic shock syndrome? What is the treatment?

There are a number of symptoms of toxic shock syndrome. A woman may have all these symptoms or only a few of them, and they may be mild or severe enough to cause death. The symptoms that a woman may watch for, especially during a menstrual period, are these:

fever	dizziness
chills	fainting
vomiting	sore throat
diarrhea	sunburnlike rash

In addition, a woman may have a rash on the palms of her hands and the soles of her feet. After a few days she will notice that her palms and soles are scaling (desquamating).

If a woman develops these symptoms, and if they go away and recur when she has another menstrual period, she should see her doctor and suggest that she might have toxic shock syndrome. About 3 percent of toxic shock cases reported have resulted in death. This figure should not alarm you unduly, however, because many of the milder cases are not even reported to doctors, and even when they are, the doctor often does not report them to the local health department.

If you report toxic shock symptoms to your doctor, he or she will want to take a culture from your vagina to see if *Staphylococcus aureus* is present. Even if the doctor cannot culture out the organism, treatment with appropriate antibiotics may be prescribed.

---

632 Are vaginal injuries common? What things might injure my vagina?

Vaginal injuries, though relatively uncommon, can occur in the following situations.

Tampons. Some women develop ulcers in their upper vaginas from the use of tampons. Usually they are not aware of such ulcers and learn of them only at the time of their routine exams. Occasionally a patient will have a little bleeding from such an ulcer and the ulcer will be found when she is examined by her doctor. Such ulcers do not seem to be dangerous and clear up when a woman stops using tampons. Once the ulcer is gone, a woman may resume use of tampons if she desires, but she needs to change the direction and depth of insertion. She should see her gynecologist after a couple of months to be sure she is not producing another ulcer.

Intercourse. On rare occasions a vagina can be torn during normal intercourse. Symptoms of such a tear are pain with intercourse followed by bleeding from the vagina. The only time I have seen this in my practice was in a young woman whose upper vagina was torn because of very forceful penile entry the first time she had intercourse. A doctor may or may not need to stitch the torn area.

Rape. Injuries of the vagina can occur with rape, but this is normally a problem only in young girls who have not yet begun their menses.

Sharp objects. Falling on a sharp object can cause vaginal lacerations. If this occurs, a woman would see her doctor for evaluation. He or she would suture any torn area, if necessary. Normally such suturing requires general anesthesia.

Tears. Tears of the vagina occur most commonly during delivery. This type of injury was discussed in Q. 523. A competent obstetrician will be able to repair any vaginal tear to insure good healing and minimal loss of blood.

If you (or your daughter) have a vaginal injury, it is important that you seek medical help and that the physician do a gentle, complete examination. Such an exam, especially of a child, will often require general anesthetic. (See Q. 43–45, 595.)

Occasionally an injury to the vaginal area will result only in a large bruise, called a hematoma. It does not normally need to be drained since such blood will usually be absorbed. If the hematoma is too large, however, the doctor may need to open it to let it drain. General anesthesia may be required.

---

633 Is it normal to have pain during intercourse? Should I tell my doctor about it?

If you are having pain with intercourse (dyspareunia), tell your doctor. This type of pain is probably not an indication of a serious problem, but it should be dealt with. Pain with intercourse can usually be relieved.

Occasional pain with intercourse is normal. When your husband pushes into the upper part of your vagina with his penis, it may sometimes catch your uterus, your ovary, or your colon in just the right way to cause pain. This type of pain may be a sharp stabbing sensation, sudden severe cramping, or just a pain deep in your pelvis. The pain may persist for a while (a few minutes or a few hours), but usually goes away fairly quickly.

Often, all a man or woman needs to do to stop this type of pain is to shift position a little bit during intercourse. If the pain is more intense, more constant, and more bothersome than the above so-called normal pain, a woman should certainly have the problem checked.

A recent study showed that the most common age for women to have painful intercourse is from thirty to fifty-five years. The conclusion from this study was that as women fall into an intercourse routine through the years, they become less stimulated, have inadequate lubrication, and begin having superficial discomfort with intercourse. Women in this age group are often embarrassed by the fact that they are experiencing pain with intercourse. They should, however, tell their doctor of such pain.

Intercourse should be gratifying and pleasant; if you are having pain it cannot be all it should be. More importantly, if you are having pain with intercourse you will subconsciously avoid it. Such a problem can trigger conflict between you and your husband because he will feel that you are rejecting him, even though you explain the problem to him.

If you are having discomfort with intercourse, it is important that you discuss it with both your husband and your doctor.

634 What things can cause painful intercourse, and what can be done to solve these problems?

The problems that can cause pain with intercourse and the solutions for these problems are discussed in the next six questions. They are:

fear of intercourse
vaginal dryness
vaginal infections
physical problems
childbirth-related problems

The size of a man's penis almost never causes continued painful intercourse. The vagina can stretch to accommodate whatever size penis a woman's husband has. This is illustrated by the fact that the vagina stretches enough to allow the passage of a baby's head in delivery.

Some women also believe, because they have been told so, that painful intercourse is caused by a tipped or retroverted uterus. One-third of all women have a tipped uterus. It is a perfectly "normal" position for the uterus and is almost never the cause of painful intercourse.

635 Can fear, or aversion, actually cause intercourse to be painful?

Yes. Some women have not dealt well with their sexuality and enter marriage with a distorted view of their bodies, sex, or men. There are many reasons why a woman might enter marriage unpre-

pared for the intimacy with a man that is necessary for comfortable, enjoyable sexual activity. The independence and self-assertiveness that is so valued by our society can be a factor in this. Distorting or failing to understand the healthy biblical view of sex can color a woman's attitude toward sex. A lack of adequate sex education can inhibit a healthy sex life. Finally, doctors are finding more and more that women who have aversion to intercourse, with related problems, often have that aversion because of previous rape or sexual molestation.

Many experts who write about sexual problems often attribute such difficulties to a woman being "overly religious" and inhibited. Actually, it has recently been shown that the healthier a woman's relationship with God is, the happier will be her sex life. (See chapter 14.)

636 What can be done to help overcome fear of, or an aversion to, intercourse?

It is important that every couple planning marriage have premarital counseling and that every woman have a pelvic examination before marriage. Such counseling and exams can eliminate most of the concern about intercourse that couples have on entering marriage.

After marriage, if there is pain with each act of intercourse after several weeks, you need some help or you could end up with a serious marital problem. First, you should see your doctor and have another examination to be sure that there are no abnormalities in your pelvic structures. Your physician may suggest some logical approaches to the problem. One of these suggestions may be having your husband come to the doctor's office with you, so that the doctor can show you or your husband how to gently dilate your vagina with fingers or with progressively larger vaginal dilators. As soon as you are able to tolerate three of your fingers or the largest dilator, you may be able to resume intercourse comfortably.

If the doctor is not successful in helping you, or doesn't know how to help, you should be referred to a good sexual counselor. (See Q. 1020.)

637 If vaginal dryness is causing painful intercourse, how should this be treated?

Vaginal dryness can result from inadequate lubrication. It is normal for a woman to have less lubrication immediately after a period, after menopause, and if she is not very sexually excited. If discomfort during intercourse is only a result of poor lubrication at those certain times, you can assume that you are normal. Merely use a lubricant (Maxilube, Ortho's Personal Lubricant, Replens, Lubrin) when you need it.

If such lubricants do not solve the problem for a postmenopausal woman, she may need to use some estrogen cream (Premarin, Ogen, and so forth) in her vagina.

I usually recommend to my patients who use estrogen cream that they put one-half applicator full of the cream in the vagina three times a week at night. It may take up to nine months for this cream to make the vaginal lining as thick and healthy and strong as it was before menopause, but it will usually make a big difference with intercourse. (Vaginal estrogen cream is absorbed into the body. It is much like taking a hormone pill three times a week.) If you still have your uterus and you start using estrogen cream, you should consider taking Provera, 2.5 mg a day, to decrease the chance that the estrogen cream can cause your uterine lining to become cancerous.

Before you begin to use estrogen creams, read the section in this book on menopause and hormones to understand how hormones work.

638 When vaginal infection causes pain with intercourse, what should be done?

The vaginal infection that most often causes pain with intercourse is monilia vaginitis. (See Q. 605.) Trichomoniasis, which can cause itching in the vagina and vulva, can also cause pain with intercourse. In addition, genital warts (condyloma) located at the entrance to the vagina can cause painful intercourse.

A vaginal infection should be treated by a doctor. When the infection is cleared, the pain normally stops.

639 What other physical problems might cause painful intercourse?

1. Low-grade PID (pelvic inflammatory disease). If a young woman is having deep pain with intercourse, she may have a low-grade pelvic inflammatory disease caused by chlamydia or gonorrhea. It is vital to have this diagnosed and treated as soon as possible. If this low-grade infection continues, it can cause sterility. (See the section on PID.)

The diagnosis of PID can require a laparoscopy. (See the section in this book on laparoscopy.) The laparoscopy can be done as an outpatient procedure and can help the physician determine if there is any PID or other significant disease in a woman's pelvis. Without the use of laparoscopy a physician can fail to identify and treat PID about 50 percent of the time.

2. Other Causes.
With first intercourse, the hymen separates into small projections of tissue that are left just inside the entrance to the vagina. These segments of hymenal tissue occasionally become irritated or tender. If this irritation continues, the tag of tissue could probably be removed in the doctor's office.

A Bartholin's gland infection can also cause painful intercourse. (See Q. 591–592.)

Congenital abnormalities of the hymen and vagina can cause pain, especially with first intercourse. A doctor can find problems of this type at the premarital examination.

An IUD can cause painful intercourse. (See Q. 909.)

Some of the most common causes of deep pain with intercourse are constipation, irritable colon syndrome, or spastic colon syndrome. As I talk with women who have pain with intercourse, I often find that they are having problems with their colon (see Q. 147). Usually these women have been told that they have abnormalities of their internal female organs and that they should have surgery. After they see a colon specialist or gastroenterologist and get their problem of constipation and/or irritable colon solved, their painful intercourse often goes away.

Deep pelvic pain can be the result of problems with the female organs deep inside a woman's body. It is relatively common for a sudden onset of severe pain during intercourse to be the first major sign of an ectopic (tubal) pregnancy. Occasionally women who have painful intercourse are found to have a growth on an ovary or in their uterus. There are at least three other pelvic problems that can cause painful intercourse.

Loss of uterine support. (See Q. 613.)

Endometriosis and adenomyosis. (See Q. 692–693.)

The treatment of a physical problem causing painful intercourse is, of course, based on the nature of the problem. The important thing is to see your doctor for a consultation and a pelvic examination.

If painful intercourse is related to prolapse of the uterus, or to tears in, or varicose veins of, the supporting ligaments of the uterus, hysterectomy may be necessary. Such a hysterectomy is done only for comfort and only when the patient asks for it. A patient certainly should not have a hysterectomy for this reason alone until she has had all the children she wants. If a woman does not want more children, a hysterectomy is the best treatment for most of these problems, assuming the pain is severe enough to warrant it.

If a patient wants more children and does not want a hysterectomy, the doctor may be able to provide some less effective treatment that can at least be a stopgap measure. A fallen uterus, for instance, can be suspended with a pessary. (See Q. 617, 697.) Tears in the supporting structures of the uterus can be sewn up with surgery through an abdominal incision; and endometriosis can normally be removed, leaving the uterus and usually at least part of an ovary and tube intact. If the pain is only intermittent, pain pills can be useful and may be all that is necessary.

640 What problems associated with pregnancy and childbirth can cause painful intercourse?

Many women find intercourse during the last two or three months of pregnancy uncomfortable and at times even painful, but it is not dangerous. Discomfort is due to the swelling of the vaginal and vulvar tissues and the fullness of the pelvic structures because of the presence of the baby and the enlarged uterus.

Episiotomies or tears of the vagina from delivery heal with some scarring. This can cause pain with intercourse and is usually worse if a woman is nursing (see below). If such pain persists for more than a year or two, it might be necessary for the doctor to cut out an area of scarring and try to sew it in such a way that there will be less scar remaining in the area. This is unusual, however, and I have done it on only one or two patients in my entire time of practice.

One of the most common causes of painful intercourse related to childbirth is that which occurs when a woman is nursing. While a woman is nursing, the pituitary gland suppresses the production of estrogen from the ovaries and stimulates the production of milk from the breasts. This inadequate estrogen causes the vagina to become dry and sensitive. In fact, this happens so often that I warn every nursing mother that she will probably have painful intercourse and should use a vaginal lubricant with sexual intercourse.

Problems of the Cervix

The cervix is the mouth—lower part, entrance—of the uterus. It is not just a "mouth," however. In newborn babies the cervix makes up five-sixths of the entire uterus! During adolescence, because of hormone stimulation, the upper part of the uterus (called the fundus) grows proportionately more than the cervix. By the time a girl starts her first period, the fundus is approximately equal in size to the cervix. When a woman reaches adulthood, and before menopause, her cervix represents the lower one-third of her uterus.

The cervix is not as passive as it might seem. When the cervix allows the flow of menstrual fluid from the uterus it is being passive, but its production of cervical mucus is an active process. Cervical mucus is the fluid through which the sperm swim up into the uterus to allow fertilization to occur. Through a wonderfully selective process, sperm are allowed passage through the cervix while most germs are not. Once ovulation is over, the cervical mucus becomes thick and sticky, sealing off the outside world so that, if a pregnancy occurs, it is safe from outside interference. (See Q. 62–66, 238–239.)

When pregnancy does occur, the cervix is able to stay closed until labor causes it to dilate. Before dilation, the cervix is so small that nothing larger than a small straw can normally go through its opening. It is so elastic, though, that labor can stretch it enough to allow the passage of a full-term baby.

The elasticity of the cervix allows it to close back up after delivery so that within just a few days, nothing—not a tampon, a penis, or anything larger than one-eighth of an inch in diameter—can normally get into the uterus through the cervix!

Both before puberty and after menopause, the cervix is relatively inactive; it does little more than protect the inside of the uterus by the small amount of thick mucus it produces. (For more information on the cervix see Q. 14.)

641 Do I need to do anything in particular to keep my cervix healthy?

There are three things you can do to help insure that your cervix stays healthy and normal.

Have intercourse only with your husband. Since precancerous and cancerous changes of the cervix, herpes, gonorrhea, and many other problems are sexually transmitted, you will probably not contract these if you and your husband have intercourse only with each other. (See Q. 657.)

Have a pelvic exam and Pap smear done yearly. The Pap smear is a screening procedure that can help prevent your developing cancer of the cervix, and the examination can make sure that you do not have polyps or growths on the cervix. (See Q. 652–660.)

Have your doctor leave your cervix alone if it doesn't need treatment. If treatment is necessary, make sure as little as possible is done to your cervix. (See the next question.)

642 What conditions of the cervix might better be left alone?

Three fairly common conditions better left alone are: cervical erosion (ectropion), leukoplakia, and Nabothian cysts. These are discussed in the following three questions.

643 What is cervical erosion?

The technical terms are *ectropion* and *eversion*. When a doctor looks at your cervix, he or she will often see a reddish discoloration immediately around the opening of the cervix. This is most commonly called an erosion and is a normal finding; it is the lining from inside the cervix spreading out from the cervical opening onto the external surface of the cervix. The color of this epithelial lining from the inside of the cervix (columnar epithelium) is more red than the lining of the rest of the external cervix (stratified squamous epithelium) because it is more delicate and its small blood vessels are closer to the surface. The juncture of these two linings (squamocolumnar junction) is usually a distinct and abrupt line that makes a circle around the opening, or just inside the opening, of the cervix. It is the red color of the columnar epithelium that led to this tissue being erroneously named *erosion*. It is more properly an *ectropion* or, if a woman has had a baby in the past and the cervix tends to gape open, an *eversion*. However, erosion is in common usage, even by physicians.

Let me repeat, though, that this finding is normal and does not need any treatment so long as the Pap smear is normal and there is no cervical infection producing excessive, bothersome amounts of mucus. Routine treatment of a normal ectropion, therefore, accomplishes little, and most physicians who have studied this situation feel that routine freezing or cautery of a cervix that is otherwise normal is a waste of a patient's money and is not the best practice.

644 What is leukoplakia of the cervix?

Leukoplakia means "white patch." Occasionally a woman will have an area of the cervix that looks as though someone has painted it white. When this occurs, the same approach should be taken as is recommended for cervical erosion—nothing.

In years past, leukoplakia was thought to be premalignant, but we now know that it is not. A Pap smear will ordinarily be able to scrape off the white patch and enough underlying cells to assure you and your doctor that the white patches are normal. The doctor may want to use the colposcope to look at the area, and may even want to biopsy it. This is good practice. Your doctor does not need to do a conization (excising a wedge of tissue) or hysterectomy because of these white patches. As a matter of fact, he or she does not need to do anything to get rid of leukoplakia permanently. At most, the patches just need to be evaluated each year.

645 What is a cervical Nabothian cyst?

It is fairly common for a woman to find a small hard nodule on her cervix. It may be discovered in feeling around in the vagina for a "lost" tampon, in checking for an IUD string, or in making sure a diaphragm is in the right position. If you feel a nodule, you can be fairly sure that it is a Nabothian cyst. I have never found a nodule discovered by a patient to be anything else except a Nabothian cyst or, rarely, a wart of the cervix.

Nabothian cysts on the cervix are extremely common. They are like acne of the face in that they are glands, in this case mucous glands, with their openings stopped up, trapping the mucus and forming small, round nodules. Since these are not precancerous, dangerous, or painful, they do not need to be treated. They may vary in size from pea-sized to a half inch in diameter.

Cervical cancers, by the way, are usually soft growths that bleed easily. It is unlikely that a woman would be able to feel a cervical cancer until it had gotten extremely large, perhaps as much as half the size of a hen's egg. By this time she would have had abnormal vaginal bleeding for weeks.

646 Can my cervix become infected? What should be done if it does?

Yes, the cervix can become infected. Such an infection is called cervicitis. A discharge of mucus (similar to what you might have from your nose with infected sinuses) might indicate a cervical infection. This type of discharge does not ordinarily cause itching but it may have an unpleasant odor.

The only way that you can know for sure whether or not you have a cervical infection is to see your doctor. When you are examined, it may be found that your cervix is slightly swollen, red, and producing infected mucus. Often when the doctor touches the infected cervix, it will bleed easily. In fact, you may have had bleeding after intercourse as a result of this infection.

The doctor will usually want to do both a Pap smear and cervical cultures. The most common cause of cervical infection is sexually transmitted disease. (See chapter 13, "Sexually Transmitted Disease.") The most common infections that will cause a cervicitis are gonorrhea, chlamydia, and trichomoniasis. If you are not married and have had sex, or if you or your husband have had sex with someone else, tell your doctor because you could have been infected with a sexually transmitted disease. It is important that sexually transmitted infection of this type be found because these germs can grow up into your uterus, tubes, and ovaries and cause major problems.

If your cervical infection persists for weeks in spite of good care, your doctor may want to do a biopsy because cervical cancer can look like, and produce the same type secretions as, cervicitis. A Pap smear is occasionally unreliable when taken from a cervical cancer that is far enough along to produce infected-looking discharge because the Pap smear may pick up only the mucus and no cancer cells.

After the physician has completed the evaluation of your cervical infection, you will be treated according to what has been discovered. If the doctor has found a sexually transmitted infection, that will be treated. If the cultures are negative, and if

Cervical Biopsy

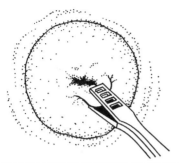

If the colposcope reveals an obvious abnormality of the cervix, small pieces of it may be removed for microscopic examination.

the doctor is sure there is no cervical cancer, your infection will probably be treated with a vaginal cream containing an antibiotic. If the infection persists, he or she may need to treat your cervix with an instrument that kills the infection by freezing the area (a cryocone). The doctor may prefer using the laser on your cervicitis, especially if you have not had all the children you want. This is because the laser leaves less scar on the cervix as it heals. Occasionally doctors will use cautery on the cervix. This is an acceptable but slightly outdated treatment. In unusual circumstances, a new procedure called LEEP might be used. (See Q. 663.)

If your cervix is markedly infected, the doctor would almost always treat you with medication first. To use the cryo, laser, LEEP (loop electrosurgical procedure), or cautery on an inflamed cervix could cause the infection to flare up, producing a dangerous cervical infection.

---

647 What types of benign (nonmalignant) polyps and growths can be present on the cervix?

There are four: cervical polyps, endometriosis, fibroid tumors, and genital warts.

These conditions are discussed in the following four questions.

---

648 What is a cervical polyp? How is it treated?

The most frequent type of benign abnormality that occurs on the cervix is a cervical polyp. These polyps are usually small (up to one-fourth inch in diameter); they are red and usually bleed easily when touched; and they are not usually dangerous. Most of the time women do not even know that they are present, and the doctor may discover them protruding from the cervical opening at the time of an annual exam. Occasionally a woman will experience bleeding with intercourse as the first indication of a cervical polyp.

Benign polyps are normally a result of mild and unimportant infection in the glands of the cervical canal. This type of infection does not need to be treated, is not dangerous, and is merely producing an irritation of the glands in that area of the cervix.

To treat a polyp, all a doctor needs to do is to grasp the growth with an instrument and snip it or twist it off. There is almost no bleeding or pain with this procedure. Such polyps may or may not grow back. If they do recur, it is not an alarming sign. They merely need to be removed again.

Premenopausal women seldom have cervical polyps that are malignant, although they can occur. A cervical polyp that is found in a postmenopausal woman is more likely to be a malignant growth because cancer of the inside of the uterus (endometrium) is more likely to occur in postmenopausal women and to show up as a polyp at the cervical opening.

---

649 What is cervical endometriosis? How is it treated?

Women normally do not know they have endometriosis of the cervix unless told so by their physicians.

Diagnosis and treatment consists of a biopsy, to be sure it actually is endometriosis. Such a biopsy usually removes the entire growth. Occasionally a biopsy must be followed by use of the freezing machine, cautery, or laser to destroy all the abnormal tissue.

This condition is not common and is usually not a problem, though extensive cervical endometriosis can be a factor in a woman's infertility.

650 What are cervical fibroid tumors? How are they treated?

If a woman has fibroid tumors growing inside her uterine cavity, the uterus will try to "deliver" that fibroid by contracting and working it down and out of the uterus, resulting in abnormal vaginal bleeding. The fibroid may even finally protrude from the cervical opening. When this happens, its blood supply may be partly pinched off, causing the fibroid to swell.

This type of problem frequently requires a hysterectomy. The fibroid may be attached so high in the uterus that it is impossible to take it out without doing a hysterectomy. Occasionally, however, a fibroid will be so small that the doctor may be able to put a wire loop around it, run the loop up to the base of the fibroid inside the uterus, and pinch the base off. This must be done under general anesthesia in the operating room. Bleeding can be so heavy from an attempted vaginal removal of such a fibroid that a hysterectomy is necessary.

If your doctor suggests a hysterectomy for this problem and you have all the children you want, it is probably best to have it done. If you definitely want to remain fertile, and the doctor cannot get the fibroid out through your vagina, he or she may be able to use a hysteroscope to look up inside your uterus to cut the fibroid at its base, or if that is not possible, to make an incision in your abdomen, cut your uterus open, and remove the fibroid at its base. (See Q. 681.)

651 What are cervical genital warts?

Genital warts (or condyloma) can grow on the vulva, vagina, or cervix. Most of the time condyloma are a sexually transmitted disease caused by HPV. Sometimes a patient will have condyloma that are not transmitted by sexual intercourse. (See Q. 968–972.)

652 What is a Pap smear?

A Pap smear is a scraping of the surface of a woman's cervix or vagina transferred to a glass slide. The scrapings are taken by the doctor with a blunt wooden or plastic stick or with a brush after visualizing the cervix and vagina with a vaginal speculum. A chemical solution (fixative) is put on the smear before it dries and this preparation is sent to a pathologist.

There are cells from a woman's cervix or vagina in the material that was scraped off, preserved, and sent to the laboratory. If the surface from which the scraping was taken was normal, the cells will look normal to the pathologist. If the cells have been affected by trichomoniasis, or are inflamed by some other infection, the pathologist can often tell that. If there is a premalignant (see Q. 584) or malignant growth, the pathologist can usually recognize this type of cell.

The Pap smear is named after the late Dr. G. N. Papanicolaou who found, in 1943, that cancerous and precancerous cells could be discovered with a screening test of this kind. The annual Pap smear became a reality for most women during the 1950s, and it has served to prevent cervical cancer in many women since then.

The surface cells of the body are continually sloughing off as new cells from underneath are growing. The cells that are sloughing off are the ones that are picked up by a Pap smear. If there is a precancerous or cancerous growth present, this area sloughs off cells at a much higher rate, perhaps ten or fifteen times as many cells as the normal tissue around it. This explains why even a small precancerous or cancerous growth on the cervix or vagina can be picked up by a Pap smear.

653 Will a vaginal or cervical Pap smear show if I have cancer in any other part of my body?

No. A vaginal or cervical Pap smear is useful only for identifying cancer of the cervix or vagina. It does not usually discover cancer of the uterus (endometrium). Abnormal cells of the cervix almost always start at the squamocolumnar junction, where the lining of the vagina meets the cells that line the inside of the cervix. This small area, often a ring of no more than one-half inch, is the origin of almost all the precancerous and cancerous cervical growths that women develop.

To understand the tremendous amount of cellular growth and activity going on in the cervix, compare the fact that this area (about the size of one of your fingernails) is responsible for cancer in 2 percent of the female population, while the breasts, which are many hundreds of times larger by comparison, are responsible for cancer in 9 percent of the female population.

654 Does a Pap smear hurt?

For many patients a Pap smear is painless. For some women a Pap smear will be painless one year and uncomfortable another year. For others, it will always be uncomfortable. Whether or not it is painful has more to do with the degree of sensitivity of a particular woman's cervix or with how nervous a woman is than it does with the technique that a doctor uses in obtaining the Pap smear.

A Pap smear should be taken from both the outer part of the cervix and from the cervical canal (the opening into the uterus). If the doctor does not scrape both places, he or she is likely to miss a precancerous growth. It is the scraping from the canal that is most likely to be uncomfortable, but it is a vital part of a good Pap smear.

655 How often should a Pap smear be done?

A Pap smear should be done annually. If you have had a hysterectomy, however, a Pap smear every three years is adequate, because a hysterectomy removes the cervix, the most likely source of cancer detectable with a Pap smear.

If you had an abnormal Pap smear for which you were treated, your doctor may suggest that you have Pap smears more frequently for a while. For instance, if I have treated a patient's cervix for precancerous changes with the laser or with freezing, I will have her get a Pap smear every three months until she has had three normal Pap smears. Then I will do one six months later and, if that one

is normal, I will have the woman come back every year for a routine Pap smear. If I have a patient who had a precancerous growth on her cervix resulting in a hysterectomy, I will follow the same pattern, and I do a Pap smear at every annual exam indefinitely.

Having annual Pap smears is wise because the number of women developing abnormal Pap smears is increasing markedly, especially among younger women. This is directly related to the sexual spread of HPV. (See Q. 657, 973.)

About 5 percent of precancerous growths on the cervix will be aggressive, fast-growing tumors. This 5 percent group will be so aggressive that within a year or two these growths can progress from the very earliest precancerous stage to invasive cancer. In 1980 we were unaware that such a large percentage of patients could have such fast-growing tumors.

If a woman has had a hysterectomy, a Pap smear at least every third year is a good idea because it can detect vaginal cancer. If a patient has had a hysterectomy, the doctor would scrape the upper vagina, an area much less likely to develop cancer than the cervix.

656 Can a Pap smear be done while I am having my period or bleeding from the uterus?

Most of the time Pap smears are quite reliable if taken while a woman is bleeding. The fixative that is put on the smear breaks down the red blood cells so that they do not interfere with the pathologist's study of the slides. Because of this, if a patient is having her period when her appointment for a Pap smear rolls around, she can keep her appointment. Many women are a little embarrassed to see their gynecologist while they are having their period, but your doctor sees much more vaginal bleeding when a woman is having a miscarriage or having a baby than with your menstrual period. If you can tolerate an exam during your period, it surely will not bother your doctor.

657 Is cervical cancer related to sexual intercourse?

Yes, it often is. Precancerous or cancerous changes of the cervix are usually a result of the sexually transmitted virus, HPV. It has now been shown that the risk for a woman's developing cervical precancerous or cancerous change is directly related to the number of sexual partners that she has had. If she has had two sexual partners, she has doubled her chance of having this type of change of her cervix. If she has three sexual partners during her lifetime, she has three times the normal risk. This risk pattern continues up to as many sexual partners a woman might have, increasing the chance of having abnormal cells of the cervix by the number of sexual partners a woman has had.

More than 93 percent of cancerous and precancerous growths of the cervix are caused by (HPV) human papillomavirus. (See Q. 973.)

There is a difference between abnormal Pap smears that show truly precancerous or cancerous cells and abnormal Pap smears that show some irritation or inflammation. These Pap smears are not "truly abnormal" indicating precancerous change. Many women who have Pap smears reported as mildly abnormal do not have any precancerous changes (this is discovered with colposcopy and biopsies). This type Pap smear is not associated with sexual activity or HPV at all and is not dangerous. If your cervix has had some inflammation present and a healing process is going on, the healing cells that are produced are growing quite rapidly and can also appear to the pathologist to be somewhat abnormal.

658 If I have not had intercourse, do I need to have a Pap smear done?

Virginal patients can develop a cervical cancer. This is very rare but because of this possibility most doctors advise all women to begin having Pap smears at about the age of twenty.

I recommend a yearly pelvic exam and Pap smear for virginal women beginning at about age twenty (just as I do for married women who have never had sex with anyone but their husbands and their husbands only with them). We do not know all there is to know about this subject yet and there are always factors to consider, such as whether or not a partner is unfaithful or untruthful. In addition, the yearly Pap smear is a good reason to see your doctor on a regular basis. It is just one part of the complete physical examination that is recommended for maintaining good health.

659 What should be done if I have an abnormal Pap smear?

Fortunately, today the investigation of an abnormal Pap smear is much simpler and involves surgery much less often than in the past. For an abnormal Pap smear, the following plan for diagnosis will be followed by most gynecologists and is the plan that I feel is best.

Colposcopy. The doctor will insert a vaginal speculum and will swab your cervix with acetic acid. (This is the same acid at about the same strength as in vinegar.) The acetic acid will cause the abnormal areas of the cervix, vagina, and vulva to become whiter than the surrounding tissue and make them easier to see. With a colposcope the doctor will be able to find the area of your vagina or cervix that is producing the abnormal cells in this way.

When this area is identified, the doctor will use biopsy instruments to take a small piece of the worst part of the abnormality and will also often scrape the lining of your cervical canal (an endocervical curettage). This procedure checks for abnormal cells in the cervical canal, an area that cannot be seen with the colposcope.

There is usually some mild bleeding. The doctor may put a swab against your cervix to compress the area and slow the bleeding.

Colposcopy is not a very painful procedure for most women. Since the cervix is magnified so greatly, it is possible for the doctor to take only minute pinches (biopsies) of tissues. The endocervical scraping hurts a little, but it requires such a short time to do that most women tolerate the brief discomfort.

Conization. Most of the time a colposcopy is all

368

that is needed. There are several situations, however, in which a conization might be necessary:

If the doctor cannot see all areas of your cervix adequately or has some question about what is actually seen.

If the squamocolumnar junction (where the linings of the vagina and cervix meet) cannot be seen.

If there is any question on the pathologist's report following a colposcopy.

If the scraping from inside the cervical canal shows precancerous cells.

If there is any suspicion that invasive cancer is present.

All these things would make a colposcopy unreliable and make a conization necessary. (See Q. 662.)

660 If I continue to have abnormal Pap smears but the colposcopy and biopsy findings are normal, what should be done?

Often when a woman's Pap smear is only slightly abnormal, the colposcopy and biopsies will be normal. In this case the problem is probably just inflammation. If this condition persists for many months, the patient should have a cryoconization, vaporization conization, or LEEP therapy (see next question) to get rid of the inflammation. When this is done, the Pap smear usually reverts to normal, ending all the worry.

661 If my colposcopy is considered reliable and shows that I have a precancerous condition of my cervix, what should be done?

In this case, the cervix can be treated with several techniques.

Cryoconization. This procedure is called a *cryocone* because the area killed with the freezing probe is similar to that which would be excised by knife with conization (as described in Q. 662).

Cryoconization involves freezing the cervix for about seven minutes. This is done in the doctor's office without anesthetic and is a painless process for most women. After the cervix is frozen, there is a fairly heavy, messy discharge for about a month. I usually have patients refrain from intercourse for three weeks after cryoconization.

Occasionally, as a cervix heals from cryoconization, the cervical opening gets very small (stenotic). This tight cervical opening can make it difficult for a repeat colposcopy to be done if abnormal Pap smears develop again. This can make it necessary for a surgical conization to be done if such abnormal smears develop in the future, and all of this surgery on the cervix can interfere with future fertility.

Laser therapy. This is called a "vaporization conization" because a cone-shaped area of tissue is removed from the cervix by vaporization with the laser, just as a cone-shaped piece of tissue is removed from the cervix with a knife with surgical conization. In the past the laser seemed to be the best method of treatment for the cervix. The disadvantage of the use of the laser is that laser therapy is more expensive and is not universally available in the United States.

I suggest that my patients who have precancerous cervical cells choose laser or LEEP therapy (see Q. 663) if they have not had children or have not completed their families whenever they have a CIN III, (severe dysplasia or carcinoma in situ: equivalent to a Pap III, IV, or V) or if they have a less severe precancerous growth that covers a large area of the cervix. I recommend the laser and LEEP rather than freezing because the cure rate with a single treatment seems to be higher and there is less damage to the cervix.

Vaporization conization (laser treatment) and LEEP heal quickly. Normally there is very little discharge and a patient can usually begin having intercourse after three weeks.

I recommend that a husband and wife not have intercourse for about three weeks after either cryoconization, laser therapy, or electro-surgical loop procedure of the cervix. This allows the cervix a chance to heal some before intercourse takes place.

662 What about surgical conization?

If the cells that were scraped out of your cervical canal at colposcopy were shown to be abnormal, or if there is any question about whether or not there is actually an invasive cancer, or if there exist any of the other problems mentioned in Q. 659, a conization should be done. A conization can usually be both diagnostic and therapeutic (in other words, can tell whether or not invasive cancer is present and, by excising the abnormal tissue, can cure the problem).

Conization (see illustration) is a simple procedure in which the doctor removes a cone-shaped wedge from around the opening of the cervix, including the cervical canal from the outer half to two-thirds of the cervix, and then sutures the cervix to stop the bleeding. To allow proper healing, it will probably be suggested that you not have intercourse for about a month following the procedure. Some doctors use the laser as a knife to cut out the cone. This requires fewer sutures.

The cone of tissue is sent to the laboratory for diagnosis. Ordinarily a doctor will do a D&C with a conization to make sure there is no cancer inside the uterus; that tissue is also sent to the pathologist.

About 10 percent of women who have a conization done will have some fairly heavy bleeding about two to three weeks after the cone is removed. Occasionally this bleeding will be heavy enough to require a transfusion and admission to the hospital for resuturing of the area. Do not think your doctor has done anything wrong if this happens. No matter how the procedure is done, or who does it, a conization will occasionally result in postoperative bleeding. It is not dangerous if you take care of it. All you need to do is let your doctor know if you start having heavier-than-normal bleeding any time after a conization. If you have bleeding heavier than the bleeding of a normal period, consider your bleeding to be abnormal and call your doctor.

A conization can result in such tight scarring (stenosis) of the canal of the cervix that problems can develop. Occasionally this can even interfere with fertility, although this problem is rare. Such tight scarring can cause a slight problem with dilation of the cervix when a woman is in labor. Again, this is unusual and can normally be taken

Conization

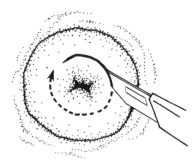

A conization removes a cone-shaped piece of tissue from the cervix for microscopic examination. The core is taken from the area around the opening of the cervical canal.

care of by the doctor stretching the cervix with his or her fingers during labor. Tightness of the cervix can also make it difficult to evaluate the cervix later if another abnormal Pap smear develops. In that case, a second conization may be necessary for a recurrent abnormal Pap smear.

After a conization is done, it is important that your doctor probe your cervix the next few times you are in the office to make sure it is staying open. There is the occasional patient whose cervix scars totally shut so that menstrual flow cannot get through. If this happens, further surgery may be necessary to get the cervix opened. This can be a frustrating problem that occasionally necessitates a hysterectomy.

A new procedure called loop electro-surgical excision procedure (LEEP) has replaced surgical conization in most situations.

663 What is the electro-surgical loop operation that is now being done for abnormal Pap smears?

In the past few years, the laser and freezing techniques for abnormal Pap smears have been almost totally replaced by electro-surgical loop excision of abnormal cells of the cervix. This procedure is called by different names, including LEEP (loop electro-surgical excision procedure) and LLETZ (large loop excision of the transformation zone). Whatever the procedure is called, it has great advantages over the previous treatments for abnormal Pap smears.

The loop electro-surgical technique can be done at the same time as colposcopy or after colposcopy results are back. When a woman has an abnormal Pap smear that needs to be evaluated, the doctor can do a colposcopy and, if needed, a loop procedure in the office. After staining the cervix with acetic acid and examining it with a colposcope if abnormal cells are found, a local anesthetic will be injected into the cervical tissues. Then the electro-surgical instrument (a thin loop of wire [an electrode] attached to an insulated handle) is used to cut out a relatively thin part of the cervix (a small "cone") that includes the squamocolumnar junction. There may be a small amount of bleeding, which can easily be stopped with simple cautery. A woman should be prepared for an unpleasant odor as the electrode cuts through her tissues. The doctor will probably use a smoke evacuator but some fumes can escape. The tissue that is removed is sent to a pathologist to be examined. Most of the time, all of the abnormal cells will be removed, and no other biopsies or treatment are needed.

The loop technique is an exciting breakthrough. It means that a woman no longer has to go to an outpatient surgical facility to have a laser procedure or a conization of her cervix. It saves time and money, and it does not have the disadvantages that accompany freezing the cervix. There is very little bleeding with the loop technique and it does not usually cause the cervix to scar shut.

Some studies show that this procedure cures 95 percent of women with abnormal Pap smears. If a woman still shows an abnormal Pap smear after the loop procedure, further evaluation and treatment are necessary. Another loop procedure could also be done.

664 What if my doctor suggests a completely different approach to an abnormal Pap smear than what you have outlined?

Treatment by your doctor should be compatible with the method of treatment listed in Q.

662. If it is not, you probably should get a second opinion.

Cervical cancer is serious enough to warrant taking the necessary precautions to avoid it or to have it treated correctly. On the other hand, the cervix is an important part of your body, and it is best to have as little done to it as possible. You should not let a doctor do conizations or other treatments to your cervix unless they follow thorough diagnostic techniques (colposcopy) and a straightforward plan of treatment is outlined.

665 What are some common errors that doctors make in relation to the cervix?

Because of their lack of understanding or because they let patients push them into doing things they do not want to do, doctors often make errors in their treatment of the cervix. Some of the most common of these are:

Overtreatment of cervical erosion, ectropion, or "red spots." Most of the time these areas are normal and need no treatment. Any doctor who has questions about them should do a colposcopy to view the cervix, biopsying if necessary. Only if true abnormalities are found is treatment necessary.

Allowing a Pap to stay abnormal. Many doctors do nothing about a mildly abnormal Pap smear. Cervical cancer, however, can be present when only a mildly abnormal Pap smear is found because of the debris and mucus that often overlie it. If you have even a mildly abnormal Pap smear, you should have it evaluated and treated until it becomes normal.

Treating for an abnormal Pap smear without prior colposcopy. Without colposcopy, a doctor cannot know where or how bad are the cells that have produced an abnormal Pap smear. It is most important that you not allow a doctor to freeze, cauterize, or laser your cervix because of an abnormal Pap smear without having first obtained a reliable colposcopy of your vulva, vagina, and cervix and biopsies of abnormal areas to be sure that you do not have invasive cancer. If you do have an invasive cancer overlooked and have it frozen, cauterized, or treated in some inappropriate way, it could spread farther in your body than it would if proper treatment had been started without delay.

Overtreatment of "severe dysplasia" or "carcinoma in situ." In years past, anytime a patient was found to have severe dysplasia or carcinoma in situ (CIN III), her doctor felt that she needed a hysterectomy. At that time colposcopies were not done, and conization was the standard diagnostic procedure for abnormal Pap smears. After a "cone," a patient would usually not have any more abnormal cells on her Pap smears. However, it was believed that a hysterectomy was necessary because the cells had been on the verge of invasive cancer.

We know now that a woman is no worse off having so-called severe dysplasia or carcinoma in situ (CIN III) than she is having mild dysplasia (CIN I). Both need treatment and both can develop into true invasive cancer if not treated. But if either condition is totally removed by treatment, there is no greater chance of recurrence on a woman's cervix for the more severe form than for the mildest precancerous condition (CIN I). A woman does not usually need to have a hysterectomy or a conization for the more severe forms of cervical intraepithelial neoplasia (CIN III).

Hysterectomy for cervical intraepithelial neoplasia (dysplasia). Hysterectomy is useful for a woman who has an abnormal Pap smear that has been reliably evaluated by colposcopy and biopsies, but only if she wants no more children and wants to have the hysterectomy. Such a woman can certainly request, and legitimately have, a hysterectomy. In any case, colposcopy should be done to make sure that she does not have invasive cancer and that her abnormal cervical cells have not spread off her cervix onto her vaginal walls. If she has invasive cancer, a simple hysterectomy is not adequate treatment. Even though it is not invasive cancer, if the precancerous cells have spread to the vaginal walls and a simple hysterectomy is done, the incision might cut across the area where the abnormal cells are, leaving some of them on the vaginal walls. With colposcopy the doctor knows exactly where the abnormal cells are growing and can either remove the lining of the upper part of the vagina at the same time he or she does the hysterectomy or use some other combined approach, perhaps the laser and hysterectomy.

666 What are the stages of invasive cervical cancer?

Once cervical cancer has become invasive, it is no longer a "skin cancer" of the cervix but has started growing down into the substance of the cervix. When this occurs your doctor will want to determine exactly how extensive this cancer has become in your body. There are four stages of cervical cancer.

Stage I. The cancer is confined to the cervix.
Stage II. The cancer has grown from the cervix into the surrounding tissues but has not yet extended out to the pelvic bones or into the lower third of the vagina or into the bladder or rectum.
Stage III. The cancer has grown to the pelvic bones or to the lower third of the vagina.
Stage IV. The cancer has grown outside of the areas involved in Stage III to involve other parts of the body, such as the intestines in the pelvic area or other distant parts of the body, or has grown into the bladder or rectum.

667 How is invasive cervical cancer treated?

The treatment of cervical cancer depends on which stage the cancer is in when it is discovered.

Most of the time the treatment for cervical cancer consists of radiation therapy. This is usually "combined therapy," which involves the use of radium in the cervix and uterus and then, either before or after that, external treatment with cobalt therapy or some similar source of external radiation given over a period of several weeks.

Radiation therapy of this type should be administered by someone well trained in its use. Even in the best of hands it can produce some annoying complications, such as a chronic irritation of the bladder due to the effect of radiation on the bladder wall. Irritation of the rectal wall can also occur. Even then competently used radiation therapy can produce some serious complications, such as holes between the vagina and either the rectum or bladder. The chance of this happening is much greater if you are not being treated by an expert in radiation therapy.

668 Is surgery ever used to treat invasive cervical cancer?

If a woman's cervical cancer is very early and has grown into her tissues less than 3 mm (about 1/8 inch), a simple hysterectomy can usually be done. It is very unlikely that the cells of this early cancer have spread anywhere else in her body. Surgery is occasionally used for cancer of the cervix that has invaded more deeply into the tissues, but only with Stage I or carefully selected Stage II cervical cancer.

The choice as to whether to use radiation treatment or surgery is made by a woman and her physicians. Normally the doctors will use radiation therapy, but they may have some good reasons for using surgery. The issues involved are so individualized and so numerous that it is impossible to discuss them fully here. It is vitally important, though, that any woman with cervical cancer be in capable hands.

669 Is it possible to cure invasive cervical cancer?

Yes. A woman can be cured, meaning she is free of any cancer after treatment. Overall cure rates with radiation therapy vary from 55 to 60 percent. Stage I cancer has an 80 percent chance of cure (but there is a much better cure rate if the cancer is very early [Stage IA]), Stage II, 60 percent chance of cure. For Stages III and IV there is much less chance of cure.

In spite of the availability of Pap smears, colposcopies, biopsies, and all the early detection procedures that we have talked about, cancer of the cervix is still the fifth leading cause of death from malignant disease among American women. Approximately 5,000 women die each year in the United States from this disease.

Problems of the Uterus

The clearest way to think of your uterus is to imagine that it is a large paper sack whose sole purpose is to hold a baby while it develops! Thinking of the uterus in this way cuts through all the mystique about the uterus (womb) and its role in a woman's life.

The uterus performs its one job, childbearing, well. We can rightly be amazed at God's creative genius in producing a body part that functions so perfectly in the performance of its task. The lining of the uterus (the endometrium), for instance, must develop daily in a precise way during a woman's menstrual cycle to receive and nurture a fertilized egg. It must allow the fertilized egg to implant itself, and this must occur without excessive bleeding since that could interfere with implantation. In addition, the uterus must be elastic enough to allow the growth of the baby and strong enough to perform the labor that will result in its delivery. Further, the contractions that cause delivery must not start too early or too late, and after delivery the lining of the uterus, which has had enormous amounts of blood flowing through it to provide nutrition and oxygen for the baby, must immediately stop all significant bleeding or the mother would die from blood loss. Finally, the lining of the uterus must heal quickly, so that the whole cycle can begin again.

The uterus is a receiver of hormones. These hormones, produced by the ovaries, enter the body's general circulation and are brought back

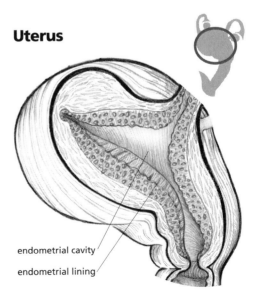

Uterus

endometrial cavity

endometrial lining

to the uterus after being pumped through the heart and blood vessels.

So far as we know today, the uterus itself produces only two hormones: prostaglandins and prolactin. Prostaglandins produce many of the symptoms that women feel with their menstrual periods: uterine cramping, bloating, and irritability. Prostaglandins also produce the uterine muscle contractions that help control the amount of menstrual blood flow during a period and are also involved in the contractions of labor.

Prolactin, which is secreted by the lining of the uterus, is produced in significant amounts only during pregnancy. The function of uterine prolactin seems to be confined to the uterus for local action. No one knows exactly what it does, but it may be responsible for allowing implantation of the fertilized egg on the wall of the uterus. Since the body's usual source of prolactin is the pituitary, a blood test done for prolactin checks the amount of prolactin from your pituitary gland (located at the base of your brain), not the amount produced by your uterus.

As the uterus is involved in such varied activity, it stands to reason that it is subject to medical problems. We will discuss these problems in this chapter. (See also Q. 124–137. Because hysterectomies often involve operations on organs other than just the uterus, a discussion of that surgery best fits into chapter 4.)

670 Do I need to give my uterus any special care?

The uterus requires no special care. It is self-cleaning, self-regulating, self-programmed. If you are maintaining sound whole-body health care and hygiene (including monogamous sex), if your menstrual periods are in the normal range (see Q. 672–675), and if you are conscientious about seeing your doctor for problems and annual check-ups, you are doing all you need to do to keep your uterus in good working order.

Some studies suggest that if women douche they are more likely to develop pelvic inflammatory disease. An excellent article on this subject was published in the *Journal of the American Medical Association* (1990, 263.1:1936). A woman may decrease the chance of developing PID if she does not douche.

671 Is there anything I should do for a tilted uterus?

There is only one thing to do about a tilted uterus—do not worry about it! One-third of all women have a uterus that is tilted back toward their backbone (retroverted); the other two-thirds have a uterus tilted forward. A retroverted uterus is no more different from a uterus that is tilted forward than a long nose is from a short nose; both are normal variations in the way a body can develop.

I frequently see new patients who are worried about a tilted uterus, usually because a previous physician told them their uterus was tilted. I reassure them that this is neither an abnormality nor a medical problem.

You should not let a doctor operate on you simply because your uterus is tilted back. If you are having painful intercourse or pelvic conges-

Positions of the Uterus

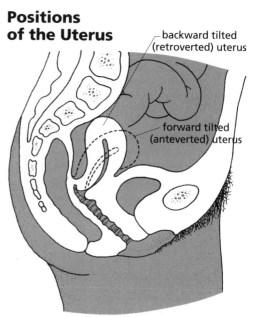

Positions of the uterus. About one-third of all women have a uterus tilted toward their backbone (retroverted). The remaining women have a forward tilted (anteverted) uterus. Both positions are normal.

tion and have been told it is due to a tilted uterus, be skeptical about such a simple answer. These things occur whether or not a woman's uterus is tilted backward.

Obviously, if a woman has pelvic pain that is caused by a problem of her uterus, she may need to have surgery. Even if her uterus is involved in her pain, however, it is almost never because the uterus is tilted. If your physician is convinced that you have a markedly retroverted uterus and that it is causing (or contributing to) your pain, you can have a uterine suspension. Don't be surprised, though, if you still have pain since a tilted uterus is generally a normal condition that does not cause pain. If you are going to have surgery for this condition and you have had all the children you want, I think it would be best to have a hysterectomy rather than a uterine suspension.

Infertility is almost never caused by a retroverted uterus. Although during the years I have practiced I have operated on a few infertile patients who had a retroverted uterus (to suspend the uterus), I did so after years of otherwise unexplained infertility. I made sure the patient understood that it was unlikely that the infertility was caused by the retroverted uterus but that I had no other reason to explain the infertility. One of these patients did become pregnant after such a procedure. If I were working with these patients today I would probably recommend that they have an in vitro type procedure instead of a suspension procedure. (See the chapter on infertility.)

I believe the retroverted (tilted) uterus acquired a bad name in years past because some doctors used it as a catchall diagnosis for numerous unexplained problems. Women are occasionally infertile and do sometimes have pelvic pain and painful intercourse. Before the 1960s these things were difficult to diagnose, and doctors found it convenient to blame otherwise unexplained problems on a retroverted uterus. Physicians always like to come up with a reason for problems! Of course, patients want to be given a specific reason for a problem, too. As time went by, newer techniques for diagnosing pelvic problems were developed and now a retroverted uterus does not have to be used as a scapegoat.

If you have a pelvic problem you can be 99 percent sure that it is not due to a retroverted or tilted-back uterus.

672 Should I worry about irregular periods?

Do not worry about menstrual irregularities if they are within the "normal" limits described in the next three questions. If your bleeding pattern seems to be more abnormal than these guidelines suggest, see a physician.

Frequently patients ask if a cortisone shot will cause irregular periods. Several of my patients receive cortisone shots occasionally because of severe allergies. Some of them will have irregular periods for several months as a side effect of that shot. Neither the woman nor her doctor should ignore this type of bleeding. If it persists beyond three or four months, the woman should notify her doctor to see if further investigation is warranted. This bleeding might be caused by a growth in the uterus and not by the cortisone.

673 How much blood loss is normal?

If the pattern of blood loss with your periods is consistent each month and you are not becoming anemic, you almost certainly do not have abnormally heavy bleeding.

The average woman loses from two to eight tablespoons of blood (30 cc to 120 cc) with each menstrual period, although it always seems more than this.

Some women must change sanitary pads every couple of hours for two or three days and will even bleed through onto their clothes and bedsheets occasionally. If they do not become anemic, this is a normal menstrual pattern for these women.

Some patients who have always had very heavy periods, and do not want any more children, get tired of such heavy bleeding and want a hysterectomy. This is a legitimate request and I will comply with their request if I feel it is not frivolous. Most women do not need or want a hysterectomy for this situation, but they do want to have less bleeding. Birth-control pills can be tried. If a woman does not smoke, she can take birth-control pills until she goes through menopause. There also is a procedure called endometrial ablation (see Q. 705). This can be done as an outpatient procedure. It can stop a woman's heavy bleeding and yet let her avoid major surgery and a hysterectomy.

If a woman has to use two large pads every hour, and if that protection is not enough to prevent staining of clothes or bed, she is having truly abnormal bleeding and needs to see a doctor. Also, if a woman with heavy periods becomes anemic, she should talk to a gynecologist about controlling her menstrual flow. Birth-control pills, endometrial ablation, and hysterectomy are the only cures for such bleeding.

Some women have a light flow. Most gynecologists feel that if a woman has some spotting and bleeding for even one day she is having a normal period. This type of flow is often present if a woman is on birth-control pills. Women who have light periods should not worry. They should just enjoy having so little inconvenience with their menstrual bleeding.

674 How long is a normal period?

Menstrual flow can last from one to ten days and still be in a normal range. If a woman's menstrual pattern has become established and occurs every month, it is usually normal, no matter what length it is. However, if the pattern changes suddenly— a "three-day" woman has a period that lasts ten or twelve days, for instance—she should at least talk to her physician. If a woman who usually has a normal menstrual flow has a very light period, she should get a pregnancy test. Bleeding in early pregnancy can be a normal event but it can also be a sign of a miscarriage or a tubal pregnancy. It is best to know as early as possible if a woman is pregnant so that she can be watched for a tubal pregnancy or miscarriage.

It is also normal for a woman to have spotting for two or three days before her period and/or spotting for two or three days after. Spotting that comes just before and just after a period is a part of menstruation and is not a sign of disease of the uterus.

675 What does the blood of a normal period look like?

Color or texture of menstrual blood do not indicate abnormalities. The color and consistency can vary from bright red blood to a muddy, brownish-black material. It is also normal for the blood to be in liquid form or in clots. Neither does a woman need to worry if her flow changes from one form to another. These variations do not indicate malignancy or abnormality in the uterus.

676 What should I do if my periods are infrequent?

It is normal for a woman's cycle, the days from the start of one period to the start of the next, to vary from twenty to thirty-five days. However, if a woman's cycle has become regular outside these guidelines, that too may be normal. For instance, I have some patients who have had menstrual periods every eighteen or twenty days on a regular basis for a long time. They have no sign of any medical problem and are obviously normal.

If a woman has menstrual periods farther apart than thirty-five days, they are usually also irregular. They may be thirty-five days apart one time and fifty-five days apart the next time. If your cycles are of this type and you occasionally go for two to three months without a period, you should talk to your doctor. Everything may be normal, but it is best to be checked out.

When a woman has a pattern of infrequent periods, farther apart than thirty-five days, that goes on for many years, she has a higher than average chance of developing cancer of the uterus later on in life. Because of this most gynecologists feel that this woman should take progesterone (Provera) every other month if a period has not begun. This increased risk applies to women who skip periods repeatedly, not those who have this happen occasionally or who temporarily, even for a year or two, have such patterns. Provera must not be taken during pregnancy, as it might cause abnormalities in the baby. I have found that most women who have periods that are less frequent than normal prefer an alternate method of treatment. Using birth-control pills is as effective as using Provera to help regulate the menstrual periods, and if a woman does not smoke, she can now use birth-control pills until she goes through menopause. (If she does smoke, she can use birth-control pills until she is thirty-five.)

Birth-control pills are conveniently packaged and only moderately expensive. They will usually control a woman's bleeding, and because they do allow a woman to bleed each month, they have been found to decrease by 50 percent the chance of cancer of the uterus even after she stops using them. (For more information about birth-control pills, see the section on contraception.)

When a woman in her forties starts having less frequent or more frequent periods, she may be entering premenopause and she may want to get a follicle-stimulating hormone (FSH) blood test to see if that is what is happening. (See Q. 200–206.)

In summary, if your menstrual periods fall into a normal pattern, there is nothing you need to do unless some persistent change occurs. If this happens you should talk to a physician to see if he or she feels that diagnostic tests need to be done. After this decision you and your doctor can decide whether or not to regulate your periods.

See Q. 702–706 for a discussion of the problem of increased or excessive bleeding of the uterus.

---

677 Why do so many women have cramps with their menstrual periods?

Most of the time menstrual cramping (or dysmenorrhea, as physicians call it), is a result of the normal function of the woman's body. This normal cramping that is not due to disease or abnormality is called "primary dysmenorrhea." It is true that women can have "secondary dysmenorrhea"—cramping caused by physical abnormalities, such as a cervical opening that is too small to let menstrual blood out, or because of some other abnormality of the uterus, or because of endome-

triosis. Most menstrual cramping, however, is primary dysmenorrhea.

Prostaglandins cause menstrual cramps. Research physicians who injected pure prostaglandins into women found that all the symptoms of menstrual cramps resulted: uterine cramping, diarrhea, vomiting, headache, irritability, difficulty with concentration, and dizziness.

The prostaglandins produce uterine pain by causing the uterus to contract just as it does when a woman is in labor. Such contractions come and go. During a contraction blood is prevented from circulating through the uterus. This lack of circulation deprives the uterine muscle of oxygen, causing it to hurt. The woman senses this pain as cramping.

As mentioned, prostaglandins can affect various other body organs. For instance, they can affect the colon and cause diarrhea, or they can affect the brain and decrease the ability to concentrate. If a young woman has these symptoms and they are severe, she should see a doctor to be sure that no abnormality of her female organs is producing secondary dysmenorrhea. If she is normal on exam, she can be quite sure that her bad cramps are a result of the normal functioning of her body.

See Q. 82 and 84 for more information.

---

678 What can be done about menstrual cramps? (Medical term "dysmenorrhea")

There are several methods of treatment available. When I advise a woman about treatment for her cramps, I tell her that my goal for her is to be able to continue normal activities throughout her menstrual period.

Exercise. A woman who is in good physical condition and gets enough sensible exercise will occasionally have less cramps than if her body is in poor condition. If you have cramps, try to improve your physical condition to see if you feel better. Try to stay in shape, both for your general health and to decrease menstrual cramping.

Pain medication. Tylenol, aspirin, Midol, codeine, and other such medications can relieve cramps. Except for codeine, these can be obtained without a prescription and can provide sufficient relief from cramps in most women. They can be taken when the cramps are painful, are not expensive, and are fairly free of side effects.

Prostaglandin inhibitors. These medications were first used for people with arthritis. Later it was found that they relieved dysmenorrhea symptoms. There are several different forms of these medications. One of these (ibuprofen) is available (in a very weak strength) over the counter as Advil and Nuprin. The normal dosage prescribed is 800 mg each time it is taken. Take four Advil or Nuprin tablets at a time before you conclude they do not work.

Theoretically one would think that these drugs would relieve all menstrual cramps, but that is not so. About half of my patients respond favorably to these drugs. The other half receive little or no relief. If your doctor gives you a prescription for one of these drugs and it does not work after one or two months, ask if you can have a prescription for a different form of this type of medication.

If you are one of the fortunate ones on whom these drugs work, you will probably have almost total relief of your discomfort, no matter how bad it is. It can be almost like magic. If the drug works, be certain to use it correctly: As soon as you feel any cramping with your periods, start taking the drug. Once you begin taking it, do not use it as you would aspirin, one here and one there. Take it regularly, just as the doctor has prescribed (normally 800 mg of ibuprofen every eight hours during the time you have bad cramping). These pills do not work the way you are accustomed to having pain pills work. Therefore, taking more than is prescribed will not help and could make you sick, although overall, these drugs are safe. If you have cramps that bother you, try this medication.

Birth-control pills. If other methods do not help, birth-control pills can be tried and will usually work. When a woman is taking birth-control pills, the lining of her uterus stays thinner than with her own normal hormone cycle. When she has a period and is on birth-control pills, she will usually have lighter bleeding because there is less lining to shed. Since there is less lining, there is less prostaglandin production and less cramping.

See the discussion of birth-control pills in Q.

890–905. By reading that material you will see that birth-control pills are safe for most females, even teenagers. If you have dysmenorrhea that is not controlled in any other way, I encourage you to ask your doctor if you may try them. But do not use birth-control pills as a license to have sex before marriage. The risk of contracting a sexually transmitted disease is high.

Heating pads or warm baths. Many find that heat relieves cramps. No one knows why. It may be that heat to the pelvis improves the blood flow through the uterus during periods of cramping and in that way decreases uterine pain. The disadvantage of this treatment is that you cannot continue normal activities while using it.

Fluid pills (diuretics). Most women will not be relieved of their cramps by using diuretics, but they will be less bloated when using these medications. If you feel bloated with your periods, cut down on your salt intake, and drink more water. If this does not stop the problem, ask your doctor to prescribe diuretics for the time just before and during your period. They might make you feel better and just might help your cramps.

---

679 **If I am having severe menstrual cramps, should I have any kind of testing to be sure that I do not have endometriosis or some other pelvic disease?**

Some women will have such severe pain with menstrual periods that it is wise to check to make sure there is no pelvic disease causing the problem. The primary disease that might cause severe cramps is endometriosis. (See Q. 138, 849.)

If a woman has severe menstrual pain, she should see a gynecologist for both a consultation and an examination. The doctor may find that everything appears normal, and may suggest birth-control pills to control the bleeding and cramping. If the physician thinks that something might be wrong, he or she might feel that it would be wise to do a diagnostic laparoscopy. This can be done as an outpatient procedure and the woman can go home the same day as the surgery. There is very little postoperative discomfort.

With the laparoscopy, the doctor can examine

the female organs for signs of endometriosis or other disease. I usually do a hysteroscopy also, which can be done immediately after the laparoscopy while the woman is still asleep to make sure there is no abnormality of the uterine lining or inside the cavity of the uterus. Hysteroscopy involves passing a pencil-size telescope through the vagina, through the cervix, and into the uterus to check the uterine cavity.

I usually recommend a D&C with these procedures so that a pathologist can examine tissue from inside the uterus to make sure no inflammation or infection is present.

The doctor may find endometriosis, pelvic adhesions, low-grade pelvic inflammatory disease, tumors, etc.

Also, it is possible to do some therapy with the laparoscope. There are two ligaments that come up into the underside of the uterus called uterosacral ligaments. At laparoscopy, the doctor can use a laser to cut these ligaments. This does not affect a woman in any way except to decrease her cramps. Cutting the ligaments only works in about 50 percent of the cases, but since it is a relatively safe procedure, it is worthwhile to try it. Adhesions can be cut and endometriosis treated with the laparoscope. (See the section on endometriosis.)

There is an operation called a presacral neurectomy that will occasionally stop menstrual pain. In the past a major incision and three- or four-day hospitalization was necessary for this surgery, but new techniques have been developed that make it possible to do the surgery on an outpatient basis with laparoscopy. If you have painful and truly disabling cramps, you may want to have a presacral neurectomy done either with an abdominal incision or with laparoscopy. Of course, if you are older and do not want more children, you can legitimately have a hysterectomy.

---

680 I have been told that I have fibroid tumors of my uterus. What are these?

Fibroid tumors, or leiomyoma, are not cancer and almost never become cancer. They are growths made up of muscle tissue. No one knows what makes uterine muscle grow so abnormally. The most common current theory of the source of fibroids is that they grow from the small muscle cells in the walls of blood vessels in the uterus. Fibroids apparently grow in response to stimulation by estrogen from a woman's ovaries because they never appear in females before the onset of menstrual periods. After menopause, any fibroids that are present usually get smaller if a woman does not take estrogen.

Fibroid tumors occur in 5 to 10 percent of all women. Black women are seven or eight times more likely to have uterine fibroid tumors than white women. As a woman grows older, her uterus is more likely to have fibroids. As previously mentioned, uterine fibroids almost never occur in children, but they are present in 40 percent of women who are over fifty years old.

Fibroids can occur anywhere in the uterus. They can be present in the wall, they can protrude from the wall on a stalk, or they can grow into the interior cavity of the uterus and cause bleeding. Fibroids can even hang on a stalk out of the cervical opening and can grow from the cervix itself.

Since fibroids probably start from a single cell, they can be as small as only a few cells, much too small for a physician to detect on a pelvic examination. They can also get very large, filling the abdomen as much as a pregnant uterus.

---

681 What are the symptoms of a fibroid?

A woman is not usually aware of small fibroids. If and when they grow larger, however, they can cause several symptoms. If the fibroid is growing under the inside lining of the uterus (the endometrium), it can cause heavy periods or bleeding between periods; it can become so large that it puts pressure on the bladder and the rectum, causing a woman to feel the continual need to urinate or making her feel constipated. Large fibroids, by exerting pressure on the veins that come back into the body from the legs, can produce leg swelling.

A fibroid will occasionally outgrow its blood

supply and start degenerating, causing a woman's uterus to become tender. This does not necessarily require surgery, but if the tenderness is too marked she may need to have surgery to make sure that it is a fibroid and not some other, more dangerous, problem such as appendicitis or PID.

If a fibroid is growing inside the cavity of the uterus, the uterus will try to expel it by contracting, working the fibroid down into the lower part of the uterus and "delivering" it through the cervix. When a doctor looks into the vagina of a woman with such a fibroid, he or she will see a reddish-purple, swollen mass protruding through the cervix.

682 How is a fibroid diagnosed?

A doctor's pelvic examination is the most useful technique for diagnosing a fibroid. The doctor can tell if the uterus feels enlarged and irregular and if it can be moved around. In addition, a fibroid will not usually be tender on the pelvic exam. If a cancer is present, the uterus will usually be stuck to some inside organ and will not be movable.

An ultrasound study is very helpful in evaluating fibroids. An ultrasound done with a vaginal transducer is a more accurate way to evaluate the uterus than is the abdominal method. It is important to determine that the growth in your uterus is a fibroid and not a growth on an ovary. A growth on an ovary is treated in a completely different way than a fibroid. (See the sections on ovarian growths, and also the next question.) Your physician may order a sonogram. Since a uterus with fibroids could also be enlarged because of pregnancy, it is important that you and your doctor consider the possibility that you may be pregnant. An ultrasound can be especially helpful for this. (See Q. 398.)

One technique that a doctor might use to evaluate fibroids is to pass a probe up through your cervix into your uterus. If you have a large fibroid present, it often distorts the inner cavity of your uterus. A probe can tell that the cavity is enlarged and distorted, proving that there is a fibroid present. Such probing, called "sounding" of the uterus, must not be done if you are pregnant.

An X-ray of the uterine cavity (a hysterosalpingogram) can show the presence of fibroids if they are distorting the inside of the uterus. (See Q. 808.) It is rare that a CT scan or an MRI study is necessary for fibroid tumors. (These are specialized types of studies done by the radiology department in a hospital.)

683 How are fibroids treated?

If you have small fibroids and have not yet had all the children that you want, you must make sure that your doctor examines your fibroids on a regular six-month basis. If your fibroids are large or are growing, you should have them removed. Such an operation is called a myomectomy. There is usually no real urgency, but if you let your uterus get as large as a four-month pregnancy before you have the fibroids removed, your chance of subsequently conceiving and carrying a normal pregnancy is greatly diminished. If you have the fibroids removed when your uterus is smaller (the size of a three-month pregnancy or less), your chances of becoming pregnant and carrying a healthy pregnancy are much greater.

If your fibroids are not growing very fast, are not as large as a three-month pregnancy, and you are not worried about pregnancy, you do not need surgery. Many women have fibroids for years with no problem; after menopause fibroids will usually shrink and become almost nonexistent if a woman does not take estrogen. Taking estrogen does not usually make fibroids grow, but the fibroids may not shrink either.

If you are having heavy bleeding because of fibroids, you may need a D&C to be sure there are no premalignant or malignant cells in the uterus, especially if you are over forty. If the D&C is normal but the bleeding persists, you need to have either a myomectomy or a hysterectomy. If you have had all the children you want, I would advise a hysterectomy in this situation, but you may choose not to have one. If you want to preserve the possibility of a pregnancy for the future, or if you do not want your uterus removed, don't consent to a hysterectomy: Find a doctor who will do a myomectomy.

Having a hysterectomy for fibroids is not done

because of the possibility of developing cancer, but because it becomes increasingly difficult to remove the enlarging uterus. Common sense would say that if you are going to need surgery, you may as well have it done at a time when it is easiest for the doctor to do it. This can decrease the chances of complications from the surgery, although most competent gynecologists rarely have a problem doing a hysterectomy for fibroids.

684 What if a doctor cannot determine that a growth in my pelvis is a fibroid?

Occasionally, in spite of your having a growth that feels like a fibroid tumor, a doctor may not be able to tell for sure whether or not you have a fibroid. If the fibroid is growing out from the side of the uterus or in the supporting structures of the uterus, the doctor often cannot tell whether there is a fibroid growing or whether there is a growth on your ovary.

It is vital to differentiate because an ovarian growth can be malignant and a fibroid almost never is.

If this situation exists, a laparoscopy—viewing the internal organs through a small abdominal incision—is usually necessary. This procedure can be done in forty-five to sixty minutes on an outpatient basis. At laparoscopy a doctor can look directly at the internal organs, will be able to see where a growth is coming from, and can usually tell what it is. (See Q. 810–812.)

You and your doctor may decide that if you are going to have surgery, you may as well have the growth removed. In that case a regular incision would be used and a laparoscopy would be unnecessary.

685 What kind of surgery is done for fibroids?

The incision made for fibroid surgery is the same as for a hysterectomy. That incision can be either bikini-type or up-and-down from the umbilicus to the pubic bone. Hysterectomy incisions are discussed in Q. 124–137. Since the incisions are the same, it is necessary for you to be hospitalized for the same length of time.

If you are having a myomectomy, the doctor will make an abdominal incision and then cut across the surface of the uterus over the fibroids so they can be removed. He or she takes the fibroids out of the uterus, just as the yolk is removed from a hard-boiled egg. Sutures are used to close the holes and to stop the bleeding. If you have more than one fibroid, this procedure is repeated over and over until all the fibroids are removed. The doctor will close the incision in your uterus with small, delicate sutures to try to prevent any adhesions, which could interfere with your future fertility.

A doctor cannot guarantee that all the fibroids have been removed, because there can be fibroids that are only a few cells in size. The chance of developing fibroid tumors again is probably about 10 percent. Most women, however, are able to have all the children they want after a myomectomy, even if they eventually grow a few small fibroids again.

Some smaller fibroids can be removed with a laparoscope. You can ask your doctor about this.

686 Will a cesarean section be necessary for delivery after fibroids have been removed?

If the doctor had to cut into the interior (endometrial) cavity of the uterus to get the fibroids out, a cesarean section might be necessary later. Since this is not usually the case, most women who have had fibroids removed from the uterus do not need a cesarean section and can go through normal labor. If you have surgery to remove a fibroid ask the surgeon if you will need a C-section for future pregnancies. This is important information to give to your obstetrician if you should change doctors.

687 What are endometrial polyps?

A polyp is a piece of tissue that hangs from a stem. An endometrial polyp is an overgrowth of an area of the lining of the uterus that projects from the wall of the uterus. Such polyps do not occur often.

Endometrial polyps may vary in size. They have been measured from less than one-eighth of an inch to more than three inches across.

688 What are the symptoms of an endometrial polyp?

Bleeding or spotting from the uterus between periods is the most common sign that a polyp is present; bleeding after menopause can also indicate the presence of a polyp. Sometimes there are no symptoms of polyps. Polyps are occasionally found by a hysterosalpingogram (see Q. 808), and polyps are sometimes found by the pathologist who examines the uterus after a hysterectomy. Obviously, polyps can be present without causing any problems.

689 How are polyps diagnosed?

If you have persistent abnormal bleeding, your doctor will probably do a D&C. The scraping of the uterus will frequently remove any existing polyps. Occasionally, though, the instrument that is used in the uterus will merely push the polyp to the side and scrape the wall of the uterus without sensing the presence of the polyp. If a woman continues to bleed, the doctor may suggest a hysteroscopy, a newer technique done with a small telescope inserted through the vagina, through the cervix, and into the uterus. This procedure is quite useful for diagnosis and treatment in women who have continued uterine bleeding. Hysteroscopy lets the doctor see inside the uterus to identify not only polyps of the uterine cavity but also other uterine abnormalities. While doing the hysteroscopy, the doctor can almost always snip away polyps, and therefore avoid more major surgery. The procedure may be done either in a doctor's office by using a paracervical block or in a hospital under paracervical or general anesthesia. (See Q. 823.) If a hysteroscope is available, your doctor may recommend that a hysteroscopy be done along with the D&C. I suggest you follow that recommendation.

690 How are endometrial polyps treated?

A D&C will often get rid of any endometrial polyps that are large enough to cause bleeding. If not, hysteroscopy with excision of the polyps will solve the problem. Although polyps usually do not recur once they have been removed, a hysterectomy is a good method of treatment when polyps become bothersome and the woman has had all the children she wants.

Endometrial polyps are not premalignant growths. However, just as premalignant or malignant cells can occur anywhere on the lining of the uterus, so they can occur on the surface of these polyps. Also, since cancer of the uterus can grow in such a way that it produces polyps, a polyp can be a sign of malignancy in the uterus. It is important, therefore, that a polyp growing inside the uterus be removed, the wall of the uterus be scraped, and all the tissue sent to a pathologist to make sure that none of it is malignant.

691 I have pressure and discomfort in my lower abdomen, and my doctor says my uterus is sensitive and a little enlarged. What can cause this, and what can be done for it?

There are three problems that can produce this kind of discomfort. The first two conditions, adenomyosis and pelvic congestion, have no danger potential and should be treated only if they are bothering a woman enough to be treated. The third problem, endolymphatic stromal myosis, an extremely rare condition, will cause uterine bleeding that is abnormal enough to require a D&C. Since the D&C will definitely confirm the presence of this problem, there is no danger of confusing endolymphatic stromal myosis with adenomyosis or pelvic congestion.

The ultimate treatment for all three problems

is a hysterectomy. But, while a hysterectomy is absolutely necessary if endolymphatic stromal myosis is present, it is never necessary for adenomyosis or pelvic congestion unless the discomfort is bad enough to make a woman want the hysterectomy. (See Q. 141–151.)

692 What is adenomyosis?

Adenomyosis is endometriosis of the muscular wall of the uterus. (See Q. 138–140, 849–859.) I picture adenomyosis as a condition in which pieces of the endometrium (lining of the interior of the uterus) are growing as islands of tissue within the muscle of the uterus. Since this tissue is the same as that which lines the uterus, it still responds to the hormones from the ovaries. It builds up and then bleeds at the time of the period. Adenomyosis, however, bleeds into the muscle of the uterus instead of from the vagina. This bleeding into the uterine muscle causes the uterus to be sensitive, especially at the time of a period. It can cause the uterus to be enlarged, although adenomyosis can be present when a uterus is normal in size.

The symptoms of adenomyosis are severe cramps, excessive uterine bleeding with periods, and spotting before or after periods. Pain with intercourse can be present, and there may be an infertility problem.

Adenomyosis occurs in as many as 20 percent of women in the reproductive age. As with endometriosis, it is active during childbearing years and becomes inactive as menopause occurs, subsequently causing no further discomfort. If a woman takes estrogen after menopause, adenomyosis can remain active. Even if it resulted in a hysterectomy, I would continue to recommend estrogen for a postmenopausal woman.

693 How is adenomyosis treated?

Hysterectomy is the best treatment for this problem, but is necessary only as a matter of comfort. If a doctor feels that adenomyosis is contributing to a woman's infertility, he or she may suggest hormones such as Lupron or Danocrine. These hormones will suppress both endometriosis and adenomyosis and increase the woman's chance of becoming pregnant if these problems are causing infertility.

The doctor can never know for sure that adenomyosis is present until the uterus is removed and the pathologist has examined it. This can be frustrating for an infertility patient, but if adenomyosis is suspected the doctor will probably suggest taking Lupron or Danocrine "just in case."

For patients who are having significant pelvic pain or bleeding problems, and who have all the children they plan to bear, it really does not matter whether or not the doctor can tell her for sure that she has adenomyosis. If she is having enough discomfort to need a hysterectomy, surgery is done because of the discomfort, not because of the possible presence of adenomyosis. Of course the hysterectomy would remove adenomyosis if it is present and therefore solve the problem.

694 What is pelvic congestion syndrome?

Pelvic congestion syndrome is a condition in which the pelvic tissues are swollen, boggy, and congested with fluid; the veins in the supporting structures of the uterus become like varicose veins. These swollen veins ooze fluid into the tissues and cause tenderness. Dr. Masters of the Masters and Johnson team has described breaks in the tissues supporting the uterus. These have come to be known as "Masters windows." He feels that these breaks in the supporting structures allow the tissues to swell and are partly responsible for the pain of pelvic congestion.

A patient with pelvic congestion syndrome usually has discomfort low in the pelvis before and during menstrual periods and occasionally at ovulation. This may consist of pain, a feeling of pelvic pressure, or both. The discomfort may be aggravated by intercourse. There can also be low back pain.

695 How is pelvic congestion syndrome treated?

Treatment for this condition is normally hysterectomy. If a woman has not had all the children she wants, she may find that birth-control pills can help her symptoms.

Some doctors feel that a markedly retroverted uterus is associated with pelvic congestion syndrome. Retroversion of the uterus causing pain is extremely rare. If your doctor is convinced of this, however, he or she can insert a device called a pessary into your vagina to hold the uterus out of the retroverted position. This is not often done these days because the device can be bothersome and often does not help. If a woman is having a great deal of trouble and wants no more children, she is better off with a hysterectomy. If she has not completed her family, a pessary might be worth a try. (See Q. 697.) If a woman with this problem is not in good physical shape, I encourage her to exercise. Being in good condition may lessen pelvic congestion.

Some sex therapists feel that pelvic congestion is caused by repeated episodes of sexual arousal without orgasm. They feel that lack of orgasm allows the pelvic structure to become congested, and they encourage patients with the problem to see a sex counselor and learn techniques for developing orgasmic intercourse.

696 What is endolymphatic stromal myosis?

This uterine growth is extremely rare. It is apparently an overgrowth of the connective tissue of the uterus. It produces heavy periods, bleeding between periods, and even bleeding after menopause. It can also produce discomfort in the low pelvis and cause the uterus to enlarge.

If a woman has these symptoms, she would almost always have a D&C done because of the bleeding. After studying the tissue scraped from the uterus, the pathologist would make the diagnosis.

The only treatment for endolymphatic stromal myosis is surgery. A woman must have her uterus, tubes, and ovaries removed. Although endolymphatic stromal myosis is not considered a true malignancy, the growths can spread to other parts of the body, and 10 to 15 percent of the women who have this problem die as a result. Therefore, after a hysterectomy for this condition, a woman should have continued medical observation and care. If there are further signs of the problem, specialized consultation will be necessary.

697 Can the uterus "fall down"?

The condition in which the uterus is "falling" is usually referred to by doctors as uterine prolapse or uterine decensus or procidentia. This is a situation in which the ligaments that hold the uterus in place are no longer strong enough to hold it where it belongs. This is usually a result of the stretching and tearing of these ligaments during childbirth, but the ligaments can also be abnormally weak (apparently an inherited weakness) in women who have never been pregnant.

Often a doctor will tell a patient that her uterus has fallen and she is totally unaware of it. In this situation, the patient does not need to do anything about it and can usually ignore any suggestions a doctor might have about surgery. It is a problem only if it is bothersome.

Occasionally a uterine prolapse will cause a woman to have low abdominal and low back pain. If a woman begins having trouble with uterine prolapse and has had all the children she wants, she should consider a vaginal hysterectomy. Uterine prolapse is often associated with a prolapse (relaxation) of the vaginal walls known as cystocele and/or rectocele. (See Q. 614.) If the vaginal walls are becoming weakened and these problems are bothering her and she has decided to have a hysterectomy, she should also have vaginal repairs. (See Q. 124–137.)

If a woman wants more children or does not want to have surgery, she can either ignore the problem or have her uterus pushed back up the vaginal canal with a pessary. A pessary is a plastic or rubber device that is inserted into the vagina for the purpose of holding up the uterus on a temporary basis. With some pessaries a patient can

Prolapsed Uterus

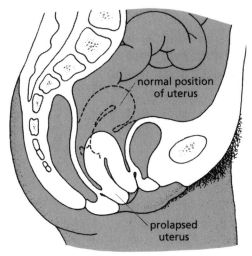

normal position of uterus

prolapsed uterus

have intercourse; with others intercourse is impossible.

If a woman has prolapse of the uterus, has not completed her family, and cannot wear a pessary, she needs to have an abdominal operation in which the doctor would make an incision, grasp the ligaments of the uterus and shorten and tighten them to hold her uterus higher up in the vagina. Some doctors are now doing this with the laparoscope.

Occasionally doctors will fit a woman with a pessary when they feel that she is too old or too ill to have surgery. I have never seen a woman alert enough to be bothered by vaginal relaxation who was not also healthy enough to have vaginal surgery. Most women can have vaginal surgery because it does not stress a woman's body very much and can be done relatively quickly. Often older women who try to avoid surgery by using a pessary tire of it after a few months and go ahead with surgery.

698 What is a D&C?

D&C stands for "dilatation and curettage." This means that the cervix is dilated, or stretched open, to introduce an instrument into the uterus to scrape, or curette, the lining of the uterus. Forceps are usually introduced into the uterus to explore its inner cavity for polyps. If a D&C is being done with a suction instrument, this instrument will often suck a small polyp into the opening of the instrument and pull it out.

All removed tissue is sent to the pathologist to be examined for malignancy.

For this procedure a patient is admitted to an outpatient surgical facility or to a regular hospital and given general anesthesia. An alternative method, which does not require a surgical facility, is the office curettage discussed in the next question. There is only mild low-abdominal discomfort after a D&C, caused by the uterine cramping that often follows the procedure. The recovery time is related primarily to the anesthesia. Women are often tired and a little groggy for a few days after anesthesia but they usually feel completely well again within a week.

After a D&C, if a woman develops fever, increasing pain in the deep pelvis, or bleeding that is heavier than a menstrual period, she needs to call her doctor immediately. This usually indicates an infection in the uterus from the D&C.

Some bleeding or spotting a few days after a D&C is normal. I recommend that my patients not have intercourse, douche, or use tampons for one week after a D&C. Exercise or regular activity, however, is fine if you have recovered from the anesthetic enough to do such things.

A D&C is a simple procedure that does not require any cutting of a woman's tissue. It does, however, require either paracervical anesthetic or general anesthetic.

Even a carefully done D&C, using good technique for scraping and careful exploration by forceps, can miss a growth in the uterus. Because of this, many physicians (myself included) now do a hysteroscopy at the time of a D&C routinely if general anesthesia is being used for the D&C. The patient doesn't feel it, and hysteroscopy only takes a few minutes if everything is normal. Adding hysteroscopy to a D&C makes evaluation of the uterine lining and uterine cavity essentially 100 percent accurate. This is a simple procedure that allows a physician to look around the inside of a woman's uterus to make sure there are no polyps or other abnormalities present. (See the section on hysteroscopy in the infertility chapter.)

Dilatation

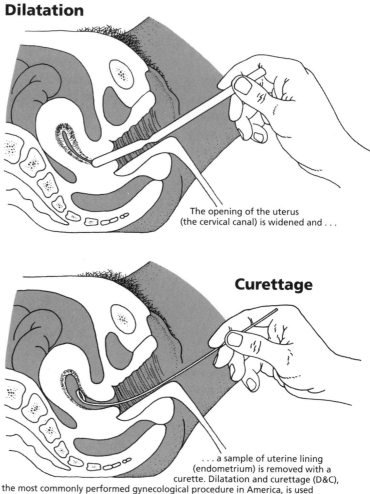

The opening of the uterus (the cervical canal) is widened and . . .

Curettage

. . . a sample of uterine lining (endometrium) is removed with a curette. Dilatation and curettage (D&C), the most commonly performed gynecological procedure in America, is used primarily to diagnose the cause of uterine bleeding or to empty the uterus after a miscarriage.

699 Are there alternatives to a D&C?

Yes. These are:

Endometrial biopsy. If a woman is having bleeding that needs evaluation but the doctor does not suspect cancer, he or she may suggest an endometrial biopsy. This technique, which can be done in the office, is not truly a D&C but is merely a sampling of the tissue that lines the uterus. From the tissue taken the pathologist can tell if infection, hormone imbalance, or some other problem is causing the bleeding. This technique is often used to see if a hormone imbalance is causing infertility.

A small round tube with an open end is inserted into the uterus, scraped around three or four times, and pulled out. The open end of the tube usually has a sharp lip that will scrape away tissue from the wall of the uterus. While scraping, the doctor usually applies a little suction with a syringe to pull the tissue that is scraped off into the tube. This material is squirted into a preservative and sent to the pathologist for evaluation.

An endometrial biopsy is normally done without any pain medication. It is painful but takes less than one minute. I usually give my patients nitrous oxide during the procedure and at times will use a paracervical. An alternative to this is their taking pain medication before coming to the office for an endometrial biopsy.

Remember, an endometrial biopsy can totally miss an early cancer of the endometrium. To be absolutely sure no cancer is present, a hysteroscopy or suction curettage must be done.

Office curettage. Curettage in the doctor's office is now being done by many gynecologists as a substitute for the traditional D&C. For this procedure, an injection of local anesthetic (a paracervical) is given on both sides of a woman's cervix. This injection, which is only mildly uncomfortable, numbs the cervix and the lower uterus. After the paracervical has become effective, the doctor introduces a small plastic tube into the uterus. This tube has an opening in the tip, with a lip on it that will scrape the uterine wall as the device is moved back and forth. Powerful suction is applied with a large syringe or some other device as the doctor scrapes the uterus. This scraping is done much like the scraping for a regular D&C.

Studies have shown that the accuracy of this type of curettage is even greater than that of the traditional D&C done in an operating room. In addition, it eliminates the necessity for general anesthesia and the cost of the operating room.

A further advantage of the office curettage is that a woman can return to work after leaving the office, and she can even resume marital relations the same day if she wants to. There is generally less cramping with this procedure than following the traditional D&C. For the patient who has heart disease or some other reason for avoiding more major surgery or anesthesia, this procedure can be done with very little risk.

Hysteroscopy. This procedure allows a doctor to look into a woman's uterus to be sure no growths or polyps are present. Then an endometrial biopsy can be done to be sure no abnormal cells are developing in the lining of the uterus. The procedure is very simple. The cervix is dilated a little. A lighted telescope is pushed through the cervix into the uterus. The uterus is distended with carbon dioxide or with different types of fluid. The doctor looks through the telescope into the uterus. If an abnormality is present it can often be repaired or removed with forceps or scissors.

700 Why can't a Pap smear be done instead of a D&C if a doctor suspects cancer?

The Pap smear and the D&C are looking for two completely different disease processes in the body. The Pap smear detects precancerous or cancerous cells of the cervix, the mouth of the uterus. The D&C is looking for precancerous or cancerous cells or other abnormalities of the endometrium, high up inside the uterus. The D&C tells almost nothing about the cervix, and the Pap smear tells almost nothing about the part of the uterus above the cervix.

701 What is meant by temporary irregularity of the menstrual cycle, and what causes it?

One of the most common reasons for women to see their gynecologists is because of temporary irregularity of their menstrual pattern. These women usually come in worried, complaining that they have never had an abnormal period before but that during the last month they have had irregular bleeding. Such irregularity may include any of the following:

Bleeding again only a few days after a normal period ends, with the "extra" bleeding sometimes being heavier and lasting longer than a normal period would.

Five or six weeks with no period, then a heavy and abnormal period (reported by a woman who knows that she cannot be pregnant).

A "normal" period that never stopped and is still going on at the time of the office visit.

These situations are almost always a result of failure of ovulation, and they can occur when a woman is in her teens or forties or in between. Almost every woman will have an episode of this type during the reproductive years of her life. After about three months a woman's body will almost always stop this abnormal-type bleeding as normal ovulation once again occurs. By the third month the woman will begin having regular, nor-

Endometrium during a Menstrual Cycle

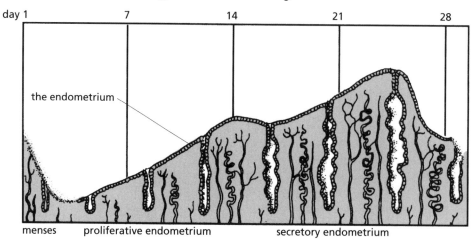

day 1   7   14   21   28

the endometrium

menses   proliferative endometrium   secretory endometrium

mal cycles again. In other words, a woman's body has done its own D&C.

Unless the bleeding persists for more than three months, or is so bothersome that a woman wants it treated, she needs no therapy. There is certainly nothing wrong with taking birth-control pills for two or three months to stop this bleeding and to regulate it, but it is usually not necessary. (A smoker over age thirty-five should never take the Pill, even for this problem.)

If you are not using contraception and have even mildly unusual bleeding, you need to get a serum pregnancy test. This type of bleeding can indicate early pregnancy, tubal pregnancy, or threatened miscarriage. If you have not had a sterilization procedure and there is any possibility of your being pregnant, get a blood pregnancy test whenever bleeding of this type develops.

702   **What should I do if I have truly abnormal uterine bleeding: much more in amount and/or lasting much longer than that mentioned in Q. 701?**

You need to see a doctor who will determine what the pattern of your bleeding is. He or she will then do a pelvic examination to check for abnormalities of your vagina, cervix, uterus, tubes, or ovaries.

In addition, since pregnancy is the most com-mon cause for uterine bleeding in women in the reproductive age, the doctor will want to determine if you are pregnant.

These diagnostic tests will often follow.

Pregnancy tests. If there is any possibility of pregnancy, the doctor will want to do a blood pregnancy test to see if you are pregnant and whether or not your bleeding is a complication of that pregnancy. This type of bleeding may be the first signal of a miscarriage or tubal pregnancy.

Sonogram of the pelvis. A sonogram helps detect whether or not there is a tubal pregnancy, a growth on your ovary, or a growth in your uterus. Although a sonogram may help determine if there is a pregnancy in the uterus itself, a sonogram alone generally cannot diagnose a tubal pregnancy. (See Q. 304–308.)

Sonograms done through the vagina have made sonography much more accurate. They are more reliable than the sonogram done through the abdomen with the woman having a full bladder. A physician can insert a small tube into the uterus and inject saline (salt water) through the tube into the uterus as he or she does the vaginal sonogram. This procedure allows a growth to be "outlined" on the sonogram screen. (See Q. 726.)

A strong warning regarding sonograms is in order, however: They can present misleading information. They can look normal even though a woman has a large growth in her pelvis or they may indicate a growth when there is none. A

388

Uterine Tests

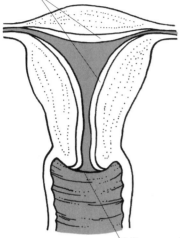

A D&C checks for abnormalities of the endometrium (uterine lining).

A Pap smear detects abnormalities of the cervix.

sonogram is a lab test, and it can be inaccurate when relied on as the only test to find growths in the female organs. Don't let a doctor scare you or operate on you on the basis of a sonogram alone. The doctor's pelvic exam is often more reliable in determining whether or not you have a growth in your pelvis. When the doctor has found a growth, the sonogram can be useful in helping decide what kind it is. Occasionally a sonogram will find a growth a physician cannot feel. At times only a laparoscopy can determine what is really going on.

D&C. A D&C is done to evaluate the lining of the uterus not only for cancer but also for other problems that might cause bleeding. (See Q. 698–699.) The best procedure is to combine a D&C with a hysteroscopy.

Other tests. Various diseases and disorders of the body can cause uterine bleeding. For example, a woman who has a blood clotting deficiency can have abnormal and heavy bleeding; stress can cause a woman's periods to become temporarily irregular; and hepatitis can produce irregularity of the menstrual pattern.

An increasingly common cause of unusual bleeding is sexually transmitted disease. If a woman has a low-grade pelvic inflammatory disease (PID) from chlamydia or gonorrhea, she may

have bleeding between periods as a result of the inflammation of the inside lining of the uterus. If there is any possibility that you might have a sexually transmitted disease, tell your doctor so chlamydia and gonorrhea cultures can be done. Other tests, therefore, would be directed toward any suspected disease process that might be going on.

703 How is abnormal bleeding treated? Should I be concerned about bleeding less often than every month?

Once the uterus has been found free of precancerous or cancerous cells, and if no other body disease is found, the cause is almost always hormone irregularity produced by or producing irregular ovulation. Once this is known, treatment can be started. If a growth or other problem of the uterus is found, it would be treated as necessary. Check the index for the various uterine problems and their treatment. Remember, though, that treatment of irregular menses is usually necessary only if the irregularity has been going on for many months, if it is bothering you enough for you to desire such treatment, or if it is causing you to be anemic.

Having a period as infrequently as every other month is not a cause for concern, but if you have periods that are three months or farther apart for many years, you have an increased chance of developing cancer of the uterus sometime in the future. This is because the estrogen from the ovaries is produced on a daily basis, whether or not a woman has a period, and this continued stimulation of the uterus by estrogen from the ovaries without the balance of hormones provided by regular periods increases the chance of uterine cancer.

The most effective treatment for abnormal bleeding due to hormone irregularity is the use of birth-control pills, but if you are over thirty-five and a smoker you should not take them. (See Q. 892–902.)

An alternate approach to treatment may be recommended by your doctor and is necessary for women who cannot take oral contraceptives. This treatment is the use of a progesterone pill (usually Provera) to take the place of the progesterone that a woman's body should be producing each month starting with ovulation. If a woman with this problem will take 10 mg of Provera for ten days every other month, it will usually bring on her period. Provera, by producing regular bleeding in this fashion, reduces a woman's chance of developing cancer of the uterus in later years. A period every other month is usually enough for this purpose.

704 Will a D&C stop my abnormal bleeding?

A D&C rarely stops abnormal bleeding, even though in years past it was used for that purpose. Prior to the development of the birth-control-type hormones that are now used to stop abnormal uterine bleeding, there was absolutely nothing to stop spotting and irregularity between periods, nor anything to stop heavy menstrual periods. Women who did not want a hysterectomy or could not have one for health reasons would often have multiple (as many as six or eight) D&Cs. Doctors had nothing else to offer the patient, and occasionally a patient's bleeding would seem to be better after a D&C.

These days D&Cs along with hysteroscopies are done for diagnosis: to find out if there is cancer or precancer present in the uterus or if there are other uterine abnormalities. If a patient has bothersome abnormal bleeding, doctors now often handle that with hormones.

The most efficient hormones for abnormal bleeding are birth-control pills. If these are not effective or if a woman cannot use them, Provera given ten days each month can sometimes regulate a woman's cycle. If these measures do not work and a woman continues to bleed heavily, endometrial ablation (see next question) or hysterectomy is usually indicated.

705 What is endometrial ablation?

Endometrial ablation is a procedure that some women are choosing over hysterectomy as a solution for their excessive bleeding. The technique removes the inner lining of the uterus, the endometrium, which produces a woman's monthly periods. This procedure became possible with the development of surgical hysteroscopy (see Q. 699 on hysteroscopy), which allows a clear view of the interior of the uterus and a channel through which instruments can be passed.

For the woman whose excessive bleeding each month has not responded to other treatment (such as birth-control pills, a D&C, antiprostaglandin drugs, etc.), endometrial ablation offers a permanent solution that means the end of troublesome bleeding yet does not involve major surgery and does not remove her uterus or ovaries. A further benefit is that many women have also stopped having symptoms of PMS (premenstrual syndrome) and have stopped having severe cramps after endometrial ablation.

An additional advantage of endometrial ablation is that the procedure does not require a hospital stay. It is done in an outpatient surgical facility and rarely takes more than thirty to forty minutes. A woman normally has very little discomfort afterward and is able to go home the same day as soon as she feels well. The procedure is done with either general anesthesia or with a paracervical block with sedation as needed.

Women who might benefit from this procedure include those who are:

bleeding excessively each month or who have unusually long periods

taking estrogen after menopause and continue to bleed year after year

medical risks for major surgery, yet need a solution for excessive bleeding

bleeding because their blood does not clot well due to leukemia, idiopathic thrombocytic purpura, and so on

Endometrial ablation does not replace hysterectomy in all cases. While it is excellent for stopping excessive bleeding, it must not be done if there is cancer (or precancerous changes) in the uterus. If a woman has large fibroid tumors of the uterus, severe endometriosis (endometrial tissue growing outside the uterus), or other similar medical problems, it is probably best to have a hysterectomy instead of an ablation because a hysterectomy will probably be necessary later.

This procedure destroys the lining of the uterus, which is necessary for maintaining a pregnancy. A woman should be certain therefore that she has had all the children she wants to have before having this procedure. (A tubal ligation could be done at the same time for contraceptive purposes to be absolutely sure of sterility.)

If you are troubled by excessive bleeding that has not responded to treatment, endometrial ablation may be a solution for you. It is a safe and sensible alternative to hysterectomy in this situation.

706 What type of bleeding might signal cancer of the uterus and indicate the need for a diagnostic D&C?

Most women who have abnormal bleeding worry about the cause being cancer, especially if it occurs when they are forty or over. It is important that a woman realize, however, that the cause of such bleeding is not usually cancer.

Remember, cancer is basically a "sore." As it grows it begins oozing a little fluid and then a little blood. Then, as time passes—perhaps weeks and months—that sore begins oozing more and more blood. This pattern of bleeding is quite different from the sporadic episodes of bleeding that almost all women occasionally have (see Q. 701). The real key, though, is whether or not abnormal uterine bleeding is persisting.

If a woman is over forty and her uterine bleeding persists off and on for more than three months, she should see a doctor and expect that diagnostic tests will be done. Most doctors feel that a woman does not even need to see a doctor until the bleeding has lasted three months or unless there is some aspect of the problem that really worries her. If a woman is under forty, it is unlikely that uterine cancer is the cause of her bleeding. Therefore, there is less urgency in diagnosing the cause of her bleeding, but neither she nor her doctor should delay diagnosis and treatment for too many months.

Types of bleeding that indicate the need for a D&C, and hysteroscopy classified by ages, are the following.

Younger than the age of forty. Bleeding between periods that persists month after month usually needs to be evaluated by D&C and hysteroscopy. Most of the time the doctor will find that the woman is not ovulating regularly. This type of bleeding is not dangerous and is not caused by cancer.

There are some conditions, however, that can increase your chance of having uterine cancer earlier than the age of forty. For example, if you are twenty-five to fifty pounds overweight, you are three times as likely to develop cancer of the uterus as other women; and if you are fifty pounds overweight, you are nine times as likely to develop cancer of the uterus as an average-weight woman; if you are a diabetic, you are more likely to develop cancer of the uterus; and, if you have had infrequent menstrual periods for many years, you are more likely to develop endometrial cancer. If you fit into one of these categories, you should be sure your doctor knows it; and if you are having abnormal bleeding, you might suggest to him or her to consider a D&C and hysteroscopy at an earlier age than might otherwise be done.

Bleeding over the age of forty. If you have an episode of bleeding between periods and start having regular periods again after a month or so, you do not usually need a D&C and hysteroscopy. If, however, you start having bleeding between periods that persists for more than three months, you need a D&C and hysteroscopy. Also, if you start spotting between periods, excluding just after or just before a period, and this spotting continues for three or four months, you need a D&C and hysteroscopy.

After menopause. Any unexplained bleeding after menopause requires a D&C and hysteroscopy. *This is an absolute rule* and you and your doctor should never violate it unless the bleeding is proven to be from the vulva or from the vaginal walls. Even then most gynecologists will suggest going ahead with a D&C and hysteroscopy except where they can actually see the bleeding coming from a scratched or scraped place on the vulva or vagina.

Nothing in life is perfect, and this includes a traditional D&C. A study done in 1979 showed that only 75 percent of such D&Cs were accurate in showing cancer. This means that, if the doctor had done a D&C without doing a hysteroscopy and found no irregularities, and you continue bleeding, then you need to have a D&C with a hysteroscopy. If the doctor suggests another D&C because you are continuing to bleed, it is a reasonable suggestion, but it should be done with a hysteroscopy. Many doctors now routinely combine these procedures, especially if the D&C is being done with anesthesia.

Although a D&C and hysteroscopy is an inconvenient and somewhat expensive procedure, it is a safe procedure and is an invaluable test providing vital information for a woman.

707 After a D&C and hysteroscopy done for bleeding, my doctor said that I had endometrial hyperplasia. What is this, and what should be done?

Hyperplasia merely means overgrowth of the tissue of the lining of the uterus. Hyperplasia of the endometrium can be broken down into four groups.

Hyperplasia. In this condition, the lining of the uterus is simply overgrown, but has no precancerous cells. A woman having this change of her uterine lining should be cautious. She should be given hormones that will absolutely regulate her if she has irregular periods. This treatment can cause hyperplasia to revert to normal. A woman with hyperplasia should have another endometrial biopsy or D&C done after a few months to make sure that her uterine lining is not becoming more abnormal. There is an increased chance of developing cancer of the uterus during the next ten years if she has hyperplasia of the endometrium. If her cycles cannot be regulated or the follow-up testing of the lining of the uterus continues to show hyperplasia and the woman has had all the

family she wants, it would probably be best for her to have a hysterectomy.

Adenomatous hyperplasia. This abnormal form of hyperplasia has no cancer cells present, but about 25 percent of women who develop it will have cancer of the uterus sometime in the next ten years. In spite of this a woman does not need to have a hysterectomy immediately. She should make sure that she has absolutely regular menstrual periods and should be tested again in a few months to see if the cells are continuing to be abnormal. If they are, or she cannot regulate her periods, she should go ahead with a hysterectomy if she has had all the family she wants.

Atypical endometrial hyperplasia. With this more severely abnormal form of uterine hyperplasia, about 80 percent of women will develop cancer of the lining of the uterus at some time during the following ten years if not treated. A woman ordinarily needs to have a hysterectomy if this condition exists.

Severely atypical endometrial hyperplasia. This abnormality is considered to be cancer, but it is confined to the surface of the uterine lining. All women with this problem will have continued change in the uterine lining progressing to actual invasive cancer (cancer growing down into the tissues of the body) unless they have a hysterectomy.

Treatment with hormones will often cause hyperplasia of the endometrium to revert to normal. However, if the endometrium has cells that have become atypical, it is generally best for a woman to have a hysterectomy unless there is some specific reason to avoid a hysterectomy. The hormone treatment used to reverse hyperplasia is Provera or birth-control pills and repeated uterine scraping for testing on a long-term basis. You and your doctor can discuss this and decide what is the best treatment in your situation.

708 If cancer of the uterus is diagnosed, what procedure is followed?

First let me state that "cancer of the uterus" or "uterine cancer" is an inexact term that gynecologists often use to refer to cancer of the lining of the uterus. This is actually cancer of the endometrium. If a patient has cancer of the cervix, that is referred to as cervical cancer, not uterine cancer, even though the cervix is part of the uterus. These are two distinctly different types of cancer and are treated in almost totally different ways. (See Q. 666–669.)

Once endometrial cancer is diagnosed, the condition is "staged" to classify the extent of the cancer in the body. The different stages of endometrial cancer are:

Stage I-A. The cancer is just on the surface that lines the inside of the uterus.

Stage I-B. The cancer has grown into the wall of the uterus but no more than halfway.

Stage I-C. The cancer has grown into the wall of the uterus and is more than halfway through.

Stage II. The cancer has grown from inside the uterus down into (but not outside) the cervix. The doctor finds this extension of the growth by scraping the inside of the cervix at the time of the D&C. This cervical scraping is included as part of a D&C done to diagnose possible endometrial cancer.

Stage III. The cancer has grown out of the uterus into other areas of the pelvis, such as into the ovaries or down into the vagina (but not outside the pelvis).

Stage IV. The cancer has grown into the rectum, or bladder, or outside the pelvis into other parts of the body.

709 How significant is the type of cell that makes up the cancer?

All cancer cells are not the same; some grow faster than others. "Grading" a cancer means classifying the aggressiveness of the cells that make up the cancer. The grade is assigned by the pathologist who studies the cancer cells from the uterus.

The following simple grading system is used by doctors.

Grade I. The architectural pattern of the growth is primarily glandular. This is a "better" tumor than the next two grades.

Grade II. The architectural pattern is a mixture of glandular and solid-type cells.

Grade III. The architectural pattern is primarily solid. (This is the worst and most aggressive type of cancer.)

710 What things besides stage and grade affect the way endometrial cancer will act in my body?

There are several things that affect the way the tumor will act in your body.

Depth of the cancer. The less deeply the cancer has grown into the wall of your uterus, the better off you are. Previously the only accurate way this could be determined was with a hysterectomy. If X-ray or radium treatment was necessary before a hysterectomy, the pathologist often could not tell how deeply the cancer had grown into the wall of your uterus because of the distortion of the uterus from radiation. That information is vitally important. However, it has been found recently that a sonogram (ultrasound) done vaginally can show the extent of the cancer growth. This may not be a totally accurate technique but it is helpful.

The location of the cancer. If the cancer started and is growing in the upper part of your uterus, you are better off than if it started or is growing in the lower part of your uterus.

Cancer cells in abdominal fluids. If the cancer cells have broken loose and are floating freely in the fluid in your abdominal cavity, you are not as well off as if that fluid contained no cancer cells. The doctor can determine this only at the time of the hysterectomy.

Lymph nodes. If the lymph nodes inside your abdomen at the time of the hysterectomy are free of cancer, you are better off than if they have cancer in them.

Age. The younger you are when you are found to have cancer of the uterus, the better off you are.

The type of cancer cell. You are better off if you have a cancer that is adenoacanthoma or adenocarcinoma. A cancer cell that is adenosquamous cancer, clear-cell cancer, squamous-cell cancer, or papillary adenocarcinoma is more aggressive and more likely to recur after treatment.

711 How are these different stages of cancer treated?

Each of the stages of endometrial cancer calls for medical care tailored to that specific stage. But the grade of the cancer (the aggressiveness of the cells) does influence the treatment.

Stage I. If the cells of endometrial cancer are not very aggressive-type cells (Grade I) and the cancer has not deeply invaded the walls of the uterus (Stage I), a woman may be able simply to have her uterus, tubes, and ovaries removed for the treatment of her cancer. If the cancer is this early and this mild, she has a fairly good chance of a 100 percent cure. If, however, the cancer has invaded the muscle of the uterus or if the cells are more aggressive-type cells (Grade II or III), a woman with Stage I cancer may need to have not only a hysterectomy with removal of the tubes and ovaries but also removal of some of the lymph nodes in her abdomen to check them for cancer. Knowing whether or not the cancer has spread to the lymph nodes helps determine the follow-up treatment mode, for example, whether radiation or chemotherapy is necessary after healing from surgery.

Stage II. A woman with this type cancer may need removal of her uterus, tubes, and ovaries, and removal of some of the lymph nodes in her abdomen. She may need to have a radical hysterectomy, which means removal of the uterus, tubes, ovaries, most of the lymph nodes in the pelvis, and the stripping away of the tissues that surround the ureters (tubes from kidneys to bladder). Often radiation and surgery is recommended with Stage II cancers of the uterus.

Stage III. When cancer has grown outside the uterus, treatment depends on where the cancer has grown. If it has grown into the ovaries or onto the surface of the tissues in the pelvis, after the hysterectomy the physician may recommend that a woman have chemotherapy. If the cancer has not grown onto the surface but is merely into the supporting structures of the uterus, radiation may be recommended.

Stage IV. When the cancer has grown into the rectum or bladder or other areas of the body, individualized treatment is necessary. Treatment depends on what kind of tumor is present and where it has spread. Ordinarily, treatment will be primarily with radiation and chemotherapy. Stage IV cancer often occurs in women who are much older and often in poor health. Women who are in this condition may be too sick for aggressive therapy.

The treatment of uterine cancer has changed a great deal during the past few years. Your physician may have an approach to uterine cancer that is different from the things stated above. For instance, your doctor may not recommend that the lymph nodes be tested if the uterine cancer is very early because this requires a larger incision and often makes the patient sicker after surgery. I recommend that if you trust your physician, follow the procedure recommended, but never hesitate to get a second opinion. It can help you determine what type treatment is best for you.

712 Which chemotherapy is useful for cancer of the uterus?

Chemotherapy is usually begun when all the cancer cannot be removed at surgery or when the doctor thinks that cancer may still be present in the body after treatment. These drugs will also be given when a woman has seemed to be free of cancer, but it shows up again in her body several months or years later.

Ordinarily the treatment is with progesterone in high doses. Drugs such as Megace, Depo-Provera, or Delalutin are all progesterone preparations sometimes used to treat cancer of the uterus that persists or recurs after initial treatment.

The patients who respond best to this type of treatment are those who are not elderly, who have had long periods of time from their initial treatment until a recurrent episode of cancer, whose recurrence of cancer was not in the pelvis, and whose grade of cancer was not very aggressive. About 25 to 35 percent of the patients who have this type of recurrence will respond well to therapy, many of them going several years without having further trouble with their cancer.

Progesterone drug treatment does not cause one's hair to fall out and does not have many of the toxic effects of other types of chemotherapeutic agents. In addition, progesterone preparations almost never cause nausea. Unfortunately they rarely produce a complete cure from the cancer.

713 What if the progesterone treatment stops working? Is other chemotherapy recommended?

Gynecologists who have special training in oncology are called gynecologic oncologists. This type of specialist or a medical oncologist would be an ideal choice to consult if you have cancer of the reproductive organs.

If you have a cancer that is not responding to progesterone or to other treatments, or if your doctor suggests that you start on some other type of chemotherapy, ask for a referral to a gynecologic or medical oncologist for consultation and treatment. If your doctor tells you that you have cancer growing but does not refer you to an oncologist, I encourage you to see one for a second opinion.

If you have a cancer that has come back or one that was not initially removed completely, it is certainly worthwhile to talk to a chemotherapist about his or her recommendation for treatment of your problem. Although you don't have to do what is suggested, you will at least know what your options are.

With some forms of uterine cancer, chemotherapy other than progesterone is recommended immediately after surgery. For example, Stage III cancer that has grown onto the surface of the organs in the pelvis may be treated with other types of chemotherapy. This is a dangerous situation

and aggressiveness in using chemotherapy can sometimes help.

Problems of the Fallopian Tubes

A woman's fallopian tubes, or oviducts, are about three to four inches long. They are attached to the uterus at one end and have a delicate, flowerlike opening on the other end that takes in the eggs from the ovaries. These tubes (which look a lot like and are about the same size as relaxed, medium-sized earthworms) have the same fragile, peritoneal lining that covers all the organs inside the abdomen except the ovaries. They have two layers of muscle and are lined on the inside by a soft pink lining (mucosa).

The inside surface of the fallopian tube is made up of different cell types. Some of these secrete mucus. Others are specialized, with hairlike projections that produce a synchronous sweeping motion, which is responsible for propelling the egg down the fallopian tube and eventually into the uterus. The inside diameter of the fallopian tubes varies from one-twenty-fifth to one-sixth of an inch.

When we look at the function of the fallopian tubes, we understand to some extent how truly complex they are. A fallopian tube is capable of

Fallopian Tube

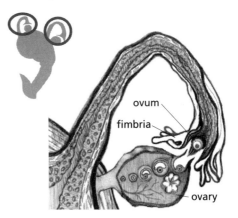

ovum

fimbria

ovary

transporting sperm and ovum in opposite directions at different times during the menstrual cycle. How this feat is accomplished is unclear. The fallopian tube is also responsible for moving the egg from ovary to uterus, but the sperm must come from an opposite direction—through the uterus into the tube—for fertilization to take place. (See Q. 237 and 238.)

714 Since the fallopian tubes are important to my becoming pregnant, is there anything I can do to keep them healthy?

There are three primary precautions to insure good fallopian tube health.

Don't have intercourse with anyone who can give you a sexually transmitted infection. Gonorrhea and chlamydia are the infections most commonly associated with fallopian tube scarring, but other sexually transmitted diseases (STD) can also cause infection of the tubes. (See chapter 13.)

Even if a man has not had intercourse with anyone else for two or three years, he can still have and pass germs to you that can cause you to develop infection in your fallopian tubes and uterus. Such infections can cause sterility. In spite of modern antibiotics and microsurgical techniques to open scarred tubes, pregnancy may be impossible after such episodes of pelvic infection.

Obviously, the best way to avoid this type of infection is for you and your husband to have intercourse only with each other.

If you enter marriage with someone who has had intercourse before, you could be infected by him. Whether or not one of you thinks there is an STD organism present, if either has had previous intercourse both should be checked and, if necessary, treated by a physician. Though some STD organisms cannot be detected, the two that can cause infection of the fallopian tubes, chlamydia and gonorrhea, can usually be detected by laboratory testing. If you or your fiancé has either or both of those infections, you should be treated so you can be free of these germs. Don't take any chances. Get treatment if there is any indication that either one of you needs it. Be sure to have a later test to determine that the infection has disappeared.

Don't use an IUD (intrauterine contraceptive device) until you have had all the children that you want. IUDs can cause an infection of the fallopian tubes that can leave them obstructed or unable to function adequately. Many people think that the Dalkon Shield was the only IUD that caused an infection in the female organs, but this is not true. Any IUD can cause pelvic infection; the Dalkon Shield just happened to be the most popular IUD when physicians noticed that IUDs could cause pelvic infection. It did cause a higher rate of infections than other IUDs, but even the newest IUDs can cause infection and should not be used if you want a future pregnancy.

Don't get your tubes tied until you know that you will not be interested in getting pregnant in the future. A sterilization procedure is done to make you permanently sterile; it is not designed to be reversed. Even though most physicians warn patients that sterilization is permanent, many patients come back wanting the sterilization reversed. (See Q. 720–721.)

Though a sterilization can sometimes be reversed, there is no guarantee that a woman will be able to get pregnant after the operation. The procedure involves major surgery and is expensive. Also, there is a greater chance of tubal pregnancy following a sterilization reversal. I strongly recommend that you use some other method of birth control until you know for sure that you do not under any circumstances want another child.

715 What is the result of infection (pelvic inflammatory disease) in the fallopian tubes? What should a woman do if she suspects such an infection?

Infections of the fallopian tubes are normally associated with infections of both the uterus and the ovaries. Such infection (called pelvic inflammatory disease or PID) can cause ulceration of the inside lining of the fallopian tube. Scarring can develop. The fallopian tubes can become blocked, and the delicate fimbriated ends of the tubes can become completely closed and destroyed. If the tubes are completely closed they may fill with fluid and become quite distended, swelling to as much as one or two inches in diameter (hydrosalpinx). If both of a woman's tubes are damaged and closed in this fashion, she obviously would be sterile.

Even if the tubes are not completely closed, scarred areas of the lining of the tube may have destroyed the tubes' hair cells (ciliated cells). In that case there is no current of fluid to bring the egg down the tube. This can result in infertility or, if an egg were fertilized in a damaged tube, the embryo might fail to pass through the tube, resulting in a tubal ectopic pregnancy.

I cannot overemphasize the danger to future fertility if you become infected with chlamydia or gonorrhea. Just one infection by one of these germs can give you up to a 25 percent chance of being permanently sterile. There is no immunity from an infection, therefore, you can get infected over and over again if men you have sex with have these germs when you have intercourse. Becoming reinfected greatly increases your chance of being permanently sterile.

I cannot adequately express to you the pain and anguish women experience when they find, years later, that they cannot get pregnant. Sophisticated, expensive infertility procedures can be done, but many women with this problem never conceive in spite of all that medical knowledge can offer, even if they can afford the thousands of dollars they cost.

If a woman has been exposed by intercourse to germs that might cause a pelvic infection and she starts developing pelvic pain and fever, she should see a doctor immediately for antibiotic therapy. The doctor will first need to make sure that she does not have appendicitis, a tubal pregnancy, an ovarian cyst, or some other medical problem.

PID (pelvic inflammatory disease) is discussed more extensively in chapter 13, especially Q. 980, 984–989.

716 Are there abnormalities of the fallopian tubes that are not due to infection?

Yes. These noninfectious abnormalities include *salpingitis isthmica nodosa*, various tumors and cysts,

and cancer of the fallopian tubes. All of these problems are extremely rare.

717 What is *salpingitis isthmica nodosa?*

This disease is so uncommon that it does not even have a common name. It is a problem involving nodular thickening of the fallopian tubes. These thickenings, when viewed under the microscope, are small cavities in the wall of the tube communicating with the central canal of the fallopian tube. It is felt, therefore, that the problem is caused when the tubal lining bulges out through the muscular layer and proliferates to form the glandlike appearance of these nodules.

Although this condition is not dangerous and does not lead to malignancy, it can cause infertility. If this problem is found and a woman is trying to become pregnant, a doctor can cut out the areas of the fallopian tubes that are involved and sew the ends of the tubes back together. Surgery of this type must be done with microsurgical technique to be successful. Fortunately only the inner half of a fallopian tube is usually involved in this process, so the outer half and the ends of the tubes with the delicate fimbria that are so important to egg intake can be left intact. (See Q. 828.)

718 Which tumors and cysts can occur on the fallopian tubes?

"Hydatid cysts of Morgagni" can occur. These cysts are normally only one-quarter to one-half an inch in diameter and are found near the open end of the fallopian tube. Apparently they are structures that would have become part of the tubes that carry sperm if the person had developed as a male. Instead they exist in the female as small grapelike structures attached near the end of the fallopian tubes. These cysts are "found" in at least two-thirds of women who have surgery for other reasons—they are not an abnormality.

Occasionally one of these growths may be several inches in diameter. When it is discovered, a doctor would not know if it is a simple hydatid cyst and would probably need to operate to determine exactly what it is. Any time a woman has a mass two to three inches in diameter in her pelvis that does not go away in a few weeks, she needs to have surgery.

Other growths of the fallopian tubes may occur. Tumors of the fallopian tubes include fibroid tumors (just like fibroids of the uterus), hemangiomas (tumors of the blood vessels), and dermoids (tumors that seem to develop from primitive cells present almost anywhere in the body and are capable of producing various types of tissue in one tumor—thyroid, fat cells, and oil glands). See the discussion of ovarian dermoids in Q. 736 since dermoids occur in ovaries much more commonly than in the tubes.

719 Can cancer of the fallopian tube occur?

Yes, but cancer of the fallopian tube is the rarest cancer of a woman's female organs. It accounts for only 0.5 percent of all the cancers of the female organs. Only about five hundred cases of this type of cancer have been reported in medical literature.

720 Is tubal ligation for sterilization a recommended operation?

If a woman knows for sure that she never wants to become pregnant again and a tubal ligation fits into her value system, it is a good operation (see Q. 949–951). If she is not sure she wants to be permanently sterile, she should use another method of birth control.

Doctors have argued back and forth through the years about whether or not a tubal ligation will cause a woman to have problems with her uterus and ovaries later on. Some doctors say that a woman is more likely to end up having a hysterectomy later on and that she will be more likely to have growths on her ovaries if she has had her tubes tied. Statistics, however, have not shown any increased chance of either of these problems. Recent statistics have shown that sterilization definitely has no effect on the future health or function of a woman's body. It appears that the tubes serve no other function than to facilitate pregnancy.

A woman who has a tubal ligation should realize that, even though her tubes are tied, she can still become pregnant. The chance is remote, varying from one in five hundred to one in two or three thousand. It does not matter whether the tubes are burned and cut, have an elastic band applied, have a clip put on them, or whether they are tied and cut; there is always a remote chance of pregnancy in the future. However, since the chance of subsequent pregnancy is so small, I advise my patients not to worry but to enjoy their newfound freedom.

Women can have their tubes tied either immediately after delivery (postpartum sterilization) or at some other time. Patients who choose to have a tubal ligation immediately after delivery must realize that a baby can be born looking totally normal but develop fatal complications the next day, or during the next few days, weeks, or months. If you think that you would want another child if your newborn died, then you should wait to have your tubes tied until some later date.

A tubal ligation done at some time other than immediately after delivery is called an "interval sterilization." It can normally be done on an outpatient basis and normally a laparoscopy sterilization or a mini-lap sterilization procedure is used. If your doctor says that he or she needs to make a large incision and keep you in the hospital for two or three days after the surgery, the doctor has probably not learned how to do one of these simpler procedures. I think it would be wise for you to find a doctor who can do a mini-lap or laparoscopy sterilization. This necessitates a much smaller incision, meaning less danger to your body and a shorter recovery time.

Most patients have the idea that a fallopian tube extends from the uterus like a finger from a hand; if it is cut off, it will just fall away and die. This is not true. The fallopian tube is attached to and supported by a thin sheet of tissue through which blood vessels and nerves come up to the tube along its entire length. If the tube is cut in its midportion, the outer half of the tube still has an adequate blood supply and is still present in the body. This explains why doctors are able to cut the scarred portion of the tube ends away and sew the tubal segments back together in patients who want to have a sterilization reversed.

721 Is reversal of a sterilization possible?

Yes. Such an operation is often possible for both men and women. Most women are surprised to learn that this procedure has been available for years. I did my first successful tubal repair in 1971. Since then the techniques have improved dramatically.

If your fallopian tubes have not been terribly damaged by the sterilization technique used and you and your husband are otherwise normally fertile, there is a 75 percent chance of your getting pregnant after having the reversal surgery done. In stating this high success rate I am assuming that your doctor would use microsurgical techniques.

But this means that 25 percent of women who have had a tubal sterilization will be unable to become pregnant later, even with surgical reversal of the original procedure. The only help available to these women is the "in vitro" (test tube) fertilization process. (See Q. 867.) Fortunately centers that do in vitro fertilization are having increasingly good success in helping women become pregnant.

The operation to repair fallopian tubes is much more involved than the original sterilization. It requires a major abdominal incision, because the doctor must do the procedure meticulously, using the microscope. These procedures can take from two to four hours for the repair. Up to three days hospitalization is usually required, with a three- to five-week recuperation period afterward. The cost, including the surgeon's fee, normally is in the thousands of dollars. Most insurance companies do not pay for a sterilization reversal.

I always counsel my patients who want reversal of their sterilization to approach the surgery with the attitude that since they cannot get pregnant the way they are, they might as well give it a try. If they do become pregnant, that's great! If they don't, at least they have done all they could and will have no regrets later.

Problems of the Ovaries

The human ovary is another of God's miracles. Its complexity is seen in its anatomy, its function, and its effect on a woman's menstrual cycle and on her total life process. Most women rarely think about the significance of their ovaries, although these organs are responsible for major changes in their lives: the development of breasts, of menstrual periods, and of the ability to conceive. The normal

Ovary

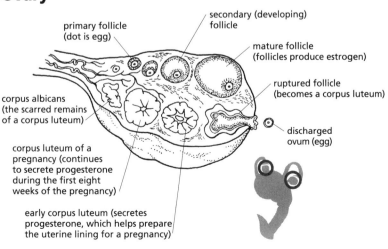

primary follicle
(dot is egg)

secondary (developing)
follicle

mature follicle
(follicles produce estrogen)

ruptured follicle
(becomes a corpus luteum)

corpus albicans
(the scarred remains
of a corpus luteum)

discharged
ovum (egg)

corpus luteum of a
pregnancy (continues
to secrete progesterone
during the first eight
weeks of the pregnancy)

early corpus luteum (secretes
progesterone, which helps prepare
the uterine lining for a pregnancy)

function of the ovaries can be seen in the regularity of a woman's menstrual cycle, a process that continues until the "death" of the ovaries at menopause, determined by the ovaries' internal time clock. God has beautifully orchestrated this process, and when a woman realizes this it can make her appreciate God's greatness even more.

722 What is special about the anatomy of the ovary?

The ovary is suspended on ligaments that extend from the uterus to the side of the pelvis (utero-ovarian ligaments and infundibulopelvic ligaments). These ligaments are capable of "moving" the ovary, making it more accessible to the fallopian tube for egg pickup. During pregnancy these ligaments are able to stretch dramatically, lifting the ovaries as the uterus enlarges.

The ovary is about one and a half inches in diameter and is made up of an external envelope (the cortex) inside of which is a core (the medulla). The ovary is much like a golf ball in that it is white, its surface is irregular, and it has an outer covering and an inner core.

The outer covering of the ovary contains the egg cells, and all the activity responsible for the maturation of an egg each month is in that layer. The inner core of the ovary is primarily supportive. It contains blood and lymph vessels and connective tissue.

For an in-depth understanding of the ovary's development and function, you might want to review chapters 1 and 2.

723 How are ovarian cysts "normal"?

Each month the ovary forms a follicle around an egg. At the time of ovulation, this follicle breaks open and releases that egg. This follicle is a fluid-filled cyst, and it can be felt by a doctor during a pelvic examination done just before ovulation. Normally such cysts will be two to three centimeters, or about an inch, in diameter. They are normal and occur every month and should cause neither you nor your doctor any concern.

Occasionally a follicle cyst can fail to break open at ovulation time. It then absorbs more fluid and becomes larger. Such a cyst can sometimes be mildly painful. This enlargement can be felt by a doctor during a pelvic exam. A follicle cyst can also secrete excess estrogen. This excess estrogen is not dangerous, but it can prevent ovulation the next month and can cause the menstrual periods to be irregular for two or three months. It can also cause breast tenderness. If this happens and there is a possibility you could be pregnant, you should have a pregnancy test to be sure you do not have a tubal pregnancy.

724 When a follicle cyst enlarges, what should be done?

If your doctor tells you that you have an ovarian cyst and that you need surgery "now," you should get a second opinion from a gynecologist. Exceptions to this would be:

1. If you are through menopause. A doctor should not be able to feel a woman's ovary if she is postmenopausal. If the ovary can be felt it may have a growth. You probably need surgery if your doctor tells you that the ovary is enlarged and may have a growth.
2. If the ovary seems "unusual" in some way to the doctor: unusually tender, unusually hard, unusually big (larger than three inches).
3. If you know your doctor well enough to be confident that he or she is well trained and will not recommend unnecessary surgery.

A reputable doctor will often recommend conservative therapy rather than turning immediately to surgery if your ovary is only about two inches in diameter or smaller. My routine is to put a patient on three weeks of birth-control pills, starting the pills on the fifth day of the next period that comes up, and then to examine her just before she finishes that three weeks' supply of the pills.

Birth-control pills "de-activate" the ovaries, allowing the fluid in a simple follicle cyst to absorb away. The ovary will usually return to normal size with just three weeks of birth-control pills, though it can occasionally take three to four months of birth-control pills for a cyst to go away.

If you cannot take birth-control pills, your doctor can watch the cyst for three or four months to see if the ovary will absorb the fluid out of the cyst on its own.

If the cyst goes away, either with birth-control pills or after three or four months of observation, you have a normal ovary. You have no increased risk of developing cancer, and you can think of that ovarian cyst as a normal part of the function of your body. You will also have avoided ovarian surgery that could have caused scarring of your ovaries and possibly decreased your fertility in the future.

725 What if the cyst does not go away?

If your doctor has said that the cyst is five centimeters (two inches) or larger, or if it is smaller than that but does not go away under either of the conditions listed above, surgery may be necessary. Unfortunately a doctor cannot tell by looking at a cyst whether or not it is a true growth, a malignancy, or a simple follicle cyst. Because of this a laparoscopy is usually inadequate for evaluating an ovarian growth. It is generally necessary to have a major incision made in your abdomen so that the doctor can remove the growth. This can usually be done with the side-to-side, bikini-type incision, about six inches long, in your low abdomen along the top of your pubic hairline.

Surgery is not done to get rid of a simple cyst, which is normal for the ovary. It is done because a cyst that does not go away can be an ovarian growth; and growths on the ovary have a 5 to 50 percent chance of being cancer, depending on a woman's age.

If you have an ovarian enlargement that is smaller than five centimeters but does not get smaller over a period of several months, you probably need to have surgery. When this situation exists, there is usually something wrong with the ovary. It is often a growth.

726 Will sonograms (ultrasound studies) or X-rays tell if surgery is needed for a pelvic mass?

Sonograms have become a major method of evaluation of the ovaries. If a physician thinks he or she has found a growth on an ovary during a pelvic exam, an ultrasound done through the vagina is usually recommended. This is not a painful procedure. The ultrasound transducer is a device that fits comfortably in the vagina of most women. Because the tip of the transducer gets within an inch or two of the ovaries, it gives a very good view of them. If an ovary is enlarged due to a simple, fluid-filled sac (a simple cyst or follicle), the enlargement of the ovary will disappear as the cyst is absorbed. If the enlargement is greater than two or two and a half inches, or if on sonogram it seems to be fairly complex with many partitions and cystic areas, it needs to be watched more carefully. If your gynecologist feels that the ultrasound picture of the ovary is worrisome, he or she will probably recommend that you have surgery.

An ultrasound done through the abdominal wall is not as reliable for ovarian growths as the vaginal ultrasound. X-rays are almost never used anymore to evaluate an ovarian growth, though a physician may occasionally want an X-ray to see if bone or teeth can be seen in an ovarian growth. If there are, it confirms a dermoid cyst of the ovary. (See Q. 736.)

727 Is laparoscopy of value in evaluating ovarian enlargement?

A competent gynecologist will often use the laparoscope to evaluate an ovary that has remained enlarged. As stated in the previous question, if an ovary is five centimeters or larger, it usually needs to be removed, not just looked at.

If your ovary is smaller than five centimeters but remains enlarged, the doctor will probably want to look at it with a laparoscope. Such an enlargement can be due to endometriosis, or it can just be scarring or adhesions in the area of the ovary that does not involve the ovary at all. It could, of course, be a tumor. A presurgical sonogram can give guidance at the time of laparoscopy.

With laparoscopy a doctor cannot look into the ovary to see what is causing it to be enlarged. The doctor can, however, put a needle into the ovarian enlargement to see if there is fluid present (aspiration). If there is, the fluid will be sent to the pathologist for examination. The doctor can sometimes biopsy an ovarian cyst to make sure it is just a cyst and not a tumor. The problem with this is that if a tumor or cancer is present, it would be best for the growth to be taken out intact and not broken open by a biopsy first. Biopsying can allow leakage of the material from the growth, and if that material were cancerous, that would not be good. However, careful irrigation of the pelvis with fluid can wash out most of the cancer and virtually eliminate the possibility of danger from the leakage. Studies done during the early 1990s seem to indicate that leakage of material from an ovarian cancer does not make a patient's condition worse and therefore is not dangerous. With the laparoscope the doctor will occasionally be able to tell that the enlargement of the ovary is not significant. This would prevent a more major operation.

Modern laparoscopic techniques have become a wonderful tool for the care of ovarian growths. More and more gynecologists are beginning to use these techniques. For instance, if a woman has an ovarian growth that does not involve any other tissues in the pelvis and does not look grossly malignant, a doctor can often remove the ovary with the laparoscope. He or she can use the laparoscope with two or three extra, very small holes in the abdomen to put sutures around the base of the ovary, cut it away from its attachments, and take it out through a small incision in the low abdomen or an incision in the upper part of the vagina. When this type of procedure is done, a woman can usually go home the same day.

Gynecologists are finding more uses for the laparoscope. It is enabling women to have surgery that would have required major incisions and would have required hospitalization in the past. Most physicians and patients feel that this is a great advance in the area of gynecology.

---

728 What type of major surgery is necessary if I have a growth on my ovary?

First, let me state that while a growth on a woman's ovary is most likely not malignant, the only way she can know for sure is with surgery.

This type of surgery can be with either the laparoscope or with an abdominal incision. An abdominal incision can be the bikini-type about six inches long, if the doctor thinks the enlargement is not cancer. If the doctor strongly suspects cancer, he will want to do a vertical incision in the middle of the abdomen to have more room to work. The surgery is done under general anesthesia or occasionally spinal or epidural anesthesia. During the surgery, the doctor can do one of three different types of operations on the ovary if no cancer is present.

Shelling the growth from the ovary. A growth may be taken out of an ovary in much the same way a pit comes out of an avocado, especially if it is a dermoid cyst. Such a growth is not totally "free," but with careful dissection it can be removed, leaving most of the ovarian tissue still intact. With very small sutures the doctor can sew the ovarian edges back together so that no raw surfaces are left along the edge to adhere to the surrounding tissues, preventing adhesions that might later cause fertility problems or pain.

Removal of the entire ovary. If the growth has destroyed most of the normal ovarian tissue, it cannot be separated from that tissue. In this case the doctor will probably remove the entire ovary. This is a simple operation most of the time; the doctor merely clamps the base of the ovary, cuts it away, and sutures the tissue from which the ovary came so that it does not bleed.

Removal of both ovaries, the tubes, and the uterus. (See Q. 731.) This is usually done if a woman does not want any more children, is in her forties, and does not want to have any more surgery on her female organs.

729 What is the recovery from ovarian surgery like?

Recovery is the same as after hysterectomy. See Q. 137.

730 Why do you recommend that a gynecologist do ovarian surgery?

Most general practitioners and general surgeons are unaware that 75 percent of women who have surgery on their ovaries will later have adhesions and scarring that can cause either pain or infertility. In addition, several of these doctors are not aware that many ovarian growths can be "shelled out" of the ovaries, leaving them normal in both hormone and egg production. For example, I know of a sad case in which a teenager had dermoid cysts on both ovaries. Although dermoid cysts are the kind that are most easily shelled out of an ovary, the general surgeon who discovered the growths removed both the girl's ovaries, leaving her sterile and without natural hormones for the rest of her life.

My suggestions are these:

Permit only a gynecologist to operate on your ovaries, and then only a gynecologist whom you feel will be gentle and careful in doing the surgery and who is thinking of your future fertility during the procedure.

If you are below the age of forty, encourage your doctor to shell out the growth if possible. Shelling out a growth from an ovary takes more time than removing the ovary, but you never know when your other ovary might require removal. It is best to keep your ovaries, if you can, up to the age of forty. (See the next question regarding the reason that removal of the ovaries may be wise at this age.)

731 I have a growth on my ovary, and my doctor says that he will probably do a hysterectomy and remove both ovaries during surgery. Is this necessary?

If you are going to have surgery for an ovarian growth, removal of the uterus, the tubes, and both ovaries is a good idea if the following circumstances exist:

1. Ovarian cancer is present.
2. You do not want more children.
3. You don't want to have further trouble with ovarian growths or take the chance of having ovarian cancer in the future.
4. You are over forty and do not mind taking a hormone pill every day starting now.

You would definitely need to take hormones until about the age of fifty if you had your ovaries removed before your menopause. If you did not do this, your chance of developing osteoporosis, heart disease, and stroke later on would be very high.

Having your ovaries removed at forty would make you different from women who have not had their ovaries out, as far as hormones are concerned, but only until the age of menopause. At menopause there is no difference in a woman who has had her ovaries removed (surgical menopause) and a woman whose ovaries stop working on their own (natural menopause). If you have your ovaries removed at forty and take estrogen, you are just like women who still have their ovaries. Then at the age of menopause (from about forty-eight to fifty-five) both you and they will have to decide if you want to continue taking hormones for the rest of your life as is now recommended by most gynecologists. (See Q. 207–225.)

Although you have to take hormones if you have both ovaries removed, there is good rationale for the four points mentioned above. If you have a growth in one ovary, there is about a 15 percent chance that a similar growth might develop on the other ovary. If you have had all the children you want and are nearing menopause anyway, you may as well go ahead and have both your ovaries removed to avoid the possibility of another ovarian growth. Having both ovaries out would, of course, eliminate the possibility of ever developing ovarian cancer.

A doctor who is going to remove both ovaries would almost always recommend removal of a woman's uterus and tubes too; unless she were young and wanted to keep her uterus, hoping that one of the new infertility techniques would allow her to be the recipient of an embryo from another woman.

If a woman has both ovaries removed, most of the time she will immediately start taking hormones. If she has her uterus removed, she can take her hormones without ever again having vaginal bleeding. Also, if the uterus is removed, that eliminates any future chance of a woman developing cervical or uterine cancer. A woman feels no worse during the hospital stay if she has only her ovaries removed or has ovaries, tubes, and uterus removed.

When I talk to patients who are forty or over about this procedure, I give them the choice of removal of the uterus, tubes, and ovaries or surgery only on the affected ovary. Recovery from either surgery is essentially the same. Some women are quite glad to be finished with having menstrual periods and free of any chance of ever having an ovarian, uterine, or cervical growth. Others are quite adamant in wanting only the ovary with the growth taken out.

Most thoughtful gynecologists are not absolutely sure how to advise a patient who is from forty to forty-five years of age. I have changed my recommendations back and forth through my years in practice. I now feel that if my wife had an ovarian tumor and were forty years old or older and we did not want any more children—and she did not have any big emotional problem with having her uterus, tubes, and ovaries removed—I would want her to do just that.

I have seen many women develop ovarian cancer later in life after having ovarian surgery when they were in their forties without having both ovaries removed. They and their families could have been saved the agony of cancer if both ovaries had been removed at the earlier surgery.

I am not implying, however, that a woman who has had cysts, growths, or surgery on her ovaries has a greater chance of developing ovarian cancer in the future. She does not.

Since it is now felt that almost all women need to take estrogen continuously from menopause on, removing the ovaries at the age of forty to forty-five only means that a woman would need to take oral hormones a few years longer. This same reasoning also applies to almost any surgery done through an abdominal incision on the pelvic organs in women over forty. (See Q. 124–137.)

732 If 85 percent of ovarian growths are not malignant and are not cysts, what are they?

Let me clarify. About 85 percent of ovarian growths in women below the age of forty-five are not malignant. If a woman is over the age of forty-five she has an increased chance that an ovarian growth will be malignant.

If a woman is between the ages of fifty and fifty-nine, and she has a growth on an ovary, 23 percent of the time it will be malignant. Between the ages of sixty and sixty-nine, there is a 30 percent chance that an ovarian growth is malignant. Between the ages of seventy and seventy-nine, there is a 40 percent chance that an ovarian growth is malignant. Above age eighty, if a woman has a growth on her ovary, there is a two-thirds chance it will be cancer.

The size of an ovary is also related to the likelihood of its being malignant. If it is less than about two inches in size, only about one in thirty-two such enlargements will be malignant. About 11 percent of growths between two and four inches across will be malignant. If the growth is larger than four inches across, there is a 60 percent chance of malignancy.

The ovary can produce more than twenty different varieties of ovarian tumors, including both nonmalignant and malignant tumors. A woman's ovarian growth may be absolutely benign (nonmalignant), it can have borderline malignancy, or it can be overtly cancerous. In addition, a growth on an ovary may have no capacity for producing abnormal hormones. On the other hand, some growths may produce hormones in such quantities that a woman's body will undergo dramatic changes, such as increased body hair growth, baldness, and an enlarged clitoris. Both benign and malignant ovarian growths can be hormone-producing tumors.

For the purpose of clarity, nonmalignant ovarian tumors will be divided into two groups: those that do not produce hormones and those that do. I will primarily point out the facts that make them different from other tumors. For an in-depth discussion, you would need to see a medical textbook. Most doctors are quite willing for a patient to sit in their waiting room and read from one of their textbooks about this very complex subject.

733 Which nonmalignant tumors do not produce hormones?

There are five benign tumors that do not normally produce hormones. I say "normally" because any tumor of the ovary can irritate that ovary, causing the ovary itself to produce increased amounts of hormones. These increased hormone levels can make a woman have irregular or abnormal periods. Those five tumors are: serous and mucinous cystadenomas, dermoid cysts (teratomas), fibromas, Brenner's tumors, and endometriosis.

734 Are mucinous cystadenomas dangerous?

Yes, because if a mucinous cystadenoma is allowed to remain in the abdomen, it can rupture. If this happens, portions of the tumor can begin growing on other organs in the abdomen, producing mucus in the abdominal cavity. Although this is not a malignancy, it is difficult for a gynecologist to remove all of the mucous-producing tissue from the abdominal cavity. Even after surgery for removal of this material, it is common for women to continue to produce this mucous material, resulting in abdominal fullness, discomfort, adhesions, and other medical problems. The medical term for this unusual condition is "pseudomyxoma peritonei." It can cause death but is fortunately rare.

The primary problem with cystadenomas of

the ovary is that they can be malignant. If a woman has an enlargement of the ovary and that enlargement is due to this type of tumor, it must be removed to prevent serious complications. The older a woman is, the more likely one of these growths will be malignant.

735 How are cystadenomas treated?

Removing a cystadenoma of the ovary almost always means removal of the entire ovary. Because a cystadenoma does not develop a capsule it cannot be shelled out of an ovary and is difficult to dissect from the ovary. Occasionally, if a cystadenoma is quite small, it can be cut out.

If a cystadenoma is found in one ovary, there is a 10 to 15 percent chance it will also be present in the opposite ovary. Although this is not a reason for removal of both ovaries in a young woman, a woman in her forties would probably be best treated by the removal of both ovaries, the tubes, and the uterus. (See Q. 731.)

736 What are dermoid cysts?

Dermoid cysts (benign cystic teratomas) make up 30 percent of all nonmalignant tumors of the ovary. They occur most often during the reproductive years, though they have been found in newborn babies and in women after menopause.

A dermoid cyst, or a teratoma, is a tumor of the egg cells of the ovary. An egg cell will occasionally begin growing without fertilization. A fertilized egg, of course, has the potential of developing into a human being, but a tumor growing from an unfertilized egg has the limited capability of developing only various tissues that make up a human body. A dermoid cyst, therefore, will typically contain hair, teeth, oil and sweat glands, cartilage, and other body tissues.

Because of the presence of these various tissues, a doctor may be able to diagnose a dermoid by taking an X-ray of a woman's abdomen. For some reason dermoids often have teeth growing in them, and these teeth seen on an X-ray can be the tip-off of a dermoid's presence.

This type of tumor can normally be shelled out of an ovary and the ovary closed with fine sutures, allowing resumption of normal ovarian function. Because dermoids often occur in the reproductive years, a gynecologist must do this procedure carefully so that fertility remains intact.

There are important reasons for removing dermoids. First, about 2 percent of them can be malignant. Second, a dermoid could rupture, spilling its contents into the abdomen. Also, any tumor in an ovary can interfere with regular ovulation and can affect otherwise normal fertility. Finally, since any of the body's tissues can be present in a dermoid, there can occasionally be enough active thyroid tissue to cause a woman to be hyperthyroid. This condition is called struma ovarii. It is not common, but it can occur.

When a dermoid is present in one ovary, there will also be one in the other ovary about 12 percent of the time.

737 What are fibromas?

A fibroma of the ovary is a tumor made up of fibrous connective tissue. This solid, firm tumor does not become malignant, but if neglected, it can get quite large.

A woman having a fibroma will occasionally also have fluid in the chest cavity around the lungs and excessive fluid in the abdominal cavity. This condition is called Meig's syndrome. Removal of the fibroma causes this fluid accumulation to go away spontaneously. Removal of the fibroma usually requires removal of the entire ovary because the fibroma often causes the ovarian tissue to disintegrate completely.

When a fibroma is present in an ovary, there will also be a fibroma in the other ovary approximately 25 percent of the time.

738 What are Brenner's tumors?

Brenner's tumors, so named because of the doctor who described them in 1907, interest physicians because they are not sure from which cell in the ovary they arise. Part of the tissue of a Bren-

ner's tumor is fibrous connective tissue, but there are also cells present that are similar to the surface cells of the ovary.

Most Brenner's tumors are benign, which is fortunate because they can occur in young women. Because they rarely occur in both ovaries and are rarely malignant, simple removal of the affected ovary seems to be adequate treatment in a young woman, but the entire ovary must be removed. If a woman does not want any more children, the best treatment is removal of the uterus, both ovaries, and tubes, because this eliminates most of the tissues to which the tumor would spread if it is malignant.

739 Can I have endometriosis of the ovary?

If endometriosis is present in the substance of the ovary, it is called an endometrioma. A doctor cannot determine without surgery if an enlargement of an ovary is due to endometriosis, although a vaginal sonogram can suggest that an endometrioma is present. A laparoscopy allows the doctor to diagnose the endometriosis. When the doctor does look into a woman's pelvis and finds an endometrioma, he or she will almost always find implants of endometriosis in other areas of the pelvis. (See Q. 138–139, 849–859 for more information on endometriosis and endometriomas.)

740 Which nonmalignant ovarian tumors do produce hormones?

There are two, both of which are discussed in the following questions: granulosa-theca cell tumors, and tumors that produce male hormones.

741 What are granulosa-theca cell tumors?

This tumor of the ovary, which produces female hormones, can occur in young girls at birth and also in women well past menopause. About 50 percent are found in women after menopause and 5 percent in children before they start their puberty.

Because these tumors produce increased amounts of female hormones, they can do unusual things. In prepubertal females they can cause premature puberty, including the development of breasts, pubic hair, menstrual periods, and shortness of stature. If a woman develops one of these tumors during her reproductive years, it can cause her to have irregular periods, or even a lack of periods. If a tumor of this type occurs after menopause, it can cause a woman to resume bleeding from the uterus and to have sensitive, enlarging breasts.

Another unusual characteristic of this tumor is that it can occasionally produce male hormones that can cause a woman to have increased hair growth, decreased breast size, and other symptoms of male hormones. Additionally, these tumors can rupture, bleed into the abdomen, and cause severe abdominal pain, necessitating emergency surgery.

Only about 5 percent of these tumors occur on both sides. Approximately 3 percent of them are malignant.

Treatment for a young woman, if the tumor is not malignant, is removal of the entire ovary. If the woman is older and has had all the children she wants, the best treatment is removal of the uterus, tubes, and ovaries.

742 Which tumors can produce male hormones?

Tumors that produce male hormones are rare. In my entire experience as a gynecologist, I have seen only one. The outstanding characteristic of these tumors, which have strange names such as gynandroblastoma, Sertoli-Leydig cell tumor, and lipid cell tumor, is that the male hormones they produce will cause significant changes in a woman's body. A woman may stop having menstrual periods and develop a beard, acne, baldness, deepening voice, and an enlarged clitoris.

These tumors ordinarily do not occur in both ovaries. If a person is young, removal of a single ovary is probably adequate. Because these tumors can be malignant, however, if a woman has had all the children she wants or is age forty or older and wants to have both ovaries removed, she should have that done along with a hysterectomy.

743 I had an ovarian tumor that my doctor said was "low malignant potential." What does that mean?

During recent years doctors have come to realize that they cannot tell whether or not some tumors will "act" malignant, or in other words, will spread. They call these tumors "low malignant potential." As many as 4 percent of ovarian tumors may fall into this category. They occur in all ages of women.

If women with borderline malignancy of an ovarian tumor have the affected ovary removed, they will usually not develop any spread of that tumor to other parts of their body. It is estimated that only 1 percent of these tumors will have any spread after the tumor is removed. If it has spread, it may be to the other ovary or to the intestines, or to other areas of the abdominal cavity. Since the chance of this type of tumor spreading is so small, if a woman wants to maintain fertility, she can have only the affected ovary removed. If she does not have the more extensive surgery, she must have more frequent examinations than she would otherwise, and she must understand that she is taking some slight risk.

Some women will feel better having both ovaries and the uterus removed. Statistically this may only slightly decrease her chance of recurrent cancer, but ovarian cancer is so dangerous it may be worthwhile.

744 Are there any techniques available for early detection of ovarian cancer?

Gilda Radner, who was a favorite comedienne on *Saturday Night Live*, died of ovarian cancer in May 1989. She wrote a book, *Gilda Radner, It's Always Something*, which told the story of her ovarian cancer and of her life almost to the time of her death. The frightening part of her story is that this world-famous woman began having medical problems almost a year before doctors were finally able to detect her ovarian cancer.

Gilda's story has frightened many women. My patients seem to feel that if Gilda's physicians could not detect her ovarian cancer, the chances of any doctor finding the same type cancer before it's too late are small.

I believe that Gilda Radner, because of her boldness in writing about her illness, has saved many women from a similar fate. Many women are now more disciplined about seeing their physicians on a regular basis.

Gilda Radner's problems during the year before her cancer was found were very unusual. Most of the time an ovarian cancer that is large enough to cause any symptoms will be found during a pelvic examination. (Encourage your doctor to do a rectovaginal exam when you have your annual checkup. This is a very important part of detecting any type of ovarian growth.)

Unfortunately, there are no tests that can be done on an annual basis that will detect ovarian cancer early. This is one of the reasons that cancer of the ovary is a frustrating problem for both patients and doctors. There is no way to detect it early, and even if there were an early-detection technique, five thousand women would have to be screened by that technique every year to find eight to twelve women who had cancer of the ovary. Because of the problem of early detection, a woman often does not even know that she has an ovarian cancer until it has progressed fairly far. When a diagnosis of cancer of the ovary is made, 75 percent of the time it will have already spread out of the pelvic structures into other parts of her body.

There are some suggestions that will help find an ovarian cancer before it gets too far along.

1. Have an annual examination.
2. If you have any unusual bloating or low abdominal discomfort, see your gynecologist for a pelvic exam. Unfortunately, some women will see a physician who is not a gynecologist for this problem, and that doctor will not do a pelvic exam.
3. If the physician thinks you have an enlarged ovary, or if the physician is not able to do an adequate examination, he or she will usually want you to have a vaginal ultrasound scan. If you have not gone through menopause, your physician may want to watch the ovary for two or three months to see if it gets smaller. An ovary can be enlarged because of a simple cyst or because of an attempted ovulation that resulted in some bleeding into the ovary (a hemorrhagic corpus luteum), which is a normal situation. If you have gone through menopause and your ovary is enlarged two inches across (five centimeters) or more, you should probably go ahead with surgery if your physician recommends it.
4. If you are going through menopause or are postmenopausal, a test of a specific monoclonal antibody can indicate an ovarian growth in your body. If your level of Ca-125 is greater than 35 U/mL, you may have ovarian cancer. Unfortunately, the level of Ca-125 can be elevated if a woman has endometriosis, is having a menstrual period, is pregnant, has PID or liver disease, pancreatitis, renal failure, inflammation, or any of several other problems. (This is why the test is not usually useful in women who are younger than menopause age.) If a woman has an enlarged ovary that looks abnormal on sonogram and the Ca-125 is elevated, it is very likely that the ovary is malignant.
5. Be aware of your family history and tell your physician if you have two or more close relatives who have had ovarian cancer. For instance, if you have a sister and a mother who have had ovarian cancer, you have a greater than average chance of developing cancer of the ovary. In this situation, I recommend that you have a vaginal ultrasound and a Ca-125 test every six months. You might even consider having your ovaries removed when you have had all the children you want.
6. If a tumor develops in one ovary, if you have completed your family, and if you are age

forty or older, let the doctor remove both ovaries and the uterus.

7. If you are having a hysterectomy for some other reason and are forty years or older, have the doctor remove your ovaries too. If you do not want both ovaries removed, at least have one removed. The less ovarian tissue there is in your body, the less likely you are to develop cancer of the ovaries.

8. Be suspicious. If you have had breast cancer and you develop a growth on an ovary, you have a 50 percent chance that the ovarian growth will be malignant (J. P. Curtin et al., *Obstetrics and Gynecology*, 1994, 84:449–452). Be sure to remind your doctor that this is your situation if he finds a growth on your ovary.

745 Why be so aggressive about detecting ovarian cancer?

Ovarian cancer is a dangerous disease. It is the second most common malignancy of the female genital tract in the pelvis (endometrial cancer is first), and it is the most common cause of death from malignancies of women's pelvic genital tract. About 13,000 women die of this cancer every year. While it does not occur as often as cancer of the uterus, it does occur more often than cancer of the cervix. About one in seventy women will develop cancer of the ovary at some time in their lifetime, and in 75 percent of these women the cancer will have already spread out of their pelvic structures into other parts of the body by the time it is found.

The death rate from cancer of the ovary is now equal to that of uterine cancer and cervical cancer combined. Even though far fewer patients actually develop cancer of the ovary than develop cancer of the uterus and cervix, the cure rate for cervical and uterine cancers is better because they can be detected earlier than ovarian cancer.

As mentioned in Q. 199 it seems that ovarian cancer occurs too infrequently to make routine transvaginal sonograms of all women past the age of menopause a reasonable procedure. This would make the annual exam more trouble and more expensive. As time goes along, it may be that this will become a routine part of the exam of postmenopausal women just as a Pap smear is now a routine part of the examination of every woman who has a pelvic exam no matter what age. One of the problems with this, though, is that ultrasound scans will show on the ovaries cysts that doctors would not have been able to feel on physical exam and that are "normal" cysts. When this happens, unnecessary worry and surgery might result. However, you should be going to a doctor who is able to use good judgment in evaluating such a finding.

The Ca-125 blood test is not likely to ever be used on all women on an annual basis as a test for ovarian cancer because of its limitations. It is elevated only with certain types of ovarian cancer. As mentioned in the previous question, it is elevated at times when there is no ovarian cancer present. If a woman does not have ovarian cancer and yet the Ca-125 is elevated, she could be unnecessarily worried and might insist on surgery that she did not need. As suggested in the previous question, if you have even one close relative who has had ovarian cancer, you should probably get an ultrasound and a Ca-125 every year—perhaps even every six months.

746 What will be done if my doctor strongly suspects, before surgery is done, that I have cancer of the ovary?

Your doctor will order a complete blood count. Several units of blood may be prepared in case you lose a moderate amount of blood during surgery. The doctor will probably order kidney, colon, and chest X-rays to be sure that other organs are not involved in the cancerous process. Your doctor may want a CT scan, a sophisticated X-ray that shows a picture of a cross section of the body, instead of the usual X-ray view. He or she may want an ultrasound examination of your abdomen. These procedures provide additional information about the location of any tumor tissue that might already be out of the ovary. Your doctor will probably want you to have a Ca-125 test done.

Your doctor will tell you that if cancer is present, an incision will be made from your pubic bone to your umbilicus and then around your umbilicus upward for another three or four inches. A large incision is necessary for a complete evaluation of the abdomen, to see whether or not the tumor has spread from the ovary, and to allow removal of as much cancer as possible.

You will need to prepare yourself for this surgery by being healthy in mind and body. The operation can take from three to five hours, because the surgeon will want to be especially careful and thorough.

747 What is done during surgery for ovarian cancer?

After the incision is made, the doctor will irrigate various parts of your pelvis with salt water (saline) and then retrieve the fluid. A pathologist will check the fluid for free cancer cells.

Next, the doctor will look and feel all through your abdomen, including the under surface of your diaphragm and over your kidneys, as well as the apron of fat (the omentum) that hangs from your colon and stomach. He or she will look around your pelvic structures carefully.

The purpose of this careful examination is to determine first, if cancer is present, and second, how far the cancer has gone. Finally, the goal of this surgery is to remove as much of the cancer as possible. Unless your abdominal cavity is examined carefully, the doctor will not know what percentage of the cancer he or she has been able to remove. The success of chemotherapy treatment is partially based on the amount of cancer left in your abdomen at the completion of surgery.

748 What surgical procedures will the doctor perform if I do have ovarian cancer?

If you still want to have children, if your cancer is totally contained inside the ovary, and if it is a low malignant potential type of cancer, the doctor may remove only the ovary where the cancer is grow-

ing. In every other situation the doctor will remove your uterus, tubes, and ovaries and as much of the cancer as possible.

The gynecologist will normally remove the omentum and any cancer implants found growing anywhere in your abdomen, as well as any lymph nodes that are enlarged, to see if they contain cancer.

Nodules of cancer can also grow on the intestines. If a large nodule cannot be cut off the surface of the intestines, a portion of the intestines may need to be cut out to remove the growth. Since ovarian cancer is usually a surface growth, this is not often necessary. When it is necessary, either a colostomy (rarely needed) or an intestinal resection would be done. (A colostomy is a procedure that routes the colon to the outside through the abdominal wall instead of through the anus. Bowel movements, therefore, must come through the colostomy instead of through the anus. An intestinal resection means removing a segment of bowel, then sewing the ends back together.)

When the gynecologist has removed as much of the ovarian cancer as possible, he or she will close the incision and you will go to the recovery room. If the surgery took several hours and/or required blood transfusions, you may go to intensive care for a day or two.

If your cancer has spread outside the ovary, you will almost always need chemotherapy afterward. If your doctor is not a gynecological oncologist, you will probably see an oncologist for this therapy.

In the past, radiation therapy was used to treat ovarian cancer. Today it is used sparingly in the United States and then only with specific, specialized problems. If yours is one of these situations, your physician will discuss that with you.

749 Is chemotherapy effective for ovarian cancer?

There are several chemotherapy drugs that are used for treatment of ovarian cancer; these drugs may be used alone or in combination with each other. The choice of drug therapy will, of course, be in the hands of a specialist who understands the use of these drugs, their benefits, their side effects, and how these relate to your condition.

In years past the outlook for patients with ovarian cancer was fairly hopeless, but with today's drugs and techniques, many patients treated with chemotherapy are free of ovarian cancer for many years, and some seem to be totally cured.

Many patients object to the idea of the use of chemotherapeutic drugs, and I can understand their feelings. For ovarian cancer, however, these drugs are useful. I strongly encourage my patients to take them in this situation. Taking them is unpleasant, of course, but you do not have to take them forever, and they give you a much greater chance of a cure or at least a longer life. Without them the cancer will almost always continue to grow, even after the best surgery. Fortunately, specialists who give these drugs today are usually able to help patients be much more comfortable during chemotherapy than in the past. This makes chemotherapy a much less dreaded procedure today.

750 What does "staging" mean in relation to ovarian cancer?

The "stage" of a cancer refers to how extensive it has become. It is a technical term, and there is a precise definition for each stage. Staging a patient's cancer helps the doctor to define clearly how far along the person's cancer is. It is also useful when doctors with different treatment techniques compare notes in an effort to find the most effective method.

751 What are the different stages of ovarian cancer?

The stages of ovarian cancer are:

Stage I. The cancer is confined to the ovary; it has not spread.

Stage II. The cancer is confined to the pelvis. It may involve, in addition to the ovary or

ovaries, a fallopian tube, the uterus, or some of the lining tissue of the pelvis (peritoneum).

Stage III. The cancer has grown outside the pelvis but is still inside the abdomen. It may involve lymph nodes in the abdomen or the lining of the intestines or other areas of the abdomen.

Stage IV. The cancer involves the liver or areas outside the abdomen, such as the lungs or lymph nodes in other parts of the body.

752 What chance of living do I have after my ovarian cancer is found and treated?

You are fortunate to be living at this time; treatment for ovarian cancer is much better than it once was. In past years doctors often opened patients up, biopsied the growth, and then closed the incision, telling the patient that the cancer was incurable. This was in earlier days when chemotherapy was not as good as it is now, when the best surgical procedures for ovarian cancer had not been determined, and when general surgeons often did this type of operation. Today most patients with ovarian cancer are operated on by a surgeon/gynecologist team or by a specialist in gynecologic oncology. This insures expert surgery and an increased chance for cure.

Your chance of cure is based on the type of cancer you have and in what stage it is when the surgery is done.

Type of cancer. A few types of ovarian cancer have special characteristics that make chances for survival better. For instance, if a *dysgerminoma*, an ovarian cancer that occurs often in young women, has not spread outside of the ovary, removal of the ovary can cure the patient. If tumor tissue is later found elsewhere in the body, this recurrent cancer can be treated with X-ray therapy and often cured. In addition, some ovarian cancer is quite sensitive to chemotherapy. This type of therapy will usually be tried in these cases.

Grade of cancer. The degree of malignancy of the cells is important. Aggressiveness of cancer cells varies from person to person, even when the same type of tumor is involved, but that aggressiveness (or nonaggressiveness) determines how quickly the cancer spreads and how much trouble it causes. For instance, if at surgery you have a cancer that is exactly as extensive as another woman's, yet your cancer is Grade I (a mildly aggressive cancer) but the other woman's cancer is Grade III (much more aggressive cancer), your chance of living for five years is three or four times greater than the other woman's.

Amount of tumor left at first surgery. If the cancer is removed so that there is no piece of cancer remaining in the body thicker than one-eighth inch, the chance of surviving for five years is greatly increased. The reason for this seems to be that if the cancer cannot be totally removed, the cancer that is left in a woman's abdomen can be penetrated by the chemotherapeutic drugs if it is a maximum thickness of one-eighth inch.

If you or a friend or relative has surgery done and the doctor merely closes you up, saying you are "inoperable," immediately call one of the phone numbers given at the end of this chapter. Get the name of a gynecological cancer specialist in your area and contact him or her. Don't give up. You may have months or years of useful life left if you are cared for properly.

Woman's age. The age at which a woman develops cancer is also significant. The younger a woman is when she develops cancer, the greater her chance of survival.

Because all of the above factors are important, it is almost impossible to predict an overall chance of survival from ovarian cancer. In general, however, the following survival rates are quoted by those who treat cancer of the ovary (American College of Obstetricians Technical Bulletin no. 141, May 1990).

> *Stage I:* About 60 to 90 percent of women survive for five years.
> *Stage II:* About 39 to 67 percent of women survive for five years.
> *Stage III:* About 4 to 13 percent of women survive for five years.
> *Stage IV:* About 4 percent of women survive for five years.

These figures mean nothing except that the more extensive the ovarian cancer is, the less likely you are to live for five years. If you have a cancer that is a low-grade malignancy, such as Grade I or II, you are fairly young, and the doctor who operated on you removed most of the cancer, you have a much better chance of living for five years than a patient who is a great deal older, who has a Grade III or IV cancer, and in whom the doctor had to leave large pieces of the cancer behind at the time the surgery was done.

753 How will my doctor know if chemotherapy is successful?

If your cancer was the kind that produced an elevated Ca-125, your physician will probably have you get a Ca-125 blood test just before your chemotherapy and every three or four weeks during your therapy. If your Ca-125 level continues to drop, the cancer is probably responding to chemotherapy; if it stays elevated, your cancer may not be responding. (Even if your Ca-125 level does go down to normal, you still have no guarantee that all cancer is gone.)

To evaluate the success of your treatment, your doctor may suggest a "second-look" operation about a year from your initial surgery. His decision to do this will be influenced in part by the Ca-125 level in your blood. This can be a vital part of your care so I encourage you to let your doctor perform this surgery if he or she thinks it is important.

This second-look operation is major surgery, of course. As large an incision will be made the second time as was made the first time. Biopsies will be taken from all areas of your abdomen. If there is cancer present anywhere in your abdomen, the doctor will try to cut all of it out, even if it requires taking out a part of the colon, the small intestines, or some other structure that can be removed at such surgery.

No one likes the idea of a second operation, but this type of surgery can be extremely helpful in getting you well.

754 I have ovarian cancer and I am scared. Can you help me?

In our darkest times we can find comfort in God's Word:

Because of the LORD's great love we are not consumed, for his compassions never fail. They are new every morning; great is your faithfulness. I say to myself, "The LORD is my portion; therefore I will wait for him."

Lamentations 3:22–24

It is absolutely vital for a woman to fight as hard as she can to overcome all the obstacles that life may present, including ovarian cancer. It is important to have surgery, take chemotherapy, and to have the second-look operation, but all this can be done without bitterness and anger. Becoming bitter and angry ruins the quality of life you have left and also makes those around you unhappy, uncomfortable, and unsure of how to relate to you.

Talk freely with your physician about your chances for survival. It is important to ask what type of therapy is recommended and what side effects you might have. Many doctors are uncomfortable discussing these things so you may need to lead your doctor into telling you what you need to know.

Of course you want a doctor who believes he or she can cure you and who will not easily give up. But if your doctor cannot give you good emotional support, talk to your pastor, priest, or rabbi, or see a psychologist or psychiatrist. Such counseling can be of great help in hard times. More important than this is your talking to God himself. He loves you. Pray. Open your heart to him. He can provide the comfort that no one else can.

755 Where can I get more information about ovarian cancer?

A woman normally has a one in seventy chance of developing ovarian cancer at some time in her life, but with two or more close relatives having ovarian cancer, her chance increases to as high as one in fifty. That is why it is so important that women with this history be watched carefully for ovarian cancer. They need to start this vigilance in their early thirties. If you have this family history, it may be best for you to have your ovaries removed after you have completed childbearing.

For more information about this problem, contact the Gilda Radner Familial Ovarian Cancer Registry, c/o Dr. M. Steven Piver or Dr. Trudy R. Baker, Department of Gynecologic Oncology, Roswell Park Cancer Institute, Elm at Carlton Streets, Buffalo, NY 14263, phone 1-800-OVARIAN.

A toll-free number has been established by the National Cancer Institute. The number is easy to remember: 1-800-4-CANCER. If you call, you will be connected with the Cancer Information Service in your area.

Since this service was established in 1976, it has responded to more than three million inquiries from the general public. The response to these calls is confidential, and you will receive, if you wish, free publications on specific cancers and also on techniques for cancer prevention, cancer treatment, and for coping with cancer.

In addition, the public library will have books, magazines, and further information on cancer. Many libraries offer access to the Internet, where you can obtain the latest information.

Finally, you might call a hospital that specializes in cancer and ask for the gynecology department. The cancer hot line can tell you how to reach the nearest cancer hospital in your area.

Problems of the Breasts

The human breast is obviously important to human beings since we are classified as a mammal (*mammae:* Latin word meaning those who nourish their young with milk) species. Also, not long ago human breast milk was necessary for the continuation of the human race. Now, although mother's milk is still the best food for a baby, there are alternative methods of feeding our young. The breast is not exclusively nurture-related, however.

A woman's breasts have great psychological, social, and sexual significance, especially, it seems, in today's society. Actually, breasts have probably always had this prestige.

Because of the importance of the breast in all these areas, there is a great deal of concern when something seems to be wrong with them. Parents are concerned if a daughter's breasts do not seem to be developing properly, and the girl herself is often concerned if her breast development does not equal that of her friends. Women are extremely concerned about breast lumps. The specter of cancer, with its potential for causing the loss of a breast, always makes the discovery of such lumps a frightening event.

In the questions that follow, we will discuss various diseases of the breasts. Other aspects of the breast are discussed elsewhere in the book: In chapter 1 we discussed the basic anatomy of the breasts; in chapters 2 and 3 we discussed developmental abnormalities of the breast in baby, child, and adolescent; and in chapter 11 we will discuss the problem of galactorrhea (milky secretions from the breasts). Refer to those chapters and to the index for further information.

756 If I develop a problem with my breasts, will my gynecologist or primary care doctor treat it?

If you have suspicious breast lumps or probable breast cancer, your doctor will usually refer you to a general surgeon. This is because most doctors who are not surgeons come from specialized educational programs that provide little training in the treatment of breast growths and breast cancer.

The information I am providing in this section about breast problems is the type of information you would receive from a gynecologist; we will not attempt to delve in great detail into breast surgery or breast cancer.

The gynecologist's (or other primary care physician's) limitation in the care of your breasts does not mean he or she is unimportant in the care of your breasts. Gynecologists do more breast exams, in fact, than general surgeons do, because of the number of patients they see for annual examinations. And, because gynecologists are familiar with the administration of hormones, they are much more likely than a general surgeon to be able to help you avoid aggravating and recurring breast nodules by use of appropriate hormones. This alone may help avoid many biopsies that a general surgeon might otherwise need to do. In addition, a gynecologist will usually be more knowledgeable and understanding if you have a problem with breast pain and will often have suggestions for relieving such discomfort.

757 Is there anything I need to do between annual examinations to keep my breasts normal and healthy?

Yes. You should do regular breast self-examinations (BSE), since 90 percent of breast lumps are discovered by women themselves, using this technique. Remember, even though you may have very recently had a breast examination by your physician, you could have an early breast cancer growing in your breast right now. If you wait twelve months for another exam, that cancer could have grown to a dangerous stage before it is found.

Since it is unrealistic for you to see your doctor often enough to feel safe about your breasts, you should do breast self-examinations once a month, right after your period. It is important to do the exam at that time, because then your breasts are the least swollen and knotty. If you have a breast nodule, your doctor may want you to check your breasts more often than once a month. Choose a special way to help you remember when to check your breasts. For example, check them on the fourth day of your menstrual period; if you are on birth-control pills, do a BSE on the day you take the first pill each month; or if you have had a hysterectomy or have gone through menopause, check your breasts on the first day of the calendar month.

Many of my patients will not check their breasts. Some are afraid that they might find a lump; others say they just forget. Both reasons, while understandable, are dangerous thinking. Failing to examine the breasts will not keep breast cancer from developing; it will only allow it to become dangerously enlarged before it is found.

You should continue to check your breasts even if you are pregnant or nursing. There have been many sad cases in which women found a breast lump during pregnancy or while nursing, but they or their physicians assumed those lumps were caused by the hormones of pregnancy or lactation, only to find out later that they had been neglecting a breast cancer.

Many women feel that they would not know a "significant" breast lump from an insignificant one. As one who has felt many breast cancers, I can say with conviction that if you have a breast cancer in your breast, you will almost certainly know it when you feel it. There is something "different" about the way it feels. Just do the exam. Don't worry about whether or not you would feel a breast cancer—you would. Such a lump will be different from the lumpy, irregular-feeling places you have previously felt. I tell my patients that they are looking for something that feels like a "Texas pecan" or a big marble. I hope you never feel it, but if such a lump is in your breast, I can almost guarantee that you will know it is different from anything you've felt in your breast.

Obviously all those who encourage you to do a regular BSE, such as your doctor and the American Cancer Society, know that you are not a professional "breast checker." In spite of that, we still encourage you to do BSE because we know that if you have a breast cancer, you will detect it sooner than if you were not examining your breasts regularly.

758 How is a breast self-examination done?

The classic technique for BSE is illustrated on p. 416.

If you feel any lumps anywhere be sure to let your doctor know.

I find that many women will not do the entire BSE procedure. If you are one who absolutely will not do all of it, at least check your breasts in the shower with soapy fingers, or check them in bed, lying on your back.

In addition to the instructions on p. 416, it is a good idea to get your doctor to show you how to do a breast examination. I use a movie in my office that gives BSE instructions. In addition, I have models of the female breast, complete with various-sized lumps, so that my patients can get an idea of what a breast lump feels like. Your doctor may have these instructional tools available. If so, take advantage of them. If not, encourage your doctor to get them.

759 Which symptoms might indicate breast problems?

There are several important danger signs that should be checked by your physician:

a lump in the breast or in the axilla (armpit)
discoloration of the skin of the breast
bleeding or discharge from the nipple
lumpiness of the breasts that makes one breast look different from the other
dimpling of the skin of the breast
retraction of the nipple
prominent veins of the breast that have not been present before
thickening of breast skin
area of the breast that is hot or warmer than the rest of the breast or than the other breast
sore on the breast or nipple that does not heal
unusual pain in the breast

760 Is it normal to have painful breasts?

Yes, it can be quite normal to have painful breasts. Pain that fluctuates with the menstrual cycle is almost always due to normal changes in the body and not to breast disease.

Breasts are made up of cells that are sensitive to estrogen and progesterone. As the estrogen level increases during the menstrual cycle, and as pro-

Breast Self-Examination

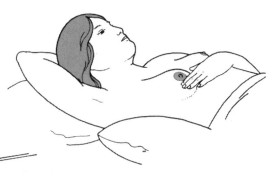

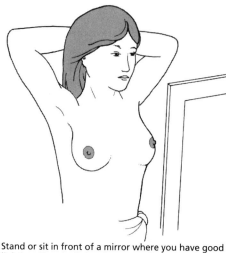

Lie down on your back. Examine your left breast with your right hand and your right breast with your left hand. It is best to do this with a small pillow under the shoulder of the breast you are examining.

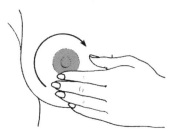

Stand or sit in front of a mirror where you have good lighting. Place both hands on top of your head and pull your arms back. Observe your breasts carefully, looking for indentations of the skin (retraction), puckering, and any irregularities or thickening of the skin. Look at the nipples to be sure that they are the same as they were in previous months. Don't be surprised if your breasts are not the same size; no woman's breasts are exactly symmetrical.

Examine your breasts with your fingers together flat against your breasts, with gentle but firm pressure. Work from the outside toward the nipple, or from the nipple out, in a circular, spiral pattern.

Also feel the area around the nipple. Squeeze the nipple gently to see if there is any discharge.

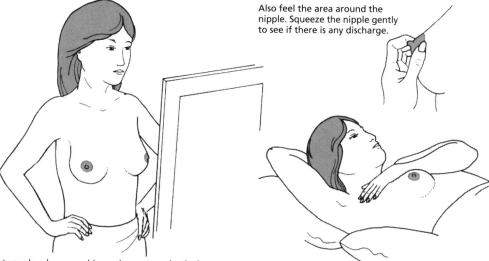

Put your hands on your hips and press to make the breasts "stand out." Then do the visual check again.

Feel up under your arm in your armpit (axilla).

416

gesterone adds to the already stimulated breast tissue, the breasts will become sensitive, especially during the days just before the menstrual period.

Some women have breasts that are unusually sensitive to these hormone fluctuations of the menstrual cycle. Their breasts can become so tender just before their periods start that they cannot sleep on their stomachs. This is normal for them. The woman who has this type of pain does not need to worry, since it is not a sign of cancer or of any other disease process.

If the breasts hurt, the problem is usually not cancer. It is most likely due to normal hormonal changes of the breasts or fibrocystic breast change. If you do have unusual breast pain, however, see your doctor. Breast cancer *can* hurt. Cancer is so slow in growing that it does not normally cause breast pain, but if you have a lump, whether or not it hurts, see your doctor.

761 Can breast pain be due to an abnormality?

Yes, breast pain can be caused by several different problems.

Pain due to nerves of the chest wall. A woman who has had a neck injury can have resulting irritation of the nerves that go to the wall of the chest. Women may think the pain they are having is in their breast tissue, but an exam will show that it is actually in the wall of the chest.

Pain from structures in the chest wall. It is not uncommon for patients to have pain in a rib, or in cartilage between the rib and the breastbone, and assume it is breast pain. An examination will usually identify this pain across the wall of the chest. If one of the muscles of the chest wall or its attachment to the bone becomes irritated, pain can develop under the breast and seem to be breast pain. Careful examination usually identifies the source of such pain.

Blood clot in a vein of the breast surface (Mandor's disease). Occasionally a vein of the skin over the breast will become clotted, causing tenderness and pain. It takes careful examination by a physician to make this diagnosis. This condition is not dangerous, but it must not be confused with inflam-matory cancer of the breast, which is an extremely malignant process.

Fibrocystic change. (See next question.)

762 What is fibrocystic disease of the breasts?

This problem, now called "fibrocystic breast change," is present in so many women that it is not called "disease" anymore. Some degree of fibrocystic change of the breasts occurs in more than 50 percent of all women, and some authorities say that all women have some elements of this change in their breasts. This is not a disease, since it is neither an infection caused by a germ, nor is it a growth, such as a tumor. Fibrocystic change is merely the overreaction of the breast tissue to normal female hormones. The cells of your breast tissue have estrogen receptors. This is how your breasts are able to sense the presence of estrogen and to respond to it with thickening and growth, and how they originally developed.

A great many women have breast tissue that overresponds to normal estrogen and progesterone production. When this happens, their breasts "thicken up" too much during the week or two before a period, then, when the hormone levels naturally decrease and the breasts lose the stimulation, too many of the cells in the overstimulated breasts break down, filling the ducts of the breasts with excess cellular debris. In addition, the ducts of the breasts are narrowed with fibrocystic change, slowing the exit of this debris even more and forming pockets of fluid that cause the pain and cysts of fibrocystic change. Since fibrocystic change can make BSE (breast self-examination) confusing, it is best to check the breasts right after the monthly period when they are the least swollen. (This is also the best time to get a mammogram.)

763 What problems can fibrocystic breast change cause?

Fibrocystic change can cause several problems.

Pain. The fluctuation of hormones in a woman's normal cycle cause fibrocystic breasts to swell and change more than they otherwise would, and these fibrocystic changes can cause pain. The pain from these changes normally increases during the premenstrual time and decreases after the period has ended. As stated previously, such pain is usually not a symptom of cancer because cancer is unlikely to put enough pressure on the breast tissue to cause pain, at least until it has been growing for a long time.

Lumpiness. Fibrocystic change causes breasts to be lumpy. Many women think that normal breast tissue should feel soft like fat. They think that any nodularity or firmness in their breasts is fibrocystic change or a tumor. This is a misconception. Normal breast tissue is embedded in the fat of the breasts. Breast tissue itself is gland tissue and is firm, just as most other gland tissue of the human body is firm. A man's testicles are glands and demonstrate the firm nature of gland tissue. The firm tissue you feel embedded in the fat of your breast is breast tissue. When you examine your breasts, it is not this firm, glandular tissue that is significant; rather it is change in that tissue that you are looking for.

Some nodularity of breast tissue is to be expected with the monthly changes in the breasts. When you do a BSE you are looking for something different such as a discrete (distinguishable) firm or rubbery nodule or a discrete cystic area. I describe them to my patients as being separate, distinct areas not actually embedded in the surrounding tissue, something like a small peeled grape that moves easily.

If you do find a breast lump, it is much more likely to be fibroadenoma than a cancer. These breast nodules are a result of fibrocystic change in the breast. If you do have these nodules in one breast, there will be similar lumps in the other breast 12 to 25 percent of the time.

764 What should I do if I find a lump in my breast?

You should make an appointment to see a doctor for evaluation. There is no need to panic, however. If a breast cancer is present, it has already been growing for several years before it became large enough to feel. A few days' delay will not make any difference in your chance of recovery even if it is cancer.

It is most important to see a doctor who will give you proper consultation and will give thorough consideration to your problem. This is far more important than for you to rush madly into the first available doctor's office.

765 What will a doctor look for when checking a breast lump?

There are several things a doctor will look for when checking a breast lump.

Changes in the skin or nipples. Changes of this type mean that a growth is more likely to be cancerous. They might include dimpling of the skin over the lump or discoloration, perhaps reddening, of the skin or nipple. Don't let an acne-type bump in the skin of your breast or nipple scare you, though. These are almost always insignificant. If a nipple is "pulled off" in one direction, this may indicate a breast cancer under the nipple area that is distorting the nipple.

An isolated lump. If your lump is isolated and not a part of a thickened area in the breast, it is slightly more likely to be cancer. A lump that is part of a group of other lumps, or part of a generally thickened area in the breast, is more likely fibrocystic change.

Attachment of the lump. If the lump seems attached to the skin or to the chest wall, it is more likely malignant. Benign lumps in the breast do not usually attach in this fashion.

Hard consistency. If your lump is hard, it is more likely to be cancer than if it is soft and easily compressed.

Bloody discharge from the nipple. Blood from the nipple can indicate a cancerous growth. This problem should be thoroughly evaluated.

Lymph nodes under the arm. If you feel some lymph nodes under your arm (in the axillary area), this can indicate a breast cancer that has spread into those lymph nodes. If you have had a lymph node in your axilla for several years, don't panic. If a node was cancerous, it would have already grown, so don't worry about one that has been there for a long time.

766 When I see my gynecologist because of a breast lump, what will he or she do?

If you have a distinct breast lump, your gynecologist will probably try to aspirate it. If the doctor can get fluid out of it and the lump then disappears, you can forget about it, the lump is not cancer.

Aspiration is an essentially painless procedure in which a doctor injects a local anesthetic into the skin and then inserts a needle into a breast lump in an attempt to draw off the fluid. You do need to have follow-up exams, and you do need to continue monthly BSE.

If the aspirated fluid is bloody, or if the mass does not go away after aspiration, your physician will probably ask you to get a mammogram and go to a general surgeon for evaluation.

If no fluid can be aspirated the mass is probably a fibroadenoma; it could, however, be cancer. If the doctor cannot get fluid, he will usually pull back on the syringe in an effort to get some cells from the tissue to send to a pathologist. If the pathologist sees cancer on the slide, a biopsy will be unnecessary. The woman can then consult a surgeon about her cancer.

If the slide does not show cancer cells, that does not necessarily mean there is no cancer present. The needle could have bypassed the cancer if it is small.

If the mass in your breast is not distinct, your doctor may suggest that you return after one or two menstrual periods to see if it has become less nodular. If time results in a less noticeable lump, it is almost certainly fibrocystic change. Even if your doctor feels confident that you do not have cancer, he or she will probably want you to have a mammogram just to be sure. If your physician is uncertain about the nature of your problem, he or she will almost certainly want you to have a mammogram and will probably recommend that you see a general surgeon for consultation.

767 Are there high-risk categories for breast cancer?

Certain situations make you more likely than the average person to develop breast cancer sometime in your life. This is not meant to scare you, but to help you. You can, of course, have all of these factors and never develop cancer, but women with some of them need to watch their breasts more carefully, consult their doctors a little sooner, and have biopsies a little more often than other women. The higher-risk categories for breast cancer are:

Being a woman. Breast cancer occurs in less than 1 percent of the male population.

Women over thirty-five. If you are over thirty-five, you are more likely to develop breast cancer. Less than 4 percent of breast cancer occurs in women under thirty-five.

Family members with cancer. If you have a close family member who has had breast cancer (mother, sister, or aunt), you are two or three times more likely to develop breast cancer than the average woman. This appears to be a genetic problem fairly often. If your family carries an abnormality (mutation) of the BRCA1 gene, you may have an increased chance of developing breast cancer. A recent study showed that 1 percent of American Jews have this problem ("Genetics," *Nature*, September 29, 1995).

Previous breast cancer. If you have had breast cancer already, you are more likely to develop breast cancer in the remaining breast than the average woman.

National origin. If you are Jewish, you are more likely to develop breast cancer. (See above—"Family.")

Menstrual cycle record. If you started menstrual periods before the age of twelve or began menopause after the age of fifty, you are more likely to develop breast cancer.

Childbirth record. If you did not have your first child until after you were thirty years of age or if you have never had a child, you are more likely to develop breast cancer than a woman who had her first child before she was thirty years old.

Alcohol consumption. If you drink alcohol daily, whether it is wine, beer, or hard liquor, you are more likely to develop breast cancer than if you do not consume alcohol that often.

Weight. If you are 10 percent above the average weight for your height and age, you are more likely to develop breast cancer.

Fibrocystic change. If you have fibrocystic change of the breasts, some studies show you are more likely to develop breast cancer. These studies are not completely reliable, however, because almost all women have fibrocystic changes. If you have this problem, let the possibility of a slightly increased risk for breast cancer motivate you to be regular about BSE and mammograms.

Diet. Recent studies have indicated that women who eat the typical American diet, which is high in meat and fat and low in fiber, have an increased risk of breast cancer.

Abortion and miscarriage. Studies done in the early 1990s show that you may have a slightly increased chance of breast cancer if your first pregnancy ended with a miscarriage or an abortion.

768 If a biopsy is the only truly accurate method of diagnosis for breast lumps, what is the value of the other tests?

Occasionally tests can indicate the presence of cancer even when you and your doctor do not otherwise suspect the possibility. For instance, 45 percent of the breast cancers that are found by mammograms are so small that they cannot be found on examination by you or your doctor. If a breast cancer is found by mammogram before it can be felt on exam, a woman has an 80 to 95 percent chance of being totally cured. If, however, her cancer is not found until it can be felt by examination, she has a 50 to 70 percent chance of cure.

Routine mammograms can show a breast cancer on the average of two years before it would be large enough for a woman to feel on breast self-examination. Obviously, therefore, if your cancer is found before it is large enough for you to feel it, your chance of cure is excellent.

769 What is a mammogram?

A mammogram is simply an X-ray of the breasts. (The examination itself is called a mammography.) The purpose of this X-ray is to find abnormalities inside the body that cannot be found in any other way.

There are two types of machines for performing mammograms. One is made by the Xerox Corporation and it does Xero-radiography (xeromammograms). The other is film screen mammography. Both of these techniques have reduced radiation levels from mammograms to about one-twentieth of what they were years ago.

Most mammogram machines expose a woman to less than one rad of X-ray, which is only about 0.1 percent of the level of radiation she receives from sunlight and the natural radiation around her each year. This amount of radiation is so minimal that a woman really does not need to worry about it. She should have mammograms done as recommended by the American Cancer Society and her physician.

A mammogram is a simple procedure. Because it takes a moderate amount of pressure on the breasts to obtain a good "picture," the procedure is a little painful. Try to tolerate a little pain since the better the mammogram, the more likely it is to find a small growth in the breast. To do the mammogram, it is necessary for a woman to undress down to her waist, but she can wear a gown to cover part of her upper body while the X-ray is being done.

770 What are the American Cancer Society recommendations for mammograms?

Most physicians, myself included, strongly support the recommendations of the American Cancer Society for mammograms. We feel that all patients should follow these guidelines unless there is a reason to have mammograms more often:

35 to 40 years of age: At least one mammogram during these years.

40 to 50 years of age: A mammogram every one or two years.

50 years of age and up: A mammogram every year for the rest of her life.

Studies have shown that if women would follow these recommendations, the number of women who die from breast cancer would decrease by at least 30 percent, and perhaps up to as much as 50 percent. A mammogram can detect breast cancers that are less than one-half centimeter in size (about one-eighth inch across). When a breast cancer is this small, there is very little chance that it has already spread out of the breast and, if treated at this stage, there is only a slim possibility that the cancer will return later.

771 Do mammograms show all breast cancers?

When discussing mammograms with my patients, I tell them that there are two types of breast cancer—the kind that shows up on mammograms and the kind that doesn't. (This is not completely scientifically correct, but it helps clarify the explanation!)

Mammograms will show about 90 percent of breast cancers, but they will not show about 10 percent of them even if they are quite large. This is because some breast cancers do not produce certain "signs" that are indications of cancer. Therefore, physical examination of the breasts is still important in detecting breast cancer.

If a woman has a breast lump that a mammogram indicates is benign, she should still have it biopsied if her physician recommends it because the lump could be cancer.

In a study reported in the journal *Cancer* (1987, 60:1979–1983), Dr. Frankl showed that if a breast cancer was found by the patient or the physician on palpation (manual exam), 32 percent of the patients died from the breast cancer. If the cancer was found by mammography, only 16 percent of the women died of the cancer, and if the cancer

was found by mammography when it was very small, only 2 percent of those patients died.

Dr. Frankl's study emphasizes the importance of mammography. This X-ray can find breast cancer much earlier than it can be felt and can help determine if the lump has malignant characteristics.

772 What problems make a mammogram necessary?

Mammograms should be done in the following situations.

Women of any age who have such irregular, lumpy, firm, or enlarged breasts that an adequate breast examination is impossible should have a mammogram done on a regular basis. They should, however, continue doing BSE. Even though it is difficult to do on certain types of breasts, BSE is still a vitally important examination.

Patients who have suspicious breast symptoms, such as a lump, nipple discharge, bleeding from the nipple, severe pain, or persistent redness of the skin of the breasts need to have a mammogram done.

Patients who have no symptoms or problems but who are in high-risk categories (see Q. 767) need more frequent mammograms on a schedule recommended by their physicians.

773 What other screening tests of the breasts are done?

At the present time, the only screening test besides mammography useful for evaluation of breast problems is ultrasound. An ultrasound machine sends out sound waves and receives them back with an echo-receiving device called a transducer. The transducer then "draws a picture" on a screen for the radiologist to evaluate. Ultrasound is a safe procedure, and there is no X-ray-type radiation involved.

Ultrasound is used primarily as a backup to mammograms, to help make breast evaluation more accurate. For instance, if a mammogram shows a lump, an ultrasound exam may be able to tell if the lump is solid or fluid-filled. If the lump is fluid-filled it is almost never a cancer. Also there are some abnormal ultrasound patterns that can suggest the presence of breast cancer.

774 What is involved in breast biopsy?

A breast biopsy is ordinarily a simple procedure. It is normally done through a small incision. More and more surgeons are doing such biopsies in an outpatient setting, although your doctor may not have access to such an operating situation and may need to admit you to the hospital.

The surgeon injects a local anesthetic, or an anesthesiologist gives you general anesthetic. A small incision is then made, and through it the suspicious portion of the breast is removed. Stitches are used to stop bleeding and the incision is closed. Healing is usually complete within three weeks.

There are great advantages to having a breast biopsy. If a woman is worried that she has breast cancer, a breast biopsy can reassure her that she does not. If she does have cancer, the biopsy insures treatment as soon as possible, giving her the best chance of cure.

775 What is needle localization for a breast biopsy?

If a mammogram shows a suspicious area in the breast but the area is too small to feel, the surgeon and radiologist can use a technique called needle localization to find it so a biopsy can be done. Using a special mammography machine, with local anesthesia, the radiologist will direct the tip of a needle into the suspicious area under the guidance of the X-ray. The needle has a small barb on the end to hold it in place for the surgeon who operates. You are then moved to where the surgeon will take out the tissue around the needle tip along with the needle. This bit of tissue will then be X-rayed to be sure this tissue is the suspicious area seen on the original mammogram. From there the tissue goes to a pathologist for evaluation.

776 If the doctor does a breast biopsy and finds cancer, will my breast be removed while I am asleep?

Almost never. Most breast biopsies are now done in an outpatient setting. The pathologist will usually not do a frozen section but will do permanent slides, which will yield results in a few days. The patient is then informed that she does or does not have cancer of the breast. If she does have cancer of the breast, she has time to decide which form of therapy she prefers.

Studies have shown conclusively that when a cancer is present, a breast biopsy does not cause that cancer to spread, provided that the mastectomy is not delayed for more than about two weeks.

Occasionally, especially with an older patient, it may be best for a woman to go to the hospital and have the biopsy done under general anesthesia. The pathologist can do a frozen section while the patient is still asleep. This takes only a few minutes, and if the pathologist finds cancer, the surgeon can proceed with a lumpectomy or mastectomy. In this way a woman can get the entire procedure over at one time. She avoids having two operations (first a biopsy, and later a mastectomy) and she does not have the anxiety of waiting one or two days for the pathologist's report. Some women prefer having their breast lump biopsy done this way.

777 If a breast lump is not cancer, what else can it be?

Eight out of ten breast lumps are benign. Those nonmalignant breast lumps might be:

Thickening or cysts. Such thickening or cysts may be the result of fibrocystic change of the breasts.

Fibroadenomas of the breast. This is usually a solitary mass in the breast, occurring in women between the ages of fifteen and thirty-nine. These lumps are usually easy to feel, are smooth and firm, and tend to move around when palpated. The problem is that a doctor cannot tell for sure by feel alone whether a lump is a simple fibroadenoma or

Special Concerns

an early breast cancer. If such a lump does not have any fluid present when a needle is used to aspirate it, a breast biopsy is almost always required to determine whether or not cancer is present. Mammography and ultrasound can often help with the diagnosis.

Intraductal papillomas. This problem is caused by an overgrowth of normal duct lining. Papillomas can cause oozing of fluid, often bloody in nature. This, of course, scares a patient and concerns her doctor. The doctor's caution is to avoid being too radical with a situation that is usually not malignant and at the same time to not overlook a cancer. Mammograms help make sure there is no cancer present. Follow-up exams are recommended. Sometimes resection of a portion of the breast from which the ducts come is necessary to stop the bleeding problem and to confirm that there is no malignancy present.

The doctor will often get a Pap smear of the fluid from the nipple for the pathologist to check for cancer cells. This is useful, but not totally reliable. If bleeding persists, your doctor will almost certainly want you to have a biopsy, even if the mammogram is normal.

Other lumps may be accumulations of fat, scar, or other less common tissues.

778 Why do I hear so much about breast cancer?

Breast cancer is a very serious malignancy affecting women in the United States. It is the number-two cancer killer of American women, and, according to the National Cancer Institute, the incidence of breast cancer has reached an all-time high in the United States. Breast cancer is the most common malignancy among women, striking an estimated one in nine women.

In 1984, the Centers for Disease Control estimated that breast cancer victims were robbed of more than 227,000 years of potential life. This means that these women were robbed of the life they would have had if they lived to age sixty-five. Stated another way, breast cancer accounts for more than 25 percent of all the life years lost prematurely by U.S. women to cancer, more than any other specific cancer reported.

Breast cancer is the second leading cause of all cancer deaths, regardless of age, among U.S. women. It follows lung cancer. Fewer women develop lung cancer, but more women die of lung cancer than of breast cancer. One sad fact is that breast cancer robs young women of years of life because it so often occurs in younger women than lung cancer.

Survival rates of breast cancer patients depends on early detection. The sooner a woman finds a breast cancer, the better. For instance, if all women over fifty had mammograms every year, the death rate from breast cancer would drop by one-third. Finding the cancer when it is small, even before it is large enough to feel, means it is less likely to have spread.

These statistics are not cited to scare you but to encourage you to do two things: be faithful about doing your breast self-examinations, and follow the American Cancer Society guidelines for mammography.

779 What surgical techniques are used to treat breast cancer?

Four techniques are used for the treatment of breast cancer.

Radical mastectomy. This procedure involves removing the entire breast, the underlying chest muscles (pectorals), and the lymph nodes under the arm. There are variations of this type of operation, but all of them are drastic, leaving the chest wall quite disfigured. In addition, these procedures can restrict movement of the arm and cause edema, or swelling of the arm.

This procedure is not done routinely in this country anymore. About the only indication for its use is a cancer that has invaded the muscles under the breast. In this case, those pectoral muscles must be removed to get around the cancer.

Simple (total) mastectomy. This operation is called a modified radical mastectomy if the entire breast is taken and, at the same time, a dissection of all of the lymph nodes under the arm is done. It is called a simple or total mastectomy

Types of Mastectomies

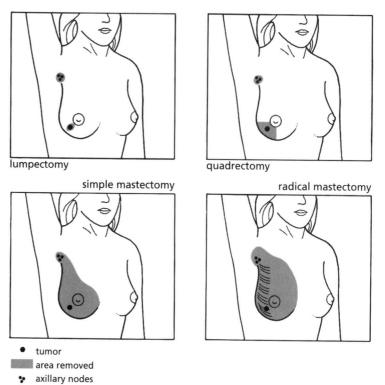

lumpectomy

quadrectomy

simple mastectomy

radical mastectomy

● tumor

▮ area removed

❧ axillary nodes

if the operation removes the entire breast and samples a few of the lymph nodes under the arm (or takes no lymph nodes). The pectoral muscles are not removed. Because of this, disfigurement is not so drastic, swelling of the arm is uncommon, and arm movement is not restricted. This is the operation most commonly used by U.S. surgeons now.

The only absolute reason for even simple mastectomy is if the tumor involves a large portion of the breast and trying to cut the cancer out would leave the rest of the breast so deformed that it might as well be removed. Studies have shown, however, that the cure rate for simple mastectomy is no better than when only a part of the breast is removed and radiation therapy given.

Segmental resection of the breast and quadrant resection of the breast. These two operations involve cutting around the breast cancer widely, taking out as much as a fourth of the breast tissue. These operations are normally accompanied by a separate incision under the arm, through which the

doctor removes at least some of the underarm lymph nodes. Tests of the lymph nodes give some idea of how far the cancer has spread in the body and how likely is a cure, since the fewer involved lymph nodes under the arm, the more likely the cure. Radiation is usually used after these operations.

Excision of the cancer lump itself (lumpectomy). It is possible for the doctor to merely cut the lump itself out of the breast. A lumpectomy is normally done only when the breast cancer is early and small and always involves removal of axillary (underarm) nodes. Radiation therapy is often used. Radiation can cause swelling and stiffness of the breast and skin discoloration. (See Q. 782.) Several studies have shown that women are just as likely to survive breast cancer with a lumpectomy as with a mastectomy.

Physicians who care for women realize that all women are very concerned about breast surgery. Therefore, various methods of treatment have been devised; these options have been used long enough now to know how successful they are. The surgical management of breast cancer is no longer automatically a mastectomy, but can now be tailored to a woman's particular situation.

780 Do you have any suggestions about how to decide on the best way to treat my breast cancer?

Breast cancer is found at different stages, different women have different situations, and there are many different attitudes among surgeons. Therefore, the approach to treating breast cancer can be somewhat confusing.

In general, it is felt that if a breast cancer is Stage I (smaller than three-fourths of an inch across and not spread to the lymph nodes) or Stage II (from three-fourths to two inches across and may or may not have spread to the lymph nodes), the lump itself can be removed and the breast treated with radiation.

Some women prefer to have a mastectomy so they can feel more confident that the cancer has been totally removed. As a matter of fact, most women today are still having mastectomies for breast cancer. You and your physician will need to discuss the best approach for you and your cancer.

With either of these operations, it is necessary that the underarm lymph nodes be removed to see if the breast cancer has spread into them.

In the following situations, mastectomy might be the procedure of choice:

1. If a breast tumor is so large that removing it would leave the breast deformed
2. If a woman has two cancers in the same breast, and they are fairly far apart
3. If a mammogram shows multiple suspicious areas
4. If a woman's breasts are very large (because high radiation doses would be required to penetrate the breast tissue to reach the cancer)
5. If a woman lives in a location where she cannot get radiation therapy easily (to avoid travel back and forth from her home to a distant radiation center over a period of several weeks)

Your physician will discuss these and other options with you so that you can come to a decision you are comfortable with.

781 I have heard it is best to have chemotherapy after surgery for breast cancer. Is that true?

If you have found your breast cancer very early, it is smaller than one-third of an inch, and there is no lymph node involvement, you probably do not need chemotherapy. If you do have lymph nodes with cancer in them, most experts feel that you should have chemotherapy if you have not yet gone through menopause. The type of drugs and the length of treatment would be an individual matter determined by you and your physicians.

If you have lymph node involvement with breast cancer and you have gone through menopause, it is unclear whether or not you should use chemotherapy. One approach is that if your cancer cells have estrogen receptors (the ability to perceive that estrogen is present), you should receive a drug called Tamoxifen. (This is an anti-estrogen drug.) The reason for using this is because any cancer cells left in your body after surgery might grow because of estrogen. (A woman still has a small amount of estrogen in her body, even after menopause.) Tamoxifen can neutralize the presence of estrogen in your body and keep that kind of stimulation from affecting any breast cancer cells in your body.

If you have estrogen receptor-negative breast cancer and you are postmenopausal, your physicians may recommend chemotherapy.

Ironically, Tamoxifen seems to stimulate the lining of the uterus in a way that increases the chance of uterine cancer. If a woman takes Tamoxifen for a long period of time, it is important for her to have an endometrial biopsy (scraping of the uterus) every few years to be sure there is no precancerous or cancerous buildup developing in her uterus.

The addition of chemical therapy to the treatment plan for breast cancer—whether it is through chemotherapy, Tamoxifen, or both—is extremely helpful. It definitely lowers the chance of a recurrent cancer.

The initial dose of chemotherapy is very important. It is apparently even more important than the total amount of chemotherapy that a woman receives. Although larger doses increase the toxicity to a patient, the ultimate results are worth it.

A hopeful comment was made by the editor of *OB/GYN Survey* (34.8) in a 1989 article in the *New England Journal of Medicine:* "It is indeed encouraging to know that this devastating cancer does seem to be slowly coming under control, but it is also important for the physician to remember that the smaller the lesion, the better the results. So don't let your patient procrastinate, and don't you procrastinate. Small tumors can be treated with excellent cosmetic effect and with a highly improved survival."

782 My doctor's standard operation is total removal of the breast for any breast cancer, and he will not talk to me about more limited surgery. Where can I get more information?

The National Cancer Institute has set up a hot line for cancer information. Through this hot line you can get information about all aspects of breast cancer: surgery, treatment, and prevention.

The telephone number for the cancer hot line is (800) 4-CANCER.

783 Is breast reconstruction a good idea after mastectomy?

Because the emotional impact of breast surgery is so great, reconstructive surgery for the breast is a major breakthrough in the overall treatment of patients with breast cancer. A Gallup Poll revealed that 60 percent of women felt that their womanhood would be impaired if they had to have a breast removed, 18 percent felt that the loss of a breast would be more important to them than the

loss of a limb, and 9 percent said they would "rather die" than have a breast removed! Obviously, then, a woman's breasts are an integral part of her femininity and sexuality, and losing a breast can cause significant psychological trauma.

Having a breast reconstructed can be an important step in adjusting to breast cancer. Not only will a woman look and feel better and therefore be less self-conscious, but she will also be more comfortable.

In addition, if women do not fear the disfigurement of breast cancer so much because they know they can have a breast reconstruction, they will, hopefully, examine themselves more regularly, have necessary surgery done more quickly, and therefore have a better chance of never having the cancer return.

784 If I know I am going to have a mastectomy, and I am considering breast reconstruction, should anything special be done in preparation for that?

If you are going to have a mastectomy, it is important that you discuss with your surgeon the fact that you plan to have breast reconstruction done. Increasingly more breast reconstruction is being done as a part of mastectomy surgery. The procedure would be carefully planned in advance as your surgeon, a plastic surgeon, and possibly a radiologist consult with each other. During the surgery, your surgeon would then make incisions in your breasts in the least visible areas, allowing the plastic surgeon, who would be on hand during the surgery to "take over" following the mastectomy, to do the best possible reconstruction.

Plastic surgeons are able to construct breasts that are very acceptable cosmetically, allowing a woman to dress as she did before surgery. When the surface skin and nipple are "salvaged," the result is completely natural; when skin must be grafted, as is necessary following radical mastectomies, and nipples are fashioned using tissue from the inner thigh, the labia, and other parts of the body—the result is still quite acceptable. In both cases, form and comfort, the two major considerations to most women, are established.

Research has shown that breast reconstruction reduces a woman's anxiety about subsequent sexual relations. The same research indicates that women have less feeling of loss, less grief, and less depression following mastectomy if they have breast reconstruction done. Such surgery also seems to lessen the fear of recurrence of the cancer. Breast reconstruction today is done either without implants or with saline (salt water) implants. You therefore do not need to worry about the silicone controversy if you desire reconstruction.

While mastectomy is emotionally traumatic, studies have shown that the severe trauma is fairly short-lived. Even without reconstruction, most women are able to accept the loss of a breast after a few months. Unfortunately, during the transition time, many women present a false attitude of casualness about their breast surgery. If you have had a mastectomy and you are hurting emotionally because of it, be sure to discuss this with your physician or have him or her refer you to a counselor with whom you can discuss and resolve your anxiety. Contact Reach for Recovery (800) ACS-2345 or The Susan G. Komen Breast Cancer Foundation (800) I'M AWARE. National Headquarters, Occidental Tower, 5005 LBJ Freeway, Suite 370, Dallas, TX 75244, (972) 855-1600.

785 I have breast pain, breast nodularity, and breast lumpiness that bother me a great deal. What should I do?

Many women are continually bothered by breast pain and breast lumpiness. These women may or may not have had several breast biopsies (all benign) or are constantly under surveillance by their physicians for their lumps, with the warning that biopsies must be done if the lumps persist. Such lumps cause a great deal of worry and concern.

I strongly recommend that a woman who continues to have this problem do her best to get that discomfort ended so that she does not have to live under a cloud of worry about her breasts. There are several things that seem to be effective.

Good breast support. A woman who has breast pain may feel better if she wears bras that give especially good support. For years I have recommended Pennyrich bras because they can be custom-fitted to a woman's particular needs. There are other bras that also do a good job. Many women have found that if they wear a comfortable sleeping bra at night, they will have less breast pain.

Restrict caffeine. Caffeine contains the chemical methylxanthine. Although carefully controlled studies have not conclusively proven the effect of the caffeine-free (methylxanthine-free) diet on the breasts, some studies have indicated that 70 percent of women have less breast tenderness and less nodularity if they get off these products.

Eliminating caffeine from the diet means no coffee, tea, chocolate, or soft drinks containing caffeine. Fortunately each of those items except chocolate is now manufactured "caffeine free." Caffeine is also an ingredient in many other regularly used products, including prescription drugs (Percodan, Soma Compound, Synalgos, Emprazil, Fiorinal, Cafergot, Empirin with codeine, Repan) and in numerous nonprescription drugs (Anacin, Sinarest, Stanback Analgesic Powders, Triaminicin, Vanquish, Anorexin, Bromo Seltzer, Cope, Dexatrim, Dristan, Empirin, Excedrin, Midol, NoDoz). Check the labels to be sure the products and prescriptions you use do not contain caffeine.

I encourage patients who have breast pain or fibrocystic change to maintain a caffeine-free diet. Although there is a slightly increased chance of having breast cancer in women with fibrocystic change, the main reason to cut out caffeine is not to prevent cancer but to lessen the problems of fibrocystic change and the worry it produces. After getting off caffeine, it may take three or four months to detect any difference in the breast symptoms. If, after that length of time, there is absolutely no change in your breast discomfort, you may use caffeine again.

Take vitamin E. I have been telling patients for years about the use of vitamin E. I suggest they use up to one thousand international units per day. I know of no reliable study that "proves" a positive effect, but vitamin E has been widely recommended for this problem by competent physicians all over the country. We have found that it significantly helps many patients. Vitamin E used in this way is more than just taking a vitamin in the usual way. It is using a vitamin as a medicine. On this large dosage you may feel bloated, have oily skin, become irritable, and have other side effects. If you have such problems you would want to stop taking the drug. You may find that taking 400 international units of vitamin E a day will be adequate help for breast discomfort. At this dosage, you are much less likely to have any side effects.

Birth-control pills. Many studies now have shown that women who are on birth-control pills have less fibrocystic change and fewer breast lumps, require fewer breast biopsies, and experience less breast pain. The studies suggest that you have to be on the pills for more than two years to have the greatest effects. The use of birth-control pills may be the best long-term treatment for this particular problem. If you can and want to take birth-control pills for your breast problem, I strongly suggest that you ask your doctor about using them.

Danocrine (danazol). This drug will stop breast pain and breast nodules in up to 80 percent of women who use it. This is probably the most underused technique for helping women with breast pain and nodularity. It works most of the time, and most women have no significant side effects from taking the drug in the smaller dosage used for this problem. In my experience, general surgeons do not usually even mention this drug to their patients. I have many patients who are seeing general surgeons regularly for breast pain and nodules and who have had biopsies of these masses, and yet have never even heard that Danocrine might help them avoid this problem. I believe the reason general surgeons do not mention Danocrine is that they rarely use hormones in their practices and are uncomfortable prescribing them. Gynecologists, who use and discuss hormones all the time, are more comfortable prescribing a drug like Danocrine.

Danocrine has been approved by the FDA for breast problems. A dose of 200 mg twice daily for two months then 200 mg daily for four months can stop a woman's problem for years. It can stop pain and make breast lumps go away, allowing a woman to avoid biopsies. I encourage you to consider using this drug if you and your doctor think it can help you. I have never had a patient have a significant problem with it when she took it according to this schedule. (See Q. 138 and 852, where we discuss the use of Danocrine for endometriosis to learn more about this drug.) Do not misunderstand: If you have a *specific* lump and your doctor recommends a biopsy, have it done. Then start on Danocrine to help avoid future lumps.

Parlodel. A hormone called prolactin is secreted by a woman's pituitary gland. It is this hormone that causes a woman's breasts to produce breast milk after she has a baby. The pituitary produces a small amount of prolactin into a woman's body all the time, even when she is not pregnant and not nursing. The breasts of some women are very sensitive to this small amount of prolactin. If a woman is having breast tenderness and the other measures we mentioned in this section have not helped her, she can try taking Parlodel 2.5 mg once or twice a day for several weeks to see if her breast discomfort lessens. If it does, she can continue to take Parlodel indefinitely for the discomfort. Parlodel causes nausea in some women. These women can try using the oral tablet vaginally instead of orally. It often works just as well but without the side effect of nausea.

786 What is a subcutaneous mastectomy?

A subcutaneous mastectomy is surgery in which a woman's breast is hollowed out, leaving a skin sac with a nipple, into which a breast implant can be placed. Subcutaneous mastectomies are recommended for women who have a high risk of developing breast cancer. These include women with a strong family history of breast cancer and those who have already had breast cancer in one breast. Subcutaneous mastectomies are also recommended for women who have continual major problems with fibrocystic change.

Although this operation can eliminate these problems, it should not be entered into lightly. In the first place subcutaneous mastectomy does not remove all risk of having breast cancer because some breast tissue is always left behind. Second, it is major surgery and can result in loss of the breasts completely. For example, a patient of mine had this procedure done and, as a result, developed infections under the skin of both breasts. She had to have the implants removed and subsequently had five more operations, which finally resulted in removal of both nipples and of some of the chest skin.

The fact that such things can happen should not scare you away from surgery that you need, but it should warn you that having your breast hollowed out, and an implant put in to replace it, is not necessarily a simple and uncomplicated procedure. Choose your surgeon carefully; you want a doctor who will not only make wise recommendations but who will also do excellent surgery.

Do not confuse this surgery with the much simpler and far less dangerous "breast job" (augmentation mammoplasty) that many women have done. Both of these operations are done by plastic surgeons.

787 Can anything be done to prevent breast cancer?

The possibility of a link between diet and cancer is a much-debated and frequently discussed subject. While a correlation has not been definitely proven, there is enough evidence to strongly suggest a positive link in many cases. A National Cancer Institute study provides the following data, based on the dietary histories of 577 women (aged thirty to eighty), with breast malignancies, and of 826 disease-free women: the more frequent the consumption of beef and pork, the greater the risk; the more frequent the eating of sweet desserts, the greater the risk; and using butter at the table, and frying with butter or margarine as compared with vegetable oils increases the risk.

It has been discovered recently that eating certain foods seems to decrease the chance of a woman developing breast cancer. Foods that contain these anticancer chemicals include broccoli, cauliflower, cabbage, brussels sprouts, soybeans, and the grains rye and flax.

Another study showed that it may be the total number of calories women eat that increases the chance of breast cancer. Other research seems to indicate that it is the fat in a woman's diet that increases the chance of breast cancer. Some American women may literally eat too much for their own good! It might be a good idea to limit calorie and fat intake to decrease the chance of breast cancer if you are taking in too many calories or too much fat.

Exercise seems to decrease the risk of breast cancer. Walking thirty minutes three times a week is a small price to pay for cancer prevention. I encourage you to do it.

Since these guidelines are conducive to overall good health anyway, with or without the cancer link, it makes sense to incorporate them into an "every day, for a lifetime" diet regimen.

An Afterword

It is evident from the material in this chapter that women do develop problems in their sexual and reproductive organs. I have seen many different responses from patients when I tell them they have a medical problem. Some women get angry; some are frightened. Others try to ignore the problem. These are normal responses. It is important, however, for a woman with a medical problem to overcome these initial reactions and resolve to do all she can to eliminate her problem. Fortunately, today women have access to medical care that was undreamed of a few years ago. Take advantage of these medical breakthroughs. There are medications available today, including certain hormone-type drugs, that can easily solve difficult problems of the female sexual and reproductive organs.

The availability of modern-day medicines does not always mean that a woman can avoid a surgical procedure. However, problems that required major surgery in the past can now often be taken care of with minor surgery, such as laparoscopy or hysteroscopy. Even if a major operation is needed, such surgery is now safer than ever before. Women who do have major surgery today are usually released from the hospital after only a few days' stay.

If you have a problem, consult a doctor who is medically excellent, is honest, and is communica- tive. Pray about it, and take advantage of the sup- port of your family and friends. You should get the problem taken care of as soon as you reason- ably can.

11

Infertility

There is, I believe, no stronger stress in a couple's life than their continued longing for a child. This chapter will be of vital importance to those couples whose fondest wish—the conception of a child—has, to this point, been denied.

A psychological evaluation of infertile couples released in 1985 showed that 50 percent of the women and 15 percent of the men felt their infertility was the most upsetting experience they had ever had.

The emotions stirred by childlessness run strong and deep. They always have. Hannah, mother of the biblical prophet Samuel, remained infertile year after year despite intense longing for a child. The anguish shared by Hannah and her husband, Elkanah, mirrors the heartache of thousands.

"Hannah," Elkanah entreats tenderly, "why are you weeping? Why don't you eat? Why are you downhearted? Don't I mean more to you than ten sons?" (1 Sam. 1:8). Poor Elkanah. He was only trying to help. In fact, he was hurting as much as she was.

This particular story had a happy ending. Hannah steadfastly continued to approach God with her problem, going year after year to the temple to pray for a child. Eventually God answered her prayer, blessing Hannah and Elkanah with a son.

Unfortunately not all infertility stories have the same happy ending. Not everyone who wants a child will have one. However, exciting new advances in the treatment of infertility make it possible for an ever-increasing number of infertile couples to achieve pregnancy.

I strongly encourage any infertile couple to pray, as did Hannah and Elkanah, asking God to grant the desire of their hearts for a child. In the final analysis, I believe that it is God who opens and closes the womb; it is God who makes the final decision about pregnancy.

True, a couple may not conceive, but then God's wisdom must be respected and trusted. He is to be praised no matter what—because every aspect of his plan for us is in our best interest.

God has made it possible for us to develop new understanding and treatment for the causes of infertility. Those with infertility problems have at their disposal some of the most modern and up-to-date medical care available in any field of medicine. All this technology gives you a fighting chance of achieving pregnancy.

Every year new tests and treatments are being developed. The techniques of microsurgery have brought fertility to thousands of people during the past twenty years; and the laparoscope, metrodin, and in vitro fertilization (test-tube babies) bring realistic hope of fertility to thousands today.

This chapter contains a wealth of information for infertile couples. There are also some important facts for those who are planning to delay starting their families for several years. A third group who will benefit from this chapter are those whose infertile friends and relatives have shared with them their anguish. The lives of this third group of people will be blessed by sharing with their childless loved ones information that may prove to be a solution to their infertility problem.

Those couples who seem to be infertile need first of all to know whether or not they are, in truth, infertile. Next they need to know what to do about it.

I urge you strongly not only to read the chapter but also to keep in mind that the sooner you get an infertility problem treated, and the more appropriate that treatment is, the more likely you are to have success: a healthy, normal baby!

The questions that follow are those that I am asked most frequently by infertile couples.

The Scope of Infertility

788 What does the word infertility mean?

Infertility is defined as one year of unprotected intercourse without conception. This assumes, of course, that a couple is having intercourse with reasonable frequency—about once or twice a week. (If a couple has intercourse only once or twice a month, that may be the problem rather than infertility.)

A woman who habitually miscarries or continually delivers so early that she cannot deliver a baby mature enough to survive is also considered to have an infertility problem. (See Q. 284–297.)

789 What is the difference between "infertility" and "sterility"?

Sterility means that either the man or the woman is totally incapable of achieving pregnancy. For example, if a woman has had a hysterectomy, or has some major deformity or disorder of her female organs that prevents her from becoming pregnant, then she is truly sterile. A sterile man is one who has no sperm, who has had a vasectomy, or who has other problems that prevent fertilization.

790 How often is infertility a problem?

Infertility exists in about 15 to 20 percent of marriages. After attempting for one year to conceive, approximately 80 percent of couples will have achieved pregnancy. After eighteen months of attempted conception, that figure increases to approximately 85 percent. Those couples unable to achieve pregnancy after that length of time are considered to have an infertility problem.

As of 1991, there were 67.5 million people of

childbearing age in the United States. Since 15 to 20 percent of these people are infertile, there are an estimated 13 million infertile people (or 6.5 million infertile couples) in this country.

In the eighties, the number of people who consulted physicians about infertility greatly increased. There are probably several reasons for this. One may be that there are fewer babies available for adoption now, due to the approximately 1.2 million babies that are aborted each year. Second, there seems to be a decline in fertility among Americans.

The decline in fertility is not fully explained, but it seems in part to be because so many men and women are delaying marriage and pregnancy until later in life. The statement was made in *Clinical Gynecologic Endocrinology and Infertility* that "It is safe to say that about one-third of women who defer pregnancy until the mid or late thirties will have an infertility problem" (Drs. Leon Speroff, Robert H. Glass, and Nathan G. Case, 4th ed., Williams & Wilkins, 1989). They also point out that this increased infertility rate is not due simply to age. They show that "the percent of married couples who were infertile increased significantly among women 20 to 24, from 3.6 percent in 1965 to 10.6 percent in 1982. Probably a reflection, at least in part, of increases in sexually transmitted disease, but the percentage did not change significantly in the other groups."

Also, men's sperm counts are lower now. Doctors have been observing a gradual decline in sperm counts during the past thirty or forty years. In the early 1900s sperm counts were normally greater than eighty to a hundred million per cc of ejaculate. Now the average male's sperm count is in the range of forty million, and we consider twenty million to be normal.

Lowered sperm counts may be due to pollutants in the atmosphere, to diet, or to general lack of, or excessive exercise. It may also mean that because people are delaying their attempts to get pregnant, when they finally come to see a doctor for an infertility problem, the male's sperm count has already dropped, since age can affect sperm production.

When and Where to Seek Help for Infertility

791 When should I consult a doctor if I am unable to become pregnant?

If you are under thirty and have not become pregnant during eighteen months of trying, you should see a physician knowledgeable in infertility evaluation and treatment. If you are over thirty, I suggest that you see a doctor after only a year of trying to conceive. Infertility evaluation and the resulting treatments take time, and even more time is required to achieve pregnancy after the problem has been diagnosed and solved. Also, the longer a couple has an infertility problem, the more likely it is to get worse. As time goes by, chances of becoming pregnant decrease even more. It is particularly important that a woman over thirty not delay seeing a doctor if she suspects that there is a fertility problem.

792 If I delay pregnancy until after I am thirty-five, could I have difficulty becoming pregnant?

Yes. Women who put off childbearing run the increasing risk of not ever becoming pregnant.

A study, done in France and reported in a 1984 issue of the *New England Journal of Medicine*, showed that a woman's fertility rate starts dropping from the age of thirty on. Up to age thirty a woman's chance of conceiving was reported to be 74 percent.

It is certain that a woman who delays trying to get pregnant until after the age of thirty-five is greatly increasing her chance of having to go through infertility evaluation and treatment. This process can be expensive, frustrating, time-consuming, and emotionally demanding.

I often talk to couples who are delaying pregnancy until they have enough money or until their schedules are convenient. What most people who have already become parents know, however, is that there is never enough money and the time is never perfect to have a child! Most parents would advise another couple contemplating future pregnancy to go ahead and have the baby while they can instead of waiting for ideal circumstances, because ideal circumstances never come.

793 If there are, as people tell me, things I might do to stimulate a pregnancy—for example, "just relaxing," having sex only during ovulation, adopting a child—why do I need to see a doctor?

First, all of those things are popular misconceptions. Many factors can cause infertility, and only a competent physician can determine the source of your own or your husband's infertility.

One of the most popular myths concerning becoming pregnant is that "if you'll just relax and quit worrying about it, you will become pregnant." However, the *reason* you are not relaxed is that you are not getting pregnant: not the reverse! Several studies on this subject show that this type of tension almost never inhibits fertility. It is normal for you to feel upset each month when you find out that you are not pregnant and you want to be. This concern will rarely interfere with your chances of becoming pregnant.

There is an exception to this rule, however. Severe emotional and physical stress can cause ovulation to become erratic or to stop. If your ovulation becomes irregular, you will then begin having irregular periods. If that occurs it will lessen your chance of becoming pregnant. If your periods are regular, however, there is no reason to "worry about worrying."

Another myth is that if you adopt a baby, you will become pregnant. There is no increased chance of becoming pregnant after adopting. Researchers have compared childless infertile women with those who have given up hope of pregnancy and have adopted. The incidence of subsequent pregnancy is no greater in the adopting group.

The third myth concerning overcoming infertility is that it is best to avoid having sex until ovulation occurs, so that the man can "save up" his sperm and have a higher sperm count.

Most urologists believe that this may be wrong. When a male goes for several days without intercourse, the stored up sperm start getting "old," possibly resulting in lessened fertility. One hint for being as fertile as possible is for the wife not to take aspirin-containing products and prostaglandin inhibitors (like Advil) during ovulation time because they can interfere with the release of the egg by the ovary.

Recent studies have shown that caffeine, moderate alcohol use, and cigarette smoking can also increase infertility. I recommend that a woman stop all three before trying to become pregnant. I recommend a man stop cigarettes and alcohol. (Caffeine may make sperm more active.)

Another myth concerns so-called fertility pills. These pills, such as Clomid, are used for a specific problem: to make a woman who is not ovulating establish regular ovulation. They are helpful only in such cases. They are not the miracle cure for all infertility problems, as some people seem to believe.

Other misconceptions about cures for infertility include undergoing a D&C or taking thyroid medication and/or hormones. One of these treatments may solve an existing infertility problem, but none of them is a universal solution to infertility. These procedures are effective for many patients, but they only treat specific problems. For example, thyroid medication will help a woman become pregnant only if tests show that she has a thyroid problem.

794 What kind of physician should I see for an infertility problem?

You should go to a physician who is skilled in evaluating and treating infertility problems. Valuable time can be wasted seeing a doctor who is only mildly interested or slightly knowledgeable about treating infertility.

Some physicians have not developed expertise in handling infertility problems. Many physicians are not really interested in fertility but do not want to have their patients go to another physician. If you have a fertility problem and your physician is working with you, the care you receive should follow the general guidelines given in the infertility evaluation section of this chapter. If not, see another doctor for a second opinion.

795 How can I know if a doctor is skilled in handling infertility and its treatment?

There are several things you can do.

Ask the doctor if he or she does much infertility work. If the doctor does only a small amount, you should probably find someone else to do your evaluation.

Contact the following groups for a reference:

1. Resolve, Inc. This national lay organization has compiled a directory of infertility specialists. (Address given at end of chapter.)
2. Stepping Stones. 2900 North Rock Road, Wichita, KS 67226; phone (316) 688-4400; Lynn Behnke, Leslie Snodgrass, Janet Malcom. A national Christian information and support group, they publish an excellent newsletter on infertility.
3. The American Society of Reproductive Medicine. Most U.S. doctors interested in infertility are members. (Address given at end of chapter.)

Use your common sense. If your doctor does not appear organized, does not have a step-by-step plan for your evaluation, or is doing little to help you achieve pregnancy, you probably need to change doctors. Remember, if you have gone eighteen months without becoming pregnant, you have an infertility problem and need testing now.

Your testing should be progressive over a reasonably short (six months) period of time. Having one test done now, another in three or four months, and another a few months later is not an adequate infertility evaluation. Remember, your evaluation should correspond with the guidelines in this chapter. If it does not, you probably need to find another physician.

There are three types of physicians who are well trained in infertility care: (1) those who take advantage of the hundreds of infertility training programs and workshops held each year; (2) reproductive endocrinologists; (3) reproductive surgeons.

The first group, those who attend infertility training programs, learn about the entire field of infertility evaluation and treatment. They are almost always members of the American Society for Reproductive Medicine and may also be members of the advanced reproductive sections, such as Society of Advanced Reproductive Technologies (SART) and/or fellows of the Society of Reproductive Surgeons or the Society of Reproductive Endocrinologists.

The second group, reproductive endocrinologists, are gynecologists who have gone through an organized two-year program of training in the area of reproductive hormones and infertility care. These programs teach in an organized, concentrated course what is just as available in the courses and workshops around the country.

The third group are those who have gone through a new infertility training program that is specifically for reproductive surgeons. This two-year fellowship produces infertility doctors with expertise in the most modern surgical procedures for infertility patients. They would also be very adequately trained in the care of other infertility problems.

A physician from any of these groups has the qualifications to give you excellent infertility treatment. Remember, though, that if you do not like working with the physician you have chosen, because you do not feel that he or she is attentive or caring enough, no matter how well trained he or she is, you should consider changing doctors, but be sure to change to another competent doctor.

The Initial Infertility Evaluation

796 Should my husband accompany me on the first visit to the doctor?

Definitely. He should be involved with you during the entire process. Conceiving and raising a child is a joint effort, and infertility care is a joint effort also.

The evaluation cannot take place without your husband's cooperation, since he is involved in not only the questioning and testing but possibly also in the treatment phases of the process. If your husband is present at the first interview, he will have a better understanding of the entire program.

Additionally, some of the procedures may require that you change your normal sexual routine. This will require his support and cooperation. His attitude is much more likely to be positive and helpful if he understands it from the start.

Finally, if your husband has met your doctor, he will feel more comfortable about calling him or her if he has any questions.

797 What can a physician do to help me with my infertility problem?

A competent physician in fertility evaluation procedures will provide accurate information about the causes and treatment of infertility and dispel any misinformation you may have on the topic. He or she will also have an intelligent and systematic approach to your problem, be able to project how soon pregnancy might be possible, assuming there is a solution or treatment for your problem, and be able to counsel you about adoption if you choose that means of having a child.

There are two things your physician should communicate to you on your first visit:

1. Your doctor should assure you that he or she or an associate will be available to you anytime you have questions or are confused about any aspect of your infertility care: how to do a test, when to be at the laboratory, or what to do next. Communication in infertility evaluation and treatment is vital.

2. Your doctor should reassure you that it is normal for you and your husband to become upset and worried during your infertility workup and treatments. You can expect frustration, tears, and anxiety, but it will help a great deal if you are able to express those emotions to an understanding physician.

798 What kind of advice might the physician give us on the first visit to his or her office?

After obtaining your history and doing an examination, the doctor will offer you some general advice to enhance your chances of conceiving. During the first visit, for instance, I make several suggestions.

If the man wears jockey-style underwear, I advise him to switch to boxer shorts. The reason for this is that the testicles need to be cooler than the rest of the body to achieve optimum sperm production. Testicles normally hang outside of and away from the body for that reason. Close-fitting underwear holds them much closer to the body than does a pair of boxer shorts. The type of underwear a man wears may not make much difference if he has a normal sperm count. If the testicles are somewhat cooler and produce better sperm, however, he may be able to get his wife pregnant more easily even if she does have a fertility problem.

I instruct a woman patient to begin taking her temperature (BBT—basal body temperature) every morning with a basal thermometer. This thermometer is necessary because it detects a narrower range of temperature than a regular fever thermometer. The thermometer should be shaken down and put at the bedside every night. First thing each morning the thermometer is put under the woman's tongue for five minutes before the results are read and recorded. A temperature chart should be kept faithfully for three months and brought back on a subsequent visit to the doctor. After three months it is usually not necessary to continue taking one's temperature. Ask your doctor what he/she wants you to do. This chart presents a graphic demonstration to infertility patients of the timing of their ovulation. It shows whether or not they are ovulating and helps them to schedule intercourse accordingly. However, recent studies have shown that the ovulation time

Sample Temperature Record

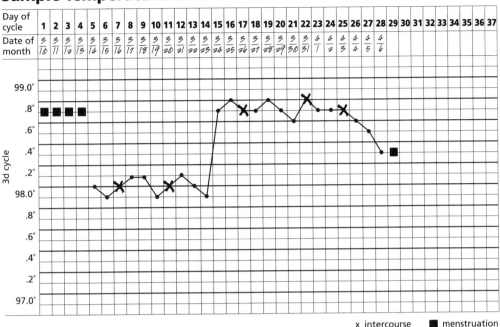

Day of cycle	1	2	3	4	5	6	7	8	9	10	11	12	13	14	15	16	17	18	19	20	21	22	23	24	25	26	27	28	29	30	31	32	33	34	35	36	37
Date of month	3/10	3/11	3/12	3/13	3/14	3/15	3/16	3/17	3/18	3/19	3/20	3/21	3/22	3/23	3/24	3/25	3/26	3/27	3/28	3/29	3/30	3/31	4/1	4/2	4/3	4/4	4/5	4/6									

x intercourse ■ menstruation

Instructions:

1. Immediately after waking in the morning and before arising, eating, drinking, or smoking, place the thermometer under your tongue for at least five minutes. (Do this every morning except during menstruation.)
2. Record the reading on the graph by placing a dot at the proper location (be accurate). If intercourse has taken place during the previous twenty-four hours, cross the dot (X).
3. Insert the date at top of column in space provided for date of month.
4. Consider the first day of menstrual flow as the start of a cycle. It is not essential to record the temperature during menstruation. However, indicate menstruation with a ■ on the graph starting at extreme left under number one day of cycle. As flow diminishes resume temperature recordings.
5. Any obvious reasons for temperature variation such as an infection, insomnia, or indigestion should be noted on the reading for that day.
6. If you detect ovulation by a twinge of pain low on one side of the abdomen or by a few drops of vaginal bleeding about midcycle, indicate it on the graph.

indicated by BBT charts can be wrong one-third of the time.

A very useful but different technique allows a woman to check her urine for her body's production of luteinizing hormone (LH), the so-called "ovulation predictor kit" (see next question). This technique allows a couple to schedule intercourse or insemination much more reliably than with a BBT chart. Your physician will show you which brand kit he or she prefers and will also show you how to use it. (See next question.) If you have irregular ovulation, that poses a different problem; your physician will discuss that with you.

Next I recommend proper frequency and timing of intercourse. No matter how fertile you are, if your sexual timing or habits are off, you will probably be slow to achieve pregnancy. For ex-

ample, I have had several couples as patients who were having intercourse only once a month, and this randomly. The conception window is apparently smaller than was previously thought, according to a study reported in the *New England Journal of Medicine* (1995, 331:1517–1521), by Wilcox et al. This study showed that the chance of a couple achieving pregnancy was greatest if they had intercourse every day during the six days before ovulation. The less intercourse, the less chance of pregnancy that month. These researchers laid to rest one misconception. They found that frequent intercourse did not decrease sperm potency.

Finally, I recommend that a woman remain in bed on her back, for at least thirty minutes after each act of intercourse during the ovulation period. (She should lie on her stomach if her uterus is tipped or retroverted.) This allows the semen to pool around the cervix and facilitates the sperm's access to the uterus. There is no reason for extreme positions such as standing on one's head or getting into the knee/chest position to achieve pregnancy. Although staying down for thirty minutes after intercourse may not improve your fertility if you have a major problem, there are some women who seem to be helped by this technique. Be sure not to use vaginal lubricants (even Vaseline and KY Jelly) because they can kill sperm.

799 I keep seeing advertisements about ovulation predictor kits. Are these legitimate?

Yes, they are. I recommend that people who want to get pregnant as soon as possible use these ovulation predictor kits. These kits, which test the urine for luteinizing hormones (LH), are available in most drugstores.

Luteinizing hormone is the hormone that is released by the pituitary to go to the ovary and cause the egg to be released. When the pituitary senses that there is enough estrogen being produced from the ovary, it assumes that there is an egg ready to be released. The pituitary then produces a surge of luteinizing hormone into the bloodstream, which goes to the ovary. Thirty-eight hours later, the ovary releases its egg.

The luteinizing hormone (LH) that is released into the bloodstream is then passed into the urine and leaves the body through the kidneys. When LH is detected by the test kit, a woman then knows that she will probably ovulate within twelve to twenty-four hours (depending on when she collected her urine, when she last urinated, and so on). When the test becomes positive, she and her husband should have intercourse a couple of times over the next eighteen hours.

Some guidelines for using an ovulation predictor kit are:

1. If you have a regular twenty-eight day cycle, you should start testing your urine on day eleven and continue until the test becomes positive. If you have shorter cycles, you may need to start testing your urine earlier. If you have longer cycles, start somewhat later.

2. Urine should be collected at the same time every day. If it is impossible to test the urine within one hour of collection, it can be refrigerated for up to twenty-four hours before doing the test. If the urine has been refrigerated, it should stand at room temperature for thirty minutes before testing.

3. Urine that is very dilute may not have an adequate concentration of LH for detection. It is important, therefore, not to drink too much fluid during the three or four hours before the urine is collected for testing.

4. Once the test has shown positive, it is no longer necessary to test the urine. The unused tests left in the kit can be saved for the next month if pregnancy does not occur.

These ovulation predictor kits are astoundingly sophisticated tests. It is amazing that they are available over-the-counter, can be used so easily, and can give such accurate results.

One drawback of these kits is that they are fairly expensive. If you have a question about whether or not you should try one, talk to your physician.

800 Is there anything else my husband and I can do to improve our chances of conceiving?

Good general health and sound lifestyle habits can have a positive effect on a person's fertility. If the woman diets excessively, is extremely obese, or exercises too strenuously, the functions of the body are changed enough to prevent normal secretion of hormones and a normal menstrual cycle.

I always advise my patients to avoid the following things while they are trying to get pregnant.

Cigarette smoking. Chemicals in cigarette smoke combine with red blood cells, preventing them from carrying a normal load of oxygen. This is one reason that smokers are less likely to gain weight. If body tissues are so starved for oxygen that they cannot grow properly, it is reasonable to assume that the reproductive system may not function properly either. Studies have conclusively shown a significantly decreased fertility in smokers.

Furthermore, once pregnancy occurs, it is imperative for the well-being of the child that the mother stop smoking. The best time to stop is before pregnancy occurs, especially if you have infertility problems.

Alcohol. A recent study clearly showed decreased fertility in women who drank moderately (one drink a day or less) (Grodstein et al., *American Journal of Public Health*, September 1994, 84.9). It is well known that alcohol is detrimental to the baby once a woman is pregnant. (See Q. 434–435.) Much more is known about alcohol used during pregnancy. As with cigarettes, for the baby's health and your own, you need to stop alcohol intake, preferably before you get pregnant. This may help you to achieve pregnancy sooner. It is my recommendation that there be either no drinking or drinking only in highly controlled moderation (no more than two drinks per week) for both the husband and wife who are trying to achieve pregnancy.

Other drugs. Less is known about the effect of other drugs on fertility. Research suggests that marijuana can affect the production of a normal egg, inhibit ovulation, and lower sperm count. When no longer used, there seems to be no effect of the drug on fertility later in life. Heroin, cocaine, and barbiturates used excessively are known to cause malnutrition, poor health, irregular ovulation, and therefore some degree of infertility. Some tranquilizers can cause the cessation of periods and thus interfere with fertility.

Men and drugs. A man's sperm production and sex drive may be affected by all these substances too. Cigarettes can have a significant effect on sperm production. I advise all the husbands in infertile couples to stop smoking. Alcohol can lead to impotence; marijuana can affect production of sperm; heroin, cocaine, and barbiturates can affect both libido (sex drive) and general health; and tranquilizers or antidepressants reduce sperm production in animals and may do the same in men.

Sperm production that begins "today" in a man's testicles does not appear in his ejaculate for about seventy-five days. Whatever he does today, therefore, will not affect his sperm count or his sperm fertility for seventy-five days. To improve his sperm he must start right now for sperm that will be ejaculated two-and-a-half months from now.

General suggestion. The maxim concerning infertility and the use of any drug is, "Don't use the drug." If you are going to the inconvenience and expense of diagnosing your infertility and having it treated, maximize your chances for pregnancy by stopping all drugs, including cigarettes and alcohol.

(In the chapter about pregnancy we discussed preconceptual planning. Please read that section. There may be some suggestions about important matters to discuss with your infertility specialist. For example, if you are diabetic or have some other medical problem, you may want to talk to your infertility doctor about getting those things under control before you proceed with your treatments.)

801 What reasons for infertility might the physician discover during the examination on the first visit?

The following abnormalities, each of which can interfere with fertility, are evaluated during the initial physical examination.

Vaginitis. If a vaginal infection is found it must be treated, as it can delay the occurrence of a pregnancy.

STD. Your physician may want to do cultures for chlamydia and gonorrhea if either you or your husband has had sex with anyone else before. I have all my infertility patients take 100 mg of doxycycline twice a day for two weeks (both husband and wife) just in case these or other infections are present. Chlamydia cultures can fail to be positive, even when the infection is present. If both a woman and her husband are treated with tetracycline, that will usually get rid of those germs that can inhibit fertility.

Growths or abnormalities in the pelvis. These may be fibroids of the uterus, ovarian tumors, or endometriosis. Additionally, if some congenital abnormalities are found on pelvic examination, these must be evaluated and may need to be treated.

Cervical stenosis. This is a narrowing of the opening into the uterus. It can prevent or make it difficult for the sperm to gain access to the uterus or it can indicate disease of the cervix that could prevent pregnancy. This condition is often due to an earlier abortion, cervical cautery or freezing, or a cervical conization (excision of cervical tissue).

DES changes of the cervix. A woman who was exposed to DES before birth because her mother took DES during that pregnancy, can have some changes of her cervix because of that. The cervix may be smaller, or have unusual ridges across it. A woman exposed to DES can also have an abnormal uterine cavity. These things can decrease a woman's fertility or cause her to have miscarriages.

Unusually heavy or abnormal patterns of hair growth and/or moderate-to-severe acne. These symptoms can be indicative of an excess production of male hormones (even in women) and may suggest the need for hormone studies.

Physical abnormalities. These can indicate abnormal growth patterns in the body that could be due to congenital problems such as chromosomal abnormalities. One of the most common of these is called Turner's syndrome or ovarian agenesis (see Q. 73), a problem that requires more extensive treatment and counseling than just dealing with infertility. However, these problems occur infrequently.

802 Which tests will the physician order for me and my husband following the first visit?

A fairly standard series of tests will be ordered. All of them are designed to evaluate the proper functioning of your body in general as well as your sexual organs and to identify problems that could be causing your infertility.

The common causes of infertility, such as a low sperm count, are first tested. The simplest, nonsurgical tests are also done first, followed by more involved tests and treatments until a cause is discovered and the proper therapy found. Often the problem can be cleared up quickly and easily, and pregnancy will occur without the need to proceed to the more advanced tests and procedures.

803 What initial tests are ordered for the man?

Most gynecologists working with infertility will order only a semen analysis.

If this test for semen quantity, sperm count and health, and semen health is normal, the husband usually needs no further testing. It is wise, therefore, that this be one of the first tests ordered for any infertile couple.

Sperm agglutination. This test to make sure the female is not allergic to her husband's sperm or that a man is not allergic to his own sperm can be helpful if infertility persists. This is felt to be a relatively rare fertility problem but it can be significant.

This test may be done either initially or later depending on medical indications. It is usually done if a man's sperm are always missing from the woman's cervical mucus even after intercourse, if the sperm all seem to be sticking together in a sperm specimen when viewed under a microscope, or when no other cause for infertility can be found.

804 What tests might be ordered for the woman during the first few weeks of evaluation?

A group of tests that any doctor would obtain during a thorough general checkup are also recommended for a woman with an infertility problem.

Complete blood count. This checks for anemia or a chronic blood problem that could affect both fertility and the health of the mother and the fetus.

Complete urinalysis. This checks for evidence of a chronic kidney disease, which could affect both fertility and a pregnancy.

SMA 21. This checks for any evidence of liver disease, gout, diabetes, kidney malfunction, and several other problems that can affect fertility in the female.

T3 & T4 and/or a TSH test. These check thyroid function. It is unusual for a thyroid problem to cause infertility, but it does occur and should be checked.

Rubella test. This tests resistance or lack of resistance to German measles (rubella) which, if contracted during pregnancy, may cause severe abnormalities in the baby. (See Q. 328–331.) If the test shows you have no resistance to rubella, immunization should be done and for the next three months you should use good contraception. You may continue testing during this time.

TB skin test. If a woman has had tuberculosis, it may have affected the female organs and caused infertility.

Prolactin test. The prolactin level needs to be checked because this hormone can indicate a small tumor in the pituitary that could be preventing pregnancy. I like to order this for every infertile woman but not all physicians do this routinely.

Progesterone testing. This is a blood test and is done a few days after ovulation and indicates that a woman's ovary did release an egg and then developed a corpus luteum that is producing progesterone, the hormone necessary for preparing the lining of the uterus for pregnancy.

Endometrial biopsy. Another method of determining whether or not a woman has ovulated is by a scraping of the woman's uterine lining after ovulation. After ovulation, the lining of a woman's uterus undergoes precise day-by-day changes that a pathologist can see. For example, if an endometrial biopsy is done on day twenty-four, the pathologist should be able to look at the tissue and say that the woman ovulated ten days ago. If the tissue is off by two days, it may be that a woman is not producing adequate progesterone from her ovaries and needs treatment for that.

STD testing. If either one of a married couple has had sex with someone else before and there is any question of the possibility of sexually transmitted disease, I recommend that a woman be tested for syphilis, AIDS, and hepatitis B. (I have already mentioned that testing for chlamydia and gonorrhea is also a good idea in this situation.)

805 How much does infertility evaluation and treatment cost?

The cost depends heavily on how soon your problem is diagnosed and which treatments will be necessary to eliminate it. The costs will increase as more office visits, medication, surgical procedures, and tests are required.

In calculating costs, two factors are important considerations. First, some insurance policies now cover these procedures. Second, while this care can add up to a sizable amount of money, remember that adopting a child is also quite expensive. Adoptions usually cost from $8,000 to $20,000 per child (1992).

It is impossible to give specific costs for the tests and treatment of infertility since they vary so much from one part of the country to another. It is important that you find out if your insurance will pay for your evaluation and treatment, and how much each test or treatment is going to cost.

Patients sometimes stop their infertility treatment because of money. I tell my patients that they should not let infertility care deplete their money to the point that it becomes a real hardship for them. It is usually "safe" to stop the care long enough to catch up, both emotionally and financially, when that becomes necessary if the delay is not too long and if the woman is not nearing 40.

806 How long does an infertility workup usually take?

The infertility evaluation can usually be completed in two to three months, but specific problems may involve an additional few months investigation.

Further Steps in Infertility Evaluation

807 What is the next step in the infertility evaluation?

After the couple has had the first consultation and the above-mentioned testing, the doctor will review the results. Any abnormality would then be clearly explained by the doctor so that the couple will understand exactly what is going on and what will happen next.

If no apparent cause for infertility was found during the first series of questions, tests, and examinations, a hysterosalpingogram (HSG) and a postcoital test (PC test) will usually be scheduled for the woman.

808 What is a hysterosalpingogram (HSG)?

This X-ray test is used to view the inside of the uterus and fallopian tubes. It is a nonsurgical procedure. An X-ray dye is squirted through the cervix, up into the uterus, and through the fallopian tubes so that these organs may be X-rayed and any abnormality will be outlined.

The test can show several things: whether or not your uterus is formed normally; whether or not there is scarring inside your uterus from a previous miscarriage or an operation such as an abortion; and whether or not your tubes are open.

A hysterosalpingogram is a reliable test for evaluating the endometrial cavity of the uterus. If the test is normal, the cavity of the uterus usually is not the cause of infertility or miscarriages. If the cavity of the uterus shows polyps or deformities, these can be the cause of infertility or repeat miscarriages.

The HSG is not so reliable for fallopian tubes. I have had many patients come to me with normal hysterosalpingograms who had been treated for infertility without a laparoscopy because of the normal HSG. When I did laparoscopy on these women, I found abnormalities of their fallopian tubes. Such abnormality can be undetected endometriosis, scarring of the fallopian tubes, and so on. Abnormal fallopian tubes can look normal on an HSG because some of the dye can "escape" from the end of the fallopian tubes seeping out through a scar that was either holding the tubes down in an abnormal position or almost closing them. On the HSG X-ray this seepage of dye would look like an open tube.

The HSG is a very important part of an infertility evaluation. Even though a hysteroscopy can help evaluate the inside of the uterus, I almost always get an HSG on infertility patients because it can detect some things that the hysteroscopy does not.

This procedure can be painful, but pain medication can be given or a paracervical block done (injecting local anesthesia into the tissues beside the cervix) to make the patient more comfortable.

There is some risk of developing PID (see Q. 827) from the HSG. If you develop pain in your low abdomen or fever a day or two after the X-ray, be sure to call your physician.

A hysterosalpingogram is usually best done immediately after a normal menstrual period. This eliminates the possibility that a woman might be pregnant.

Some researchers have found that women who have had an HSG are more likely to get pregnant during the following year, but this is not the reason most infertility specialists have the procedure done. It is done to find out what is wrong so proper medical care can be given to achieve pregnancy.

Hysterosalpingogram

dye outlines uterine cavity and channels in the fallopian tubes

dye spills from open tube

instrument inserted in cervix, using plunger, dye is released

Hysterosalpingogram (hystero-uterus; salpingo-fallopian; gram-picture)—an X-ray picture of uterus and tubes is obtained by injecting dye into the uterine cavity, filling the cavity so that the dye overflows into the fallopian tubes, and then taking an X-ray. This procedure can reveal many types of abnormalities.

809 What is the postcoital (PC or Sims-Huhner) test?

While awaiting the hysterosalpingogram, or soon after, a postcoital or Sims-Huhner test (SHT) can be done. This test examines the cervical mucus and its reception of your husband's sperm.

Your husband's ejaculate (material that comes from his penis during intercourse) is mostly mucus. True there are millions of sperm, but if all the mucus were removed and the sperm concentrated, there would be only a few drops of material left (the concentrated sperm). Once the ejaculate is in your vagina, the sperm swim out of it and into your cervical mucus. If your cervical mucus is not receptive to the sperm, it acts as a barrier to the sperm, keeping them from reaching the uterine cavity.

For the SHT, several scheduling considerations are necessary. First, most physicians recommend that intercourse take place from two to twelve hours prior to the scheduled office visit set up for the SHT. Second, the office visit must be scheduled at ovulation or one or two days before ovulation.

If the postcoital test is done at a time other than at ovulation, the cervical mucus will be thick and hazy in appearance. If it looks that way just before ovulation, it usually means that a woman is not producing healthy cervical mucus.

If your physician speaks about the "spinnbarkheit" of your cervical mucus, he is referring to its "stretchability." Healthy cervical mucus will stretch out to eight to ten centimeters, which is about four inches. (You may have noticed this stretchability if you have ever examined your vagina at the time of ovulation.) It is this stretchable, thin, healthy cervical mucus that enables your husband's sperm to swim easily into your uterus.

During the procedure the doctor will take mucus from the cervix, put it on a laboratory slide, and look at it under a microscope. There should be many active sperm, and these sperm should have good direction as they swim—as though they know where they're going.

This test produces a good indication of the condition of the husband's sperm and the woman's cervical mucus. If the sperm are immobilized or killed, the mucus is "unhealthy and hostile," and the condition probably needs to be treated. (See Q. 819.)

Normal, healthy, pre-ovulatory cervical mucus will dry in such a way that it looks like a fern under a microscope. If your doctor says your cervical mucus has a good fern pattern, it is another indication that your cervical mucus is healthy.

Actually, some recent studies have shown that a "good" or "bad" postcoital may not be as important as previously thought. In one study, a laparoscopy done at the right time of the month and after intercourse showed that sperm had actually traveled up into the uterus and tubes in some women with "bad" PC tests, and no sperm had reached the uterus and tubes in some women with "good" PC tests. Because of such information, most specialists do not rely on this test very much and often do not even do it anymore. If a patient does not get pregnant by the time the evaluation is complete, they will probably recommend bypassing the cervix and doing intrauterine inseminations anyway. Nevertheless, most doctors will try to get the cervical mucus healthy and receptive to sperm (see Q. 820), or will try to bypass unhealthy cervical mucus with the new technique called intrauterine insemination (IUI) with washed sperm. (See Q. 862.)

It is important to understand that a postcoital test is not a substitute for a semen analysis. The postcoital test does not tell a great deal about your husband's sperm specimen. To determine whether or not he is fertile, the doctor must have your husband take a semen specimen to the laboratory for a competent evaluation. Just because his sperm do get into your cervical mucus does not mean he is able to fertilize you. Having a postcoital test will not prevent pregnancy during the month it is performed.

When all the studies mentioned above have been done and abnormalities have been corrected, if pregnancy still has not occurred a diagnostic laparoscopy needs to be done.

810 What is a laparoscopy?

This is a minor surgical procedure, usually done with general anesthesia on an outpatient basis, that does an enormous amount of good for an infertile woman. After the surgery one's activities are limited only by the fatigue and weakness that ac-

Laparoscopy

In a laparoscopy a needle is inserted into the lower abdomen and a special gas (carbon dioxide) is introduced to lift the abdominal wall away from the organs. An optical telescope (laparoscope) is inserted into the abdominal cavity through a small incision (about one-quarter inch long) usually made along the lower edge of the navel. A second incision, also about a quarter-inch long, may be made just above the pubic hairline. Through this incision

laparoscope

small instruments, such as a probe, are inserted to facilitate movement of tubes, etc. A doctor can evaluate the condition of portions of the abdominal cavity and the various female organs. Many types of surgery can be performed during a laparoscopy.

company relatively minor surgery and general anesthesia.

A laparoscopy takes about forty-five minutes, unless some other procedure (laser, surgery) is done at the same time. After you are put to sleep, the physician inserts a needle through the lower edge of your navel. Three quarts of carbon dioxide gas are allowed to flow through the needle into your abdominal cavity, blowing it up like a balloon. This does not stretch a woman's muscles and make her abdomen loose, nor does it cause her abdomen to "stick out" more than it did before. The tissues of the abdomen are very stretchable and will go back to normal after the procedure.

Two incisions are usually made—one in the lower edge of the navel and another just above the pubic hairline. Neither incision is more than a quarter of an inch long.

Through the upper incision the doctor inserts a telescope with optics so refined that the interior of the abdomen can be seen as though one were looking directly at it through a large incision. Through the lower incision the doctor inserts small instruments such as a long probe, or an instrument with delicate teeth to pick things up and move them around.

About half of the time in infertile women the laparoscopy reveals some abnormality, such as endometriosis, adhesions, or congenital abnormalities. These abnormalities are often correctable. Occasionally, using the small instruments that are employed during the laparoscopy, adhesions can be cut, biopsies can be taken, and the laser can be used without making larger incisions. At other times the abnormalities are too major to be corrected through these small incisions, and a major operation must be done later.

Most doctors always arrange for a laparoscopy to be done after ovulation. They normally dilate the cervix and scrape some of the uterine lining out (D&C) at the time of the laparoscopy. The D&C done after ovulation is beneficial because it gives a sample of the lining of the uterus to send to the pathologist for evaluation. The lab report tells whether or not this lining is responding properly to the hormones from the ovary and from other glands in the body. It can also determine if any infection is present inside the uterus. The procedure likely would not remove a just-beginning pregnancy because the embryo is so small and the entire uterine lining is not curetted. To avoid that possibility, however, I have my patients use foam and condoms the month of the procedure.

Recovery from a laparoscopy takes a few days. A patient should stay in bed the evening after surgery, getting up only to use the bathroom. The next day she can get up and do anything she wants, but she may not feel like doing much for two or three days.

There is some pain as a result of laparoscopy. A woman may have shoulder pain, which is referred pain from the diaphragm where gas bubbles are causing temporary irritation. She may also have incision pain, but it is not excruciating and lasts only two or three days. Most women can return to full activity in two to four days, although some will be groggy and tired from the anesthesia for up to two weeks.

811 Is the use of the laser through the laparoscope a useful procedure?

The use of the laser during laparoscopy is an exciting and truly revolutionary technique that has saved many patients major surgery. If you are going to have a laparoscopy done, it would be ideal if you could have it performed by a physician who has the training and desire to use the laser if necessary. Of course, it is also necessary that the operating room have the laser equipment available to hook up to the laparoscope if it is needed.

With the laser hooked up to the laparoscope, the doctor can operate on your abdomen without having to make a large enough incision to get his or her hands inside. With laser laparoscopy a doctor can cut adhesions, cut fibroids off the uterus, vaporize endometriosis, open fallopian tubes, and destroy cystic structures. Of course, the laser cannot be used to do any of these things if they are too large or too extensive. It is not a panacea.

The wonderful thing about laparoscopy, however, is that it can often be used to remove a mild abnormality that may or may not be responsible for infertility. For instance, mild endometriosis can cause infertility, but because it is mild, a doctor never knows if it really is the endometriosis that is causing the infertility. Without the laser laparo-

scopic technique, a doctor often cannot adequately treat endometriosis without Danocrine, or GnRH therapy, or major surgery. But the question in his or her mind is, "Is such mild endometriosis really the problem?" If the laser is used through the laparoscope such endometriosis can be completely eliminated. This will often lead to pregnancy, but even if it does not, it will eliminate this mild endometriosis from consideration in future fertility evaluation and treatment.

812 Is a laparoscopy really necessary?

No patient has had a complete infertility evaluation until a laparoscopy has been performed. D&C alone is inadequate, because it is the less important part of this procedure. If a doctor suggests just a D&C for fertility testing and you have not had a laparoscopy, your doctor is probably unfamiliar with the best techniques for the diagnosis and treatment of infertility. You should probably get a second opinion.

For example, I once had a patient whose previous physician, except for failing to do a laparoscopy, had done an adequate infertility evaluation. The X-ray of her uterus and tubes was normal. On the basis of the evaluation the woman had undergone treatment for approximately three years. Because she continued to be infertile, however, I did a diagnostic laparoscopy on her and found that both of her tubes were almost completely closed. The X-ray of her uterus erroneously had looked normal and the physician did not investigate further. She had wasted two or three years because her original doctor had not done a laparoscopy.

My suggestion concerning laparoscopy is this: First have all the preliminary tests done. If everything seems all right and you are under thirty years of age, wait six to twelve months to see if pregnancy will occur. If it does not, have a laparoscopy and D&C. However, if you are over thirty, or if some abnormality has been detected that would be clarified by a laparoscopy, go ahead and have it done immediately.

Even though everything appears to be normal

Hysteroscopy

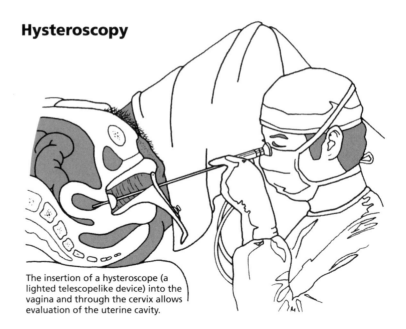

The insertion of a hysteroscope (a lighted telescopelike device) into the vagina and through the cervix allows evaluation of the uterine cavity.

on all other exams and tests, the laparoscopy is necessary to insure that the tubes and the rest of the pelvis are normal.

Many other surgical and nonsurgical procedures can be done to treat or diagnose a particular infertility problem, but the foregoing material covers most of the initial studies necessary for proper evaluation of infertility.

813 **My physician has talked about doing a hysteroscopy with my laparoscopy. Is that wise?**

I routinely do a hysteroscopy (see section in this book on hysteroscopy) when I do a diagnostic laparoscopy. A hysterosalpingogram (HSG) is a fairly reliable procedure, but it can be wrong. The hysteroscopy takes only a few minutes and it helps to do a second evaluation of the cavity of the uterus just in case the HSG missed an abnormality.

If, at hysteroscopy, a polyp or growth is seen inside the uterus or there seems to be a uterine septum, those things can be removed or repaired without the patient having a longer recovery time. A hysteroscopy has almost no more risk than a D&C. After the hysteroscopy, the uterus can be scraped so that endometrial tissue can be sent to a pathologist for evaluation. (See Q. 699.)

Male Infertility Problems

814 **When a cause for infertility is discovered, is it more often with the female or with the male?**

Problems with the male organs cause infertility about 30 percent of the time, while female abnormalities are also responsible about 30 percent of the time. A combination of factors involving both husband and wife cause about 40 percent of the problems.

815 **How should a man collect the semen specimen?**

A man will usually collect the specimen at home by masturbation into a clean container (such as a glass jar that has been thoroughly washed and rinsed well). He or his wife can then take that specimen to the laboratory. It should be kept at body temperature, and it is best to get it to the laboratory within an hour.

A man should remember two things when collecting a semen specimen for analysis:

Special Concerns

1. Do not abstain from intercourse for over four or five days before collecting the specimen because this can make the sperm count lower than it really is. Abstaining from intercourse for two or three days is adequate for a good specimen.
2. Do not collect the specimen following withdrawal during or after intercourse. This contaminates the specimen with vaginal secretions and also makes it possible to lose part of the specimen. (This makes it appear as though you have a lower sperm count than you do.)

If a man does not want to collect a specimen by masturbation, there is a plastic sleeve he can put over his penis. When he ejaculates, this sleeve will collect the specimen. (This sleeve is much like a condom, but a man can put a small hole in it if he does not want it to act as a contraceptive.) The sleeve with its semen can be taken to the laboratory for evaluation.

It is important not to use a vaginal lubricant when collecting the specimen because it can kill sperm. For the same reason, a couple should not use a lubricant when they are having intercourse on the days they might be able to achieve pregnancy.

816 What will be done if a problem is discovered with the man?

A low sperm count, unhealthy sperm, or a congenital problem are major factors in the problems that can cause male infertility.

A urologist ordinarily treats a man with an infertility problem. Here I will give only a brief overview of male infertility. As previously stated, most gynecologists specializing in fertility care can order the preliminary semen tests. Further testing and treatment will require seeing a urologist.

If the sperm analysis shows the production of few or no sperm (a sperm count that is twenty million or higher per cc of semen is considered normal), several other tests will be performed. These include hormone tests to be sure no hormone problem exists; testicular biopsies to see if sperm can be produced; X-ray vasographies (injection of dye into the vas) to pinpoint the location of blocked sperm ducts; testing the sperm to see if they will penetrate hamster eggs.

Many couples are surprised when I mention that smoking, alcohol, marijuana, and anabolic steroids can affect a man's sperm. Even if a sperm count seems fairly good, it is best for a man not to smoke, to drink no more than one or two drinks a week, and to use no marijuana or anabolic steroids during the time he and his wife are trying to get pregnant. Though the sperm count may be good, stopping the use of these things will usually increase the sperm count even more and improve the chance of pregnancy.

An infection of the semen can usually be successfully treated, whether it is from prostatitis, seminal vesiculitis, or some other type of infection. If there is an accumulation of veins around the testicle (varicocele), the urologist may want to operate to tie off the engorged veins. The rationale behind this surgery is that the enlarged veins keep the testicle warmer than it should be. Testicles produce the best sperm counts when they are cooler than the rest of the body. When the varicocele is tied off, the testicle (or testicles) gets cooler and starts producing better sperm. With a varicocele, a man's sperm count is usually adequate but the motility of many of the sperm is poor.

If a man does not have a varicocele but still has "bad" sperm, the doctor may try giving him Clomid or some other drug. Although the results are often unsatisfactory, their use may be worth a try.

If this does not work, intrauterine inseminations with washed sperm can be done. (See Q. 862.) Or, if that fails, in vitro fertilization can be done. (See Q. 867–876.) IVF procedures can include fertilizing a wife's eggs with sperm by placing sperm in the same container as the eggs or injecting a single sperm into an individual egg. If none of these techniques works, insemination with another man's sperm can be done. This is called artificial insemination with donor sperm, or AID. (See Q. 863–866.)

If a man has had a vasectomy for sterilization, he can have that vasectomy reversed. A doctor who uses microsurgical technique can open the scrotum where the initial incision was made for the vasectomy. The scarred ends of the vas can be cut open and sewn back together so that sperm can once again flow through the reproductive tract. If the vasectomy was done recently, your husband has an excellent chance of producing normal sperm that can result in a normal pregnancy for you. If it has been several years since the vasectomy, he has less chance of producing healthy sperm. If it has been more than ten years since a vasectomy was done, your husband may have only a 10 to 20 percent chance of being able to produce healthy sperm after his vas are repaired. The only way to know whether or not an operation to repair the vas will work is to try it. If your husband decides not to have this operation, or if after a vasectomy reversal no pregnancy occurs, the only alternative for you to become pregnant is to have artificial insemination done using donor sperm. (See Q. 863–866.)

IVF procedures may be useful for a man with this problem or a man who has testicles, but no sperm. New techniques allow a small portion of a man's testicle to be surgically removed and ground up. The immature sperm from that material can then be extracted and injected into a wife's eggs and pregnancy can result. For more information on this procedure call Mr. Tom Turner at (512) 370-4447 in Austin, Texas, at the St. David's-Columbia Hospital IVF program.

The Scope of Female Abnormalities Affecting Fertility

817 Which structural abnormalities in a woman could be discovered in an initial physical examination?

A thorough, competent infertility doctor may occasionally find a physical abnormality on the ini-

tial exam of an infertile woman. (A detailed description of treatment for these conditions is given in later questions.)

Abnormal vagina. A tough hymen can prevent proper penetration of the penis; a vaginal blockage can prevent deposition of the semen by the cervix, and a vaginal infection can produce short-term infertility. Surgery can correct these problems. When it comes to vaginal infections, trichomoniasis (see Q. 603) seems to be a bad offender.

Abnormal cervix. Cervical problems can inhibit fertility through abnormal cervical mucus due to cervical infection, previous cervical surgery, inadequate hormone stimulation of the cervical mucus, or a woman being allergic to her husband's sperm. Cervical stenosis (tight cervix) and mycoplasma or chlamydia cervical infections can also affect fertility. Women who have been DES-exposed will frequently have cervical abnormalities.

Abnormal uterus or abnormal endometrium (uterine lining). There are many problems involving the uterus that can prevent conception, including fibroid tumors and congenital abnormalities. The inside of the uterus is called the endometrial cavity, and the lining of the inside of the uterus is called the endometrium. There may be polyps projecting from the uterine wall, fibroid tumors distorting the uterus or its cavity, or an infection of the uterus. The endometrium reflects the function of the ovaries and other hormones in the body. If these hormones are functioning abnormally, the lining of the uterus will not undergo proper changes during the female monthly cycle and will therefore not be receptive to pregnancy.

Abnormal fallopian tubes. Problems of the tubes may result from previous infection that scarred or blocked them, a previous sterilization procedure, congenital abnormalities that caused distortion of the tubes, previous tubal pregnancies, endometriosis, or salpingitis isthmica nodosa (SIN).

Abnormal ovaries. The ovaries may not function properly because of endometriosis, scarring from previous infection, polycystic ovarian syndrome, or some abnormality of hormone production by the ovary.

Abnormal hormone functioning. Since hormones control ovulation, abnormal hormone function can cause infertility. The hypothalamus, located at the base of the brain, monitors the release of hormones. This gland is the master control gland for the female cycle. Its abnormal function can cause an irregular cycle or prevent ovulation. Abnormal function of the pituitary, thyroid, or adrenal glands can also prevent normal ovulation.

Cervical Abnormalities and Infertility

818 What can be done if there is an abnormality of the cervix?

If a cervix just "looks" abnormal, with ridges or irregularity, you were probably exposed to DES in your mother's womb. Nothing needs to be done, because that condition is probably not contributing to your infertility. If the cervical opening is too tight because you have had cautery, freezing, or a conization of your cervix, something may need to be done, such as a dilatation of the cervix (as in a D&C). This procedure may require anesthesia.

Occasionally the opening of the cervix may be so small that the doctor will be unable to find it; this is usually the result of having had a conization done in the past. If surgery is required to repair the cervix and a D&C is not possible, then the doctor may need to make an incision in the abdomen, split the uterus from above, and probe down through the cervix into the vagina to redevelop a cervical opening. A problem with the cervix that is this severe is rare.

819 How is the cervical mucus involved with fertility?

During most of the month the sticky, thick cervical mucus "defends" the interior cavity of the uterus and the fallopian tubes by preventing the passage of sperm, germs, and chemicals. Just before ovulation, however, a remarkable transition takes place: Estrogen produced by the ovaries causes the cervical mucus to develop spinnbarkheit (see information about this in the discussion of the postcoital test in Q. 809), a condition essential for the successful transport of sperm. The mucus of the cervix is made up of macromolecules. When the cervical mucus becomes watery and develops its spinnbarkheit, it means that these macromolecules have arranged themselves into parallel "rods of mucus." This physical arrangement of the molecules of the mucus allows sperm to swim freely into the woman's uterus. While allowing sperm passage, the cervical mucus continues to prevent the passage of most germs and the mucus from the man's semen into the uterus. After ovulation occurs, the macromolecules of the mucus change so that the mucus becomes thick, sticky, and resistant to penetration by sperm, germs, or medications.

820 What can be done if my cervical mucus is abnormal?

You may have an obvious cervical infection called cervicitis, which should be treated with antibiotics by mouth, with a vaginal antibiotic cream, or by treatment of the cervix with laser or freezing. If you have a chlamydia or gonorrhea infection, it must be treated. These two infections can pass through the cervical mucus into the uterus and cause pelvic inflammatory disease. PID can cause sterility. If you or your husband has had sexual activity with others that might have allowed you to become infected with one of these germs, be sure to tell your physician.

Certain cervical infections may exist without any symptoms yet still produce infertility, for example, infections with mycoplasma or chlamydia organisms. Because cultures of these germs are not always reliable, I routinely treat all first-time infertility patients and their husbands with tetracycline for two weeks to rid them of such organisms. Incidentally, the husband is treated because he can have any germ in his urethra that his wife has in her vagina.

Despite much research and testing of new and different techniques, infertility physicians do not yet know a great deal about cervical mucus and its association with infertility. The approach of most physicians knowledgeable in infertility management involves this sequence of events in the evaluation and treatment of cervical mucus problems:

1. A postcoital test is done.
2. Any infection is treated. (Some physicians treat all infertility couples with tetracycline.)
3. If the cervical mucus seems to be unhealthy other than because of infection, bypass it by doing intrauterine inseminations (IUI). (See the section in this chapter on IUI.)
4. If pregnancy still does not occur, use Pergonal therapy three or four times because Pergonal usually produces excellent cervical mucus.
5. If pregnancy still does not occur, consider using an IVF-type procedure.

It is unclear whether or not the effect of cervical mucus on infertility is a primary contributing factor to infertility.

It may be that bad cervical mucus is not truly a long-term cause of infertility. I did mention earlier in this chapter that some women who have no sperm present on a postcoital test will have sperm found when a laparoscopy is done at the same time. This would indicate that we really do not even know how to test the cervical mucus properly for normal passage of sperm. Because of all these factors, therefore, most infertility specialists will treat a problem of cervical mucus much like a problem of infertility of undetermined cause. The approach to this type of problem is, "Even though we don't know what is wrong, we can do some things to help pregnancy be achieved."

---

821 **I have heard that it is possible for a woman to be allergic to her husband's sperm, and that he can be allergic to his own sperm. Is this true?**

A small percentage of those couples who seek infertility evaluation will discover that the woman is allergic to her husband's sperm. Physicians refer to this allergy as "immunity" to the sperm and call this "immunologic infertility."

The best way to test for this immunity is the "immunobead test." One way to do this is to put a woman's blood serum with her husband's sperm in a test tube in the lab. If a man's sperm then seem to be "sticking together," the wife may have immunity against her husband's sperm. The immunobead test can be done using a man's own serum against his own sperm to see if a man is allergic to his own sperm (this will often happen if a man has had reversal of a vasectomy).

The problem of immunologic infertility is twofold. First, we don't know how significant such immunology is, even if a woman has antibodies against her husband's sperm (or he against his own). In some cases where this situation exists, spontaneous pregnancies will occur.

If a couple is unable to get pregnant, however, and no other cause for infertility can be found other than significant immunity to the sperm, treatment for the condition seems appropriate.

The second problem physicians face regarding immunologic infertility is that there is no standard, proven treatment. Three things are often suggested:

1. If a woman has antibodies against her husband's sperm, he can use condoms every time they have intercourse except on the days when pregnancy can occur. If a woman is exposed to fewer of her husband's sperm, it is possible that her body will produce fewer antibodies against those sperm, allowing pregnancy to occur. This regimen is not often helpful.
2. High doses of cortisone-type drugs can be given, but this is sometimes associated with a major complication—aseptic necrosis of the femoral head may develop (the hip "self-destructs"), a situation which leads to the need for a total hip replacement. Most doctors do not recommend this therapy.
3. In vitro fertilization may sometimes be the only solution with immunologic infertility. When a woman's eggs are removed from her

body for this procedure, they are washed free of all her serum and put directly with her husband's sperm, making it possible for the eggs and sperm to fertilize away from the presence of antibodies. If you want to get pregnant and nothing else is working, an IVF procedure may be necessary.

Immunologic infertility can be a very frustrating problem for both the couple and the physician. Thankfully, IVF-type procedures seem to offer the answer.

Uterine Abnormalities and Infertility

822 What if my doctor finds an abnormality of my uterus?

If there is something growing in your uterus that is large enough for your doctor to feel, it will almost always be a fibroid tumor—a knot of muscle growing in the wall of the uterus that almost never becomes cancerous, but can prevent pregnancy or cause miscarriages.

A fibroid tumor may not interfere with fertility, but if fibroids have caused the uterus to increase in size to that of a two- or three-month pregnancy, they should be removed. If the uterus gets larger than that, the normal muscle of the uterus can be so damaged by surgery to remove these larger fibroids that infertility can result from the surgery.

If a woman has fibroids that have increased the size of the uterus to larger than a three-month pregnancy, a physician may need to treat the patient with a GnRH agonist (Lupron) for three months to decrease the size of the fibroid tumors, thus allowing less damage when they are removed. (See Q. 858.)

Though the removal of fibroids (myomectomy) is a major operation, it is usually success-

ful unless the uterus has grown very large and GnRH did not make it smaller. An operation to remove fibroids requires an incision in the abdominal wall. If it is necessary to cut into the inner cavity of the uterus, the woman will have to have a cesarean section for delivery if she later becomes pregnant.

Fibroid tumors are very common, and hysterectomy is without question the easiest operation for fibroids. If your doctor suggests that you have a hysterectomy when you still want to have a baby, get another opinion. If your physician says that he or she will "try" to get the fibroids but is not sure that is possible, I encourage you to get a second opinion. You need a surgeon who is skilled in working with infertility patients. Such a physician can almost always assure you that all of your fibroids can be removed without a hysterectomy.

A final note on this subject: One important reason for a young woman to have annual examinations is to make sure that she is not developing fibroid tumors. Although they are not common in women in their early twenties or younger, they can be present then (as women get into their late twenties and early thirties they become much more common).

823 What if an X-ray of my uterus by hysterosalpingogram shows scarring or polyps inside my uterus?

If you have scarring or polyps inside your uterus, a D&C, diagnostic laparoscopy, and hysteroscopy may need to be done.

Scarring in the uterus (synechiae) needs to be evaluated by hysteroscopy. When I do a hysteroscopy for this reason, I almost always do a laparoscopy at the same time. If there has been enough disease or trauma to a woman's uterus to cause significant abnormality, laparoscopy may discover significant associated scarring of the tubes and ovaries.

When the X-ray shows abnormalities in the uterine cavity, it is most important that they be corrected. Scarring in the uterus can cause both infertility and miscarriage. Small polyps or growths in the uterus seem to act like an IUD (intrauterine contraceptive device) in preventing pregnancy.

Occasionally a woman may have so much scarring inside her uterus that she cannot even have a period (Aslerman's syndrome). Scarring inside the uterus usually results from a scraping of the uterine lining done because of pregnancy. This may be from a D&C, necessary because a woman is hemorrhaging after a delivery, or a miscarriage. Or it may be from an elective abortion procedure that caused enough damage to the uterus to prevent a later pregnancy. Versy C. Buttram, M.D., past president of the American Fertility Society, in his excellent book *Surgical Treatment of the Infertile Female* (Baltimore: Williams & Wilkins, 1985) states: "The most common antecedent factor for IUA [intrauterine adhesions] in this author's experience has been elective pregnancy termination by aspiration technique."

A hysteroscope can almost always be used to correct scarring or polyps inside the uterus. This instrument (see illustration on p. 446) allows visualization and surgery of the interior of the uterus. Polyps can be removed, scars can be cut apart, and congenital abnormalities can be corrected. (See Q. 699.)

The hysteroscope has become of tremendous value for women with abnormalities of the endometrial cavity. In the past, most of these problems required major surgery, but now they can usually be corrected in an outpatient surgical facility with the woman going home the day of surgery.

Occasionally, some of the abnormalities seen on the X-ray of the uterine cavity cannot be corrected with a hysteroscope. In this case, the doctor must make an incision in the abdominal wall to cut the uterus open from above to make it normal. Although this is a major operation, it is usually worthwhile for an infertile woman. After the abnormalities are corrected, normal pregnancy often results (though C-section is usually required for delivery).

824 What if the hysterosalpingo-gram shows that I have been born with an abnormal uterus?

As a female baby develops inside the mother's uterus, the baby's own uterus is formed from two halves: one from the right and one from the left side of her body. Normally these meet in the middle, fuse, and then develop a cavity in the middle which becomes the endometrial (uterine) cavity.

Occasionally the two halves of the uterus form on each side of the body but do not fuse properly in the middle. Variations of this type of abnormality occur. They may range from a woman having two vaginas lying side by side—with two cervixes and two halves of a uterus that function as two normal, separate uteri—to having only a small indentation in the top part of the uterus.

An abnormal uterus may or may not be a problem for you. If you have not had miscarriages and have had no trouble getting pregnant, you need not be worried if your doctor tells you that your uterus did not form properly.

Having two uteri (uterus didelphys) usually does not cause fertility problems. However, it can result in miscarriages or premature deliveries. When this is thought to be the problem, the two uterine bodies can be sewn together to form one cavity. This is done by making an incision in the abdominal wall, opening the two uterine bodies, and sewing them together. This does not have to be done until you have become pregnant and know that you lost a pregnancy because of an abnormal uterus.

I had as a patient a young woman who had become pregnant several years ago in one side of her double uterus. Her physician at the time told her that she should have an abortion, because he was sure she would miscarry or deliver prematurely. She took his advice and had the abortion.

After moving to our city she came to me and asked that I repair her uterus so that she could have a baby. I then had to tell this young woman that the abortion had been unnecessary and that her uterus did not need repairing, unless it was proven that she could not carry a pregnancy. Her doctor was evidently unfamiliar with infertility issues.

Special Concerns

A less severe form of abnormal uterine development is the septate uterus. The two halves of the uterus come together but do not fuse completely. As a result there is a wall either partial or complete, between the two halves of the uterus. The septate uterus does not usually cause infertility, but it can often cause repeated miscarriages. If you have this problem, operative hysteroscopy to repair your uterus will almost certainly allow you to carry a normal pregnancy. A septate uterus is one infertility problem that physicians are "relieved" to find because it can, most of the time, be so easily corrected with the hysteroscope.

Any of these abnormal situations is compatible with normal reproductive capacity. In other words, you may be able to become pregnant normally and carry babies in a normal fashion. If you are having trouble becoming pregnant and you have this type of uterine abnormality, you should have a complete evaluation for other possible problems of fertility before any type of surgery is done on your uterus. If everything else seems normal and the only abnormality is the uterine abnormality, then it is reasonable to have surgery to correct it.

After the uterine cavity has been evaluated, the tissue that lines that cavity, the endometrium, should be evaluated. This is accomplished by an endometrial biopsy, as explained in the next question.

825 Why is an endometrial biopsy done?

Endometrial biopsies are done primarily to be sure that the ovaries are ovulating and producing normal hormones after ovulation, and that the uterine (endometrial) lining is being prepared by those hormones to receive and nurture a baby. If no ovulation is occurring, this will usually be proven by the results of the biopsy. A luteal phase defect is diagnosed in part with this same test. (See Q. 843–846.)

Another way to detect ovulation is by a blood test to check the serum progesterone level. If ovulation has occurred, a woman's progesterone level, halfway between ovulation and her menstrual period, should be at least 6.5 ng/ml. This value may vary according to your own physician's laboratory, but he or she will know what value usually corresponds to normal ovulation according to that laboratory.

Occasionally the endometrial biopsy done to check for hormone changes finds an infection. If the endometrium is infected, antibiotics may be prescribed. Another endometrial biopsy may be done later to evaluate the effect of the treatment of the infection.

An infection inside the uterus could also involve the tubes and ovaries. This can be determined by performing a laparoscopy and an endometrial biopsy at the same time. I have occasionally found chlamydia in this uterine tissue even though the

Endometrial Biopsy

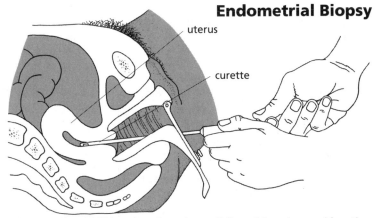

uterus

curette

When an endometrial biopsy is performed, a small piece of tissue is scraped from the lining of the uterus and removed for microscopic evaluation.

woman had already been treated for chlamydia. More intensive treatment is then required.

826 How is an endometrial biopsy done? Is it painful?

An endometrial biopsy is often done in the doctor's office, usually without anesthesia. Although the procedure is quickly accomplished, it is painful.

If a physician does not have nitrous oxide available in his or her office, the patient can be given strong pain pills to use before coming to the office. A paracervical block can also be used.

I have given patients nitrous oxide (just like dentists use) to relieve the pain. This has worked so well that I now recommend this technique for certain other simple-but-painful procedures that are done in the office.

An endometrial biopsy is done by inserting into the uterus a small, hollow, round tube with a sharp lip. As it is drawn back, some of the lining of the uterus is collected. This tissue is sent to the pathologist for evaluation.

Because this procedure hurts, I usually try to do it when I do the laparoscopy for infertility. This way, a woman does not have to experience any pain with the endometrial biopsy.

Fallopian-Tube Abnormalities and Infertility

827 What if my physician finds that my fallopian tubes are abnormal and suspects that is causing my infertility? What produces such abnormalities and how can they be treated?

Several problems may cause the fallopian tubes to be abnormal. These problems comprise the most common cause of infertility, accounting for 35 percent of infertility in couples, and over 50 percent of female-related infertility.

Sexually transmitted diseases (STD). Gonorrhea and chlamydia are spreading like wildfire among young people in the United States. They are the most rapidly increasing cause of infertility in the United States. These two organisms cause most of the pelvic inflammatory disease that occurs in this country; PID can cause so much damage to the tubes that they close completely, or to the pelvic structures that they become so scarred that an egg cannot get to the tubes. Of women who are infertile, one-third have that problem because of damage to their fallopian tubes from one of these two sexually transmitted diseases. Another problem that can result from this kind of tubal damage is ectopic pregnancy. Occasionally an egg gets partially through the tube, where it becomes lodged and fertilized, resulting in such an ectopic or "out of place" pregnancy.

To explain what is meant by adhesions and scarring of the tubes and other organs, I often use this example: If you scrape the sides of two of your fingers till they are quite raw and then bind them together for several weeks, they will grow together. Physicians would refer to the scar between the fingers that held them together as an "adhesion." This is what happens to the tubes, ovaries, intestines, and other organs inside the pelvis as a result of infection. They stick together as though glue had been poured on them. The scars that hold them together and distort them are adhesions.

Infections from gonorrhea or chlamydia cause infertility in about 11 percent of women with a first infection, about 23 percent with the second infection, and about 54 percent with three or more such infections. (See Q. 986.)

If a young woman gets chlamydia as a teenager from intercourse with her boyfriend, she may never know she has the disease until she is married and finds that she is unable to have a baby. I see this with my infertility patients frequently. About half of the women who are infertile because of damage to their fallopian tubes were unaware that they had had a fallopian tube infection. These infections are one of the primary dangers of sex before marriage. If you want to have children, you shouldn't have intercourse until you get married.

Intrauterine devices. Women who use IUDs run a greater than normal risk of pelvic infections (two or three times normal) and such infections usually occur during the first few months that an IUD is in place. Because of this increased risk of infection, I urge women not to use IUDs unless they have had all the babies they ever want. If a woman has used an IUD she has doubled her chance of being infertile.

Endometriosis. Endometriosis can cause distortion and scarring of the fallopian tubes and the surgery that is done to remove endometriosis can also result in damaged fallopian tubes. Endometriosis is a fairly common cause of infertility, and infertility may be the only symptom of her endometriosis. (See Q. 849–859.)

Elective abortion. A small but significant percentage of women who have chosen to have abortions will have infertility problems later due to infections of the tubes or damage to the uterus resulting from those abortions.

Previous pelvic surgery. Any surgery done on the pelvic structures can result in scarring of the tubes and subsequent infertility. Since some pelvic surgery is unnecessary, my advice is that you not let a doctor operate on you, especially for an "ovarian cyst," unless you know it is absolutely necessary.

Tubal (ectopic) pregnancy. Tubal pregnancies are both a result of and a cause of scarred tubes. When a tube is scarred, it can trap a fertilized egg, causing an ectopic pregnancy. That pregnancy can then severely damage the tube, and subsequent surgery for the ectopic pregnancy can cause more tubal scarring.

Appendicitis. An infected or ruptured appendix can cause so much infection in the pelvis that a great deal of scarring of the female organs can result. This scarring can be so severe that a woman cannot get pregnant except with an in vitro fertilization procedure.

Voluntary sterilization. "Band-Aid" sterilization has made female sterilization so acceptable and easy that many women are having it done. And, as the news of its successful reversibility spreads,

more and more women are requesting a reversal of a previous sterilization. Surgical reversal of a tubal ligation can often be done successfully but it also can leave some scarring of the tubes. (See Q. 829.) About 60 to 75 percent of women who have a sterilization reversal are able to get pregnant. There is a higher chance of ectopic pregnancy in these women, however, because of scarring of the tubes from the tubal surgery.

---

828 What can be done if my fertility evaluation shows I have scarred or blocked fallopian tubes?

First, if the problem was discovered with a hysterosalpingogram, a laparoscopy needs to be done to determine the probable cause and the extent of the damage. If the laparoscopy shows significant scarring, he/she will usually try to cut it loose right then with laparascopic techniques. Your health will not be damaged if the scars are left alone, but removal of them may increase the possibility of your achieving pregnancy.

At the time of laparascopy, the gynecologist may be able to open the fallopian tubes and cut all important adhesion. This would be the easiest way to have infertility surgery. If the scar is too severe, however, major surgery may be required. Even with this major surgery (or with the laparascopic procedure) you probably have only a 30 percent chance of pregnancy following surgery. Also, one thing to remember is that after such surgery there is a greater than normal chance of your having an ectopic pregnancy. If the scar is so severe it cannot be cut loose using the laparoscope, there are two choices. A major operation with a 6-inch incision can be done (results—30 percent chance of getting pregnant) or an in vitro fertilization procedure. Whether I encourage a patient to go ahead with surgery depends on the severity of the scar. Generally, if the scar can be cut loose with the laparoscope, that is best; otherwise in vitro fertilization is the only chance they have of becoming pregnant.

If you choose to have the surgery, the physician should use microsurgical technique. He or she will usually do the surgery through a six-inch "bikini" incision in your lower abdomen, made crossways just above your pubic hairline. Your surgeon should not only be familiar with microsurgery but enthusiastic about the technique and willing to take the time required to use it correctly.

Although you may feel fine within a few weeks after this surgery, it may take your pelvic tissues a long time to become normal enough to produce a pregnancy, especially the tissues of the delicate inner lining of the tube. I tell patients I have operated on that they will probably not become pregnant for a year, and possibly longer. If pregnancy does not occur after one or two years, further evaluation and treatment would be necessary. Ultimately, in vitro fertilization or adoption may be the only options available for obtaining a child.

The statistics of 30 percent chance of pregnancy following surgery apply when the problem of infertility is due to fairly serious pelvic adhesions, but the chances are better with less severe adhesions.

Some women have such severe scarring and adhesions of the pelvis that an operation to free and open the fallopian tubes is almost useless. Patients with problems this severe may have only a 5 percent chance of becoming pregnant, even after major surgery. A woman may better use her time, money, and energy by going ahead with in vitro fertilization procedure. If she cannot afford an IVF-type procedure, she may want to proceed with major surgery to attempt to free her uterus, tubes, and ovaries of the scarring, but she must realize that there is a great chance she still may not be able to get pregnant except with IVF.

If a woman has been found to have extensive adhesions and she has these repaired by laparotomy or operative laparoscopy, her doctor may feel that a laparoscopy one month later is important. Some tissues might have stuck back together. This "second-look laparoscopy" can help free up the pelvic organs again and result in a greater chance of later pregnancy.

About one-fourth of patients with blocked fallopian tubes have some type of obstruction in a part of the tube that either lies in or is just outside the uterus. Occasionally this obstruction is due to some dried secretions present in the fallopian tubes. This obstruction can be corrected if a small catheter is pushed into the tube to dislodge the material. At laparoscopy the physician can also put a hysteroscope into the woman's uterus and, while an assistant is watching through the laparoscope, thread a small catheter up into the uterus under direct visualization. He can guide the catheter into the opening of the fallopian tube and then, as his assistant watches, thread it through the portion of the fallopian tube that is passing through the wall of the uterus and out into the part of the tube that lies outside the uterus. The assistant can watch as this catheter goes through the part of the fallopian tube that was obstructed. The physician can then inject dye. The assistant can watch the dye flow through the tube and out the end to prove that the tube is open.

Therefore, if you have a tube that appears to be obstructed near or in the uterus, I recommend that you have a laparoscopy at which time your physician can use the catheter to try to dislodge the material in it.

If your tube is obstructed because of previous infection or scar, a catheter forced through it will do nothing but tear it. This will not solve the problem. Usually the scar will just re-form. Even if the scar is forced open, though, it would not be healthy enough to allow an egg to pass through and into the uterus. Catheterizing this kind of scarred and abnormal fallopian tube would only increase the chance of tubal pregnancy.

829 Tell me more about the surgery that is required for reversal of a sterilization.

A sterilization can be reversed, but frequently (25 to 40 percent) the procedure is unsuccessful. Also some sterilization techniques so totally destroy the fallopian tubes that a reversal procedure is impossible.

If your sterilization was done with the coagulation (electrical burn) technique in only one area of the tube, or if you have a Fallope ring or a Hulka Clip (or some other method of sterilization in which cautery was not used), you have a good chance of pregnancy if you have repair of your tubes.

The first test your doctor would order is a semen analysis on your husband. If he has normal semen, then your doctor may want you to have a hysterosalpingogram before doing your tubal repair. This can show how much fallopian tube is still attached to your uterus, giving the doctor some idea of how successful the tubal reanastomosis might be. If after evaluating the HSG and your sterilization records your doctor has a question about whether or not there is too much fallopian tube damage to be repaired, he or she will probably want to do a diagnostic laparoscopy to evaluate the tubes thoroughly before performing additional major surgery.

Once the evaluation is completed and it has been determined that neither you nor your husband has any other fertility problems and that your tubes can probably be repaired, you will be scheduled for surgery. The operation involves a routine abdominal incision so that your doctor can directly examine your tubes. If the doctor sees that surgery will allow the possibility of successful reversal, the tubes will be positioned so that they are visible through the operating microscope (or through magnifying lenses). Then the doctor will cut off the scarred stumps of the tubes, cauterize bleeders, and sew the two tube openings together with very fine suture. (The suture used is smaller than a human hair and difficult to see with the unaided eye.)

Few insurance companies will pay for this procedure. Because of this, some physicians have started doing this operation as an outpatient procedure on those women who seem appropriate for successful outpatient surgery (ones who are not overweight, not too nervous, and not too sensitive to pain). Outpatient surgery makes the procedure about half as expensive as it would be if it were done in the hospital, but it takes a tough woman to go through surgery that is this major and go home the same day.

Ovarian Abnormalities and Infertility

830 My doctor said I might have polycystic ovarian syndrome. What is this, and how is it treated?

Polycystic ovarian syndrome (PCOS) is an abnormality of the ovaries that produces irregular periods and infertility. Although there are numerous other causes of irregular periods, if you have had irregular periods since puberty it is likely that you have this syndrome.

Other common symptoms of PCOS are obesity and a tendency toward excessive hair growth. Although these two characteristics are not always present in PCOS cases, when they do occur the odds are ten to one that you have PCOS.

Polycystic ovarian syndrome is a genetic problem, but the mode of inheritance has not been determined. If a woman goes through a period of time without ovulation (anovulation), she seems more likely to develop this problem later. There seem to be many causes of this condition, including significant stress, significant weight gain, overactivity of the adrenal glands, and so on. When polycystic ovarian syndrome is present, there seems to be a lack of normal enzyme production by the ovaries, which causes them to produce more male hormones and less female hormones. The ovary does produce some male hormones normally. More than 85 percent of women who have PCOS have elevated levels of one or both of the male hormones—androstenedione or testosterone.

Because of the ovaries' failure to ovulate and the overproduction of male hormones, the pituitary produces too much luteinizing hormone (LH), the hormone that makes the ovary release its ripened egg, but only a normal or slightly below normal amount of follicle-stimulating hormone (FSH). This is the pituitary's ill-conceived attempt to make the ovary release its eggs. Often a vaginal sonogram of the ovaries will show that the ovaries contain multiple small cysts.

PCOS can usually be treated with medication. Before treatment, tests should be done to make sure the symptoms are not caused by abnormality of the adrenal glands, the pituitary, or the thyroid. Your doctor may have already tested you for such problems.

(See the excellent review of this problem in the *New England Journal of Medicine*, September 28, 1995, 333.13:853–861, by Stephen Franks, M.D.)

831 My doctor said Clomid or Serophene is used to treat PCOS. What are these drugs and what do they do?

Clomid and Serophene are actually the same drug: clomiphene. This drug causes a woman with polycystic ovarian syndrome to ovulate 80 percent of the time and to become pregnant 50 percent of the time. This is why the drug is known as "the fertility pill."

Clomiphene was first studied in 1960 as a possible contraceptive. Surprisingly during this research it was found to induce fertility.

The chemical structure of clomiphene is similar to estrogenic substances. Scientists think that the hypothalamus, the large control gland at the base of the brain, regards clomiphene as the body's own estrogen. Once the clomiphene is taken in by the hypothalamus, the hypothalamus cannot measure the true amount of estrogen in the body's circulation and perceives it to be low. This causes the hypothalamus to signal the pituitary to stimulate the ovaries, to make them ovulate.

In addition to inducing ovulation, the use of clomiphene often creates regular twenty-eight- or twenty-nine-day menstrual cycles, with ovulation on day fourteen or fifteen. This cycle makes it "easier" for pregnancy to occur. With regular periods intercourse can be more accurately timed to coincide with ovulation, and the endometrial lining is developed in the most normal fashion for reception of a fertilized ovum.

The ultimate goal of using clomiphene is pregnancy, and it has truly been a miracle drug in helping thousands of otherwise infertile women achieve pregnancy.

832 Are any side effects or multiple births connected with the use of clomiphene?

Yes, there are some side effects, but these are generally unimportant and not too bothersome.

About 10 percent of women taking clomiphene will have hot flashes that are similar to those experienced in menopause, although it does not cause menopause to start. Occasionally there is some abdominal swelling and bloating (5 percent experience this). There will sometimes be breast discomfort (2 percent), nausea and vomiting (about 2 percent), visual symptoms such as bright spots of light (1.5 percent), headaches (about 1.5 percent), and dryness or partial loss of hair (about 1.5 percent). The cause of these symptoms is generally unknown, but in all cases the symptoms disappear when the medicine is discontinued, leaving no permanent effects. Occasionally a patient will feel some discomfort in her ovaries as they enlarge in response to the clomiphene.

If you should develop one or more ovarian cysts while taking clomiphene and continue to take it, the ovary can become huge: as big as a softball or even bigger. This can cause pain and can also cause the release of more than one egg, which increases the possibility of a multiple pregnancy. This situation, called ovarian hyperstimulation, is not usually a problem with clomiphene as it can be with Pergonal or Metrodin. But this is the primary reason for a monthly check by the doctor before prescribing more clomiphene.

In summary, the drug seems to cause almost no health hazards, and its side effects seem to be limited only to the month in which it is taken.

Although there is an increased chance (about 8 percent) of having a multiple birth, most of these are twins. I have only had one patient get pregnant with triplets due to clomiphene, and none have had more than triplets. However, as of this writing there have been one sextuplet birth and three quintuplet births reported in the world among women who took clomiphene.

The miscarriage rate for clomiphene users is only 20 percent, which is the same rate as in pregnancies achieved without clomiphene.

833 Is there an increased risk of having an abnormal baby while using clomiphene?

Most studies show that there is a slightly increased risk of abnormalities in pregnancies produced by clomiphene. The increased risk is so small, however, that experts conclude that the benefits definitely outweigh the risks. Most researchers believe that the increased risk of having an abnormal baby is due to the already existing subfertility (decreased fertility) of the couple who must use clomiphene to achieve pregnancy rather than to the clomiphene itself.

834 How is clomiphene taken?

Patients are given a prescription for five clomiphene tablets, and each clomiphene tablet contains 50 mg of clomiphene citrate. One tablet is taken each day for five consecutive days, starting on the third to fifth day of the menstrual cycle. (Your doctor will tell you which day to start.) The cycle is always counted with the first day of the menstrual period being "day one."

Women taking clomiphene must usually be examined by their physician each month during the menstrual period. Most patients will ovulate with the first dose of clomiphene citrate. If they do not ovulate after two or three months, the dosage may be increased to two clomiphene tablets per day for five days, or even up to four or five clomiphene tablets per day for each of those days. Also, ovulation can sometimes be induced by taking clomiphene for a total of up to eight days rather than just five.

Patients on clomiphene should at first keep a daily temperature chart every month to determine when they ovulate. This is done by using a basal body thermometer. If no period comes and the temperature did not go up about the fifteenth day, ovulation did not occur. I recommend that a woman who is starting clomiphene take her temperature the first three months. If, while on clomiphene, she has a temperature change at midcycle (indicating ovulation) and she has regular periods, she is most likely going to continue to ovulate on a regular basis while taking clomiphene. In

this case, she can stop taking her temperature and start using an ovulation predictor kit to determine exactly when to have intercourse. Ovulation predictor kits are a more expensive way to determine the best time for intercourse, but they are also more accurate than taking the temperature.

If a woman who is taking clomiphene (and who has been having regular periods and ovulating) misses a period, she may be pregnant and should see her physician for a pregnancy test.

835 What if I still don't have regular periods after taking clomiphene?

If a woman is taking clomiphene and not having periods, more intensive ovulation induction is necessary. She may need to have vaginal ultrasound to see if her ovaries are developing follicles. If follicles are developing but are not rupturing and releasing their eggs, her physician may want to give her human chorionic gonadotrophin (HCG). This condition is called the luteinized unruptured follicle syndrome (LUF).

Human chorionic gonadotrophin is a hormone extracted from the urine of pregnant women or from the placentas that result from normal births. HCG is structurally and biologically similar to luteinizing hormone (LH), the hormone produced by the pituitary that "kicks" the ovary and makes it release its egg. A woman who is not ovulating properly may have poor production of LH from her pituitary. The HCG shot takes the place of the LH that the body should be producing.

HCG is usually given as a single shot in the muscle on the day that the vaginal ultrasound shows that the largest follicle on the ovary is about 18 mm across. Normally you will ovulate thirty-eight hours later. When HCG is used, you should have intercourse the evening of the shot and on each of the next two days.

If your physician gives you HCG, he or she may want you to return a day or two after the HCG injection to make sure it worked. This can be confirmed by visualizing a collapsed follicle with the ultrasound machine. If a follicle collapsed, it probably released an egg (the egg itself is too small to be seen with the ultrasound) and pregnancy is possible.

HCG is a very safe drug. I have never had a patient with an allergic reaction to it, and it does not increase the chance of having twins or triplets.

836 Is there any other treatment to try if ovulation does not occur when using clomiphene or human chorionic gonadotrophin, or if I still have not become pregnant after using clomiphene for a long time?

The next treatment tried will usually be follicle stimulating hormone (Pergonal, Metrodin, etc.). Although it is possible to give up to five clomiphene tablets a day and to use HCG, most physicians will not continue increasing clomiphene to that level. After clomiphene has been used for a few months and pregnancy has not occurred, the chance of a woman getting pregnant with it decreases significantly. If she has not conceived after six or eight months of clomiphene, she should probably proceed with Pergonal or Metrodin therapy. She can always go back to clomiphene if a one-month cycle of Pergonal doesn't result in pregnancy.

Pergonal, Metrodin, and similar drugs are hormones called human menopausal gonadotrophin (HMG), so called because they are extracted from the urine of women who have gone through menopause. (These women have an elevated amount of follicle stimulating hormone [FSH].) Pergonal contains primarily FSH, but it also contains some LH. Metrodin is pure FSH. These and similar drugs stimulate the ovaries of an infertile woman in the same way the hormone it contains stimulates the ovaries of all normally ovulating women every month. The hormone in these drugs therefore is normal for a woman's body. When we give these drugs we are giving this normal hormone in a larger amount than the normal woman's body usually produces.

837 When is the use of follicle-stimulating hormone (FSH) indicated?

There are five groups of women who need these drugs.

Women whose pituitary glands are not producing follicle-stimulating hormone (FSH) and thus are not ovulating. Problems that can cause this include growths or diseases that destroy all or part of the pituitary, thus keeping it from producing enough hormone. Surgical removal of the pituitary would also place a woman in this category.

Women whose pituitaries are producing FSH, but who are still not ovulating. Most of these women are having irregular periods and have polycystic ovarian syndrome (PCOS). They will usually try clomiphene first, but if several monthly courses of clomiphene do not cause ovulation, Pergonal can be tried.

Women who have abnormal cervical mucus. If a woman's infertility seems to be due to a cervical mucus abnormality and other methods of treatment have been unsuccessful, Pergonal or Metrodin might be tried. Pergonal almost always causes the cervix to produce healthy cervical mucus. This is an aggressive treatment for this problem, but it is often the only successful treatment. (See Q. 820.)

Others. Women with infertility problems of unknown cause are often successfully treated with Pergonal even though there is no specific reason to use it. Then finally Pergonal is used for in vitro fertilization-type procedures.

838 How are Pergonal (and similar drugs) taken?

There are many ways to use Pergonal. A common technique is for a woman to take 150 units of Pergonal a day, starting on the fifth day of her menstrual period. (Pergonal must be given as an injection into the muscle because it is not absorbed if taken by mouth.) A woman receives this much Pergonal every day until the eighth or ninth day, when she has an ultrasound scan and a blood test for estrogen. These tests will show whether or not the ovaries are responding to the drug.

The amount of Pergonal or Metrodin may be

increased or decreased, according to the way the ovaries are responding. The ultrasound scans and blood tests will be done every day or two until the woman has at least one follicle present that is about two-thirds inch across and has an estrogen level high enough to indicate a good follicle. When a follicle is large enough and the estrogen level is high enough, the physician will administer HCG to make the follicle release its egg thirty-eight hours later. (See Q. 835.)

Pergonal and Metrodin are usually very safe medications (as is HCG), but they can overstimulate the ovaries. (This is called "hyperstimulation syndrome.") If a woman's serum estrogen level is below 2500 pg/ml on the day HCG is given, however, there is little chance of hyperstimulation. These figures apply primarily to women who are using these drugs for ovulation induction and not for women who are having IVF. (Speak to your physician if you are concerned about hyperstimulation.)

839 What about complications with Pergonal (and similar drugs)?

Although it is possible for hyperstimulation to occur, these days it is unlikely that hyperstimulation will be too severe since the ovaries can now be carefully monitored with estradiol blood tests and sonograms. But severe hyperstimulation can occur.

The primary complication of Pergonal and Metrodin use is multiple pregnancy (more than one baby). This was dramatically illustrated in late 1997 by the birth of the McCaughey septuplets. In the past, before we had sonograms that could show how many eggs were developing, women would release several eggs without knowing it. This would result occasionally in conception of five, six, or more babies. Today's monitoring systems, however, enable us to know fairly accurately how many eggs a woman is going to produce. The way most knowledgeable doctors administer these drugs today, there is a 20 percent chance of a woman having more than one baby. (About 15 percent will be twins and 5 percent will be more than twins.)

The general recommendation is that if a woman has more than three or four follicles, she should use contraception to keep from getting pregnant that month. (Nor should she receive the HCG injection that forces the release of those eggs.) If a woman is older than thirty-five, she and her physician will probably discuss this situation and decide what to do. Because of the lessened chance of any individual egg fertilizing in the woman over age thirty-five, she may take some risk and attempt pregnancy with the multiple-egg release.

Although some women tire of using Pergonal after just one cycle, I encourage my patients to try at least four cycles before moving on to IVF procedures (the next step).

Concern was raised in 1993 about clomiphene, Pergonal, and Metrodin causing ovarian cancer. It is important to emphasize that these drugs are not cancer-causing chemicals like cigarette smoke. It seems the more times a woman's ovaries have produced eggs in her lifetime, the more likely she is to develop ovarian cancer. Women who have ovulated very few times in their life have very little risk of ovarian cancer. In spite of the theoretical risk of ovarian cancer from drugs that cause more eggs to be released from ovaries—drugs like clomiphene, Pergonal, and Metrodin—and in spite of some preliminary studies, there seems to be little risk of cancer from these drugs. As a matter of fact, Leon Speroff, M.D., internationally-recognized authority, stated in the January 1996 *Ob-Gyn Clinical Alert* "it is appropriate to state that there has been no definite evidence indicating an increased risk of ovarian cancer from the use of fertility drugs."

840 What are the results of using Pergonal (and similar drugs)?

If patients are properly selected (those who actually have a chance to get pregnant with Pergonal), from 50 to 75 percent will conceive. However, a slightly higher than normal number of these pregnancies end with miscarriage (28 percent), so only about half of the treated patients will carry a baby to term. Don't be too discouraged by a miscarriage. If you are able to get pregnant once, you probably can again.

Treatment with these drugs requires a great deal of time, dedication, and money. It also requires being able to get to the doctor's office frequently during the first half of the cycle.

841 When should these drugs not be used?

They should not be used if a woman is post-menopausal, whether because of premature menopause or regular menopause that occurred at the normal age. I have patients who have gone through menopause who want to take Pergonal to make their ovaries work again. If a woman has truly gone through menopause, her FSH level is already high; giving more FSH in the form of these drugs will not make her ovulate. If she has not truly gone through menopause, however, it is possible that they might help. This is a complicated situation that should be discussed with an infertility specialist.

In addition, these expensive medications should not be used until the absence of other fertility problems has been proven by a complete evaluation or until these have been treated with other techniques as extensively as possible.

Let me warn you that these drugs are being misused in a very dishonest way by some doctors. If a doctor takes excessive pride in being an infertility specialist but cannot do in vitro fertilization procedures for whatever reason (for example, no IVF program in his town), he may continue recommending Pergonal or Metrodin cycles month after month. I have actually seen a patient who had this done by an unscrupulous doctor multiple times over a three-year period. Unfortunately, by the time she came to my care she was forty-four years old, an age at which in-vitro fertilization is much less successful than at thirty-nine. In general, if Pergonal or Metrodin has not produced pregnancy with four cycles, it is best to consult with a doctor who does in vitro fertilization to find out about that.

842 What can be done if I ovulated with clomiphene or FSH drugs but did not get pregnant? What if I didn't ovulate?

Infertility care for a woman who does not get pregnant after using clomiphene or Pergonal (or who does not ovulate with these drugs) must be individualized and based on careful consultation.

If you ovulated while taking clomiphene or Pergonal but did not get pregnant, the most direct path to pregnancy is an in vitro fertilization procedure. This will give you the best chance of becoming pregnant. If you did not ovulate with the usual doses of clomiphene or Pegonal, you may be able to ovulate with the higher doses of Pergonal (or Metrodin) that are used with IVF procedures.

843 My doctor has said that I have a "bad luteal phase." What does that mean?

A woman's luteal phase is the time of her menstrual cycle from ovulation until her period starts. "Bad luteal phase" means that there is something wrong with the hormone production from the ovaries during this time. The medical term for this is "inadequate luteal phase." After ovulation, the ovary forms a corpus luteum cyst, which then produces a hormone called progesterone. The normal production of progesterone results in changes in the inner uterine lining that either prepares it for receiving the embryo (if pregnancy occurs) or causes menstruation to result (if it doesn't).

If the progesterone production is normal and the lining of the uterus is properly developed in anticipation of pregnancy, then pregnancy can occur. If the production of progesterone from the ovary is insufficient, the luteal phase is inadequate. This problem apparently stems from a lack of the cells that produce progesterone in the corpus luteum. In this situation there is nothing wrong with the lining of the uterus itself, other than that it has been poorly prepared for pregnancy by inadequate ovarian progesterone production.

844 How is an inadequate luteal phase diagnosed?

There are three methods used now for diagnosing an inadequate luteal phase. One method is to study a woman's ovulation pattern (determined from temperature charts or from the results of ovulation predictor kits). If her period starts ten days or less after ovulation, she probably has an inadequate luteal phase. If her temperature rises slowly or goes up and down during the time after ovulation, this can also indicate an inadequate luteal phase.

A second technique for diagnosing inadequate luteal phase is the measurement of the amount of progesterone in a woman's blood after ovulation. If a woman's progesterone level is not as high as it should be after ovulation, her ovaries are not producing adequate amounts of progesterone.

A third method of diagnosing an inadequate luteal phase is an endometrial biopsy. (See Q. 825–826.) The lining of the uterus undergoes precise changes every day of a woman's cycle from ovulation until menstruation starts, usually on the twenty-eighth day. On each particular day after ovulation the lining has a corresponding precise appearance with a normal luteal phase. If biopsy of a uterus is done on day twenty-three of the cycle but the tissue appears to be characteristic of day twenty-seven endometrium, there is an inadequate luteal phase. If the two are not within two days of each other, a luteal phase defect probably exists.

One problem with the diagnosis of inadequate luteal phase is that a woman may have a luteal phase defect one month and not have it the next. A luteal phase defect can be somewhat tricky to diagnose. If it is suspected, therefore, a woman may need to have her progesterone measured after ovulation during several different months, or she may require several endometrial biopsies.

845 Since an endometrial biopsy is done after ovulation, will it cause me to have an abortion if I am already pregnant?

An endometrial biopsy usually does not interfere with early pregnancy, but this is always a possibility.

A great deal of information is gained from an endometrial biopsy done after ovulation that cannot be obtained any other way. Since it is usually performed on women who are infertile, there are few who would unknowingly be pregnant. Of these few who might be pregnant, the biopsy would have a slight chance of ending their pregnancy because the embryo is so tiny at that stage of

pregnancy. Because the chance of hurting an early pregnancy is so slight, and the information gained is so helpful, almost all infertility specialists feel the procedure is necessary in certain situations. I recommend that a couple use barrier contraceptives the month a biopsy is going to be done to avoid any possibility of interrupting a pregnancy.

846 How is an inadequate luteal phase treated?

There are several treatments. The most common is the use of natural progesterone after ovulation until a period comes or until pregnancy is confirmed. In the past natural progesterone was available only in vaginal suppository form. Now it is available as oral capsules or even as sublingual troches (absorbable tablets placed under the tongue). A woman may use any one of these that her doctor prescribes. Some investigators have reported as much as 50 to 60 percent pregnancy rates in patients treated this way if they have inadequate luteal phase and no other problem.

The disadvantage to using the natural progesterone is that it is expensive. In addition, this medication may be difficult to obtain.

Most people now know that natural progesterone is safe in pregnancy. As mentioned all through this chapter, progesterone is vital for the development of the lining of the uterus after ovulation. It is also necessary after pregnancy occurs. As a matter of fact, without progesterone it would be impossible for any pregnancy to occur or survive. The natural progesterones are essentially just like a woman's normal progesterone and are safe in pregnancy. There are some synthetic progesterones, such as Provera, that should not be used in pregnancy. The molecule of the synthetic progesterones is very different from the natural progesterones now used during the preparation for pregnancy and for maintaining pregnancy.

Other methods of treatment include the use of bromocriptine (Parlodel), HCG, and Pergonal. (See Q. 835–836.) Your own doctor will recommend the treatment he or she thinks will be best for you.

Now that I have spent all this time talking about luteal phase defect, let me give you a recent

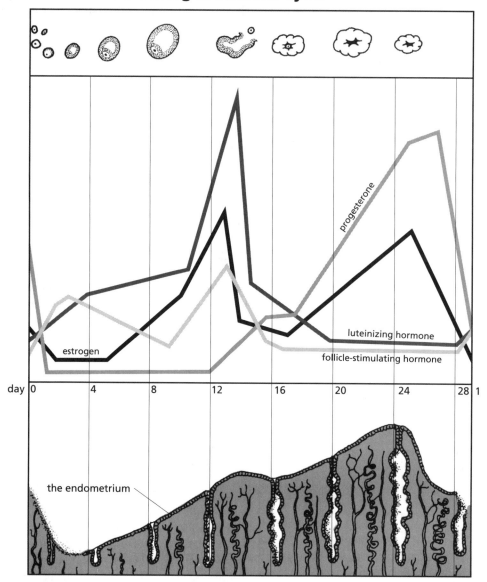

quote from Leon Speroff, M.D., a world-renowned authority on infertility: "We continue to struggle with the luteal phase defect. Not only are we not certain how to diagnose this entity, but we're not even sure it is a cause of infertility" (*Ob-Gyn Clinical Alert*, October 1994). He goes on to say that the treatment for this problem if it does cause infertility, doesn't hurt, and may help, so he advocates especially Clomid treatment, though there may be uncertainties about diagnosis.

847 **I have heard that my pituitary gland can produce too much prolactin and that can keep me from getting pregnant. Is that true?**

Yes. If the body is secreting too much prolactin, menstrual cycles become irregular and the breasts begin secreting fluid (galactorrhea). The condition can become severe enough that a woman will not be having any menstrual periods (amenorrhea) and

Special Concerns

will be secreting a great deal of fluid from her breasts. Parlodel (bromocriptine) will usually decrease the amount of prolactin and enable ovulation to occur normally.

Prolactin is secreted from the pituitary gland, a small gland at the base of the brain. If the gland becomes overactive, it will release too much prolactin. Sometimes this occurs if there is a tumor (pituitary adenoma) present in the pituitary gland.

Pituitary adenomas are the most common tumors in the human body, present in 30 percent of all people. Most of these are small and do not cause any problem. Until 1969, when a blood test was developed to find elevated levels of prolactin, there was not even a reasonable way to know that most of them existed.

If a blood test shows a very high prolactin level (usually greater than 100 ng/ml), a second test, a CT scan (computer X-ray of tissue inside the body) of the pituitary is needed to see if a tumor is present. If the CT scan shows that there is no tumor, the patient probably has an overactive pituitary gland. In that situation, treatment with Parlodel usually (in 90 percent of the women) halts the excess production of prolactin, stops the breast secretions, allows normal periods to begin, and, for many, allows pregnancy to occur.

If the CT scan indicates a tumor, treatment is usually necessary, whether or not a woman is attempting to become pregnant. If the tumor is small, treating it with Parlodel is often successful. But if the tumor is large or does not respond to Parlodel, surgical removal is usually necessary. Decisions concerning these problems and any surgery involved require consultation with specialists in endocrinology and neurosurgery.

Although high prolactin levels are not a common cause of infertility, infertility specialists occasionally have a patient with this problem. I routinely do a prolactin-level test on all infertility patients. Abnormal periods are a definite indication for such a test.

848 How is Parlodel taken, and are there any side effects?

Ordinarily Parlodel is taken in a dose of 2.5 mg, twice a day. This may be increased by your doctor if necessary.

Occasionally women taking Parlodel may experience nausea, vomiting, diarrhea, or even faintness. To keep these from occurring, a woman can start Parlodel with one-half of a 2.5 mg tablet daily. If that causes problems, she can use the tablet vaginally instead of orally, as it will absorb through the vaginal lining. When she is able to tolerate half a pill, either orally or vaginally, she can increase the dosage to one pill a day. The dosage can be increased up to whatever amount is necessary. Some women find that their prolactin level will revert to normal with just half a Parlodel tablet a day. The usual dose is two tablets daily. Follow-up prolactin tests should be done while using Parlodel to control the pituitary production of prolactin.

Usually the drug does not cause severe reactions and has not been shown to cause any congenital abnormalities in children of women who take the drug. Of course, as soon as a woman knows that she is pregnant she should stop taking it.

Endometriosis and Infertility

849 What is endometriosis, and how does it cause infertility?

Endometriosis is one of the most common causes of infertility in women. It affects an estimated 25 percent of women over twenty-five, and it causes infertility in 25 to 30 percent of all women who cannot get pregnant.

Endometriosis is tissue like that which lines the inside of the uterus (the endometrium) that began growing in the wrong place in your body. During each menstrual period it is normal for some menstrual flow to back up through the tubes and into the abdomen. This fluid contains live endometrial cells that will, in some women, attach and start growing where they do not belong: behind or in front of the uterus, on the ovaries or tubes, or on the intestines. This is endometriosis.

A problem then results because this tissue acts

as if it were inside your uterus. Since female hormones circulate in the bloodstream, they are brought to this endometrial-type tissue no matter where it is in a woman's body. The tissue thickens and responds to the female hormones as it would if it were inside the uterus. Then at menstruation time the tissue breaks down, producing bloody material just like the uterus does each month.

Bloody material released from endometrial tissue outside the uterus obviously cannot get back through the tubes and out the vagina. Instead it forms pockets of blood wherever it is growing. The irritation of this blood causes scarring and adhesions to develop. This scar tissue damages the female organs and can even become severe enough to make a hysterectomy necessary.

Endometriosis can cause the buildup of enough scar tissue to create a blockage in the fallopian tubes and can scar ovaries and tubes so that it is difficult for the egg to get from the ovary to the tube. It can even envelop the ovaries so that an egg cannot get out.

Also, endometriosis apparently is the source of excessive production of hormones called prostaglandins. These prostaglandins may be released into the peritoneal fluid that bathes the internal organs and cause spasms of the uterus and tubes, inhibiting their ability to transport the egg properly. Prostaglandins can even affect the ovaries' ability to produce normal hormones or to release the egg normally. This may be how even mild endometriosis causes infertility.

850 How is endometriosis diagnosed?

A doctor usually discovers endometriosis during a fertility evaluation, but the only way the doctor can know conclusively that endometriosis is present is to do a laparoscopy.

Laparoscopy is essential to the diagnosis of endometriosis and vital for an infertility evaluation. If you have not become pregnant in an appropriate length of time, and other infertility tests do not show your problem, you should proceed with a laparoscopy.

851 Are there symptoms of endometriosis that I might notice myself?

Endometriosis sometimes, but not always, causes:

pain with menstrual periods
deep pain with intercourse
pain with bowel movements
pain in the central part of the lower abdomen
pelvic pain with exercise
painful urination
blood in the urine and/or stools
spotting prior to periods
heavy periods
infertility

In the early stages and occasionally even with extensive endometriosis you may not have any of these problems. Endometriosis usually does not develop quickly, and it may take years to become widespread and to worsen. If you know you have endometriosis and are interested in becoming pregnant, you should be under the care of a doctor well versed in endometriosis. You never know at what stage it will affect your fertility. You also never know when it will progress to the point that you can no longer have "fertility surgery" and will need a hysterectomy.

852 How is endometriosis treated?

When a woman has laparoscopy for an infertility problem, her endometriosis can usually be treated during that laparoscopy. When the doctor sees the endometriosis and determines its severity, he or she can attach a laser to the laparoscope and remove the endometriosis by vaporizing it away with the laser. At the same time he or she can often cut most of the adhesions and even remove large areas of endometriosis from the ovaries. If an ovary has been totally destroyed by endometriosis, it can often be removed at laparoscopy if that is necessary. (See Q. 811.) Whether or not all the endometriosis can be completely removed depends on how severe it is and at what stage it is. I recommend that if you are going to have a laparoscopy for infertility, you should have it done by a physician who is capable of using the laser with the laparoscope and also can do operative laparoscopy.

If a woman's endometriosis is minimal, mild, or moderate (Stage 1, 2, or 3) and is completely removed by the laser at laparoscopy, she can then attempt to get pregnant with no further therapy for endometriosis (at least for a few months).

If the physician is not sure whether all the endometriosis has been removed, he or she will probably want the patient to use either danazol (Danocrine) or GnRH agonist (Lupron or Syneral) for a few months before trying to become pregnant. (These drugs block the normal estrogen stimulation of endometriosis and cause it to dry up.)

If a patient's endometriosis is found to be severe at laparoscopy, three to six months of medical treatment, with danazol or GnRH agonist and then major surgery, may be recommended. At this surgery, using microsurgical technique, the doctor will remove as much endometriosis as he or she can. This series of procedures seems to give a patient with severe endometriosis the best chance of becoming pregnant.

If a woman with endometriosis does not get pregnant after a few months, her doctor may want to do another laparoscopy to see if the endometriosis has grown back. If it has, she may need either more endometriosis treatment or an IVF-type procedure to get pregnant (depending on the situation).

If you need major surgery for your endometriosis, be sure it is done by a doctor skilled in fertility surgery. Some gynecologists are not interested in spending the tedious time it takes to cut out (or laser) each little spot of endometriosis. It is much easier to do a hysterectomy, so be sure you do not give permission for that unless your doctor has explained beforehand why it might be absolutely necessary. If you want to get pregnant in the future and your doctor is talking about hysterectomy, get a second opinion.

853 How is endometriosis treated surgically?

The operation requires an incision like that used for a hysterectomy (either "bikini" or up-and-

down). Time in the hospital after surgery is usually two to four days, followed by a two-week recovery period at home.

The concept behind such surgery is fairly simple, but the surgery is not. The doctor cuts out, or vaporizes with the laser, all endometriosis that can be safely removed. If it requires cutting an ovary open, the gynecologist does that. If he or she can leave one ovary and tube fairly normal, the other ovary and tube may be taken out if they are badly scarred.

Also, if the uterus is retroverted or leaning back, the surgeon suspends it (sews it forward). The laser may be employed to remove hard-to-reach areas of endometriosis.

The doctor may also do a presacral neurectomy. This involves cutting the network of nerves from the uterus, tubes, and ovaries, hoping to further relieve any residual spasm of the uterus or tubes and make it easier for the egg to get down the tube. Cutting these nerve fibers can also help alleviate the cramps that so often accompany endometriosis, but it does not affect sexual responsiveness or feeling. If you become pregnant after a presacral neurectomy, however, you will usually not feel labor pains as strongly as normal.

It is sometimes necessary to remove part of the colon or part of the bladder in order to get all the endometriosis. This in no way affects your ability to urinate or have bowel movements after recovery from the surgery. The idea is to remove as much endometriosis as possible without damaging the pelvis.

854 How effective is this surgery?

The chance of spontaneous pregnancy following this type of surgery depends on how advanced and extensive the endometriosis was. If it was not too bad, there is a 75 percent chance of getting pregnant. If, however, the endometriosis was fairly severe, the chances decrease to 40 percent or less. If pregnancy does not occur, an IVF procedure would probably offer the only other chance to achieve pregnancy.

The severity of endometriosis is classified from Stage 1 to Stage 4. If your doctor finds that you have endometriosis, you should ask what stage your disease is in. This will help you understand your situation and more intelligently participate in treatment decisions.

855 Can endometriosis keep coming back?

Doctors can never be sure that all endometriosis has been removed. Some can be left in areas of scar tissue, and there can be microscopic implants that are impossible to see at surgery. There is always, therefore, the possibility of endometriosis growing back. Approximately 13 percent of patients who have had surgery for endometriosis will require a second operation. Only a small percentage will require a third operation.

When a patient has had endometriosis surgery and still does not become pregnant, a repeat laparoscopy should be done to see if she has recurrent endometriosis. A laser laparoscope might then be used to get rid of any endometriosis still present.

856 Can endometriosis occur in the uterus itself?

When endometriosis exists in the muscular wall of the uterus, it is called adenomyosis or "internal endometriosis." When that occurs, it is as though the lining of the uterus has developed roots that have gotten cut off from the surface endometriosis. These areas of endometriosis then grow, bleed, and form a scar in the wall of the uterus. This causes the uterus to be irritable and can result in infertility.

Unfortunately the diagnosis for adenomyosis is difficult and unreliable. However, the following pattern often suggests the presence of the disease. An infertile patient, who has been totally "worked up," including laparoscopy, and treated for whatever problems were found, still does not become pregnant. Months later, at a second laparoscopy, there is some suggestion that her uterus is more boggy and vascular, perhaps slightly larger than a normal uterus. On revisiting the office, a vaginal sonogram may suggest a growth in the wall of the uterus. Only then is adenomyosis suspected.

The only treatments for this disease for the woman trying to achieve pregnancy are danazol and GnRH agonists (Lupron or Syneral) or an IVF-type procedure. If adenomyosis was actually the cause of her infertility, the woman may be able to achieve pregnancy with one or both of these treatments.

857 What is danazol (Danocrine)?

Danazol is a synthetic testosterone-like hormone. It works primarily to stop the pituitary's production of gonadotrophins. The pituitary produces FSH and LH. These hormones are called gonadotrophins. They circulate to the ovaries and make them produce estrogen and eggs. If the pituitary does not produce gonadotrophins, the ovaries will not produce estrogen. If estrogen is not produced from the ovaries there is much less estrogen in a woman's bloodstream, which means endometriosis and adenomyosis do not grow. (Breasts will also be less tender because they are sensitive to estrogen.)

Because danazol, in a sense, "puts the female reproductive system to rest," endometriosis is "put to rest" too. It becomes increasingly thinner and more inactive.

Danazol is a good drug. The side effects are few, and it relieves the pain of endometriosis in 90 percent of the patients. (About 10 percent are not helped significantly.) Danazol works best on endometriosis that has spread across the surfaces of the pelvic tissues and poorest on accumulations of endometriosis in the ovaries.

After Danocrine has been used for several months (it is rarely used for more than six months), it can be stopped, and the woman may become pregnant. If a woman's endometriosis is too extensive for danazol alone, the drug can be used in preparation for surgery, since it can make surgery easier and more effective.

Some women do not feel well while using danazol. The primary side effect is weight gain, but women on danazol also tend to feel bloated and heavy. It may also cause women to feel irritable, it can decrease their breast size, make their skin oily, and cause acne. The worst side effect of danazol is that it can cause a woman's voice to deepen and her body hair growth to be heavier and darker. These two complications are rare if danazol is used properly.

858 You have mentioned GnRH agonist several times in this chapter. What is that?

GnRH is gonadotrophin-releasing hormone produced naturally by a woman's hypothalamus into her pituitary gland. (See the chapter on the female hormone cycle.) GnRH stimulates the pituitary to produce the gonadotrophins FSH and LH.

The hypothalamus normally produces a short burst of this hormone into the pituitary about every ninety minutes. If the pituitary gets too much GnRH, it stops producing FSH and LH.

Lupron and Syneral are drugs called GnRH agonists. This means that they are similar to natural GnRH. When Lupron and Syneral are given to a woman, they shut the pituitary down so that it no longer produces gonadotrophins (FSH and LH) because the pituitary thinks it is receiving too much GnRH. This means the pituitary no longer stimulates the ovaries to produce estrogen and progesterone.

When no estrogen and progesterone are secreted, the endometriosis thins and dries up and causes fewer symptoms. The advantage Lupron (given as an injection) and Syneral (given as a nasal spray) have over danazol is that the side effects are not as bad. The primary side effect of GnRH agonists is hot flashes, but occasionally insomnia and mood swings occur.

Since GnRH agonists work in much the same way as danazol, most infertility specialists feel that either can be used for treating endometriosis.

859 Where can I find more information about endometriosis?

There are two organizations that can be of great help in learning more about endometriosis. They are:

The Endometriosis Association
8585 North 76th Place
Milwaukee, WI 53223
(800) 992-3636
Canada: (800) 426-2363

RESOLVE
1310 Broadway
Somerville, MA 02144-1731
(617) 623-1156

There may be a local chapter of RESOLVE in your town. Check the phone book for the address and phone number.

860 If all the preceding avenues of evaluation and treatment are exhausted, what means remain for having a child?

There are three topics yet to be covered in this chapter. All of them are pertinent to our discussion of infertility and of interest to those couples who want to pursue every means available to have a child.

These three topics are artificial insemination (by husband or donor sperm), in vitro fertilization (test-tube babies), and adoption.

Artificial Insemination

861 Why can't my husband's sperm be concentrated by freezing many of his specimens and then taking the live sperm from them?

Collecting and freezing sperm specimens to provide enough healthy sperm to produce a pregnancy might seem a logical solution to the problem of a low sperm count. This technique is not useful, however, because when a specimen with low sperm count is frozen, many of the already limited number of sperm are killed. Intrauterine insemination (IUI) is therefore usually used. If this doesn't work then either IVF or donor inseminations can be done.

862 What is intrauterine insemination, and why is it used?

Intrauterine insemination (IUI) is a commonly used technique for treating infertility. This procedure involves the insertion of washed sperm (from husband or donor) directly into a woman's uterus.

To prepare the sperm for IUI, the semen is mixed with tissue culture media (culture media that is used to grow living cells) and then centrifuged. The sperm are drawn off, often washed again, and then suspended in more tissue culture media. This procedure results in sperm that are free of all the mucus from a man's ejaculate. They can be injected directly into a woman's uterus with a small plastic tube with no significant danger to her. (There is always a small chance of infection when anything is put into the uterus.)

IUI is now being used in the following situations:

1. The husband has a low sperm count, poor sperm motility, small volume of semen, excessive volume of semen, or semen that is too sticky.
2. The wife has cervical mucus in which sperm do not survive: "bad" postcoital test. (See Q. 809, 820.)

3. Wife has cervical stenosis (cervix that is too tightly closed).
4. Pregnancy does not result from other infertility therapy and no obvious cause for continued infertility is known.
5. The husband has retrograde ejaculation.

I normally do this procedure one time each month, as close to the time of ovulation as possible. (I like for patients to use an ovulation predictor kit to determine the ideal time for IUI.) The actual insemination is usually a simple procedure, both for the doctor and for the patient. It usually causes no more discomfort than a regular pelvic exam.

Positive aspects of the procedure, other than the fact that it does not hurt, are that there are few complications, and patients tend to have a higher pregnancy rate with IUI than with normal intercourse.

Although there are no figures to give percentage chances of successful fertilization with IUI, statistics do show that it increases the chance of pregnancy for many infertile couples.

863 When is artificial insemination with donor sperm used?

Donor insemination (AID) is useful if a husband has no sperm. It may also be used if he has abnormal sperm or an extremely low sperm count, and has been unable to get his wife pregnant. If he has

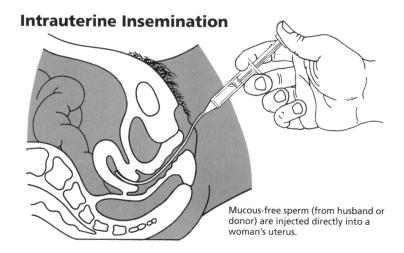

Intrauterine Insemination

Mucous-free sperm (from husband or donor) are injected directly into a woman's uterus.

Special Concerns

a genetic disease he does not want to pass on to a child, he and his wife may choose to have insemination by another man's sperm.

In addition, if a woman has Rh-negative blood that has resulted in previous stillbirths, she could be inseminated by an Rh-negative donor, thus bypassing the Rh problem. This is rarely necessary today because of the use of Rho-GAM. (See Q. 465.)

864 What are some of the objections to the use of AID?

There are arguments against artificial insemination using donor sperm (AID). Many religious faiths oppose this type of conception, and many individuals are uncomfortable with it.

Many husbands feel that having their wives inseminated by another man's sperm is a reflection on their own virility, or they do not like the idea of their wives being pregnant "by another man." Some people will not consider AID because they feel it is "unnatural."

Many couples are now rejecting AID because of the fear of the wife being infected by the AIDS virus that could be in the donor's semen. Most programs that do AID freeze semen, hold it for six months, and then test the donor again for AIDS before using the semen. This procedure has decreased the possibility of AIDS transmission via AID. There are other problems that can be transmitted by the donor sperm: genetic abnormalities, Hepatitis B, cytomegalovirus, chlamydia, gonorrhea, and so on. An AID program should be sure that all donors are questioned and tested for these problems. The American Society for Reproductive Medicine has an excellent set of guidelines for AID. You should review them if you are interested in this procedure. (See address at the end of this chapter.)

I believe that no couple should consider donor insemination unless both parties feel totally confident that it is what they want.

865 Does AID always work?

No. Donor inseminations produce pregnancies in only about 70 percent of the women in whom they are used. Those who are under the age of thirty are a little more likely to achieve pregnancy by inseminations (about 75 percent) and women who are over the age of thirty are a little less likely to become pregnant with AID (50 to 60 percent).

866 Are there legal problems with AID?

The courts have not settled all legal questions about donor inseminations, but it is agreed that a husband who consents to his wife's being inseminated by a donor is legally that child's father from then on. Currently, the legal problems resulting from the transmission of viruses and diseases via AID have not been addressed.

Assisted Reproductive Technology (IVF, GIFT, ZIFT, etc.)

867 What are assisted reproductive technologies?

Louise Brown's birth in 1978 marked a milestone in infertility technology: Louise was the first in vitro fertilization baby ever born.

Mrs. Brown's doctors had removed one of her eggs, fertilized it outside her body, and put it back into her uterus. The pregnancy was carried in a normal way from that point. This event opened the eyes of physicians and scientists to possibilities they had never thought of before.

Since Louise's birth, many variations of the "test-tube baby" technique have been designed. These plus other infertility procedures are now called "assisted reproductive technologies"

(ART). While ART procedures were still considered somewhat experimental until a few years ago, many of them are now standard care for infertility patients.

In vitro fertilization was initially designed for completely sterile women—women whose fallopian tubes were destroyed and could not be repaired surgically. (Problems that produce this condition include PID, severe endometriosis, and severe scarring from appendicitis.) ART is now used for women whose tubes may still be open but who have not become pregnant after endometriosis surgery; for cases when the man's sperm quality is so poor that he cannot produce a pregnancy; for women who have poor cervical mucus or who have antibodies to their husband's sperm; for couples for whom no reason for their infertility is found, and for various other problems.

Many infertile couples do not take advantage of ART procedures. There are several reasons for this:

1. ART procedures are usually expensive.
2. Patients are often not referred to an ART specialist or to an IVF program even though either might be useful for their infertility. Occasionally physicians who do less complicated infertility care will not refer their patients to an IVF program because they don't want to lose control of those patients. Some of my patients have had many more infertility operations or Pergonal treatments than I would have advised. (See Q. 841.) They probably should have been referred for an ART procedure long ago both for the best chance of pregnancy and to eliminate months of surgery and treatments that had almost no chance of success.
3. Some people consider ART procedures experimental or "weird." Again, many ART procedures are not experimental and are a standard part of infertility care.

I encourage couples to at least learn something about ART to see if one of these procedures would benefit them.

868 I have heard that assisted reproductive technology programs (ART programs) are not honest about how many pregnancies they have produced. How can I find a good ART (IVF) program?

While some ART programs may be dishonest about their results, they are a small minority. A primary problem in the past may have been one of standardization of reporting. In the United States there has been an IVF-ET registry since January 1987, which monitors almost all of the assisted reproductive technology programs in the United States. You can get a report from the IVF registry by writing to:

American Society of Reproductive Medicine
1209 Montgomery Highway
Birmingham, AL 35216-2809
(205) 978-5000

Ask for The Specific Data Report on the assisted reproduction programs in the United States. (Call to verify fee before you order.) The key statistic to look for in these reports is the overall live birth rate (what percent of couples took a live baby home after having had an ART procedure).

All programs vary in their statistics. One year there may be a higher live baby rate than another year, which can make one program look better than another temporarily. It is probably best to look at a program's statistics over a period of two or three years to assess its possibilities for you.

869 The pregnancy rates of ART seem low. Is it really worth my time and money when there is only a 25 to 50 percent chance of pregnancy from one of these procedures?

When a normal, healthy, fertile couple has intercourse for one month with no contraception, there is about a 25 percent chance of pregnancy. Since 12 percent of those will miscarry, however, there is only about a 22 percent chance of a successful pregnancy. As you can see, ART-type procedures at times exceed normal pregnancy rates for a fertile couple. So ART programs are relatively successful for couples who have long-term infertility problems.

As years go by, it is likely that there will be even better pregnancy rates with these procedures than a normal fertile couple has. Most of us involved in this work feel that the benefit is definitely worth the time and expense for a couple who wants to do everything possible to have a child.

870 Once fertilization occurs, I consider the embryo to be a human being. Don't ART programs destroy human embryos?

It is not necessary for an in vitro fertilization program to destroy or throw away human embryos. The program I helped found at St. David's Community Hospital in Austin, Texas, has never destroyed or thrown away a single healthy embryo. The only embryos we have not put back in their mothers have been eggs fertilized by more than one sperm (a condition incompatible with life of more than a few weeks in the uterus).

Because of the embryo's immaturity of development up to the fourteenth day, the ethics committee of the American Society of Reproductive Medicine coined the term *preembryo* and made the decision in 1986 that the "preembryo" could be treated differently than an embryo that has reached fourteen or more days of development. I resist using the term *preembryo* because I do not agree with the committee. I believe that the embryo from the day of fertilization deserves protection. The term *preembryo* implies that embryos can be destroyed at will until after fourteen days of life.

The late Dr. Jerome Lejeune, who discovered the genetic cause of Down syndrome, held the same position I do. A booklet published by The Center of Law and Religious Freedom contains testimony concerning the 1989 Maryville, Tennessee, court case over custody of "seven frozen embryos."

As to the term *preembryo*, Dr. Lejeune was of the opinion that there is no such word. In support of his position, Dr. Lejeune cited to the court the definition of embryo ". . . the youngest form of a being. . . ."

Dr. Lejeune went on:

. . . we had no need at all of a sub-class which would be called a preembryo, because there is nothing before the embryo. Before an embryo there is a sperm and an egg, and that is it. . . . And the sperm and an egg cannot be a preembryo because you cannot tell what embryo it will be, because you don't know what sperm will go into what egg, but once it is made, you have got a zygote and when it divides it's an embryo and that's it (pp. 43–44).

In our in vitro fertilization program, we have never destroyed an embryo from the moment of conception (with the one exception I gave). In the early days (before cryopreservation of embryos), we would fertilize only as many eggs as a couple wanted put back into the wife's uterus. The remaining eggs would be discarded without being fertilized.

Now that we do cryopreservation, we do it only for couples who will agree to eventually return to have all the frozen embryos put into the wife's uterus, even if she gets pregnant with the initial ART procedure. If she is unable to come back to receive the rest of the embryos, the couple agrees beforehand to donate those embryos to a program that can use them for women who need embryo donation.

A national organization of Christian physicians and dentists (Christian Medical and Dental Society) has a medical ethics commission that has carefully considered this whole issue. The members of the commission have produced ethics statements concerning many of today's medical issues, and they have written a well-reasoned statement on reproductive technology. If you are interested in reading that (or any other ethics statements), you can contact them by calling the Christian Medical and Dental Society, (615) 844-1000 in Bristol, Tennessee. I believe the ethics statement they have produced on this subject is one of the finest available in the world today.

871 How is an assisted reproductive technology (ART) procedure of the IVF-type accomplished?

The procedure is theoretically fairly simple. Here is an example:

The week before a woman's menstrual period is due to start, she takes daily GnRH agonist (Lupron) shots. (This drug shuts down her pituitary so that it doesn't interfere with the ART process.)

On the second day of her menstrual period, a woman starts daily Pergonal (see Q. 838) shots (or Metrodin or a combination of the two).

After four days, the woman has a blood test for estradiol (estrogen) and an ultrasound scan to see if the ovaries are developing follicles and eggs. The dosage of Pergonal is adjusted up or down, depending on how responsive the ovaries are. Estradiol blood tests and vaginal ultrasound are done every day or two until there are at least two follicles that are 18 millimeters across (about three-fourths of an inch) and an estrogen test that shows whether or not these follicles are producing adequate estrogen. (It is normally expected that about 300 pg/ml per large follicle will be secreted.)

When at least two good follicles are present and the estradiol seems adequate, a woman will be given HCG to cause the eggs to mature and ovulation to occur thirty-eight hours later. The two largest follicles help guide the doctors but there are almost always a number of smaller follicles—most of which will contain good eggs.

About two hours before ovulation, the eggs are removed (before they are released by the ovaries). This retrieval of the eggs is accomplished by laparoscopy or through the vagina with an ultrasound machine that has a needle guide on it.

The eggs that are removed are identified under a microscope. Sperm are put with them, and they are placed in an incubator, usually for two days.

The embryos that have developed after two days are drawn up into a thin plastic tube. This tube is inserted through a woman's vagina, through her cervix, and into her uterus. The embryos are then gently placed into the woman's uterus. They will float around for two or three days before, hopefully, implanting and producing the desired pregnancy. (The embryos do not usually fall out of the uterus before implantation because they have the same weight as the fluid in the uterus, much like a scuba diver is weightless while underwater.)

If pregnancy does not occur, the couple can repeat the process whenever they want to. Most couples like to wait at least a month before trying again. This gives them a chance to relax, both emotionally and physically.

872 Describe the different ART procedures that are commonly done today.

There are several assisted reproductive technology procedures commonly in use. They are:

In vitro fertilization/embryo transfer (IVF/ET). This procedure follows the outline I gave in the previous question using the Lupron/Pergonal/HCG formula. The goal is to produce as many eggs as can safely be produced (without hyperstimulating the ovaries). Since IVF/ET is done for women whose fallopian tubes are not capable of reproduction, there is no reason to do a laparoscopy; the eggs are almost always removed through the vagina with the transvaginal ultrasound and needle guide if possible. This procedure can be done with only sedation and local anesthesia. (Local anesthesia is injected into the vaginal walls, and the needle is pushed through the upper vagina, behind the uterus, and into each ovary.)

Fluid is aspirated from each of the follicles until they have all been emptied. The fluid is examined, the eggs removed, and sperm is put with the eggs to be fertilized. Generally, three or four embryos are transferred back to the woman's uterus two days later. A pregnancy test is done about two weeks after the procedure.

If the couple wants to do cryopreservation of other embryos (in case they do not get pregnant) for future pregnancies, the number of embryos they want are produced by fertilizing that number

In Vitro Fertilization and Embryo Transfer

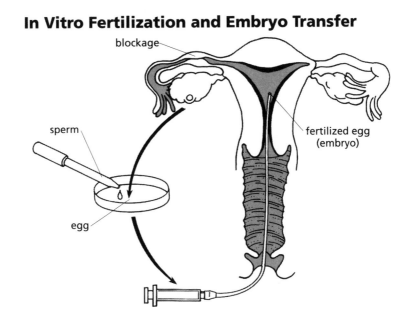

of eggs and extra eggs are discarded without fertilization. The resulting embryos that are not going to be put back in the uterus two days later are frozen usually the morning after they are fertilized.

Gamete intrafallopian transfer (GIFT). The initial steps of this procedure are the same as with IVF. When the follicles are ready, however, they are removed by laparoscopy instead of by vaginal retrieval. The eggs are removed from each follicle and put with the husband's sperm while the woman remains asleep on the operating table. The eggs and sperm are then drawn up into a small plastic tube and it is brought to the operating table. The tube is threaded through a small incision and then into one or both of the woman's fallopian tubes. The mixture of eggs and sperm are ejected and the tube withdrawn. No other treatment is necessary with the exception of the usual use of progesterone shots or vaginal suppositories until it is determined whether or not pregnancy has occurred. With GIFT, pregnancy occurs spontaneously in the woman's fallopian tube where it normally occurs, and the embryos pass into the uterus in the "normal" way where they become a growing pregnancy.

This procedure is somewhat more expensive and more time-consuming than IVF because it must be done with laparoscopy.

The GIFT procedure can be used if a woman has at least one functioning fallopian tube. It is useful for a woman who has endometriosis, an ovulation problem, or a problem with cervical secretions. It is useful for a man with low sperm count or low sperm motility, and for couples with unexplained infertility.

Zygote intrafallopian transfer (ZIFT). ZIFT procedures progress much like the standard ART procedures described in previous questions. The eggs are removed with a transvaginal ultrasound machine, fertilized, and the fertilized eggs are transferred into the woman's fallopian tube(s) by laparoscopy the next morning. If the procedure works as desired, the embryos remain in the fallopian tubes a day or two and then implant in the uterus, resulting in the desired pregnancy.

The ZIFT procedure requires that a woman have at least one functioning fallopian tube. It is useful for couples who have endometriosis, low sperm count, problems with cervical mucus, and unexplained infertility. (This procedure is sometimes called tubal embryo transfer or TET.)

Combination procedures. Some ART programs combine procedures if a woman has at least one healthy, functioning fallopian tube. For instance, if a woman's eggs are removed at laparoscopy, one or two of those eggs and some sperm can be put back into a fallopian tube, as is done with GIFT. To further increase the chance of conception, one or two eggs (or more) can be fertilized in the laboratory and transferred into the woman's uterus two days later. This is an IVF/ET/GIFT combination procedure.

Intracytoplasmic sperm injection (ICSI). This procedure involves the direct injection of an individual sperm into the inside of an individual egg. The procedure is done in the lab after eggs have been removed from the woman's body with sperm the husband has collected by masturbation. A microscope is used to pick up the sperm with a small glass pipette and to push the tip of the pipette into the egg. Fertilization is often achieved no matter how low the sperm count, no matter what their shape, and no matter how slow-moving the sperm. This procedure has already revolutionized the fertility treatment of couples with infertility because of low sperm counts or abnormal sperm. It is an expensive procedure, but except for using sperm from a sperm donor or adopting, it may be the only hope a couple has for pregnancy.

New horizons. The possibilities for new procedures using assisted reproductive technology seem almost endless. "Natural cycle" IVF could possibly be done in physicians' offices in the future. "Natural cycle" IVF does not require drugs to produce controlled ovarian hyperstimulation (COT—the term for the use of clomiphene or Pergonal or other drugs to make the ovaries produce more than one egg a month). With natural cycle IVF, a physician would merely remove the one egg a woman matures each month, put sperm with it, and then transfer it into the uterus. The transfer of only one embryo each month would have a lower chance of pregnancy than with regular IVF/ET. However, because it could conceivably be done at a much reduced cost in the doctor's office, it might prove a good technique. Technical problems and very low pregnancy rates are the primary reasons these procedures are not now being routinely done in doctors' offices.

Another technique on the horizon is doing the GIFT procedures through the vagina. For example, the eggs could be removed through the vagina with ultrasonographically guided aspiration of follicles. These eggs could be mixed with sperm and introduced into the woman's fallopian tube through her vagina, cervix, and uterus using fluoroscopy, ultrasound, or hysteroscope to locate the opening of the tubes for insertion of the catheter with the eggs and sperm. This procedure has been done and has produced pregnancies though the pregnancy rates have been very low. Whether it will become a popular, useful technique, no one knows at this stage.

Egg donation. If a woman has no ovaries or has ovaries that do not produce eggs, she and her husband can have egg donation from another woman. The other woman may be a relative who is willing to use Pergonal or other drugs for controlled ovarian hyperstimulation (COT) to produce several eggs, or the eggs may come from a woman who has done an IVF procedure herself and is willing to "share" her eggs. The couple desiring pregnancy can use the husband's sperm to fertilize the donated eggs. The eggs and sperm can then be transferred to the wife's uterus by the usual techniques for IVF/ET, GIFT, or ZIFT.

Embryo donation. A couple unable to produce eggs or sperm but still wanting a child can receive embryos from an embryo donation program. The most likely source of these embryos are from a program that has "extra" frozen embryos. These embryos can be transferred into the uterus of an infertile woman, where they can grow as her own pregnancy. (This can be compared to adoption in that the child is not "biologically" the husband's or wife's, but it differs from adoption because the woman actually carries and delivers the baby.)

Surrogate parenting. If a woman has no uterus but she still has ovaries and her husband has sperm, the sperm and eggs can be collected from the couple, fertilized in the laboratory, and the resulting embryos transferred to a surrogate mother—a woman willing to carry a pregnancy for the couple. This procedure is fraught with ethical and legal problems and is rarely used.

---

873 Tell me about the freezing of embryos.

With IVF procedures, drugs are given to stimulate the ovaries to produce as many eggs as is safely and reasonably possible (controlled ovarian hyper-stimulation). Most women who take fertility drugs produce more eggs than they need for the one month in which they are doing the procedure. At this point cryopreservation (freezing) provides an alternative.

With cryopreservation, embryos can be preserved for future transfer into a woman's uterus. If pregnancy occurs with the original cycle, a couple still has embryos saved and can have subsequent children as a result of the initial IVF procedure. Without cryopreservation, there is no way to preserve embryos for later pregnancies. If extra eggs have been collected at IVF, they must be discarded. In some programs, all eggs are fertilized and the best embryos selected for transfer. If cryopreservation is not done, the poorer embryos are discarded. (Destroying embryos raises major ethical problems for many people, including myself.)

Embryos can be kept frozen for years and survive thawing as though they had been frozen for only a short time. Studies indicate that babies born after cryopreservation do not have an increased incidence of congenital abnormalities.

When embryos are thawed, about 70 percent of them survive. As technology progresses, it is very likely that that percentage will increase. (It is also likely that many of the embryos that do not survive are defective in some way and would not have produced a pregnancy.) Each time frozen embryos are transferred to a woman's uterus, there is up to approximately a 10 percent chance of achieving pregnancy.

The advantage of cryopreservation is that it decreases the amount of medical care a woman needs to receive to get pregnant with an ART-type procedure. For example, if a woman goes through stimulation for an ART procedure and produces a large number of eggs, she can have some of those eggs used for the initial ART procedure and the rest cryopreserved. If she does not get pregnant with the initial cycle, the frozen embryos are available for attempts at getting pregnant in subsequent months but without her needing Pergonal or egg retrieval. If she gets pregnant with the first cycle, she will have embryos preserved to use when she wants to have a baby again.

874 What problems are associated with the transfer of frozen embryos?

There are three problems most couples will think about if they are considering cryopreservation:

1. Freezing human life seems "unnatural." I think most of us feel that freezing human embryos is a little "weird" or unnatural. The late Dr. Jerome Lejeune, a French professor of fundamental genetics, who believed that unique human life begins at the moment of fertilization, clarified this problem. In testimony at a custody trial for seven human embryos in Tennessee in 1989, he stated his opinion that temperature is merely a measure of the speed at which molecules move in a given medium. He said that if temperature is progressively diminished, the speed and the number of collisions of the molecules are progressively slowed. Time is frozen, not the embryos. Life is not arrested at freezing, and life is not started again when thawed. Dr. Lejeune felt that cryopreservation does not change that unique human life other than to slow down the molecules during the time of cryopreservation. I agree.

2. All embryos will not survive cryopreservation. Some people are uncomfortable with the fact that all embryos will not survive the freezing/thawing process. When considering embryonic life, however, it is important to remember that approximately 50 to 75 percent of the embryos formed naturally in a fertile woman's body do not survive the entire fertilization, implantation, and pregnancy process. It is also important to remember that the entire motivation in programs that do not destroy embryos is to preserve as many as possible and to allow as many of these embryos as possible to become growing babies inside a mother's uterus. Most embryos do survive thawing, and as technology improves, an even higher percentage will probably survive.

3. Widely publicized cases involving frozen embryos have brought up ethical questions regarding the practice of cryopreservation. One case was the death of an Australian couple who had embryos cryopreserved; another was a Tennessee divorce case in which a custody battle for seven frozen embryos resulted. (The husband wanted

the embryos destroyed; the wife wanted to save them for future pregnancies.) The ethics commission of the Christian Medical and Dental Society wrote a statement (available from them at P.O. Box 5, Bristol, TN 37620-0005) that I believe deserves consideration by couples who are considering cryopreservation. The statement, approved by the 1990 House of Delegates of the society (sixty-three in favor—one opposed) is a consensus of a large number of conscientious physicians and dentists. CMDS basically stated that it could not advise couples to use cryopreservation, but that it did not advise against it. The group said that if cryopreservation is used, it should be used with specific safeguards to avoid the possibility of destruction of embryos or of preservation of excessive numbers of embryos. They presented these practical guidelines for cryopreservation:

1. Cryopreservation of embryos should be done with the sole intent of future transfer to the genetic mother.
2. Embryos should be produced from the husband's sperm and the wife's eggs.
3. A limited number of embryos should be produced to eliminate cryopreservation of excessive numbers of embryos.
4. There should be prearrangement by the couple that if the wife becomes pregnant, all remaining frozen embryos will be transferred back to her at future times of her choice.
5. There should be prearrangement that in a situation where embryos could not be transferred to the wife (e.g., where the wife dies or has hysterectomy), they will be adopted by another couple who desire to have a child for themselves by having the embryos transferred to the adoptive mother.

The St. David's Community Hospital In Vitro Fertilization and GIFT Program adopted these guidelines for its cryopreservation program. Unfortunately, few fertility programs in the United States follow these specific guidelines, but a couple considering cryopreservation can adopt the guidelines for themselves. They can insist that the program with which they are working follow these guidelines for them. In this way, a couple can insure that any embryos they produce will not be destroyed.

It is my opinion that American society will eventually hold ART programs responsible for embryos they produce and will insist that the programs stop producing excessive numbers of embryos that will eventually have to be destroyed.

875 What is selective termination (selective reduction) of a multiple pregnancy?

There are several major problems with assisted reproductive technologies. One of the biggest problems is that about 25 percent of the pregnancies that occur will be multiple pregnancies.

Fortunately, when a multiple pregnancy does occur, it is usually just two babies. Occasionally, though, women will become pregnant with three, four, five, or even more babies. Most women can carry twin pregnancies with no trouble, but with triplets, premature delivery occurs about 75 percent of the time. In addition, about 50 percent of the babies will have some form of respiratory distress and about 20 percent will die either just before or just after delivery. (There is almost no information available concerning pregnancies of four or more babies, but they are significantly more dangerous than a triplet pregnancy.)

A pregnancy with four or more babies produces tremendous anguish. A couple is finally pregnant with the babies they have wanted for a long time, but they know that there is a great chance that they could lose all of them. The couple is faced with a real dilemma: to try to carry all the babies to birth or to terminate the lives of all but a couple of the babies to insure better odds for the remaining babies being healthy and normal.

The process used to terminate multiple pregnancies is called "selective termination" or "selective reduction." Doctors that do this procedure prefer doing it during the first three months of the pregnancy. Generally, a chemical such as potassium chloride is injected into one of the babies, killing it. The procedure is usually repeated with other babies until the mother is carrying only two or three live babies.

It is possible for a woman to lose an entire pregnancy as a result of selective termination, but if she carried the multiple pregnancy of four or more babies, there is also a high chance she would lose the entire pregnancy.

All ART physicians and team members hate this dilemma. Their goal is to have as high a pregnancy rate as possible with as low a multiple pregnancy rate as possible. To accomplish this doctors have been putting fewer embryos inside the mother at the time of an ART procedure. This has greatly decreased the number of multiple pregnancies but has slightly lowered pregnancy rates.

Cryopreservation has also helped with the problem of multiple pregnancies. Using cryopreservation takes the pressure off the initial ART procedure. Fewer embryos can be put inside a woman each time because she can return in a month or two to get cryopreserved embryos transferred again if necessary without having to go through further medical treatment to get more eggs.

The ultimate solution to the multiple pregnancy problem will be freezing human eggs. If eggs could be removed, not fertilized, and taken straight to freezing, there would be almost no objection to destroying them later if they were not needed. These eggs would be basically like the thousands of eggs that every woman carries in her ovaries until menopause except they would be held in the liquid nitrogen instead of in her ovaries.

Unfortunately, eggs that have been frozen and thawed do not usually fertilize when exposed to sperm. (It is not impossible for this to happen, however; babies have been born from the fertilization of frozen eggs.) I have no doubt that the technology for successfully freezing human eggs will be developed. When it is, the problem of multiple pregnancy and cryopreservation of embryos can be virtually eliminated.

876 How do you feel about the use of these three techniques to achieve pregnancy?

It is my personal commitment to do all I can, within my ethical and moral limits, to aid infertile couples in achieving pregnancy. In the process I remind myself and the couple that there are higher goals in life—the protection of the dignity of an individual, the preservation of the family as ordained by God, and the maintenance of healthy relationships within those families. Despite the intensity of their desire to have a child, I believe infertile couples must not and should not be coerced into using any technique they cannot wholeheartedly accept. Nor should a doctor engage in procedures that violate his or her ethical or moral beliefs. However, it is important for all of us not to lose perspective and realize that just because a procedure is new or unprecedented does not make it "wrong." When penicillin was new, there were people who felt it should not be used because it interfered with the "natural" process of life and death.

Adoption

877 Do some couples who come to you with a fertility problem decide to forego infertility evaluation and treatment and try to adopt a child?

Yes. Many couples do not want to expend the time and money or go through the frustration and inconvenience involved in the evaluation and treatment of infertility. For those couples adoption is the answer, unless they find themselves pregnant before the adoption process is complete.

878 How long should we persist in infertility treatment before we consider adoption?

My general recommendation is this: After you have had a full evaluation and have had a year or two of treatment without becoming pregnant, you might consider starting the adoption process.

I encourage you to continue your infertility

therapy, however, because the adoption process often requires two or more years of waiting before a child actually arrives in your home. It is possible that during this time you could become pregnant.

Adoption agencies generally do not mind if you continue your attempts to become pregnant while working with them on an adoption. If you become pregnant, you can always cancel the adoption process.

Trying to adopt a child has an additional advantage if you have been attempting to become pregnant for quite some time. It can be a pressure-relief valve for you and your husband, even while you continue infertility treatments, because you will know that one way or the other, at the end of two years, you should have your new baby.

A doctor can be of great help, not only in working out a plan for your infertility evaluation and treatment but also in assisting with the adoption process. The three of you should maintain communication as you proceed through every step of the fertility evaluation and as you consider adoption.

879 We don't want to adopt a baby. Is that abnormal?

It is quite normal not to want to adopt a baby, and many couples feel this way. Just as no couple should undergo an infertility workup unless they want to, no one should adopt a child who does not want to.

If you feel that you cannot, without reservation, accept an adopted child as your own, it would be foolish to adopt. It would not be good for you or the child and might result in more anguish than being childless. I also believe, for the same reason, that one mate should not push the other into adopting if he or she is not comfortable about adoption.

880 How do we begin the adoption process?

Contacting adoption agencies in your area may facilitate the visitation process, but it is not necessary

to limit yourself to those agencies. Many adoption agencies do not limit adoptions to their own geographic area.

I suggest that you find out what limitations and regulations an agency has before making application to them. Stipulations regarding age, religion, race, or marital status may preclude your being able to adopt a child through that agency.

It may be helpful to maintain regular communication with an agency so that they will know you are sincerely interested in adoption. You could call or write periodically, and you may even wish to have your physician write an unsolicited letter of recommendation. Don't be overbearing, insistent, or impatient, but be tenaciously persistent. Courtesy and tact along with your persistence are essential.

Don't give up! Most of my infertility patients who are unable to become pregnant eventually are able to adopt a baby.

To get information on all aspects of adoption, contact the National Adoption Information Clearinghouse, 11426 Rockville Pike, Suite 410, Rockville, MD 20852, phone (301) 231-6512.

881 Is it possible to adopt a baby through a doctor or lawyer?

When adoptions are carried out through an agency, there is little risk of you ever being forced to return the baby to the natural mother. Although a judge can reverse the adoption on certain specific grounds, such as the biological mother having given up the child because of fraud or coercion, it rarely happens.

About 75 percent of adoptions are conducted through agencies. This is primarily because most pregnant women will go to an adoption agency, rather than to a doctor or a lawyer, when they want to give up a baby. Also, independent adoptions are illegal in some states and limited in others.

If you are unable to get a baby through an agency, you might want to try a private adoption. There is a greater chance of disappointment with a private adoption, however, because the birth mother can change her mind and get the baby back before the process is complete. Even after completion of the adoption, if there is any evidence of fraud or coercion, she may be able to get the child. This situation is much more likely to occur with a private adoption than with an agency adoption.

Before you attempt a private adoption, be sure to check with an experienced adoption attorney concerning your state's laws for this type of adoption. Some states have stringent private adoption limitations.

882 What about adopting foreign, impaired, or older children?

Foreign adoptions are possible, but they involve many delays and obstacles. There are American agencies that specialize in foreign adoptions. You can get their names and addresses by writing the National Adoption Information Clearinghouse. (See Q. 880.) One organization specializing in foreign adoptions is Los Niños International, 1600 Lake Front Circle, Suite 130, The Woodlands, TX 77380-2189, phone (713) 363-2892.

If you are interested in adopting biracial, impaired, or older children, you might contact orphanages in your area or your local child-and-family service organization. One word of advice: Be sure to get adequate counsel about problems you might face in the future as a result of such an adoption. By the way, all states except Hawaii have subsidy programs for parents who adopt hard-to-place children.

883 Where can I get more information about adoption?

Since there are so many issues involved in adoption, I feel it is wise for a couple to get as much information as possible. These issues include "open" or "closed" adoption, the rights of the birth father, laws for interstate adoption, how and when to tell a child he or she is adopted, and what to do if your child wants to know (or meet) the birth mother. Check with your local or church library for books

on the subject. The following are some excellent sources of information.

Focus on the Family has a booklet called *A Guide to Adoption* by Douglas R. Donnelly that gives some excellent general information about adoption.

Organization for United Response (OURS), Inc., 3307 Highway 100 North, Suite 103, Minneapolis, MN 55422, is an adoptive support group with many state and local chapters.

Stepping Stones and RESOLVE are sources of information about adoption. (See Q. 886.)

Should You Adopt by Christine Moriarty Field (Revell, 1997) is written by an adoptive parent who is a former attorney. This book explores the process of dealing with infertility to the actual adoption. There are also many resources listed in the appendixes.

Tapestry Books, P.O. Box 359, Ringoes, NJ 08551, has an adoption book catalog published by Laurie S. Wallmark. It lists books about adoption for children and adults. It is an excellent resource. The phone number is (908) 806-6695.

The National Council for Adoption, 1930 Seventeenth Street NW, Washington, D.C. 20009-6207, phone (202) 328-1200, has published *The Adoption Fact Book*. It might be a useful resource.

Adoption Law and Procedure, edited by Joan H. Hollinger, published by Matthew Bender & Co., December 1988, has information that might be helpful with your technical concerns about adoption.

For those who desire to adopt children with problems, an organization called Aid to Adoption of Special Kids (AASK) at 3530 Grand Avenue, Oakland, CA 94610, can be helpful. The phone number is (415) 451-1748.

884 Is it possible for me to breast feed an adopted baby?

It may be possible! As many as 50 percent of women can at least partially nurse their adopted babies. A woman who wants to do this must be committed to doing everything necessary to insure success, but even then, she must realize that there is a 50 percent chance she will not succeed.

I recommend that a woman who plans to try nursing an adopted baby begin preparation several weeks in advance of getting the baby. One technique is for the woman to start taking 25 mg of chlorpromazine three times a day and to stimulate her nipples every one to three hours. These techniques help to start secretions of milk from the breasts. Nipple stimulation also helps toughen the nipples for the baby's sucking.

The LaLeche League International (1400 N. Meacham Rd., Schaumburg, IL 60168, phone 847-519-7730 or 800-LeLeche) can be of great help and encouragement in this endeavor.

and to resent it when your friends ask when you are going to "decide" to have a baby.

All this is normal. The danger lies in denying these emotions.

On my initial visit with a couple with an infertility problem, I warn them that they will get upset as they go through the process of diagnosis and treatment. No matter how "together" a couple is, they almost always experience this; if they expect it, they are not taken by surprise and can handle it better. If this happens to you, talk to your doctor about it. Most of the time he or she will be able to calm your fears and worries. If that reassurance and encouragement are not enough, be sure to get counseling.

Emotional Support for the Infertile Couple

885 Why are my husband's and my own emotions running so out of hand as we consider and work on our infertility?

As stated in the introduction to this chapter, I believe that few stronger stresses come into a marriage than the continued absence of a longed-for child.

Often a couple with an infertility problem needs counsel. If you and your husband are frustrated, tell your doctor. If it seems wise he or she will help you find a counselor who will be able to help you. Counselors have a good success rate in helping people who are grappling with a single problem.

The biggest danger is for you or your husband to deny that you are upset by your current problem. Every couple who confronts a period of infertility is upset to some degree. Infertility wends its way into every part of your life: your schedule, your intimacy with each other, your finances, your comfort, and your social life.

It is normal for you to "hate" Mother's Day and your cousin who just told you she was pregnant,

886 Are there organizations that might give me emotional support during this time of infertility?

There are several. One is an extremely warm and helpful Christian group that publishes a newsletter. They can be reached at the following address:

Stepping Stones
1368 Elizabeth Street
Denver, CO 80206
(303) 333-5407

RESOLVE, Inc., is a lay organization with many chapters throughout the United States. The national office is very helpful in providing information about infertility.

RESOLVE, Inc.
1310 Broadway
Somerville, MA 02144-1731
(617) 623-1156
REFERRALS: (617) 623-0744

The following organization has a catalog of sympathy and announcement cards for miscarriages and stillbirths, booklets to help siblings and grandparents deal with their feelings, booklets on what family and friends can do, scrapbooks to preserve memories of a lost baby, and burial cradles for miscarried babies. Their newsletter includes articles, letters, and stories for those who have lost babies and lists current services offered (referrals to support groups, funeral directors, speakers, pen pals, literature, help line, and telephone volunteers).

Pregnancy and Infant Loss Center
1412 East Wayzata Boulevard, Suite 30
Wayzata, MN 55391
(612) 473-9372

An organization that offers excellent support and information to couples who have experienced pregnancy loss is:

Compassionate Friends
P.O. Box 3696
Oak Brook, IL 60522-3696
(630) 990-0010

A national organization of physicians interested in fertility problems includes both gynecologists and urologists, and it is a good source for names of physicians with this interest:

American Society for Reproductive Medicine
1209 Montgomery Highway
Birmingham, AL 35216-2809
(205) 978-5000

887 Are there periodicals that are helpful to infertile couples?

Yes. Currently there are at least two newsletters, published by Stepping Stones and RESOLVE, Inc. The addresses for these organizations are given in the previous question.

An Afterword

We are learning more about infertility all the time. It is wonderful to be able to take advantage of the knowledge about infertility that God has allowed us to gain. The use of the laser in infertility surgery, in vitro fertilization, greater knowledge about the hormones controlling reproduction—all these are exciting advances, and they herald real hope for infertility patients in the future.

The fact that these techniques are possible does not eliminate the validity of the feelings and emotions that are a part of life itself. Human beings are not meant to go through life as pawns of science, and the ultimate goal of life is not achievement of pregnancy and parenthood. Full personhood is more than that.

As future procedures for the solution of infertility come along, it is most important to evaluate them carefully before accepting or becoming involved with them.

12
Birth Control—Temporary and Permanent

The same Bible that tells us in Psalm 127 that children are a gift from God (v. 3) also speaks of the responsibilities of parenting:

> If any one does not provide for his relatives, and especially for his own family, he has disowned the faith and is worse than an unbeliever.
>
> 1 Timothy 5:8 RSV

It is wonderful to have children (most of the time!), and there are countless rewards in seeing them grow and mature and become individuals in their own right. With every privilege, however, comes responsibility, and there is an enormous responsibility in having children. A husband and wife should be willing and able to care for the children that they decide to have.

Fortunately today, most couples have the options of deciding when to have children and how many to have. Today's contraceptive choices usually make that possible. I think that it is legitimate for a couple to use the available options to control the size of the family. We do hear a great deal about "choice" today. It is my opinion that a couple has a legitimate choice before they get pregnant to use contraceptive techniques carefully. The techniques can fail, however, and once pregnancy occurs, whether on purpose or "by accident," I believe the time for "choice" is out of human hands and into God's. The Bible talks about God's creative power in Psalm 139, "You created my inmost being; you knit me together in my mother's womb," and I believe we should hold God's human creation sacred.

If you are not pregnant, there are many factors to be considered in family planning. During a time when husband and wife are extremely busy, it may be best for them to delay pregnancy. If a husband and wife need time to get their own relationship straightened out, it is often best to postpone temporarily the added stress of a newborn child. Economic factors influence almost every couple that is thinking about getting pregnant. There may be numerous other factors for prospective parents to consider as they plan their family, but often the final decision about when to have, or when not to have, a child is as much emotional as intellectual.

Contraception is a double-edged sword, however. It can allow the delay of a family until it is no longer possible for the couple to conceive.

Most physicians who care for infertile patients strongly urge married couples to go ahead with pregnancy if the wife is thirty-five or older. From the age of thirty-five, fertility decreases fairly rapidly. Contraception can also make it convenient for a couple to delay starting a family until they eventually feel too old to do so, thus cheating themselves out of one of life's most significant blessings.

Because there are such effective methods of contraception available, I feel it is vital that couples be educated about them. Since God has given us minds capable of reason, with proper thought we can decide how to use our sexuality, how to use contraception, and how to plan our families.

Each of us should let God work in our minds and actions, so that the ultimate result is God's will for us as individuals and as families.

Choosing a Birth-Control Method

888 What is the common goal of all methods of contraception?

The goal of contraceptives is to keep the sperm from meeting and fertilizing the egg. Birth-control pills, for instance, accomplish this by preventing the ovary from releasing an egg; vasectomies serve the same purpose by preventing a man's sperm from passing out of his testicles into his ejaculate. Natural family planning prevents pregnancy by keeping an egg and sperm from being in a woman's reproductive system at the same time.

Since the definition of contraception found in *Webster's New Collegiate Dictionary* is "voluntary prevention of conception or impregnation," we will not and should not discuss abortion as a technique for contraception. If an unwanted pregnancy occurs, contraception either failed or was not used. When pregnancy occurs, a totally different set of considerations is called for. (See Q. 169–183.)

889 How important is it that contraception be a mutual decision between husband and wife?

It is enormously important. Communication is vital in marriage, and mutual agreement concerning sexual activity and contraception is essential to a sensitive understanding between husband and wife.

Discussion about contraception should begin as part of a premarital examination for the woman, and the couple should have an open discussion with the physician about sexual relations and contraception. But even more important is the couple's discussion about contraception after leaving the physician's office. Any couple planning marriage should read the material in this chapter before seeing their doctor, so that they can ask better-informed questions and arrive more quickly and knowledgeably at a decision about contraception.

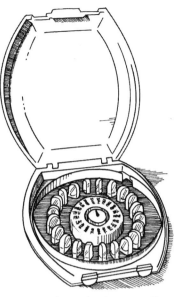

21-day package of oral contraceptives

Birth-Control Pills

890 How do birth-control pills work?

Birth-control pills contain synthetic estrogen and progesterone that produce an artificial menstrual cycle in your body. They do this by "putting to sleep" your ovaries and normal hormone system. Because your ovaries are, in effect, asleep, they do not release any eggs and you cannot get pregnant. With no egg to fertilize, the sperm merely swim into your body, die after several hours, are then absorbed by your body as small packages of protein, or they are passed out of your uterus and vagina with other secretions.

The Pill also makes the cervical mucus thick and hostile to penetration by sperm. Although literature from birth-control pill manufacturers claim that the Pill makes the uterine lining thin and hostile to the implantation of the embryo, there is absolutely no evidence of this happening.

891 How are birth-control pills used?

When you begin taking birth-control pills, you should decide what time of day you would most easily remember to take them. It does not matter whether it is morning, noon, or at bedtime. Many women like to take their oral contraceptive at bedtime to avoid any nausea that the pills might produce.

Oral contraceptives are available in two different types of packages—twenty-one-day and twenty-eight-day.

Twenty-one-day packages. The twenty-one-day packages provide a pill a day for twenty-one days. You then take no pills for seven days. You are pro-

tected from pregnancy all month long, even during the seven days that you are taking no pills.

To begin the twenty-one-day package the first time, start the pills on the first day of a period. "Day one" is the first day of a period, not counting the day or two of slight spotting that precedes the period for some women. Once you start the pills, take one a day for twenty-one days (three weeks). Then stop the pills for seven days and start a new package.

You will almost always have your period the week you take no pills. Your period will usually start a couple of days after you stop taking the pills, and it may or may not stop by the time you start your next package of pills.

If you prefer, you can arrange your schedule of pill intake so that your period always comes during the week, avoiding having a period on the weekend. Merely delay starting your next package of pills until the next Sunday, or start them a few days early so that the starting day is on a Sunday.

Twenty-eight-day packages. The twenty-eight-day packages contain the same type and same number of hormone pills as the twenty-one-day packages, but the twenty-eight-day packages also contain seven "sugar pills" (nonhormone) to be taken at the end of the hormone-pills schedule.

Do not skip any days between the end of one twenty-eight-day package and the beginning of the next.

Some twenty-eight-day packages instruct you to start the first pill on a Sunday. Therefore, the first month you take them, you should begin the pills on the Sunday after your period begins. If your period begins on a Saturday, then begin your pills the next day. If your period begins on a Sunday, start your pills that evening. If your period begins on Monday or any other day of the week, start your pills on the next Sunday. The seven sugar pills at the end are a different color. While you are taking them your period will start, because they contain no hormones.

If you have recently given birth and are not nursing, you can start oral contraceptives between the third and sixth weeks after delivery. If you are breastfeeding, however, or if there is any possibility that you might be pregnant again, you should not take birth-control pills until you know that you are not pregnant.

As soon as you start taking the pills, you are probably protected from getting pregnant. If you switch to a different brand of pill, you are probably safe as soon as you start that pill. I say "probably" because there are some physicians who feel that there is a slightly higher chance of pregnancy occurring when a woman first starts oral contraceptives or when she changes to a different brand of pill. For the best protection from pregnancy, use a contraceptive foam or condom the first ten days you are on a new pill.

If it doesn't matter to you what day of the week your period begins, the best time to start taking your first package of birth-control pills is the day your period begins. Doing this essentially eliminates the risk of getting pregnant with the first package of pills. From that point, you can take

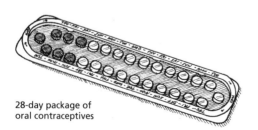

28-day package of
oral contraceptives

them three weeks, stop for a week, take them three weeks, and so on, as you usually do. (With the twenty-eight-day package, start them on the first day of your menstrual period. Whenever you finish taking one pack, begin taking the next pack on the very next day.)

892 How long can I take birth-control pills?

Extensive research has shown that women may use an oral contraceptive as long as they want without any permanent change to their reproductive and hormone systems. Except for the week off each month, the pills do not have to be discontinued until menopause except for women who smoke. Women who smoke must stop the birth-control pills at age thirty-five because of a significantly increased risk of strokes and heart attacks if they continue taking them. (See Q. 899.)

In the package insert, the FDA states that if a woman does not smoke and does not have some other health problem that would make birth-control pills dangerous (such as liver disease or very high cholesterol), it is safer for her to use birth-control pills until menopause than it is for her to use less effective contraception or to have a sterilization procedure.

893 What should I do if I miss a pill?

Don't panic! If you miss a pill, just take an extra one the next day. If you miss two pills, take an extra pill a day for two days. (You could have some breakthrough bleeding if you miss pills.) It is unlikely that you will become pregnant if you do this, but if you absolutely do not want to risk pregnancy, it would probably be best for you to use a barrier contraceptive, such as vaginal foam or a condom, with intercourse for the next ten days. With the higher-dose pills used in the past this was not so critical, but with the lower dosage now in use, missing a pill is more likely to allow a breakthrough ovulation and pregnancy. Remember, the pregnancy rate with birth-control pills is low, but

Special Concerns

the women who are more likely to become pregnant are those who take their pills erratically.

Missing pills, by the way, will not damage your body.

A recent study showed that a woman can miss as many as four birth-control pills and still be protected from pregnancy if she immediately resumes taking them. In a study reported by Gerald S. Letterie, M.D. (1991), it was found (by using pelvic ultrasound exams and by measuring serum FSH, LH, progesterone, and estradiol levels) that women did not ovulate if they resumed taking their pills after having missed taking four pills.

894 I have had bleeding during the twenty-one days that I take my pills. Is something wrong? What should I do?

One of the most common problems with birth-control pills is breakthrough bleeding, or bleeding during the twenty-one days a woman is taking her hormone-containing pills. This is almost never a sign of a medical problem, nor is it in any way harmful for a woman's body. Some women bleed while taking oral contraceptives because the small amount of hormones contained in modern birth-control pills cannot keep their uterine lining from shedding. This does not increase the chance of pregnancy.

Of course, if bleeding persists it could be due to a medical problem, such as a tumor. It could also be due to a pregnancy. If bleeding persists for more than two months, call your physician.

There are basically three methods of treatment for breakthrough bleeding.

Change to another brand of birth-control pill. Your doctor will help you decide if this is wise and will prescribe an alternate brand.

Add an ethinyl estradiol 0.02-mg tablet, a form of estrogen, to your hormone intake each day. Increasing the amount of estrogen in your body will usually build up the uterine lining enough to stop breakthrough bleeding. You would, of course, need your doctor's advice and a prescription for this hormone.

Double up on your birth-control pills. This is a good, simple technique. You already have the pills and do not need to call your doctor to do it,

although you may want to check with him or her first. Just take an added pill a day, out of an extra package, until the bleeding stops. Then take an extra pill for an additional three to four days. After that, drop back to one pill a day.

If you allow the bleeding to persist, you may start having worse cramping and heavier bleeding than you normally have with a period. When breakthrough bleeding gets this heavy, it may take several days to get the bleeding stopped when you finally do change your hormone dosage. If you start treatment for the breakthrough bleeding and you come to the end of your package before the bleeding stops, stop the pills, go one week without them, then start a new package of pills at the regular time. Remember, it is normal to bleed at the "wrong time" during the first one or two months you are on a new pill. Don't worry about this, but if it bothers you, follow one of these suggestions to control it.

895 I have bad cramps when I have breakthrough bleeding during the time I am taking the twenty-one pills. Is this normal?

Yes. Many women have worse cramps with breakthrough bleeding than they normally would have with their periods when they are not on the Pill.

Your increased cramping is probably normal. If it is severe, however, call your doctor. It is possible for you to be pregnant and to be having either a miscarriage or a tubal pregnancy while you are on oral contraceptives, so do not ignore bleeding or pain.

896 What are the chances of pregnancy occurring while taking the Pill?

The chance of pregnancy with correct use of the Pill is extremely low. Theoretically, the Pill is almost 100 percent effective.

The birth-control pill commonly called the "mini-pill" has a higher pregnancy rate. It contains only a low dose of progesterone (no estrogen). I do not normally recommend it for birth control because of this higher failure rate.

Birth-control pills would, without doubt, be

the most effective reversible contraception available today if they were always used correctly. Unfortunately, "it is generally agreed that the actual failure rate with oral contraception is about 6 percent and probably even higher in adolescents" (M. Klitsch *Family Planning Perspectives*, 1991, 23:134–138). This is a higher rate of pregnancy with birth-control pills than had previously been recognized.

Recent studies have shown that taking birth-control pills while pregnant does not increase the risk of abnormalities in the babies (M.B. Bracken "Oral Contraception and Congenital Malformations in Offspring; a review and meta-analysis of the prospective studies," *Obstetrics/Gynecology*, 1990, 76:552–557).

Some drugs decrease the effectiveness of birth-control pills; you should use additional contraceptives while taking them or increase your birth-control pills to 50 mg pills. Some of these drugs are:

Anticonvulsants
  phenytoin
  primidone
  barbiturates (phenobarbital)
  carbamazepine (Tegretol)
Antibiotics
  ampicillin
  rifampin
  tetracyclines (the small dosage most people use to treat acne does not decrease the potency of birth-control pills)

There is no perfect contraception. If you have intercourse, even if you are using birth-control pills, you can get pregnant. If you do use them, use them properly. If you do not understand the instructions in your package of pills, return to your physician or your pharmacist for further explanation.

897 Which women cannot use birth-control pills?

Women should not use oral contraceptives if they:

are over thirty-five and smoke
are pregnant

think they might have breast cancer or have had breast cancer (unless their physician approves the use of birth-control pills)
have liver damage or liver disease
think they might have cancer of the uterus or have had cancer of the uterus (unless their physician approves the use of birth-control pills)
have (or have had) deep blood clots in their legs (thrombophlebitis)
have had a stroke or a heart attack
have abnormal bleeding from their female organs that has not been diagnosed
have abnormalities of their blood-clotting system that causes their blood to clot too easily
have cholesterol levels greater than 250 mg/dL (although with proper treatment from her physician to lower her cholesterol, she may be able to use birth-control pills)

898 Which women should be cautious about using birth-control pills?

Women with certain health problems should not use birth-control pills unless their physicians are fully aware of their individual situation and recommend them. These problems include:

1. *Women with hypertension.* Generally, with their doctors' approval, women under thirty whose hypertension is well controlled can use birth-control pills.
2. *Migraine sufferers.* Some studies have shown that women with migraine headaches have a greater risk of having a stroke, which means they probably should not take the Pill. (Some younger women, however, experience fewer headaches on birth-control pills.)
3. *Diabetics.* Since diabetics are more likely to develop hardening of the arteries, they probably should talk to their physician about the wisdom of using birth-control pills.

4. *Women who are going to have surgery.* Because surgery may increase the risk of blood clots (and birth-control pills can aggravate that condition), it would be best to stop the Pill a month before surgery. Women who stop using their contraceptive pills must be very careful not to become pregnant before surgery.

5. *Women with a history of jaundice with pregnancy or jaundice with prior birth-control pill use.* Women with either of these histories should probably not use the Pill, though some women with "jaundice of pregnancy" will not develop jaundice on oral contraceptives and can safely take the Pill.

6. *Women with gallbladder disease.* Since the Pill can increase the risk of developing gallbladder disease, a woman who already has this problem should probably not take the Pill.

7. *Women with sickle-cell disease.* Women who have this disease should discuss this with their doctors before using the Pill.

899 Are there detrimental side effects of birth-control pills?

With the modern lower dose oral contraceptives, women have fewer side effects than they did with earlier pills. However, side effects may still occur. For example, a woman may feel tired, bloated, headachy, or irritable; she may gain weight; she may have a decreased desire for intercourse; she may develop tenderness of her breasts; she may be nauseated or have vomiting; she may have spotting or bleeding at times other than during her menstrual period; she may have no bleeding at menstrual time; or she may get pregnant.

Liver tumors (hepatomas) are more likely to occur in women who take birth-control pills, but they are extremely rare. I have never seen a patient with this type of tumor.

One of the major concerns about birth-control pills through the years has been whether or not using them increased the chance of cancer. Studies have now proved that they do not. They actually decrease the overall chance of a woman developing cancer. The Fetal and Maternal Health Drugs Advisory Committee of the FDA did an extensive study on this subject. They studied more than twenty published reports covering a period from 1977 to 1989. They found no overall increase in the likelihood of a woman's developing breast cancer if she took birth-control pills, and they did not recommend any change in prescribing or using the pills.

As for any link between birth-control pills and cancer of the female organs, the news is good: Birth-control pills actually decrease a woman's chance of developing ovarian and uterine cancer. (See Q. 900.)

Women on birth-control pills do have an increased chance of developing gallstones, but if a woman takes the pills for four years without developing them, she is not likely to.

It was once thought that epilepsy worsened in birth-control pill users, but this has been proven untrue.

It was also once believed that the Pill caused fibroid tumors to grow faster, but this, too, has been proven false. In a study by R. K. Ross and Associates (*British Journal of Medicine*, 1986, 293:359) research showed that women with fibroid tumors of the uterus have less risk of increased growth of the tumors if they are on low dose pills for ten years or more than women who did not take oral contraceptives.

Women who smoke and are over thirty-five should not use oral contraceptives. It is just too risky. These women have a significantly increased risk of heart attacks, strokes, and death.

900 Are there beneficial side effects from the use of birth-control pills?

Based on figures for the mid-1980s, taking oral contraceptives allows almost 60,000 American women annually to avoid hospitalization. The use of oral contraceptives is responsible for the hospitalization of about 9,000 women, but the hospitalization of the majority of these women could have been avoided if the women over age thirty-five who smoked had stopped using the Pill.

Some other benefits of using birth-control pills include:

Less chance of unwanted pregnancies. A woman using oral contraceptives will not usually become pregnant unless she wants to and therefore lessens her risking the potential dangers associated with any pregnancy, including less chance of ectopic pregnancy.

Insures routine checkups. Women cannot get birth-control pills unless they see a physician. This means that they will have such things as yearly Pap smears and breast exams. It also means that they will often get in the habit of the "annual exam" and will continue it even after stopping the use of the Pill. This one habit has probably saved far more women from cancer and other medical problems than all the problems the Pill has ever produced.

Less menstrual cramping. Birth-control pills may be the only method of helping a woman who suffers from severe cramps who has not been helped by any other medication.

Lighter menstrual periods. Birth-control pills usually make a woman bleed less with her periods. This is especially beneficial if a woman usually has extremely heavy periods. This decreases the chance of a woman developing anemia (low blood count).

Less pelvic inflammatory disease (PID) from gonorrhea. Women who are on birth-control pills are up to 50 percent less likely to get infections of the uterus and tubes from gonorrhea. Those who do get such infections generally have milder infections than women who are not on the Pill. However, they are just as (or more) likely to get pelvic inflammatory disease from chlamydia. A chlamydia infection can be even more destructive to the female organs than gonorrhea, so a woman should not rely on oral contraceptives to protect her from PID.

Fewer ectopic (tubal) pregnancies. Just as birth-control pills decrease the number of normal pregnancies, so they decrease the number of tubal ectopic pregnancies. (Ectopic pregnancies are still the second leading cause of death from pregnancy in women in the United States.)

Fewer breast lumps. Statistics have shown that women on birth-control pills have only one-fourth to one-half as many breast lumps as women who are not on oral contraceptives. This means, of course, far less chance of needing (or having to worry about) breast biopsies. If women have taken birth-control pills for an extended period of time, they have less fibrocystic changes of the breast.

Less ovarian cancer. Women who have used birth-control pills are less likely to develop cancer of the ovary, because the more times a woman has ovulated, the more likely she is to develop cancer. Since birth-control pills prevent ovulation, they decrease the chance of a woman developing ovarian cancer later on in life. The longer a woman uses birth-control pills, the less likely she is to have ovarian cancer. The benefit varies from 40 percent in short-term (three to five years) users of birth-control pills to as much as 80 percent in women who have used birth-control pills for many years.

Less uterine cancer. Women who have used birth-control pills for a few years are estimated to be half as likely to develop cancer of the uterus (endometrial cancer) than women who have never used oral contraceptives. This protection lasts for at least ten years after stopping the pills.

Less rheumatoid arthritis. Some studies suggest that women who have taken birth-control pills may have half as much chance of developing rheumatoid arthritis in the future as women who have not been on the Pill. Although some studies question this, most physicians who prescribe birth-control pills feel that they decrease a woman's chance of having rheumatoid arthritis.

Fewer ovarian cysts. Women on oral contraceptives will not develop the ovarian cysts that are a part of the body's attempt to produce eggs each month (because the body is not trying to produce eggs while the birth-control pill is used). The advantage of this is that it is much less likely that you would be told by your doctor that you have an enlarged ovary and that you need ovarian surgery. (See Q. 724.)

Less endometriosis. Birth-control pills decrease the amount of bleeding from the lining of the uterus, thus decreasing the amount of endometriosis in the body. Endometriosis is tissue similar to the endometrium and it responds to hormones in much the same way. Not all women will experience this effect, but it is generally true.

Fewer fibroid tumors and smaller fibroid tumors. Women who have been on birth-control pills for several years have fewer (and/or generally smaller) fibroid tumors than women who have not.

Decrease in the number of abortions. If women take birth-control pills carefully, they will usually not get pregnant. For those women who would abort if they got pregnant, birth-control pills prevent pregnancies that would be aborted.

Less toxic shock. Women who use birth-control pills are less likely to have toxic shock syndrome. This is apparently true because they pass less blood, thus using fewer tampons, and have thicker cervical mucus, thus preventing the passage of the toxic shock bacteria into the uterus.

Less premenstrual syndrome. About one-third of the women who take birth-control pills will find that they have less PMS. (Taking birth-control pills, as a matter of fact, is one treatment for PMS.)

901 How soon may I try to become pregnant after I stop taking birth-control pills?

There is no medical reason for you to wait to become pregnant after stopping birth-control pills. If you get pregnant immediately, it will not hurt you or the baby. The only reason most physicians suggest waiting two or three months is so that you can establish regular menstrual periods, making it easier for you to know exactly when you became pregnant.

For the very best obstetric care, you should know how far along you are in your pregnancy. If you have established a regular menstrual pattern before you get pregnant, you will have a better idea when your pregnancy began. There is no other reason to wait any particular length of time after stopping birth-control pills.

902 Do birth-control pills work by causing abortion?

Birth-control pills generally prevent ovulation. They suppress the release of gonadotrophin-releasing hormone (GnRH) by the hypothalamus, and thereby block the pituitary's release of FSH and LH in most women. A number of studies show no elevation of FSH or LH in women who are on the Pill. Ovulation, therefore, rarely occurs. Also, in most women, birth-control pills cause a thickening of the cervical mucus. This severely impairs the sperm's ability to swim into the uterus.

Some studies show that women may ovulate from 2 to 5 percent of the time when they are on the Pill. This is a very low rate of ovulation. Even then, the thickened cervical mucus will almost always keep the sperm from getting into the uterus and reaching the egg. Of course, some of the women who ovulate do get pregnant while taking birth-control pills, but the primary reason is they skipped too many pills or did not take them correctly, allowing ovulation to occur.

When a woman is on the Pill, the endometrial lining is thin but this does not mean that the embryo cannot implant. The embryo can even implant on the inhospitable lining of a fallopian tube to cause a tubal pregnancy. In addition, if ovulation does occur while a woman is taking her birth-control pills, the lining of the uterus may actually become thicker and more hospitable to the embryo.

Finally, there is no research that shows that birth-control pills work by causing abortions. Since women on birth-control pills occasionally become pregnant, common sense indicates that miscarriage also occasionally occurs. There is no scientific data to show that miscarriages happen more frequently to women on the Pill than they do to those who are not.

903 What dose of birth-control pill should I take?

A woman should take one of the new, low dose birth-control pills that contain 20 to 35 micrograms of estrogen and low dose progesterone. These pills are extremely safe and contain one-fifth the amount of estrogen and one-tenth the amount of progesterone that the original birth-control pills contained. Another similar form of birth-control pill that has an even lower amount of progesterone is the triphasic pill (Ortho-Novum 7/7/7, Tri-Norinyl, Triphasil, Tri-Levlen and others). These pills are also quite safe.

These low dose pills do not usually have as many bad side effects as the original pills. The older higher dose pills often caused swelling, depression, breast tenderness, and other symptoms. While these symptoms can happen with the newer pill, they rarely occur.

The contraceptive effect of the low dose pills is just as good as with the higher dose pills. (I am not talking about the "mini-pill," which contains only progesterone and is not as effective.)

904 Is it really safe for women over thirty-five to take birth-control pills?

The FDA says that it is safe for a woman who is over thirty-five to use birth-control pills until she goes through menopause if she does not smoke and doesn't have other reasons for not taking the pills (see Q. 897). Because studies showed that the adverse effects of birth-control pills were found to be limited primarily to smokers over age thirty-five, the FDA Advisory Committee for Fertility and Maternal Health Drugs recommended (October 1989) that the age limitation for oral contraceptives in healthy, nonsmoking older women be removed. In January 1990, the FDA accepted the advisory committee's recommendation to eliminate the "de facto" age limit on birth-control pill use and requested that manufacturers modify their labels to state that the benefits of the Pill after the age of forty may exceed the possible risks.

Most women over thirty-five who try the new pills like them and want to stay on them through menopause. Regular menstrual periods with a lighter flow and without cramps, in addition to no worry about contraception, can be a strong motivation to take the pills. Additional incentive in the form of a dramatically lower risk of cancer (ovarian, uterine, and breast) and a decreased risk of

vascular disease has made many women believers in the "new Pill."

905 If I take birth-control pills continuously, how will I know when I have gone through menopause?

If you are taking birth-control pills, your doctor will want to know when you have reached menopause because the amount of estrogen and progesterone in birth-control pills is more than you will need for a hormone replacement after menopause.

Dr. Leon Speroff, professor of obstetrics and gynecology at the Oregon Health Sciences University in Portland, stated: "One approach to establish the onset of the postmenopausal years is to measure the FSH level annually, beginning at age fifty. It is important to obtain a blood sample on day six or seven of the pill-free week. By then, the steroid levels will have declined sufficiently to allow FSH to rise. When FSH is greater than 40 mIU/mL, it is time to transfer to a hormone replacement program" (*Contemporary OB/GYN*, August 1991).

This means you can stay on birth-control pills until you are fifty. Then each year from age fifty on, you should have a blood test to check your FSH level. If the FSH level is 40 mIU/mL or higher, you have passed menopause, and you can switch from birth-control pills to a hormone replacement.

The Intrauterine Contraceptive Device (IUD)

906 What is an intrauterine contraceptive device, or IUD, and how does it work?

An IUD (intrauterine contraceptive device) is a small plastic device that can be inserted by a physician through a woman's cervix and into her uterus to prevent pregnancy. The procedure is done in a physician's office, usually during or immediately after the menstrual period so that a woman can be sure she is not pregnant.

There are only two types of IUDs in use in the United States today. One is a progesterone-releasing IUD (the only type available is the Progestasert), which is effective for one year; the other is a copper-bearing IUD (one type presently available is the ParaGard), which is effective for up to six years. (Both types should be removed at the end of their effective period.) Your physician will advise you regarding the best type IUD for you.

No one knows exactly how the copper IUD works, but it seems fairly certain that the contraceptive effect is produced in several ways. Copper IUDs either kill sperm or keep them from being able to swim through the uterus and into the fallopian tubes. Studies have shown that women without IUDs will have thousands of sperm in their fallopian tubes within fifteen to thirty minutes after an insemination, but women with IUDs in place are almost always found to have very few sperm in their tubes.

In addition, women with IUDs rarely have any eggs in their tubes. In *Fertility and Sterility* (May 1988, 49.5), Alvarez and his associates showed results of a study on women who were having sterilization procedures. They flushed out the fallopian tubes of these women, some of whom had IUDs in place and some of whom did not. While they did find eggs in the tubes of women with IUDs, the eggs were present at a lower rate and were not fertilized. In women without IUDs, over half the eggs showed signs of having been fertilized. This study indicates that both eggs and sperm are affected in some way that inhibits their ability to fertilize.

A further finding of this study showed that there were absolutely no eggs in the uteri of any of the women who used IUDs. Alvarez and his associates summarized their study by saying: "There is no evidence from this study of the presence of fertilized eggs in the fallopian tubes of women using IUDs."

It seems clear that the primary effect of a copper IUD is to provide contraception without producing abortion. The rare pregnancy that may result during IUD use can be carried to term or miscarried.

All of these facts should be considered in making a decision about using an IUD. If a woman or her husband is uncomfortable about the slight possibility that they might miscarry because of an IUD, they should not use one. An alternate contraceptive technique should be chosen.

907 How does an IUD affect fertility?

Infections of the pelvic organs (pelvic inflammatory disease, or PID) occur more often in women who use IUDs than in women who do not. When an infection occurs, the tubes can be scarred so abnormally that they cannot carry an egg into the uterus, producing infertility or absolute sterility. The risk of infection is three to five times greater for women who use an IUD. If a woman has had a PID, she is even more likely to develop infection again if she has an IUD put in.

If a woman does develop PID, the infection can not only cause sterility but may also necessitate surgery. Women with PID can develop abscesses of the tubes and ovaries that can make it necessary to have them removed.

It is possible for a woman who has an IUD to develop an ectopic (tubal) pregnancy, just as she could have a normal pregnancy. The progesterone-containing type of IUD seems to cause more ectopic pregnancies than the other IUDs.

Although you may be told that it is okay to use an IUD if you have had at least one child, I strongly urge you not to use this contraceptive technique until you have had all the children you ever want to have. I believe the IUD is a good method of birth control for a woman who has had her family but does not want to have a sterilization procedure or has not gone through menopause. The copper-bearing IUDs have low pregnancy and infection rates; I believe they are safe for a woman who is married and has her family.

908 What should I do if my IUD causes spotting or bleeding?

A woman can start bleeding the moment she has an IUD put in and continue to have it as long as the IUD is present. This is not the norm nor is it dangerous, but most women will not tolerate such bleeding.

It is more likely that spotting and bleeding will occur intermittently. It is normal for a woman to start spotting or bleeding a year or two after insertion of the IUD. Such bleeding is usually due to the IUD, and removal of the IUD usually stops the bleeding. This bleeding is not dangerous unless it becomes very heavy and persists for many weeks, at which point anemia could develop.

If a woman is forty or over, spotting or bleeding between periods may be an indication of cancer of the uterus. The IUD should be removed and a D&C or endometrial biopsy done to check for the possible presence of cancer. If you have such bleeding and are in this age group, check with your doctor promptly.

909 Will an IUD cause pain?

From the day an IUD is inserted, a woman could have pain from it. If this pain persists for several weeks, a woman usually has the IUD taken out by her doctor. I think this is wise, because such pain could indicate a low-grade infection of the uterus that could get worse.

It is common for a woman to have an IUD in place for a year or two and then start having pain. If the pain is a minor problem, it is fine to leave the IUD in place. If it becomes constant and more severe, the IUD should definitely be removed.

If you develop pain while wearing an IUD, see your gynecologist first. When I insert an IUD I warn patients that they could have pain anywhere from the lower chest to their mid-thighs from the IUD! Gynecologists have learned that IUD pain can be felt anywhere in the central part of a woman's body. I cannot overemphasize this. I have had patients who went to doctors other than gynecologists and who even had surgery for pain, only to find out later that all the pain was caused by their IUD. If there is any question about whether or not pain is due to an IUD, I encourage you to have it removed to see if the pain goes away.

910 What happens if I get pregnant with an IUD in place?

If you miss a menstrual period and think you might be pregnant, you should see your doctor as soon as possible. It is very important to establish that you do not have a tubal pregnancy. If you do, your doctor will know how to handle this potentially dangerous situation. (See the section in this book on tubal ectopic pregnancy.)

If you are pregnant (with a normal, uterine pregnancy) and your IUD string is still visible, it is usually best for your doctor to gently remove the IUD. (This action can of course cause a miscarriage.) If the string is not visible, or if the physician cannot get the IUD to move by pulling on it, a woman and her husband must make a decision. If the IUD is left in place the woman has an increased chance of later having a miscarriage, a uterine infection, and/or premature labor and delivery. Statistics show that if a woman is pregnant and her IUD cannot be removed, there is a 50 percent chance of miscarriage. If the IUD can be removed, the risk falls to 20 to 25 percent. Although allowing the IUD to remain in place if it cannot be removed increases the incidence of miscarriage or premature labor, if the pregnancy continues normally the presence of the IUD does not seem to damage the baby. The chance of an infection occurring because of the presence of an IUD with a pregnancy is small.

Some physicians will tell patients who have an IUD in place with a pregnancy that abortion is necessary. This is not true. Many women have carried a pregnancy successfully with an IUD in place. A couple in this situation must understand the risks and do what they feel is best.

The Diaphragm for Contraception

911 What is a diaphragm?

A diaphragm is a dome-shaped rubber cap with a flexible spring rim. (See illustration.) It is approximately three inches in diameter.

Actually, a diaphragm should be called the diaphragm-plus-jelly contraceptive, because the diaphragm itself does not produce any significant contraceptive effect. The diaphragm merely holds the contraceptive jelly against the cervix; it is the jelly that kills the sperm. If the contraceptive jelly is put into the vagina without a diaphragm, the jelly will "glob up" into one corner of the vagina, making it relatively ineffective as a contraceptive.

Since the diaphragm does not completely seal off your upper vagina, sperm can swim around the edges of it. When they do this, they are killed by the contraceptive jelly. Even if you have a small hole in your diaphragm, any sperm that swim through the hole are usually killed by the jelly held in position by the diaphragm.

912 How is a diaphragm obtained?

A doctor must prescribe and fit a woman's diaphragm. He or she will use a set of fitting rings, inserting them into your vagina one at a time until one is found that fits. A diaphragm should be comfortable, and it should fill the area from the back of your vagina to your pubic bone.

Occasionally patients find that the size that seems best to the doctor is not the one that is most comfortable to them. When this happens the doctor will usually give them the size they need to meet their individual comfort needs. As long as the diaphragm stays in place during intercourse, it does not really matter that the size be absolutely precise.

One of the most important aspects of getting a diaphragm is remembering to purchase the jelly to use with it. Contraceptive foam, by the way, should not be substituted for the jelly; pregnancy would be much more likely to occur.

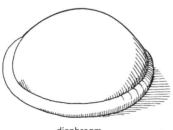

diaphragm

913 How is a diaphragm inserted?

It is most important that your doctor, or the nurse, explain carefully how the diaphragm should be used. Basic instructions include the following.

Hold the diaphragm by the rim, with the cup facing up. Spread about a three-inch strip of jelly on the soft, central part of the cup. Use a little jelly around the rim so that it will slide into your vagina smoothly.

Squeeze the edges of diaphragm together to make it long and thin, so you can insert it into your vagina. Most women find it easier to insert a diaphragm when they are standing with one leg up on the bed or the commode. The first few times you do this you may find it easier to lie on your back on your bed with your legs pulled up and apart. You can get your fingers deeper into your vagina that way.

In putting the diaphragm in place, you should insert the back edge of the diaphragm behind your cervix and the front edge up under your pubic bone. You should then be able to feel your cervix through the soft, central part of the diaphragm. Your cervix feels much like the end of your nose.

Some women prefer using a diaphragm inserter, a plastic stick with blunt hooks on it. The diaphragm is stretched out on it, inserted into the vagina, and then slipped off the inserter. Further positioning is the same as when no inserter is used. This device can be obtained at your pharmacy.

914 When should a diaphragm be inserted, and when should it be removed?

You should insert your diaphragm no more than one to two hours before intercourse. The jelly will lose some of its potency and will tend to drain out of the vagina if you wait longer than that. Most women put their diaphragms in before they start sexual play, but some couples prefer putting in the diaphragm together as part of their foreplay. As soon as the diaphragm is in place, it is safe to have intercourse.

You should leave the diaphragm in place for six to eight hours after your last intercourse so that all the sperm deposited at intercourse will be dead by the time the diaphragm is removed.

915 Is it safe to have intercourse more than once with one diaphragm insertion?

It is best for you to put an application of contraceptive foam in your vagina on top of the diaphragm if you repeat intercourse after more than an hour or two. Or your husband can wear a condom as an alternative to using the foam.

916 How is a diaphragm removed?

To remove your diaphragm, simply put your finger up behind your pubic bone, hook the edge of the diaphragm, and pull it out. If you cannot get it out the first time you use it, don't panic. Simply go to your doctor and let the doctor or nurse help you. Don't start digging around for it because you can scratch yourself and cause bleeding.

It will probably not hurt your body if you forget and leave the diaphragm in your vagina for several days. Menstrual flow goes right around the edges of a diaphragm. However, since toxic shock has occurred in women who use the diaphragm, it should not be kept in for more than twenty-four hours.

After removing the diaphragm, you should wash it with soap and water, rinse it well, dry it off, and place it back in its container. A light dusting of corn starch may be used. Avoid the use of talc; it can be dangerous. Air and light can cause the rubber of a diaphragm to become brittle. A diaphragm is usable as long as the rubber is soft and pliable and it does not have holes in it. Diaphragms often last for many years.

917 What effects does a diaphragm have on intercourse?

Most women cannot feel the diaphragm when it is properly fitted, just as most women cannot feel the presence of a tampon. A man will usually feel a difference since his penis makes contact with the rubber of the diaphragm. Most men do not find this sensation objectionable.

918 What is the chance of pregnancy with a diaphragm?

Statistics show that the chance of pregnancy with a diaphragm is in the range of four to twenty per hundred women in a year. If a woman uses a diaphragm carefully, she probably has no more than a 4 percent chance of pregnancy; if she is careless and intermittently forgets to use her diaphragm, she has a 20 percent chance of pregnancy. Many women have used the diaphragm for many years with no pregnancies resulting. From the turn of the century until the mid-1960s, the diaphragm was the mainstay of birth-control methods.

919 Are there women who should not use the diaphragm?

There are three factors to be considered when deciding whether or not to use a diaphragm for contraception.

Discomfort. Some women find a diaphragm uncomfortable. If changing diaphragm sizes does not solve the problem, choose another method.

Urinary-tract infections. Use of the diaphragm can cause some women to develop bladder infections. Apparently the pressure of the diaphragm on the bladder is the cause of this. If you continually have urinary-tract infections of your bladder or kidney, be sure your doctor knows you use a diaphragm. Even if the doctor doubts that there is an association, you might stop using the diaphragm and see if there is any improvement. Be sure to use an alternate form of contraception during that time.

Vaginal relaxation. Women who have had babies often have sagging vaginal tissues that can push a diaphragm out and make it impossible to use a diaphragm. A doctor will usually be able to tell if this condition exists when a woman is examined for diaphragm size.

Contraceptive Foam

920 What is contraceptive foam?

Contraceptive foam is a "barrier" type of contraceptive, which means that it kills sperm before they can get into the cervix. The foam coats the cervix and vagina, killing sperm that come in contact with it.

When the medication is drawn into the vaginal applicator, it foams up. The advantage of foam is that it expands and coats the vagina and the cervix effectively. A contraceptive jelly will not spread as effectively as foam and will accumulate in one part of the vagina, failing to kill all the sperm.

921 How is contraceptive foam used?

After the medication is put in the applicator, the applicator is inserted into the vagina and the medication ejected into the vagina. Ideally this should be done at least ten or fifteen minutes before intercourse so that the foam can spread around the vagina. However, the foam should not be put into the vagina more than thirty minutes before intercourse because it could begin draining out and have less contraceptive effect.

Most women do not feel the need for douching after using the foam. The medication seems to absorb into the body after intercourse and does not produce as much of a mess in the vulvar area as contraceptive jelly does.

922 Does contraceptive foam produce any undesirable effects on intercourse?

Yes, there are a few drawbacks to the use of this method of contraception, which may bother some couples.

A couple often must stop sex play to insert the foam into the vagina.

The foam is messy, and some couples do not like that.

An additional plunger of foam must be inserted into the vagina before repeating intercourse.

The odor bothers some people.

The foam may irritate the tissues of some people.

923 What is the chance of pregnancy when using contraceptive foam?

The chance of pregnancy is greater than with the diaphragm or the condom. About twenty to twenty-five pregnancies per hundred women can be expected to occur each year.

To minimize the risk, my advice to a couple who use foam for contraception is that they use it every time they have intercourse except during the menstrual period. In addition, during the week around the time of ovulation, the man should use a condom or the woman a diaphragm. If a couple wants to be sure that the woman does not get pregnant, they should use a condom plus foam or a diaphragm plus foam every time they have intercourse.

Condoms

924 What are condoms, or rubbers?

A rubber (condom) is a contraceptive device used by a man; it fits onto his penis tightly enough to stay in place during intercourse, catching his semen when he ejaculates and keeping it from getting into the woman's vagina. If a condom has a hole in it or if it breaks during intercourse, the possibility of pregnancy can be as great as if no contraception had been used.

Direct from the package, a condom looks much like a miniature diaphragm; when unrolled it looks like a wiener-shaped balloon.

925 How is a condom used?

A condom can be put on the erect penis immediately before intercourse. It is important, however, for a couple to realize that a man's penis may ooze a little semen before ejaculation, and that even small amounts of sperm deposited at the vaginal opening can result in a pregnancy. Therefore, it is extremely important that the husband's erect penis make no contact with the opening of the vagina without having the condom on. When the condom is rolled on it is important to leave a small space at the tip for the ejaculate. This will prevent the condom from rupturing.

To remove a condom, a man must hold its rim at the base of his penis until he has withdrawn his penis from a woman and before his penis becomes too small. He must then slip it off gently. If he pulls too fast, the condom can tear, semen can escape, and his wife can become pregnant.

926 What is the risk of pregnancy with a condom?

The chance of pregnancy with condoms is high, especially with young people. For instance, one study showed that for women over age thirty, up to four out of a hundred will get pregnant using condoms each year. If women are under age twenty-five, however, from 10 to 33 percent of them will get pregnant each year while using condoms. Most studies indicate that there is about a 15 percent chance of a woman becoming pregnant if condoms are used as the only method of birth control.

If a married couple wants to use condoms as their primary contraceptive, I suggest they use them with every act of intercourse except during the menstrual period. In addition, during the week around ovulation, they should use foam or a diaphragm along with the condom. If a couple wants to be the most safe, they will use a condom and foam every time they have intercourse.

927 What are the disadvantages of using condoms?

There are several undesirable side effects of condom use.

Irritation. Irritation of genital tissues is a problem for about 10 percent of users. If a couple finds a condom irritating, a different brand of condom may solve the problem. Some men and women are allergic to latex. If irritation develops from condom use, latex may be the culprit.

Effects on spontaneity. A man must wait until he has an erection before he can put on the condom. Many people do not like this interference with their spontaneity.

Lessened sensation. Men often do not have adequate sensation with a condom. They often describe it as taking a shower while wearing a raincoat!

Semen leak. After intercourse the man's penis becomes flaccid. This allows the condom to leak semen that could cause a woman to become pregnant. It is important that, once intercourse is over, the man withdraw his penis and the condom to prevent the condom from leaking its contents into the vagina.

928 There has been a lot of discussion and publicity about condoms in the past few years. Is there any new information available about their use?

Yes. A number of interesting facts have become evident:

1. Viruses can pass through lamb membrane condoms. People who depend on condoms for protection from sexually transmitted disease should always use latex condoms. (If a woman is allergic to latex, her husband can wear a lambskin condom over the latex one; if he is allergic to latex, he can wear a lambskin condom under the latex one. This may help prevent an allergic reaction but may not always be effective.)
2. Condoms should be kept cool and dry to avoid deterioration. They should not be carried around in purses or wallets or left in glove compartments of cars.
3. Oil-based lubricants such as petroleum jelly (Vaseline) can weaken latex and should not be used with condoms.

4. Some studies show that about 2 to 3 percent of condoms break during sex. Manufacturer's regulations permit condoms to be released for sale if they show an overall average of "no more than three condoms per thousand with holes in them."

Only the most disciplined people have any chance of even partially being protected from either pregnancy or sexually transmitted disease with condom use. Studies consistently show that very few men and women practice this kind of discipline. (For more information on this subject, see the chapter on sexually transmitted disease.)

929 What is a "female" condom?

A female condom is a plastic device that resembles a diaphragm/condom combination. It consists of a soft, loose-fitting, polyurethane (soft plastic) sheath and two flexible polyurethane rings similar to those of a diaphragm. One ring, which helps a woman insert the sheath into the vagina and serves as an internal "anchor," lies inside the sheath. The second ring remains outside the vagina to make it possible for the man to find the "entrance" to the vagina, which is now lined by the sheath.

Like male condoms, this device does not require any fitting, and it is disposable after a single use. The female condom provides more protection for a woman's female tissues than the condom a man uses because it covers her labia, her entire vagina, and her cervix, and simultaneously protects the base of the penis and the scrotum.

Unfortunately, studies show higher pregnancy rates with female condoms than with male condoms.

Female Condom

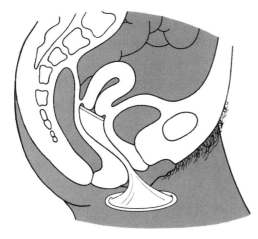

Contraceptive Suppositories and Injections

930 What are contraceptive vaginal suppositories?

Contraceptive vaginal suppositories came on the market with great fanfare several years ago. They were touted as being the ultimate contraceptive, but they have not worked out that way. The primary problem with this method of birth control is a pregnancy rate that is about 20 to 25 percent per year, no better than the contraceptive foam.

The discussion in this chapter concerning the use of contraceptive foam applies almost word for word to the use of the suppositories. (See Q. 920–923.) If a woman prefers the suppository to the foam, she should use it instead of the foam. She should not use the suppository as her only contraceptive device, unless she does not mind getting pregnant.

If the suppository is used, it should be inserted with every act of intercourse except during actual menstrual flow. To increase its effectiveness a condom or diaphragm should be used with it during the week of ovulation.

931 If I become pregnant while using foam or jelly, will this have any effect on my baby?

Studies have indicated that there is no harm to babies whose mothers conceived while using spermicide contraceptives.

932 What is Norplant?

Norplant is a highly effective birth-control method that was FDA approved in December of 1990. Once the Norplant capsules are in place, they keep a woman from becoming pregnant for five years. If a woman decides she wants to get pregnant before that time is up, the implants can be removed and fertility is restored.

Norplant consists of six small plastic (Silastic) capsules that are inserted under the skin in a woman's inner arm, just above the elbow. Each capsule contains 36 milligrams of levonorgestrel. This synthetic progesterone contained in the capsules is absorbed into a woman's body and functions much like a birth-control pill. Ovulation is suppressed, cervical mucus becomes sticky (which hinders the passage of sperm into the uterus), growth of the lining of the uterus is suppressed, and there is possibly a suppression of progesterone secretion during the last half of the month.

Studies show that Norplant capsules allow only four or five women in one thousand to get pregnant in a year. (This compares to 20–50 women per thousand per year who get pregnant on birth-control pills.) One reason for the low pregnancy rate is that once Norplant is inserted, women can forget about using other birth-control measures.

The failure rate with Norplant is higher in patients who weigh more than 150 pounds. Even then, only 8.5 women per hundred in a five-year period are likely to get pregnant. Women who use Dilantin, Tegretol, or similar drugs are also a little more likely to get pregnant with Norplant.

Norplant has the lowest pregnancy rate of any reversible method of birth control. It can be left in place for five years, providing good protection from pregnancy for that period of time. The capsules can be removed and new ones inserted after five years for continued contraception if desired.

When Norplant capsules are removed, fertility returns to normal within the first three months. (Women who have a fertility problem after having the capsules removed would probably have had a fertility problem even if they had not used Norplant.)

The primary disadvantage of using Norplant is that it causes some women to have irregular vaginal bleeding. About 82 percent of patients will have a change in their menstrual bleeding, and more than 9 percent of these women have the Norplant removed during the first year of use because of this change. This is a significant problem. Women spend over $650 to get Norplant inserted and almost 10 percent have it removed because the irregular bleeding bothers them so much. Consider this if you are thinking about having Norplant inserted. The menstrual bleeding may be irregular, coming too often or not as often as usual, or with periods being longer or shorter than usual. Occasionally bleeding is heavy with Norplant.

Other problems are some of the same ones women experience on birth-control pills: weight change (32 percent), headaches (24 percent), and acne (15 percent). Other less common problems include discharge from the breast, increased hair growth, scalp hair loss, breast tenderness, vaginal discharge, nausea, dizziness, and ovarian cysts. (These cysts usually go away spontaneously.)

The symptoms (especially the menstrual irregularities) caused by Norplant often decrease as time goes by. After the first year or so, the side effects usually disappear.

Another disadvantage of Norplant is the cost (more than $650). Although taking birth-control pills for five years is considerably more, the initial cost for Norplant may be a drawback for some women.

A final disadvantage of Norplant is that it must be removed by a physician. A small incision similar to the original incision must be made to remove the capsules. Though this sounds easy, it can be very difficult and uncomfortable. It can take up to 1 1/2 hours and is done under local anesthesia. Blood vessels and nerves have been damaged in the removal. As with any medical procedure, lawsuits have been filed against doctors because of these problems. Finally, doctors do charge for doing the removal. Before you have a Norplant put in, be sure and ask the doctor how much he is going to charge to remove it.

933 How is Norplant inserted?

After injecting a local anesthetic, the physician makes a tiny slit in the skin of the upper, inner arm, about two inches above the elbow. Each of the six capsules is individually pushed through the incision in a slightly different direction, spreading them out much like the fingers of a hand. The small cut does not require a suture; a Band-Aid or small adhesive dressing is all that is necessary. The procedure is usually done in a physician's office.

The Norplant capsules are just over an inch long and not even an eighth of an inch around. The procedure to implant the capsules takes only ten or fifteen minutes; more than 80 percent of women report either no discomfort or only slight discomfort during the procedure.

934 Should Norplant be used by unmarried teenagers?

Absolutely not. The one major concern I have about Norplant is that it will be used in unmarried teenagers. If teenagers use Norplant for birth control, this protection from pregnancy will make them feel "safe" for five years. These teenagers will then not have any protection against sexually transmitted disease. As they change sexual partners and are exposed to the multiple sexually transmitted diseases that teenagers so often have, many will later realize that they have become sterile, have developed cervical cancer, or have gotten AIDS. Though they did not get pregnant, their lives were dramatically complicated by the false sense of security Norplant provided.

Those of us in the health-care profession realize that teenage pregnancy is a terrible problem, but we also realize that the sexually transmitted diseases ravaging our teenagers are equally appalling. I feel very strongly that we must not subject our teenagers to a contraceptive technique that will make them feel "safe" and, therefore, make them feel that they can change sexual partners and have intercourse at will with no risk.

I think it is wrong for health-care providers to insert a five-year contraceptive into a child's arm and then send her out into a dangerous sexual environment. In one study, 83 percent of sexually active girls wish they had waited till they were older to have sex (Fielding, 1991). In another study, 84 percent wanted more information on "how to say no" without hurting the other person's feelings

(Marion Howard, 1990). These girls need someone to love them and to counsel with them, not to just have a contraceptive placed in their bodies.

935 What about contraceptive shots?

If a woman is given an injection of 150 mg of Depo-Provera, a long-acting progesterone, she will not become pregnant for three months. Studies have shown that the pregnancy rates with Depo-Provera are similar to the pregnancy rates with birth-control pills.

There are several problems with using Depo-Provera for contraception.

Women who have had a shot of Depo-Provera may be unable to get pregnant for much longer than three months. Occasionally a woman will not resume her periods for as long as a year after a Depo-Provera injection. If a woman has plans for pregnancy in the next few years, she should absolutely not consider Depo-Provera as a contraceptive.

Women who receive Depo-Provera may have spotting or bleeding all the time or they may have no periods for many months.

Once Depo-Provera is injected into a woman's body, there is no way to remove it. She must allow her body to complete the absorption of the drug before its effect will be gone.

Other problems occur with Depo-Provera that are much like the problems occurring with Norplant. (See previous questions.)

Natural Family Planning

936 Is natural family planning, sometimes called the "rhythm method," effective for birth control?

The term *natural family planning* is now used instead of the term the *rhythm method* to describe the use of periodic abstinence to affect birth control. This change in terminology has been made because this method of contraception employs the same techniques that are useful for helping a woman become pregnant, and it implies control over both when one becomes pregnant and when one does not.

Other terms used for natural family planning are *fertility awareness, sympto-thermal,* the *Billings' method,* and the *Creighton Model.* Each of these terms uses slightly different techniques to avoid the use of drugs or contraceptive devices in family planning.

With natural family planning, couples refrain from intercourse when they think an egg has recently been released, or is about to be released, by the woman's body. If there is no egg free in the body, there can be no pregnancy. The goal of this technique, therefore, is for the couple to determine when ovulation occurs so that no intercourse takes place around that time.

If a woman has irregular periods, she can often still use natural family planning methods. While it may require more training and diligence, if a woman is careful, persistent, and willing, she can often learn to be observant enough to use these methods to avoid (or achieve) pregnancy even with her irregularity.

It is important that a woman who is regular not become complacent about her monthly cycle. Even a woman whose periods are generally "like clockwork" each month can ovulate early or late in any given month.

The essence of this technique is that a couple must be able to predict when the wife is going to ovulate. If such prediction is not possible, then the technique will not work.

937 How is natural family planning used?

Natural family planning techniques involve determining a woman's fertile period (when she is ovulating) and abstaining from intercourse to avoid pregnancy or having intercourse to achieve pregnancy. These techniques take ad-

vantage of the body's natural rhythm of fertility and infertility.

A couple may use only one or two techniques or may need to use several techniques to help determine when it is safe to have intercourse.

Evaluation of cervical mucus. A common factor of most natural family planning techniques is the observation of cervical mucus. During the days immediately after a menstrual period, cervical mucus is either undetectable or very scant. As the estrogen levels rise after the period, the cervical mucus becomes stretchy ("spinnbarkheit," see Q. 809), more abundant, and whiter and clearer. There are various ways to check the quantity and quality of cervical mucus. A woman can simply wipe the vulva with a piece of tissue, she can remove some mucus from the vulva with her finger, or she can put two fingers into her vagina, grasp the mucus, and pull it out. If preventing pregnancy is her goal, abstinence should be practiced during the days when the cervical mucus first becomes moist or slippery and should be continued for about four days.

Recording the menstrual cycle. With this method a woman records on a calendar when her periods come. Over a span of several months she can determine how regular they are. Many women are surprised when they actually record the occurrence of their periods as they often find that their cycles are much different (more regular or more irregular) from what they had thought.

Basal body temperature. This technique involves the purchase of a basal body thermometer (available at most pharmacies) and the use of that thermometer every morning. A woman shakes down the thermometer, puts it at her bedside, and, when she awakens in the morning, takes her temperature for five minutes and records it on the chart. A Basal Body Temperature Chart makes it much easier to keep a temperature record. These charts can be obtained from your physician or pharmacist. (See Q. 798 and accompanying illustration.)

About halfway through her cycle, a woman will notice a rise in her temperature indicating that ovulation has occurred. When a woman's temperature has gone up and stayed up for three days, she can be fairly certain that the egg that was released is no longer alive. (Eggs usually live only about 24 hours.) It is safe to resume having intercourse at this point.

A woman who records her temperature, checks her cervical mucus, and watches for other changes at the time of ovulation is using what is commonly called the sympto-thermal method of natural family planning.

Pain with ovulation. Many woman feel low abdominal pain at the time of ovulation. Some women do not notice it, but many women who have not noticed it before will be aware of it when they are watching for it. This discomfort, caused by the egg coming out of the ovary, is called *Mittelschmerz,* or "mid-pain."

Cervical dilatation. When a woman is checking her cervical mucus, she can also feel the cervical opening. This opening dilates from the end of the menstruation up to the time of ovulation and then contracts down again. A woman can record this change on her chart along with her temperatures and cervical mucus changes.

Other symptoms. There are a couple of other less common symptoms of ovulation. These can be slight spotting of blood at mid-cycle and/or breast discomfort, such as a prickling or tingling sensation.

Chart for Identifying "Safe" Days for Intercourse

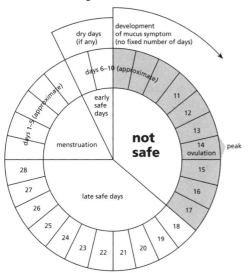

By observing the changes that occur in her body on a month-to-month basis, a woman can determine fairly accurately when she ovulates. Thereafter, by avoiding intercourse for two days before any possible early ovulation and for two days after any possible late ovulation, she can usually avoid pregnancy.

938 What effect does family planning have on a sexual relationship?

By cooperating in the effort to either avoid or achieve pregnancy, a couple functions as a team and grows together. During the days of abstinence from intercourse, a couple can satisfy each other with "nonintercourse" activity. After a period of abstinence, a couple may find that returning to sexual intercourse can be even more exhilarating because it was "forbidden" for a while.

A couple must be united in their efforts when using natural family planning. If one marriage partner responds negatively or resentfully to the restrictions imposed by this method, frustration and resentment can result. If this contraceptive technique is causing problems, therefore, a couple should talk about whether it is the best method for them.

939 What are the chances of pregnancy with natural family planning?

Studies have shown that a couple's chance of pregnancy varies greatly. The couples most likely to have an unplanned pregnancy are those who do not have good instruction in the technique of natural family planning or the discipline to abide by it.

Some studies have shown that with couples who are well trained and conscientious in the use of natural family planning, no more than one couple in one hundred will get pregnant per year. If a couple does not carefully follow instructions, pregnancy rates can be as high as fifteen to twenty per hundred women per year.

940 Who should not rely on natural family planning as a method of birth control?

There are several contraindications to the use of natural family planning. First of all, women who feel they absolutely must not get pregnant would be best served by another method of birth control.

In addition, couples who do not have the discipline to abstain from intercourse at a specific time each month should not rely on natural family planning.

Some women find it very difficult to use natural family planning techniques for contraception or as an aid to becoming pregnant. These women include those who have poor cervical mucus production, poor temperature rise with ovulation, or certain hormone problems (such as polycystic ovarian syndrome). Even with a physician's care, it is very difficult for these women to determine when ovulation occurs. Most women do not have these problems, and therefore natural family planning techniques usually work if a couple is willing to expend the time and effort required to learn and practice the techniques properly.

941 What are the effects of natural family planning on subsequent fertility?

The effects of natural family planning on future fertility are great! Not only does a couple do nothing that would interfere with future fertility, they also learn a great deal about the woman's fertile time. When they do want to have a baby, they may be more capable than other couples of achieving pregnancy when they desire it.

942 Where can I obtain further information on natural family planning?

An organization called The Couple to Couple League International, Inc. (P.O. Box 111184, Cincinnati, OH 45211-1184) can provide information about natural family planning.

The Roman Catholic church has been in the forefront of teaching natural family planning. Your local Catholic church might have such instructional classes available.

Alternative Methods of Contraception

943 What are "counterfeit" contraceptive techniques?

There are procedures many couples think of as contraception that are totally "counterfeit." Such techniques are totally ineffective, and if a couple continues to practice them, pregnancy will often result. If a couple who uses one of these techniques has not conceived, it is only because they have not used the method long enough or they simply do not achieve pregnancy easily. Any healthy, normal, fertile couple who uses these techniques will be expectant parents sooner or later—and probably sooner.

These are ineffective contraception techniques:

Douching. Douching does not protect against pregnancy. Many sperm are in the cervical mucus within seconds of intercourse. Douching cannot wash this sperm-laden mucus out of the cervix. Pregnancy can certainly occur.

Withdrawal (coitus interruptus). This term refers to a man's withdrawing his penis from a woman's vagina before he ejaculates. This is not a good contraceptive technique, since some semen is released before ejaculation and this material—even at the entrance of a woman's vagina—can cause her to become pregnant.

An additional problem with this is that a man must maintain excellent control. His penis must be totally outside of his wife's vagina, and directed away from her vulva, before he ejaculates. Obviously a disadvantage to this technique is that intercourse is interrupted by a sudden separation just at the point of maximum pleasure.

Dental dams or other material used instead of a condom. These materials (sandwich bags, plastic wrap, etc.) were not made for this purpose. The activity of intercourse can break them or they can leak, allowing either sexually transmitted disease infection or conception to occur.

Feminine hygiene materials. None of the products sold for "feminine hygiene" (douches, deodorants, or other similar products) is effective for contraception.

Breast-feeding. Women often do not ovulate during the months they breast-feed, but a woman can start ovulating during this time. Remember, a woman ovulates before she has a period. She cannot wait, therefore, for a period to occur before she begins using contraceptives. She may have already ovulated and become pregnant, without having a period since her baby's delivery.

If a woman and her husband have learned natural family planning techniques, they may be able to detect the onset of ovulation by the daily change in her cervical mucus. If a couple is not doing this, they need to use some type of contraceptive.

No orgasm. An orgasm is not necessary for pregnancy to occur. Women become pregnant with or without orgasm.

Intercourse during a menstrual period. I have implied several times in this chapter that a woman will not get pregnant during her menstrual period. To be absolutely correct, however, I must say that although I have never known a woman who conceived during her period, such a thing may be possible, especially if a woman confuses bleeding between periods as a true period. This is such a rare occurrence that I still say it is safe to have unprotected intercourse during a menstrual period. If you want to be 100 percent sure you do not get pregnant, however, it is best to use contraception even during your menstrual flow.

Please understand that I am talking specifically about whether or not it is possible to become pregnant when I say it is "safe" to have intercourse during a woman's menstrual period. There are other considerations. The Mosaic law of the Old Testament forbade couples to have intercourse during that time, and some reports show that women who do have intercourse during their periods are more likely to have endometriosis. A couple must decide for themselves whether or not they will have intercourse during the wife's menstrual period.

944 What about the morning-after pill—is there an effective one?

Gynecologists are frequently asked to supply a pill to use the morning after unprotected intercourse. Such medication taken the day after intercourse has been found to prevent conception most of the time. Recently, a combination of an estrogen and a progesterone, identical to that found in an Ovral birth-control pill and taken two times twelve hours apart, has sometimes been found to work as a morning-after pill if started within seventy-two hours of intercourse. Since no morning-after pill works every time (studies indicate it fails about 20 percent of the time), many doctors have stopped providing them. They are concerned that any medications taken at such an early time in a pregnancy could damage the child. DES was commonly used as a morning-after pill until it was found that DES caused abnormalities in children born to mothers who had taken it during pregnancy. Although DES is a synthetic estrogen, its bad record made all estrogen administration suspect during pregnancy. (Recent studies confirm that taking oral contraceptives early in pregnancy will not hurt the child if the pregnancy continues.)

The major problem with this technique is that it may produce its effect by causing an early abortion. Scientists do not know how the morning-after pill works. It has not been shown to work by causing abortions.

945 Is abstinence a viable choice for an unmarried woman?

Abstinence is the only choice that is 100 percent effective for avoiding pregnancy. I am often asked by unmarried women if abstinence is normal and healthy. I answer a resounding, "Yes." There is nothing about a woman's body that makes abstinence harmful. As a matter of fact, statistics strongly show the opposite. If a woman is not abstinent until marriage, there is a tremendous risk of becoming infected with a sexually transmitted disease because of the widespread STD infection of single males in our society. For those who are not married, abstinence has many advantages. (See Q. 973.)

If a woman has had sexual intercourse as an unmarried person, she can still choose abstinence now. Some call this secondary virginity. Remember that the more sexual partners you have in your lifetime, the more likely you are to become infected with a sexually transmitted disease and therefore to ultimately be sterile or have cancer or sores. You can choose now to be abstinent if you are single.

Sterilization

946 What is sterilization?

A sterilization procedure is an operation on a person's reproductive organs to make pregnancy highly unlikely. This method of birth control is very popular. Annually, 7 or 8 percent of married couples have a sterilization procedure done on either the husband or the wife. About one-fourth of married couples have a sterilization procedure within a year of the last desired child.

Such a procedure can be a great asset to a couple's sexual relationship. After sterilization they can have intercourse without fear of pregnancy and yet without the bother of birth-control pills, foam, condoms, or diaphragms. Many women even find that their sexual responsiveness improves after sterilization.

947 What are the methods of sterilization?

The methods of sterilization are:

Tubal sterilization. A woman may have surgery on her tubes so that an egg from her ovary and sperm in her vagina are unable to make contact.

Vasectomy. A man may have the vasa tied off, which prevents the sperm produced in his testicles from getting into the upper part of his body and eventually being ejaculated during intercourse.

Hysterectomy. Hysterectomy (removal of the uterus) is the only 100 percent effective sterilization procedure, except for removal of a woman's ovaries or removal of a man's testicles. If a woman has "female problems" and is considering hysterectomy anyway, the desire not to have more children can be the deciding factor in choosing to proceed with a hysterectomy.

948 Who should be sterilized, me or my husband?

Perhaps it is because I am a gynecologist that I tend to feel that it is best for the woman to have the sterilization. She is the one whose body bears the risks inherent in pregnancy. If she is sterilized, she no longer has to worry about the risk, even if she loses her husband by divorce or death and remarries. If the husband is the one who has the sterilization and the woman enters into a new marriage, she must again consider what she wants to do about her fertility.

Most studies show that a vasectomy is more likely to fail than a tubal ligation. These studies indicate that about one in a hundred men produce an accidental pregnancy after having been sterilized, whereas after a tubal ligation only about one in five hundred women will become pregnant.

949 How is a laparoscopy sterilization done? Why is it called Band-Aid surgery?

Laparoscopy sterilization is the most commonly used technique for sterilizing women today. It is performed by using a special viewing instrument (laparoscope) inserted into the abdomen. It is not major surgery, and the patient can usually go home from the hospital the same day the surgery is performed. The procedure can be done with a

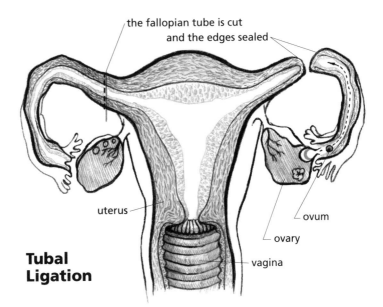

the fallopian tube is cut
and the edges sealed

uterus

ovum

ovary

vagina

**Tubal
Ligation**

local anesthetic, but general anesthesia is normally used.

Laparoscopy is sometimes called Band-Aid surgery, because the incisions required can be covered by a Band-Aid.

To do this surgery, the doctor dilates the cervix, inserts an instrument into the uterus, and lifts it, reaching behind the uterus to get to the tubes. A small needle is inserted in the lower edge of the umbilicus (navel), through which two or three quarts of carbon dioxide gas are allowed to flow into the abdomen. This lifts the wall of the abdomen off the intestines, so the operating instruments can be safely inserted into the abdominal cavity.

Most doctors use the "double puncture" technique, which requires two incisions. One (about one-third inch long) is made just above the pubic bone, and the other (about one-half inch long) is made in the lower edge of the navel. A small amount of pubic hair may need to be shaved for the lower incision. After the laparoscope is inserted through the higher incision, it is used to observe the pelvic structures. Operating instruments, which are used to work on the tubes, are inserted through the lower incision. (See Q. 810.)

After the tubes have been blocked by cautery,

clip, or band (see the following question), the instruments are removed, the gas is allowed to escape, and the incisions are closed.

I normally gently scrape the lining of the uterus at this time (a D&C) and send a sample to a pathologist. Since the cervix is already dilated and the instrument is already in the uterus, it is convenient to test for premalignant or malignant tissue in the uterus. If the tissue is normal, the woman could feel confident that any uterine bleeding she might have during the next year or

Skin Incisions for Laparoscopy Sterilization

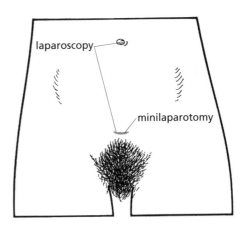

laparoscopy

minilaparotomy

two was not caused by cancer, because cancer does not develop that fast. Many doctors do not do this D&C. They feel that the cost of the tissue examination by the pathologist is not worth it, since the tissue will be normal for most women.

950 How are the tubes blocked during a laparoscopy?

There are three techniques that are used to block the fallopian tubes during a sterilization procedure.

Cautery and division. Cauterization is done to keep the tubes from bleeding when they are cut. After this electrocoagulation has been completed, each tube is cut through where the burn was made, usually about a third of the way from the uterus to the end of the tube.

Hulka clips. These are small clips with a copper spring. They are placed over the middle part of the tube and closed. Pressure keeps the blood flow from going through the part of the tube inside the clip. That part of the tube dies, effectively blocking the tube.

Falope rings. A Falope ring is a rubber-band-shaped piece of silicone that is put around a "knuckled-up" portion of the tube. Such a ring is so tight that it cuts off the blood supply, causing the part of the tube it encircles to die, thus dividing the tube.

951 What is the recovery from a laparoscopy or a minilaparotomy like?

Normally you will be able to go home the afternoon of the day you have the surgery performed. You should be on a liquid diet that evening and have someone stay with you through the evening and night. That night you should get up only to go to the bathroom. Getting up too often can cause small, residual bubbles of air or carbon dioxide gas to rise up under your diaphragm and cause fairly severe pain that you would feel in your shoulders. This is called referred pain; it comes from the diaphragm, but is felt in the shoulders. Even if you stay down as you are sup-

posed to, you may experience some shoulder pains. This is normal.

Your doctor will probably have given you prescriptions for the pain and nausea that often occur after general anesthesia. The pain pills can be helpful for the discomfort from the incisions, the shoulder pain, or for the uterine cramping that occasionally occurs after this operation.

It is normal to have a little oozing of blood from the incisions; it is also normal to bleed from the vagina for as long as a week or two after the procedure.

Starting the day after surgery, you can do whatever you feel like doing, though some women do not feel like doing much. I have had patients ranging from one extreme to the other. One patient went to a party the night of her surgery, but I have had several patients who did not feel well for two weeks after surgery. These latter women were not hurting; they were merely tired and sleepy from the anesthesia.

The average patient who has surgery on Friday afternoon will feel like going back to work on Monday. She may tire after a half-day and need to rest, and possibly do the same on Tuesday, but by Wednesday she will feel like being active a full day.

It is fine to shower or bathe the day after surgery, but I advise patients to wait one week before they resume intercourse, douching, or the use of tampons.

Some patients feel bloated the first few days after this surgery. This is because the intestines do not handle food as efficiently for a few days after surgery as they did before, not because any carbon dioxide gas is still present. All carbon dioxide is absorbed out of the abdomen in only a few hours.

Bruising is common around the incisions. It can extend all the way from the navel to the pubic area, out to the side of the abdomen, and even to the flanks. Some of this bruising is due to the instruments being pushed through the wall of the abdomen, and some is caused by the doctor grasping the skin of the abdomen to lift it up so that instruments can be inserted.

Normally the incisions cause little pain, but it is common to have a slight infection of the incisions. If you notice a little redness and pus oozing out of one or both of your incisions, apply warm, wet towels to the area as frequently as you can. If the area seems to be getting more and more inflamed and tender, call your doctor, who will probably prescribe an antibiotic.

952 What is a postpartum sterilization?

A postpartum sterilization is one that is done immediately after delivery of a baby, or during the next day or two. If you are pregnant and know for sure this baby is the last one you want to have, it is convenient and sensible to have the sterilization done immediately after the delivery.

The only warning I give my patients considering this procedure is that the most risky time in a human's life is the first twenty-four hours after birth. A baby can be born looking normal, but die within the first day because of some major congenital abnormality that was impossible to detect at birth. This happens rarely, but if you feel that you would want another child if your newborn were to die, I recommend that you delay sterilization until at least the next day—or, perhaps more wisely, for about six months. I have seen similar problems occur when husbands have had vasectomies while their wives were pregnant with what they had decided would be their last child. If your husband is considering having a vasectomy done while you are pregnant, be sure that you and he have discussed the possibility of losing your child, either before or after delivery.

Postpartum sterilization can be done following either a normal vaginal delivery or a cesarean section.

After normal vaginal delivery. Immediately after delivery, the uterus is still quite large. The top of it is usually at the level of the navel, making the fallopian tubes, which are attached to the top of the uterus, easily accessible through a small incision in the lower edge of the navel. The doctor merely makes a single incision, reaches in first to one side and then the other, picking up each fallopian tube separately and pulling it through the incision so it can be tied and cut. The small incision is then closed with sutures.

A woman who has had a vaginal delivery and then a tubal ligation may want to stay in the hospital an extra day because of the discomfort of the sterilization, but this is not usually necessary. There is little risk in having this type of sterilization done.

After a tubal ligation, a woman may do anything she would have otherwise done, including nurse her baby. There is no limitation, either in the hospital or after she goes home, that would not have been placed on her by normal recovery from delivery.

After cesarean section. This is the easiest of all sterilizations to do. After the doctor has sewn up the uterus, he or she merely reaches over, lifts each tube with a clamp, ties it with a suture, and cuts away the part of the tube that has been tied off. After tying off the tubes, the cesarean-section surgery is completed as would normally be done. After this surgery a woman may have mild discomfort in her sides, but this is not nearly as uncomfortable as the C-section itself.

953 After a sterilization procedure has been performed, what happens to the eggs a woman produces and to any sperm that enter her cervix?

Both the egg and the sperm die inside the woman's body. The egg usually dies within twenty-four hours after ovulation, and most sperm will be dead within two or three days after entering the woman's body. After they die these cells are absorbed into the body, representing no more than a little added protein. There are millions of cells in a person's body that die and are absorbed and replaced every day. The absorption of dead egg and sperm cells is no different and does not damage a woman's body.

954 What is a vasectomy?

A vasectomy is a surgical procedure that makes a male sterile. It is a fairly simple operation, and it is almost always done with a local anesthetic. A urologist or a general surgeon usually does this type of surgery.

The procedure involves an incision on the undersurface of both sides of the scrotum, about an inch to an inch and a half long. After locating the vasa (the tubes that carry the sperm from the testicles to the internal sexual organs) the doctor ties them off, cutting part of them away. The doctor may cauterize the vasa, put clips on them, or fold the ends back and tie them away from each other. No matter which technique is used, the procedure is still relatively simple.

After a vasectomy a man usually needs to rest for an hour or two and take it easy at home for the rest of the day. He should avoid hard or strenuous exercise for two or three days and should wear some support for his scrotum. Pain pills may be taken as needed. Discomfort ranges from mild to moderately severe, but almost all discomfort should have disappeared after seven or eight days.

A man may have intercourse as soon after a vasectomy as he feels comfortable doing so, but he should use some method of contraception until an examination of his semen shows that there are no sperm present. This may take two or three months.

If a man develops swelling and redness of his scrotum after the vasectomy, he should call his doctor immediately, especially if he begins running a fever.

Vasectomy

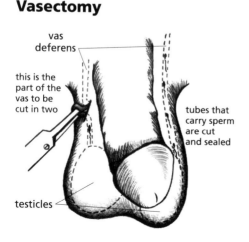

vas deferens

this is the part of the vas to be cut in two

tubes that carry sperm are cut and sealed

testicles

It is estimated that there is a failure rate with vasectomy ranging from about one in a hundred to one in five hundred men. If a couple chooses this method of sterilization, I suggest that they not worry about this extremely low chance of pregnancy. Instead they should enjoy the freedom from worry that sterility affords.

955 Is it possible to reverse a vasectomy?

The chance of fertility after a vasectomy repair is determined by three things: an accomplished microsurgeon, enough vas to repair, and the length of time from the vasectomy to the attempt at reversal (the shorter, the better).

A vasectomy reversal can be successfully performed on most men, and subsequent pregnancy rates are as high as 80 percent. (See also Q. 720–721.)

An Afterword

Good contraceptive techniques are one of the miracles of modern medicine. We can be thankful for them. I would give a warning, though. We can become so accustomed to having total control over everything in our lives that we become disoriented, upset, and angry when our planning goes awry. An unplanned pregnancy can lead to such a distorted statement as that written by a well-known professor and chairman of a major department of obstetrics and gynecology: "Unwanted pregnancy is a disease that should be treated as such."

That well-motivated physician, like many others in our society, seems to forget that it is God, ultimately, who "opens and closes" the womb. If we have done our best to avoid pregnancy and it still occurs, we need to view it as an unplanned blessing and expect a special gift from God in this "accident."

Most gynecologists, including myself, have seen couples who panicked over an unplanned pregnancy and rushed into an ill-thought-out abortion, only to come back a year or so later, unable to achieve pregnancy. Such couples often suffer an agony of self-incrimination for having destroyed a life and, in the process, having possibly destroyed their fertility. I have had many infertile couples who have terminated the only child they had ever conceived and now because of subsequent infertility very likely the only baby they will ever conceive. These people could have avoided all this heartache by accepting their surprise pregnancy as a blessing from God.

However, contraceptive techniques do provide control over most conception and can be a boon to both humankind in general and to individual couples in particular.

13 Sexually Transmitted Disease

Sexually transmitted disease (STD) is a dangerous, rapidly growing, worldwide epidemic. Its most likely potential victims seem to be blissfully unaware that they can get STD.

> It was the age of overindulgence. It was the age for tolerance of anything in anybody. It was the age of fear of imposing one's own social values on someone else. It was the age of the trivialization of sex. It was the age of anti-celibacy. It was the age when early teenage sex was commonplace. It was the age when homosexuality came out of the closet and became almost acceptable to those who once found it intolerable. It was the age of easy, irresponsible oversex, abortion on demand, chlamydia, and genital herpes. It was the age of AIDS.
>
> Not since syphilis among the Spanish, plague among the French, tuberculosis among the Eskimos, and smallpox among the American Indians has there been the threat of such a scourge. Yet, the acquired immunodeficiency syndrome (AIDS) is different from any disease previously seen.
>
> From the introduction to an editorial in the *Journal of the American Medical Association,* June 21, 1985, by Dixie E. Snider, Jr., M.D., titled "The Age of AIDS: A Great Time for Defensive Living."

AIDS is not the only STD that medical experts are concerned about. The Centers for Disease Control and the Federal Health Resources and

Services Administration recently declared war on the more than thirty known STDs infecting and ravaging the lives of Americans. Look at the statistics: One in two single sexually active Americans will acquire STD by the time they are thirty years old. Twelve million new cases of STD occur every year in the United States.

Except for AIDS, STD is usually only a minor problem in men, especially if treated early. Almost all the severe complications of STD are experienced by women. James O. Mason, the director at the Centers for Disease Control in Atlanta, has said, "Sometimes I wonder why the female population doesn't stand up and scream about this."

A woman can have intercourse with a man who has not had intercourse with anyone else for years and still get STD from him. She too can carry STD for years and pass it on in the same way.

The most rapidly increasing cause of infertility and the most common preventable cause of infertility in the United States is infection of the female organs (with resultant scarring), often caused by a usually curable sexually transmitted disease.

Precancerous and cancerous growths of the vulva, vagina, and cervix have increased alarmingly in numbers in the past few years, especially among young women. Research indicates that these conditions are almost always caused by a sexually transmitted virus, the human papillomavirus, the same virus that causes genital warts.

In the following questions we will discuss some general facts relating to STDs as well as the most common forms of such diseases. There are a number of rarely occurring STDs that will be mentioned only briefly.

General Facts about STD

956 What is sexually transmitted disease?

Sexually transmitted disease, or STD, is a term that is used now for what was called venereal dis-

ease a few years ago. Because of the changed sexual mores of our society, these diseases are now the most common reportable infectious diseases in the United States.

STD infections are passed from one person to another by intimate contact. This contact may involve the sex organs, the mouth, or the rectum. The delicate linings of these areas, plus their warmth and moisture, allow the growth of the organisms that are sexually transmitted disease. Because these germs require this type of environment, they are passed almost exclusively by intercourse and other intimate contact between two individuals.

957 Who can get sexually transmitted disease?

The person who contracts a sexually transmitted disease is usually someone who had intercourse with another person who is infected. If you have never had intercourse with anyone except your husband or wife, and he or she has never had intercourse with anyone else and never does so in the future, you are almost absolutely safe so far as sexually transmitted disease is concerned. The only exceptions are extremely rare, such as developing STD from an injection or from a blood transfusion.

No matter what your age or your status in society, you can catch one of these diseases if you violate the above rule even one time. As a matter of fact, a person can catch two, three, or more different sexually transmitted diseases at one time. And it does not matter how neat and clean you are, or whether or not you douche after intercourse; if you have intercourse with an infected person, you can become infected with a sexually transmitted disease.

958 Can a man or woman have a sexually transmitted disease without knowing it?

Up to 85 percent of people who have sexually transmitted diseases have no idea that they have these infections. For example, a classic study done in 1967 by Shapiro and Lentz reported that 85 percent of patients who were proven to have gonorrhea had no symptoms, and recent studies have shown that up to 85 percent of women and 40 percent of men with chlamydia had no symptoms. Many other studies have confirmed this problem with herpes and other STDs.

Syphilis is the second most dangerous sexually transmitted disease (STD). AIDS is the most dangerous. Initially, syphilis merely causes a painless sore. If this sore is inside a woman's vagina, she will not even know it is there. The rash that a few weeks later follows the initial sore may not be severe enough to cause a woman to seek medical help, and when the rash is gone, there may be no symptoms of the syphilis for years. During all this time, however, the woman could give syphilis to a sex partner or to her baby if she is pregnant. (One of my associates was startled when he delivered a baby with congenital syphilis. The mother had no symptoms and was completely unaware of the disease until a routine blood test was done when she was admitted to the hospital for delivery. The baby was infected from the mother and had to be given large doses of antibiotics intravenously. The mother had been infected by the man she had sex with during pregnancy.)

Herpes can be present without symptoms. A major study of herpes reported in the *New England Journal of Medicine* in late 1997 showed that most people with herpes are infectious even when no sores are visible. This means that those who have herpes have the virus present in genital tissues even when they have no outbreak, and can pass the virus to anyone with whom they have intercourse.

A person who has become infected with HIV may not develop any signs of AIDS for many months or years, yet that person can give AIDS to any sex partner from the time of the initial infection on.

In summary, it is estimated that up to 70 percent of people who have sexually transmitted diseases will have no symptoms of those diseases. There may be no way for either one of you to know if the other person is infected without extensive testing, and in this situation what you do not know can hurt you very badly.

959 Will my partner be honest about previous sexual activity from which he might have gotten a sexually transmitted disease?

Men and boys are often not honest about past sexual activity to their current girlfriends. A report in the *New England Journal of Medicine* (S. D. Cochron et al., 1990, 322:774, 821) said that in a survey of 422 sexually active college students, many admitted lying to have sex. More men reported lying than women: 47 percent of the men and 42 percent of the women said that they had not been truthful about how many previous sexual partners they had had. In addition, 42 percent of the men and 33 percent of the women said they would not tell a partner if they had a "one-night stand," and 23 percent of the men and 10 percent of the women said they would not tell a partner if they were currently involved with someone else.

You cannot always trust a person who wants to have sex with you to be honest about past sexual experiences. If a person has had sex with even one person in the past, it is possible that he or she has a sexually transmitted disease. Sexually transmitted disease is so common today that if a person has ever had sex with more than one partner, it is possible that he or she already has a sexually transmitted disease. Interviewing a man before you have sex with him may not keep you safe from STD.

960 I am seventeen years old and still a virgin. I have heard that it is dangerous for a teenager to have sex. Is that true?

Sex for a teenager outside of a mutually faithful marriage relationship is extremely dangerous. Women below the age of twenty are much more susceptible to STD germs. According to the major 1997 report called "The Hidden Epidemic—Confronting Sexually Transmitted Disease" from the Institute of Medicine, there are several reasons for this. Among those are:

1. Women under twenty have changes of the lining over the cervix (columnar epithelium) that make the cervix more susceptible to invasion by both chlamydia and gonorrhea. This is called "ectropion."
2. Young women probably have lower levels of antibodies that protect against the germs of some sexually transmitted disease.

A sexually active fifteen-year-old girl, for example, has a ten times greater chance of developing pelvic inflammatory disease than a twenty-five-year-old. Females under twenty years old who have had PID (pelvic inflammatory disease) are twice as likely to become reinfected as are older women. Tubal pregnancies are one of the leading causes of death of pregnant women in the United States, and women fifteen to nineteen have the highest risk of dying from this problem. Sexually active females under age twenty are three times more likely to have chlamydia than older women.

One study shows that as many as 46 percent of sexually active teenagers are infected with the human papillomavirus (HPV) and, therefore, have an increased risk of getting cancer of the cervix later in life, because the HPV organism causes almost all precancer and cancer of the cervix. (See the chapter on HPV infection.)

Another thing that makes "teenage sex" dangerous is that statistics show that the younger people are when they start having intercourse, the greater the number of sexual partners they will probably have in their lifetime. The more sexual partners a person has, the more risk there is of sexually transmitted disease.

961 Will condoms protect me from sexually transmitted disease?

Studies would suggest that if you have sex outside of marriage, occasionally changing part-

ners and depending on condoms for protection, you will probably become infected with a sexually transmitted disease sooner or later. Condoms give almost no protection against the most common viral STD, human papillomavirus (HPV) infection, and give unreliable protection against chlamydia, an infection that can cause infertility.

Another problem with condom use is that people rarely use condoms 100 percent of the time, and failure of use even one time can allow a person to be infected with STD.

If you are single, sexually active, and using condoms to try to prevent pregnancy and disease, you must use condoms every single time you have sex without fail. (Remember that even then, you are not 100 percent protected from all diseases.) I recently saw a twenty-two-year-old woman who had used condoms every time she had intercourse with the four sexual partners she had had since being a virgin. She still had become infected with the human papillomavirus and as a result had a precancerous growth on her vulva. This sexually transmitted disease had cost her a great deal in time, money, and worry. All experts on human papillomavirus infections agree that condoms give little, if any, protection against this viral infection, the most common STD in the United States.

Usually a couple begins a relationship using condoms, but becomes complacent as the relationship progresses. You tell yourself that this present sex partner is a "nice" person who surely doesn't have a sexually transmitted disease and is surely faithful to you. You may stop using condoms and start using birth-control pills, and, when you do, you are exposed to all the sexually transmitted diseases that person has.

Another aspect of condom use often overlooked is that even if condoms are used, syphilis and genital herpes and other STDs can be transmitted from sores not covered by the condom. In addition, STD can spread from genital/genital contact, from oral/genital contact, or from oral or anal sex. Also, skin-to-skin contact can spread scabies, pubic lice, and HPV.

962 I've heard that the very best technique for avoiding sexually transmitted disease is mutual monogamy? Is that true?

Mutual monogamy (both partners having sex only with each other) is not protective against sexually transmitted disease unless that monogomy means staying with the other person for life. Sandra Samuels, M.D., director of the Rutgers Student Health Services, Rutgers University, Newark, New Jersey, did a study on chlamydia infection that showed astounding results. Dr. Samuels found that 33.3 percent of the men cultured and 37.7 percent of the women cultured had chlamydia infection. When she questioned them about their sexual practices, this is what she found:

One hundred seventy-seven women were questioned as to the nature of their sexual relationships. The majority of women (62.7 percent) reported long-term (greater than six months) monogamous relationships, whereas nineteen of thirty-six men (53 percent) questioned reported multiple casual relationships. Reported lengthy monogamous relationships were not associated with a low incidence of infection either because the partner had been carrying chlamydia for a long time or had had sex with a "third party" at some point, unknown to the patient.

A new sexual partner every six months is not safe mutual monogamy. As a matter of fact, a person who has several sexual partners in his or her lifetime has a dramatically increased risk of getting a sexually transmitted disease.

A classic study reported in the *Journal of the American Medical Association* (1987, 256:10) pointed out that there is a quantum (huge) increased risk of hepatitis B if a person has had more than ten sexual partners in a lifetime. If there is that much greater chance of having hepatitis B, which is not one of the most common sexually transmitted diseases, there is an even higher chance of being infected with other STDs.

I urge you not to depend on your faithfulness to a sexual partner—or his to you—to protect you from sexually transmitted disease. Mutual monogamy will protect against STDs only if you stay with each other for a lifetime. This is called marriage.

963 How can I know if I have a sexually transmitted disease?

You cannot know for sure without seeing a physician. Although your body might show signs of sexually transmitted disease, STD is generally found when a woman who suspects the problem goes to a doctor for testing.

You should ask a physician to test you for STD in any of the following situations.

If you know or suspect that you have been exposed to a sexually transmitted disease.
If you have symptoms that suggest the possibility of a sexually transmitted disease.
If you are certain that you do have STD by the presence of warts, herpes ulcers, and so on.

964 What are symptoms of sexually transmitted disease that my doctor and I might look for?

Some of the symptoms of sexually transmitted disease mimic other diseases; some of them might be noticed by men, others by women. Let's take a closer look at symptoms that *might* be caused by sexually transmitted disease. Men usually have fewer symptoms of STD than women do. Because a man's sex organs are not as moist as a woman's, the STD germs do not proliferate as rapidly and therefore are less likely to present a problem for a man. For this reason, men often do not know they have an STD. Women often do not know they have an STD because their genital organs are internal and the infection can hide inside their bodies.

Some of the possible signs or symptoms of STD that a *man* might notice (or that you might notice about a man) include the following:

1. *Discharge from the penis.* Any fluid (pus, discharge, secretions) from a man's penis other

than urine or semen (ejaculate) is cause to see a doctor. This symptom almost always indicates sexually transmitted disease. Gonorrhea or chlamydia or nonspecific urethritis would usually be the cause.

2. *Burning with urination.* A burning sensation during urination often indicates a sexually transmitted disease. A doctor should be consulted because gonorrhea and even chlamydia can cause this.

3. *Growths in the genital area.* Any growth on the penis or scrotum or in the anal area may mean genital warts or other sexually transmitted infections. (*Any* new growth, *anywhere* on the body should be seen by a physician, although those in parts of the body other than the genitals are less likely to indicate a sexually transmitted infection.)

4. *Sores on the genitals.* Small, tender sores on the genitals may be herpes ulcers. If they are painless, firm, and thickened, they may indicate syphilis. Such sores should be promptly evaluated by a doctor.

Possible symptoms of sexually transmitted disease that *both men and women* might have are:

1. *Skin rashes or sores.* Both syphilis and AIDS can produce skin sores or rashes, and scabies can cause a very irritating rash. Any body rash should be evaluated by a physician.

2. *Enlarged lymph nodes.* AIDS and syphilis can cause enlargement of the lymph nodes all over the body. Some of the more unusual STDs can cause enlarged lymph nodes of the groin.

3. *Long-lasting infections.* Any infections of the skin, lungs, or other parts of the body that do not clear up quickly should be checked by a doctor. AIDS and some other STDs can cause such problems.

4. *Inflammation of a joint.* If inflammation, redness, and swelling are present in a joint (such as a knee or an elbow), a physician should be seen. Gonorrhea can cause such infections. If there is a possibility of sexually transmitted infection, this should be mentioned to the doctor.

5. *Yellow eyes, dark urine.* Signs of hepatitis include the whites of the eyes turning yellow or the urine turning cola colored. Hepatitis B is one of the most common sexually transmitted diseases in the world.

6. *Itching of the pubic hair.* Pubic lice can cause such itching.

Some of the *female* symptoms of sexually transmitted disease include:

1. *Vaginal discharge.* Although a vaginal discharge does not always indicate sexually transmitted disease, if it is excessive, it itches, or it has an odor, it *always* should be evaluated. If the discharge could possibly be caused by sexual contact, that should be mentioned to a physician. Vaginal discharge can be a symptom of gonorrhea, chlamydia, herpes, or even of HPV (cause of genital warts).

2. *Sores on the genitals.* Ulcers of the vulvar area, especially if urination causes discomfort, may indicate herpes. If a sore is slightly thickened and painless, it could be syphilis. Any sore or lump should be evaluated.

3. *Growths in the genital area.* Growths around the vulva, inside the vagina, or around the anus may be genital warts. Treatment is most important, because the virus that causes these warts is the most common cause of cervical, vulvar, and vaginal cancer.

4. *Burning with urination.* Normally, a burning sensation with urination merely indicates a bladder infection. As the urine pours out over herpes ulcers, however, the burning may be quite intense. Whether the burning is caused by herpes or by bladder infection, it should be diagnosed and treated by a doctor.

5. *Lower abdominal pain, especially with fever.* A woman with a gonorrhea or chlamydia infection may carry the germs for many months without symptoms. When either of these germs begins actively spreading in the body, pelvic inflammatory disease (PID) is usually the result, causing abdominal pain and fever. These symptoms should be

checked by a doctor immediately. The sooner an infection of this type is treated, the less likely it is that sterility will result.

965 If I have an STD, should I tell my sex partner?

If you have a sexually transmitted disease, you should definitely tell anyone with whom you are having sex. Doing this gives your partner a chance to decide what he or she wants to do. The partner may want to stop having intercourse until you have been tested not only for the sexually transmitted disease you know about but also for others. (It is possible to have more than one STD at a time.) Generally, the blood tests and cultures that are done for someone with one STD include testing for chlamydia, gonorrhea, hepatitis, AIDS, and syphilis.

A startling chain of events can occur when people do not tell their partners that they might be infected. Public health workers have found as many as two hundred people infected by a sexually transmitted disease from one person who either did not know or did not tell a sexual partner about an STD infection. Because of this, you should tell all the people you have had sex with that you are infected with STD so they can know to be tested.

966 Do I have to notify the health department if I have STD?

Your physician should notify your local health department if you have a reportable STD, and you should insist that this be done. Officials there will sometimes want to talk to you (confidentially, of course) to find out with whom you have had sexual contact, so that these people can be treated and the transmission of the sexually transmitted disease ended.

The sexually transmitted diseases reportable in most states are syphilis, gonorrhea, lymphogranuloma venerium, chancroid, and granuloma inguinale. A few states now require reporting of only gonorrhea and syphilis. Reporting of HIV infection is already required by many states, but not as an STD. This is so health authorities can help you inform past sexual contacts so they can get tested and treated.

967 If I have an STD, will my doctor find it when I have my annual examination?

No. Just as you can have other infections in your body that your doctor will not find unless you have symptoms, so you can have an STD that will not be found unless you have symptoms. Unless the infection produces abnormal discharge or growths in your body, your doctor will not usually suspect that you are infected.

Do not expect your doctor to ask you if you could be infected by STD when he or she sees you for an examination. A doctor will not ordinarily ask this if you seem normal on exam. This is not because of embarrassment. It is because doctors have found that if they ask a patient about STD, the patient thinks the doctor has found a problem that might actually be STD. The other reason is that doctors do not want to imply in any way that they suspect patients of activity that could make a sexually transmitted disease possible.

Obviously it is up to you to tell your doctor if you think you may have been exposed to a sexually transmitted disease.

If you are married and suspect that your husband may have had an extramarital affair, tell your doctor. You can be tested for STD and either have your mind relieved by having negative tests or get treated for any infection that is found.

I have had patients come to me with this problem, saying that they were terribly uncomfortable about discussing STD with me. This is understandable, but let me assure you that doctors do not feel awkward in this situation. Your physician sees and treats this type of problem every day. You should not let your embarrassment keep you from getting help.

HPV—Genital Warts—Condyloma Acuminata

968 What is HPV and how is it associated with genital warts?

Human papillomavirus (HPV) is the most common sexually transmitted infection in America today. Without question, it is the most common sexually transmitted infection that doctors see in their practices.

A study reported in the *American Journal of Diseases of Children* (December 1989, 143 [12]: 1443–1477) showed that the sexually transmitted virus was found in 38 percent of sexually active females aged thirteen to twenty-one. A more recent study reported from the Student Health Center of the University of California at Berkeley reported that 46 percent of the sexually active women attending their gynecology clinic were found to have infection with HPV.

HPV infections can be classified into three different situations. The first situation is the presence of genital warts caused by the HPV virus. The second situation is precancerous and cancerous changes of the cervix. The third situation is you can have the HPV organism in your vagina without having any warts or any abnormality of your Pap smear. When this happens, there are tests that can show whether or not the virus is present in your body. These tests, one of which is called ViraPap, look for the HPV viral material called DNA. There is usually no reason to have this test done, because there is no treatment to get rid of a virus.

If there is no wart or abnormal Pap smear, there is no advantage in knowing that the virus is present. Even when a woman is treated for warts or an abnormal Pap smear, and is well, the virus can still be present in her body for months or years, perhaps lifelong (according to some experts).

969 What are genital warts, and what causes them?

Although the warts of condyloma acuminata look and act like ordinary warts, they are termed "vene-

real or genital" because of their location (on the parts of the body normally associated with sexual intercourse), and also because they are a different type of wart from that which occurs on other parts of the body. Rarely, a person can acquire genital warts without having sexual intercourse, in spite of the implications of the name. The virus that causes these warts can occasionally be present on other parts of the body, especially the fingers, and can be spread by touch. In an adolescent or mature woman, however, infection by condyloma acuminata, or genital warts, is usually a result of sexual intercourse.

Studies now show that condoms do little to stop the sexual transmission of this virus. It gets on the scrotum, the labia, the thighs, and in all the sexual secretions. If a person has sex with someone who is HPV infected there seems to be almost no way to avoid infection.

970 What are the symptoms of genital wart infections?

A woman usually notices a small bump or several small bumps on her vulva, either on her labia between her anus and the lower part of her vagina or around her anus. As time goes by, there may be more and more growths in this area. The warts may grow together and increase in size, sometimes becoming as large as a fist, or they may occasionally clear up spontaneously for no known reason.

Warts may, and often do, grow on the walls of the vagina. They may also grow on the cervix. Genital warts, however, rarely grow outside a woman's moist, warm genital area.

Genital warts often cause a vaginal discharge, and warts on the vulva will occasionally become mildly infected and sore and will bleed if scratched or handled roughly.

971 How are genital warts treated and cured?

If the warts are ulcerated or are unusually hard or abnormal, the first thing the doctor would do is send a biopsy of one of them to the lab. Once the doctor has established that the growths are genital warts, there are several different methods of treatment.

Treatment of other existing medical problems. Certain conditions seem to aggravate genital warts. Vaginal infection is a primary offender. If you have a vaginal infection (trichomoniasis or some other type), this should be treated first to decrease the amount of vulvar moisture, allowing greater success in treating the warts.

One factor that encourages the proliferation of genital warts is having a partner with an uncircumcised penis, since a man who has a foreskin often has warts under it, especially if he practices poor personal hygiene. Other contributing factors are pregnancy, taking birth-control pills, a faulty immune system (such as in a person who has had a kidney transplant and is on drugs for that), or diabetes. Patients who have one of these conditions will occasionally find their warts more easily controlled when the associated condition is eliminated or carefully controlled.

Podophyllum. A mixture of 10 to 25 percent of podophyllum in tincture of benzoin can be dabbed on each wart. Podophyllum should be washed off the morning after treatment. In spite of this, a woman's skin can become severely irritated. Usually the severe irritation is because the warts are being killed by the podophyllum. I have found that women who have the worst reaction to podophyllum are more likely to have all their warts disappear with one or two applications than women who have almost no irritation from its use. Theoretically, the absorption of podophyllum by a wart causes the cells of the wart to stop growing and to die. This may happen with some warts but not with others.

The doctor will usually have a patient return for treatment each week until her warts are gone. If they are not gone after two to four treatments, most doctors will then use another method of treatment.

Ordinarily, only a small amount of podophyllum is used in the vagina or on the cervix because absorption of this medication can make a woman sick. It must not be used in pregnancy because of the possibility of absorption of the chemical into the mother's body, with resulting damage to the fetus. One of the following techniques is used if a patient has extensive vaginal or cervical warts or is pregnant.

Laser. The laser can be used to evaporate warts. This can be done with a local anesthetic or with general anesthesia in an outpatient operating room if there is a large number of condyloma. If a patient has genital warts that are not clearing up after several treatments with podophyllum or with any other technique, I strongly advise her to see a doctor who uses the laser.

Since use of the laser is expensive, even those doctors who use it will usually try podophyllum first. If the warts do not respond to that treatment, the doctor will then suggest use of the laser, which is quite safe, even during pregnancy.

Trichloracetic acid (TCA or Nevitol). This acid can be applied to warts on the vulva, in the vagina, and on the cervix. Sometimes it is effective and sometimes it is not. If it does not work after two or three applications, the laser or one of the following methods should be tried.

Freezing. A "freezing," or cryotherapy, machine can be used to freeze warts. A local anesthetic will be administered for warts on the vulva. Warts in the vagina can sometimes be frozen without anesthetic. I have not found cryotherapy very useful for warts, because each wart must be frozen separately down to its base. Although some doctors use this technique with some success, I prefer the laser.

Cautery. Using a local anesthetic, your doctor can burn off, or cauterize, warts. This is a good treatment, especially if you have only a few warts. If you have many, the laser works better and will leave you much less sore from the treatment. The problem with cautery is that it will also burn normal skin around and under the warts, causing soreness and scar.

5-Fluorouracil. This drug, which is used in cancer chemotherapy, can be mixed in a cream base for use in the vagina or on the skin. It can be useful for warts, but it will almost always cause a great deal of vulvar irritation. Your doctor may prescribe this for you; it is safe to use and may work, but you should expect considerable vulvar irritation while using it. Some protection from the irritation may be obtained by covering the wart-free portions of your vulva with a heavy coat of Vaseline.

Interferon. This is a protein substance produced by the human body's cells in response to viral infections. New recombinant DNA techniques have enabled manufacturers to produce interferon so that a person who is infected with a virus can be injected with a larger amount of interferon than that person's cells would ordinarily produce. Interferons seem to inhibit the production of viruses in cells. For several years, physicians have been injecting with interferon genital warts that were resistant to other treatments. It was hoped that this would be the ultimate treatment for genital warts but, unfortunately, interferon does not always eliminate all the warts. About 75 to 80 percent of such patients do get better, however, and some experience complete relief with this drug. The treatment is expensive and requires multiple injections in the skin under and around the warts.

Surgery. Occasionally, whether you have only one persistent wart or several large ones, surgery will be necessary. Local anesthetic may be used, but usually general anesthesia is necessary. Surgery of this type can involve a combination of cautery, laser, and cutting of the warts.

972 Are genital warts dangerous during pregnancy or harmful to the fetus or newborn baby?

If the warts have grown so large that they block the birth canal, a cesarean section will be necessary. If you are pregnant and your warts are growing rapidly, the laser may be useful. *Do not let a doctor use podophyllum on you while you are pregnant because it can cause problems for the baby.* Occasionally the warts grow so fast during pregnancy that cesarean section is the only method for delivery.

Many doctors now believe that a baby born to a woman with genital warts in her birth canal has a greater chance for developing vocal-cord papillomas (warts) in the first six to eight months. Since 60 percent of babies with these papillomas have been born to mothers with genital warts, if you have such warts when you deliver your baby, it is probably best to have the baby examined by an ear, nose, and throat specialist about six months after delivery to make sure there are no polyps present. If your baby develops hoarseness, chronic cough, and has trouble making sounds, he or she should definitely be examined for polyps by such a specialist. I know of two children who have had more than a hundred operations for this horrible problem. Fortunately, this is a rare problem, especially in light of the fact that HPV is so common.

Diane B. Ritter reported at the International Society of STD Research in 1987 that the HPV virus was found in the amniotic fluid in twenty-one women who were pregnant. When the babies were born, they seemed healthy and were unaffected by this virus; however, they were under observation from birth since HPV is a cancer-causing virus and it is possible that they could later develop cancer somewhere in their bodies. (Remember that women with HPV on their cervix may not get cervical cancer for years.)

973 How are abnormal Pap smears associated with sexually transmitted disease?

The evidence now seems conclusive: More than 93 percent of cancer of the cervix and precancerous changes on Pap smears are caused by HPV (1997 NIH consensus report on cervical cancer). Although there may be a slight chance that these conditions are sometimes not due to this sexually transmitted disease, most of the time they are. Abnormal Pap smears that are truly precancerous or cancerous almost never occur in women who have not had intercourse. (It is possible, but unusual, for a woman to get the wart virus from warts on other parts of her body or from, for example, a man's fingers or from some other source.)

524

If you develop a precancerous or cancerous Pap smear, it does not mean that your husband has had a recent affair. If either of you had sex with even one other person at some time in the past (even if it was twenty or thirty years ago), the HPV could have been acquired and brought into the marriage and now cause your problem.

If neither you nor your husband ever had sex with anyone else, it is very unlikely that you ever need to worry about having a Pap smear that shows precancerous or cancerous changes.

It is important to note that I am speaking of "truly abnormal" Pap smears. Many Pap smears are reported back as showing questionable cells, and most of the time these are due to irritation of the cervix. This type of mildly abnormal Pap smear is very common, and it is not a sign of any type of sexually transmitted disease. If subsequent evaluation shows there is precancerous or cancerous change, that is usually due to the HPV. (See the section about the cervix.)

There are some startling illustrations of the relationship between sexual activity and abnormal Pap smears. Some men cause every woman with whom they have sexual intercourse to develop a precancerous-type abnormal Pap smear (they are carrying a very aggressive type of HPV). The second wives of men whose first wives died of cervical cancer are more likely to develop precancerous Pap smears than second wives of men whose first wives died of some other cause. This is probably because these men are carrying an HPV organism. There are more than seventy different types of HPV. It has now been shown that a woman is more likely to get cancer if she has been infected with types 16, 18, 31, 33, and 35.

Perhaps you have had intercourse with someone other than your own mate, or you know that your spouse has had intercourse with someone else. What is done, is done; what is important now is that you have a Pap smear taken every year. Cervical cancer usually develops slowly, often over a period of one to seven years. Before the actual development of the cancer, abnormal changes can usually be detected in a Pap smear.

The goal of a Pap smear is not only to detect cancer but to detect precancerous cells before they turn into cancer.

The effect of the papillomavirus in causing cancer is not limited to the cervix. Papillomavirus also seems to be the cause of the alarming increase in precancerous and cancerous growths on the vulva of women in our society, especially in younger women. (See Q. 584–588.)

Herpes

974 What should I know about herpes?

There is not only a lack of information on this subject, but there is a wealth of misinformation. We know that 30 percent of sexually active single Americans have been infected with this common sexually transmitted disease.

A person's primary, or first, herpes infection usually follows a standard pattern of development. Tingling, itching, and burning of the infected area of the vulva are usually the first symptoms of herpes infection in a woman. After two or three days that area will become red and form one or more fluid-filled blisters that rupture over a one- or two-day period, leaving small ulcers at the site of the infection. These ulcers can be extremely painful and tender to touch. They can be so painful, in fact, that they make intercourse impossible and occasionally so severe that urination cannot be tolerated.

Almost all people will have enlarged lymph nodes in their groin with their first herpes infection. They will often develop aching muscles, fever, nausea, and headache.

Many patients with a primary herpes infection need to be seen on an emergency basis by their physician because of the severity of the pain or because of inability to urinate. Large doses of Zovirax (acyclovir, an antiviral drug) are usually given, and occasionally a catheter will be inserted into the bladder so that the patient can go home and rest until healing begins to take place.

Primary lesions of herpes usually last two to four weeks from start to total healing without acyclovir; with acyclovir, the healing time can be cut in half.

975 Can I have herpes more than once?

Most people who have had a primary herpes infection will have recurrent infections. These are not new infections but merely a reoccurrence of the original herpes. Precisely because secondary infections can continue to develop and there is no medication to permanently stop them, herpes is considered "incurable." Remember that medical science has never yet cured any virus, even the common cold. Actually, acyclovir can be taken on a daily basis and, for more than 75 percent of people with herpes, it will suppress their recurrent episodes of herpes. As long as a patient's herpes responds to acyclovir, and she continues to take it daily, she can be totally free of any outbreaks.

These recurrent episodes of herpes are often triggered by emotional events, menstrual periods, intercourse, or trauma to the vulvar area. As the years go by some patients will have fewer and fewer secondary lesions until, finally, they will have no secondary lesions. Some people, however, will continue to have secondary herpes outbreaks for years.

One unfortunate aspect of taking acyclovir on a continual basis is the expense. Acyclovir (in 1996) cost about $1.25 a capsule, and most women need to take two, three, or four a day to keep their herpes suppressed. This can become a significant financial drain.

Secondary outbreaks of herpes are almost never as uncomfortable as the first episode. Normally with secondary lesions the area becomes slightly red and forms the little fluid-filled blisters that break, leaving small, tender ulcers that clear up within a week or two.

In the past we thought that if a person had a primary infection with herpes but no secondary infections, he/she probably developed an immunity to herpes. Now we know that most people continue to have outbreaks and continue to be infected, but the recurrent sores are often too tiny to notice.

976 What organism causes herpes?

Genital herpes is usually caused by a virus called herpes simplex type II, which is almost always passed by sexual contact. Fever blisters are usually caused by herpes simplex type I, a virus usually caught in childhood.

In the past few years, research has shown that infections by these two viruses are not nearly so distinct and separate as once had been thought. About 15 to 20 percent of infections of the female genitalia are caused by herpes type I, and many of the so-called fever blisters that men and women have are caused by herpes type II.

For the one who suffers from herpes, it doesn't matter if she has type I or type II. The symptoms are the same, the frequency and recurrence are the same, and the reason she got it is the same— by having sex with someone who had that type of herpes.

Condoms do not give reliable protection from herpes because herpes sores can be present on parts of the body not covered by the condom.

977 How dangerous is herpes during pregnancy?

If a baby is delivered through the birth canal while a woman has an active herpes sore (caused by herpes type I or type II), the herpes virus can get into the baby's body and infect the child. This infection in a baby is much different than it is in an adult. Herpes normally spreads all through the baby's body, and there is a strong possibility that the baby will be severely damaged or will die from the infection. (See Q. 388.)

978 How is herpes treated?

No virus infection, including herpes, is curable, because viruses do not respond to antibiotics as do pneumonia, gonorrhea, and other bacterial infections. A number of treatments have been tried for herpes, but only one type has been found useful: Zovirax (acyclovir) and similar drugs. When a patient uses these drugs in capsule, injection, or ointment form with the first infection, it decreases the severity and duration of that infection and diminishes the possibility of a secondary outbreak.

If acyclovir or similar drugs are used with a secondary infection on a regular basis, it shortens the healing time for even these sores.

The injectable form of these drugs can be used only in the veins and is best reserved for those with a severe primary herpes attack, infants with herpes infections, or herpes patients who have abnormal immune systems. This includes people who are on drugs to suppress their immune system (such as people who have had organ transplants and AIDS victims).

The ointment form of acyclovir may be used for any herpes outbreak. It speeds healing and decreases pain, but to be most effective it must be applied every three hours day and night until the sores have healed.

If victims are being bothered by recurrences of sores more than once a month, they may find that taking the capsule form of one of these drugs daily either stops the sores from developing or decreases their frequency. People with recurrent herpes have now taken Zovirax for as long as three years. While there seems to be no danger in taking the drug for long periods of time, your doctor will want to counsel you about this.

979 Why is herpes so feared if it is not dangerous?

Herpes occurs in all strata of society, including the middle and upper classes who normally have significant control over their lives. Herpes represents a loss of control that is unlike many other sexually transmitted diseases that can be effectively cured. Herpes continues to come and go at will, bringing with it obvious external changes to a woman's body that she can see and feel.

Except for the risk to a newborn baby (a risk mostly eliminated by a C-section), there is really no more danger from a herpes infection than from a bad cold. Of course, a herpes infection usually indicates that a person has had intercourse with someone else who had herpes. The first episode of infection can occasionally be quite painful, and recurrent outbreaks can be aggravating.

In spite of the relative "harmlessness" of herpes, one study showed that 84 percent of people with herpes reported occasional episodes of depression, with half of those describing the depression as being "deep." About 70 percent of people with herpes noted a feeling of social isolation. About 53 percent said that they consciously avoided potentially intimate situations, even during periods free from herpes outbreaks, and 10 percent of this group said that they had stopped having intercourse completely.

The lesson that herpes teaches is that in spite of the fact that we would all like to be able to do anything we want to without any consequences, our actions always do have a result, sometimes an undesirable one. If you have intercourse with someone who has had intercourse with someone else, you can catch herpes.

Once herpes is a part of your life, however, there is nothing to do but accept it. There is certainly nothing to be gained by being angry about it. Accept the condition as a natural consequence of the choice you made; realize that herpes is not going to damage you physically, and go on with your life from there. If you are unmarried and do not have herpes, the best course of action is to avoid the heartache and expense of this aggravating disease by postponing sex until marriage.

If you are considering marriage, and either you or your loved one has had herpes, you need to tell the other. The one who has not had herpes may develop it after the marriage.

If you or your husband has had herpes in the past or have occasional herpes outbreaks, I recommend that you not worry about protecting yourselves from each other. If one picks up the infection from the other, it will make no difference in your relationship in the long run since herpes does not actually damage the body. It is better to "share the problem" than to spend years with the tension of trying to keep the uninfected partner from contracting herpes constantly in the back of your mind as you try to develop a normal, healthy sexual relationship. This would probably be a useless endeavor anyway.

Gonorrhea

980 What is gonorrhea?

In a book that he wrote with other specialists (*Benign Diseases of the Vulva and Vagina*, 3d ed. [Chicago: Yearbook Medical Publishers, 1989]), the late Dr. Herman L. Gardner said, "Gonorrhea is probably the most important bacterial infection in the civilized world." It is caused by a bacterium called *Neisseria gonorrhoeae*.

As many as 100,000 women are made sterile by gonorrhea each year in the United States. About 20 percent of women who contract gonorrhea and develop pelvic inflammatory disease (PID) have continuing pelvic pain for years, and there are a million episodes of PID per year in women in this country. It has been estimated that gonorrhea costs the women of our country two billion dollars per year.

Although you may have heard similar facts many times before, let me urge you to consider them carefully. Gonorrhea is not something that "always happens to somebody else."

If you are having intercourse with anyone other than your husband, or if your husband is having intercourse with someone else, you can get this infection—and it can be devastating to your female organs. It was primarily the realization of the effect of this infection on American women that caused William M. McCormack, M.D., of Downstate Medical Center, Brooklyn, New York, to write an article

titled "Sexually Transmitted Disease: Women As Victims" (*Journal of the American Medical Association*, July 9, 1982, pp. 177–178). Dr. McCormack states:

The economic costs are staggering. The direct cost of treatment of acute PID in the United States has been estimated to be more than six hundred million dollars annually. The total cost of this disease is upwards of three billion dollars a year.

The human costs, although less easily qualified, are also of enormous importance. Almost one million women are treated for PID in the United States each year, necessitating more than two hundred twenty thousand hospital admissions. Involuntary sterility, ectopic pregnancy, and chronic pelvic pain are important sequelae.

The long-term complications of PID result from the healing process. As the inflamed fallopian tubes heal, they may become completely occluded, resulting in involuntary infertility. The risks are substantial. Patients who have a single episode of gonococcal PID have a six percent chance of becoming infertile. The prospects for future reproduction are even poorer for women who have had multiple episodes.

Partial obstruction of the fallopian tubes predispose to ectopic pregnancies. Women who have had PID are six to ten times as likely to have an ectopic pregnancy as are women who have not had this infection. Adhesions that occur during the healing of acute PID can result in chronic pelvic pain if the adhesions compromise the ovaries, the bowel, or other tender pelvic structures. Chronic pelvic pain occurs in ten to twenty percent of patients.

Condoms may give some protection from this infection, but only if used consistently. This means 100 percent of the time—no exceptions. If not used in this way they are almost as useless as if not worn at all.

981 Will I know if I have contracted gonorrhea?

The incubation period for a woman exposed to a man with gonorrhea is usually from two to seven days, but it can be much longer. *Incubation* refers to the length of time from the deposition of germs into the woman's vagina to the time when symptoms of an infection appear. Women can carry the germ around for weeks, months, or years, only to develop PID later or to pass the germ on to an unsuspecting sexual partner.

The 80 percent of women who carry gonorrhea without knowing it are like human time bombs. The germs can suddenly start proliferating, several months or years after exposure.

One of the major problems of a woman carrying the gonorrhea germ without being aware of it is that she can pass it to any sexual contact that she has until her gonorrhea is found and treated.

If a woman is infected with gonorrhea her physician may or may not find that she has a slight, pus-like discharge on routine exam, but the patient herself might not know that anything is wrong at all.

If there are symptoms, they may include the following:

Vague, mild symptoms. There may be a messy, watery vaginal discharge. Burning with urination may occur. These symptoms may be present without any symptoms of infection of the uterus, tubes, or ovaries.

Symptoms of PID (pelvic inflammatory disease). The first symptoms of a gonorrhea infection often are those caused by inflammation of the pelvic organs: low abdominal pain and fever. Once these symptoms start, they usually get continually worse, with the pain increasing and the fever going higher until effective treatment is begun. The typical patient with such an infection walks into the doctor's office or the emergency room bent over at the waist because of the pain.

Combination of symptoms. A woman who has intercourse with a man who has gonorrhea often develops a vaginal discharge a few days later. This is a symptom of vaginal and cervical infection by the gonococcus organism. When she has her next period, the gonorrhea germs will start growing profusely. They will ascend into the uterus and invade the uterine lining, tubes, and ovaries.

982 Is gonorrhea dangerous during pregnancy?

The gonorrhea germ cannot ordinarily get into the pregnant uterus, but if the organism gets into the baby's eyes during delivery, it can cause blindness. Fortunately public health laws in most states now require that an antibiotic solution be put into the eyes of all newborn babies to prevent this catastrophe. Since up to 80 percent of women with gonorrhea are unaware of it, many newborns would be blinded if this law were not in effect.

983 Can gonorrhea be cured?

The gonorrhea germ can be killed with antibiotics, but antibiotics cannot erase the scarring that might have been caused by the infection before treatment. In the past, penicillin was adequate for the treatment of gonorrhea, but this is changing. Organisms resistant to penicillin have developed, and patients with gonorrhea must now be treated with more effective antibiotics that will kill these resistant strains.

The general recommendation now is that gonorrhea be treated with an antibiotic called ceftriaxone. There has been little resistance of gonorrhea organisms to this antibiotic since it was introduced in 1985. If this antibiotic is not used, and a patient has a resistant strain of gonorrhea, the infection can continue to spread until the right antibiotic is used. Also if a patient is not also treated with tetracycline (or similar antibiotic to kill chlamydia), her PID may continue to rage, since a large number of people who have gonorrhea also have chlamydia. (One study showed that 26 to 48 percent of females with gonorrhea are also infected with chlamydia.)

Chlamydia

984 What is chlamydia?

Chlamydia (pronounced cle-mid'-ee-a) is the most common reportable infectious disease in America. About 30 to 40 percent of some groups of teenagers are infected with chlamydia bacteria. There are at least four million Americans newly infected each year. It is a major cause of pelvic inflammatory disease (PID). Chlamydia is three to five times more common than gonorrhea, and it is often a "silent sexual disease."

Many women who are infected with chlamydia will have no fever and no pain, but their tubes and ovaries are being damaged just the same. As a matter of fact, a study reported in *Fertility and Sterility* (February 1990, 55.2 by H. J. Thejls, et al.) showed that of the women who had surgery and had signs of past infection in the tubes and ovaries, only one-third of the patients had ever had any symptoms of PID. Two-thirds never had pain, fever, or discomfort with the infections. Most of them had probably been infected by chlamydia and did not know it.

985 What are the symptoms of chlamydia infection?

As with gonorrhea, a woman may have a vaginal discharge, a Bartholin's gland abscess (see Q. 591–593), or infection in the pelvis (PID) that causes pain with or without fever.

A man who has a chlamydia infection, as with gonorrhea, may have a urethral discharge and burning with urination, inflammation of the prostate gland, or he may have no symptoms.

986 Is chlamydia dangerous?

The major problem of chlamydia infection is that it, like gonorrhea, can cause pelvic inflammatory disease. This germ, however, is even more likely to cause sterility than is gonorrhea. One report says that 12 percent of women who have one chlamydia infection in their fallopian tubes will become sterile; after a second infection, 25 percent of the patients will be sterile; and after a third infection, 37 percent of patients will be sterile. Additionally, 20 percent of women will have pelvic pain that persists for months and even years after only one episode of chlamydia infection. The infection is now considered so dangerous and so rampant that any woman having extramarital intercourse should have a chlamydia test each time she has a new sexual partner or anytime her sex partner has intercourse with someone else.

987 Is chlamydia dangerous during pregnancy?

Although this germ does not get into the uterus during a pregnancy, it is a common cause of infection in the uterus after delivery. A woman who has fever, pain, and tenderness of her uterus after delivery may have a chlamydia infection.

Newborn babies can develop an eye infection if the mother has chlamydia in the vagina. In fact, it is the most common cause of eye infection in young babies. It rarely causes blindness, but it can.

Babies can also develop a mild pneumonia from the chlamydia organism. For a normal baby this is not dangerous, but for a baby weakened in some way (for example, prematurity) this infection can be a problem. As many as 30,000 newborns each year develop this pneumonia. Chlamydia can also cause middle ear infections in infants.

988 Can chlamydia be cured?

As with gonorrhea, the chlamydia organism can be killed with antibiotics, but the scars that have already developed will not clear up after antibiotics have been taken. Antibiotics commonly used to kill gonorrhea germs usually do not kill chlamydia. If chlamydia is present, tetracycline is usually quite effective in curing the infection. If a woman does have pelvic inflammatory disease, even if seemingly caused by gonorrhea, she should also be treated for chlamydia at the same time since chlamydia and gonorrhea coexist so often.

989 How can I keep from getting chlamydia?

The best method of prevention is to wait until you get married to have intercourse and then to have intercourse only with your husband and he only with you. The use of foam and condoms every time you have intercourse outside of these guidelines has been found to offer unreliable protection for a woman's fertility. This means that if she has intercourse outside of marriage, even if she uses condoms carefully, she may become sterile.

Syphilis

990 What is syphilis?

Syphilis is one of the most dangerous sexually transmitted diseases. It is now at a forty-year high in our country.

Syphilis is acquired almost exclusively by sexual contact with someone who has syphilis. About 50 percent of those who have such contact with a syphilis carrier will become infected from one act of intercourse.

Because of the danger of syphilis, it is extremely important that you have a blood test for syphilis after you have had intercourse with anyone who might have a sexually transmitted disease. This test should not be done until twelve weeks after exposure because it is not until then that the test will reliably be positive. If you have the test done sooner and it shows a negative result, you will, perhaps falsely, think you are free of the disease.

991 What are the symptoms of syphilis?

Without a blood test, syphilis is extremely difficult to detect in women. The first sign is usually a painless sore, called a chancre (pronounced "shanker"). This sore is located where the infectious organisms penetrate the body and usually develops from ten to ninety days after intercourse with an infected person. It may look like a pimple, a blister, or an open sore, and it is usually not tender. This chancre usually goes away in two weeks, causing many people to think, falsely, that they are cured. This is never the case, however. The disease has only gone "underground" in the body to begin its insidious work.

A woman may have a chancre in her vagina or on her cervix where it is not visible. Since it is painless she would be totally unaware of its presence.

Once the primary syphilis stage is past, a woman will not show signs of syphilis for six weeks to six months. Secondary syphilis then develops, causing fatigue, fever, hair loss, skin rash, a warty-looking growth (condyloma latum) around the vulva or anus, and/or enlarged lymph nodes in various places around the body. Secondary syphilis can also cause hepatitis, kidney disease, meningitis, changes in the bones of the body, and eye infections.

This process can go on in a woman's body for four years before she enters the third or tertiary stage of syphilis, which develops in about 25 percent of patients who have not been treated. Tertiary syphilis is a common cause for aortic aneurysms and disease of the heart valves. It is also a common cause of insanity.

Blood tests can determine the presence of syphilis, or a smear of the secretions from a chancre or from the skin lesions of secondary syphilis can show the presence of syphilis germs.

992 Which organism causes syphilis?

Treponema pallidum, a spirochete-type microbe, causes syphilis. This organism is 100 percent susceptible to penicillin and has never developed any resistance to that antibiotic.

993 Is syphilis dangerous?

Syphilis is a horrible, destructive disease. Untreated, it can cause insanity, nerve damage, blindness, deafness, and heart disease. It can also cause miscarriage, stillbirth, congenital abnormalities of a newborn, and even death to both mother and child. (See next question.)

994 Does syphilis affect pregnancy or the newborn?

If a woman has untreated syphilis while she is pregnant, she can have a miscarriage. If she does carry the pregnancy to term, the baby can be so badly infected that it is stillborn. Even if this does not happen, the baby may be born with bone deformities, tooth abnormalities, or blindness. A baby can be born looking normal but with the syphilis organism in its body. If untreated, the baby can later become blind, deaf, paralyzed, insane, or have an early death.

There is one note of assurance, however: If you discover that you have syphilis before the eighteenth week of your pregnancy, you can be treated and the baby will almost certainly not be affected. Syphilis organisms generally cannot cross through the placenta from you into the baby until after the eighteenth week of pregnancy. It is for this reason that most states require a blood test for syphilis early in pregnancy. An untreated mother has only one chance in six of delivering a healthy baby. If your state does not require syphilis testing in pregnancy and your doctor does not order it, I would suggest that you ask for it. (See Q. 339–341.)

One of my associates had a patient who, at the start of her pregnancy, had a negative syphilis test. When she was admitted to the hospital for delivery, however, a routine hospital admission syphilis blood test was positive. After delivery, the baby was tested by having a

spinal tap and was found to have syphilis in its spinal fluid, and because of this required intravenous antibiotics.

If you suspect during your pregnancy that your husband might have had sex with someone else and brought syphilis home to you, be sure to tell your doctor so that you can be tested and treated as early in pregnancy as possible. This could decrease the medical care your baby will need after delivery.

995 Can syphilis be cured?

Yes. Antibiotics will always kill the germ that causes syphilis, although they will not reverse any damage that might have already occurred in a woman's body if treatment has been delayed.

If you have had intercourse with someone who has syphilis, it is best to go ahead and have a dose of antibiotics (4.8 million-unit shot of procaine penicillin with one gram of probenecid by mouth to make the penicillin more effective). There is no need to wait for a blood test to see if you have syphilis before you get treatment since there is a 50 percent chance of your becoming infected. If you get treatment the syphilis infection would be cured before it could cause any damage to your body. (There are alternate antibiotics available if you are allergic to penicillin.)

996 Can I get syphilis more than once?

Yes, you can. Any time there is a possibility of your having been infected a second time, you should get tested and/or treated. You do not develop immunity in your body to syphilis.

997 How can I keep from getting syphilis?

As with other sexually transmitted diseases, the way to prevent infection is to refrain from intercourse before marriage and then to have intercourse only with your husband, who has intercourse only with you.

If you do have intercourse with someone else, use foam and condoms. There is some indication that this might keep you from becoming infected with this particular sexually transmitted disease initially, but if you continue to change sexual partners—even though you are using barrier contraceptives—you will probably get a sexually transmitted disease. And remember, if the syphilis sore is on a part of the body not covered by a condom, there is no protection.

Other Sexually Transmitted Diseases

998 Are there other STDs?

Yes, there are. Three of these "minor" sexually transmitted diseases are: chancroid, lymphogranuloma venereum, and granuloma inguinale. These diseases are classified as "minor" for two reasons. One is because they occur so much less often than any of the STDs mentioned previously, and the other is because they are confined to the area where the infection starts and grows, rather than affecting the rest of the body. Because of this they are not usually life-threatening.

Chancroid. This is often a highly contagious infection caused by a bacterium called *Hemophilus ducreyi*. It was described as a "relative medical curiosity in the United States" until the past few years. Dr. Anna-Barbara Noscicki, at a 1990 meeting, reported, "Ten years ago a dramatic resurgence began. In 1989 more than 5000 cases were reported. Large outbreaks have occurred in California, Florida, Texas, and New York. Most of these infections have been in men." This is often a disease of the sexually promiscuous. It is more common in underdeveloped countries of the world, and a lack of personal cleanliness seems to be a major factor in developing the infection. The disease is first seen as a small bump (in women this is usually located on the labia, most often near the clitoris), which turns into an abscess, and finally into a tender ulcer. The ulcer is shallow and looks infected. If neglected it can spread to the inner thighs and groin areas and can be present for years. Recent studies have shown that antibiotics with sulfa in them, such as Septra or Bactrim, are effective against this organism. Erythromycin can also be used to treat chancroid.

Lymphogranuloma venereum (LGV). This infection produces enlarged lymph nodes in the groin and a rectal infection that causes a discharge of mucus and pus from the rectum. Enlarged lymph nodes around the anus may be present as the first sign of infection in a woman. This is especially so in people who engage in rectal intercourse. Occasionally these lymph nodes can break open and produce draining ulcerations. The agent that causes LGV is thought to be a form of chlamydia, but the usual chlamydia organism does not cause this disease. Antibiotics are effective against this organism. Tetracycline, sulfa drugs, and Erythromycin have been found useful.

Granuloma inguinale. This sexually transmitted disease is only mildly infectious and is extremely rare in the United States where fewer than one hundred cases are reported each year. The infection is most commonly reported among rural black people in the southeast United States.

This infection starts as a small, painless bump on the genitals. If it is not treated, it gradually enlarges over a period of months, finally developing a velvety, beefy-red growth. Tetracycline seems to be the best antibiotic for this disease.

Since a cancer of the vulva can look much like this infection, it is important that the doctor do a biopsy to make sure that the growth is not cancerous. Enlarged lymph nodes are not usually present with this infection, making it different from the previous two STDs. Granuloma inguinale is caused by a microorganism called *Donovania granulomatis*.

Chancroid, lymphogranuloma venereum, and granuloma inguinale were not often seen in this country in the past. They are more commonly seen today. Though not terribly widespread, these infections can be dangerous and destructive— they should not be taken lightly. They can cause enlargement of the sex organs, stricture of the intestines with blockage of the intestinal tract, and even, rarely, death. A person with one of these diseases will know something is wrong and should see a doctor for diagnosis and treatment.

999 What are "crabs" and pubic lice?

Crabs and pubic lice are the same thing. Unlike most of the other STDs, this condition is not dangerous, but it certainly can be disconcerting. Pubic lice are small parasites that can be seen without magnification. They live in the hairy areas of the body and most commonly occur in adults in the genital hair. Pubic lice are usually passed by direct contact with the pubic hair of an infected person. These organisms can, however, be picked up from bed sheets, clothing, or towels.

This infestation usually causes extreme itching in the area where the lice are present, but some people have no symptoms.

The treatment for pubic lice is a shampoo such as Kwell, which contains a lice-killing medication that will get rid of the organisms. Fortunately the treatment is easy and always works. The treatment should be repeated one week after its first use. Also all underwear, bedclothes, and pajamas should be washed at the same time during that week. It is important that both you and your sexual contact be treated.

The lice that live in a person's pubic area are different from those that infest the hair on the head. Generally pubic lice stay in the pubic hair and head lice stay in the area of the head. If a woman has pubic lice, she does not need to wash her hair with the same medicated shampoo that she uses in her pubic area.

If you are pregnant (or think you might be) and have lice, see the section in this book about drugs and pregnancy. You will need to take precautions in treating this problem.

1000 What is scabies?

Scabies is a condition caused by a mite, a parasite that burrows under the skin and causes itching.

The infestation can exist in the skin folds of the body, and on the genital areas, on the fingers, wrists, and nipples, and even in the navel. The primary problem associated with scabies is severe itching wherever the mite is present in the skin.

When a doctor is examining a patient who has itching and small bumps in the areas of skin typically infested by scabies, he or she will examine the skin with a magnifying lens. If the doctor finds the burrows caused by the presence of the mites, a definite diagnosis of scabies can be made.

Several types of medication can be applied to the skin to kill these parasites. This infection is not dangerous, only very annoying.

1001 Is hepatitis a sexually transmitted disease?

Most of us do not think of hepatitis as a sexually transmitted disease, but sexual contact is one of the major ways it is spread.

There are a number of hepatitis viruses. Hepatitis B is much more commonly passed sexually than are the other hepatitis viruses. In fact, hepatitis B is one of the most prevalent sexually transmitted diseases in the world. It is the ninth major cause of death worldwide. It causes cirrhosis and cancer of the liver, and it can pass from a mother to her baby during delivery.

Most obstetricians now routinely test all patients for hepatitis B during the early part of pregnancy because if the mother is a carrier of hepatitis B and that is known, the baby can be immunized immediately after birth and be protected from becoming infected. (See Q. 322.)

It has been shown that if a person has ten or more sexual partners in a lifetime, he or she has an enormously increased risk of having a hepatitis B infection.

The hepatitis B virus can be present in saliva, blood, urine, stool, menstrual blood, vaginal secretions, and other bodily secretions. It has been shown that in a group of people who have hepatitis B, one-third of their spouses will develop hepatitis, while only 2 percent of the other household contacts will develop it. There is also a high incidence of hepatitis B among prostitutes, homosexuals, and patients attending sexually transmitted disease clinics.

1002 Can vaginitis and vaginal yeast infections be sexually transmitted?

These problems can be sexually transmitted. (See Q. 602–607.)

Yeast infections (monilia vaginitis, candida vaginitis, fungus vaginitis). Monilia vaginitis can be passed from a woman to her husband. It is rare for a man to be the first to develop this infection and then transmit it to his wife. A monilia infection is not a sign that a husband has been unfaithful because the organism is often present in a person whether or not he or she has had sex.

When I treat a patient who has a monilia infection, I encourage her to continue having regular intercourse. As she uses her medication, some of it will get on her husband's penis and treat him at the same time.

Monilia infection in the man can produce an irritation on his genitalia, of his groin areas, and of his inner thighs ("jock itch"). A man can use the same medicine that his wife uses for her infection. All he needs to do is rub this cream on himself two times a day. He will normally get well sooner than his wife because his genitalia are not as moist as his wife's vulvar and vaginal tissues.

Monilia vaginitis is not dangerous, but it is irritating. The primary problem a woman will have with monilia vaginitis is itching on her vulva.

One of the first signs that a woman who is infected with HIV is progressing to AIDS is a monilia vaginal infection that does not respond to treatment. If she has had sexual activity that could have caused her to get AIDS, and she has a monilia vaginitis that she cannot eliminate, she should mention to her doctor that there is a possibility of HIV infection so that she can be tested for it. (See Q. 605–606.)

Trichomonas vaginalis vaginitis. If a woman develops trichomoniasis, she and her husband must both be treated with Flagyl because if a woman has "trich," her husband also has it. If she is treated and her husband is not, he can give the infection back to her as soon as she stops her antibiotics.

Though trichomoniasis is normally passed by intercourse, it is quite common for a woman to get this germ on her hands from someone else and then transfer it to her vagina by touching her vulvar tissues.

The important thing is that once a woman develops trichomoniasis, she *and* her husband be treated in order to get rid of the problem.

The primary symptom of trichomoniasis is vulvar itching. Three very significant new discoveries about *Trichomonas vaginalis* are first, that it probably can cause pelvic inflammatory disease (PID). (See Q. 603.) Second, it can cause premature labor in pregnant women. Third, it can cause a greater susceptibility to HIV.

Bacterial vaginosis (BV). This infection was once known as gardnerella vaginitis or hemophilus vaginitis. It is found primarily in sexually active women, and though it is not always transmitted sexually it is considered a sexually transmitted disease. There is no question, though, that if a woman has this infection, her sexual partner will have it, too. To get rid of the infection, both partners must be treated. A woman who has BV can have a profuse, thin, gray-green discharge accompanied by a foul odor. There is usually no irritation or itching of the vulva. Treatment by Flagyl (metronidazole) 500 mg, twice a day, for seven days for both husband and wife, usually works. Clindamycin, 300 mg, twice a day for seven days, is usually effective treatment. An important new finding about BV is that it is probably a cause of many premature deliveries. Because of this, obstetricians are being much more vigilant in testing for and treating pregnant women with this problem. (See Q. 604.) Also, a woman infected with BV is more susceptible to becoming infected with HIV.

Acquired Immunodeficiency Syndrome

1003 What is AIDS? What is HIV?

The virus that causes AIDS is human immunodeficiency virus (HIV). Men and women who acquire this viral infection will often have a brief, mild flulike illness that lasts for a few days and goes away. If their body has, in fact, been invaded by HIV, however, that virus will never, as far as we know, go away. There have recently (1996) been a few children whose bodies seem to have become free of the virus. If indeed this ever happens, it is rare. When people have been infected by HIV, they are said to be "HIV positive" because their blood test is positive for antibodies to HIV.

HIV will almost always begin its relentless destruction of the immune system once a person is infected. When this destruction becomes extensive enough, the immune system becomes vulnerable, and the disease AIDS begins.

The symptoms of AIDS (acquired immunodeficiency syndrome) may be vague at first. Previously healthy people begin having such nonspecific signs and symptoms as feeling listless, fever of unexplained cause, marked weight loss, diarrhea, and enlarged lymph nodes in several areas of the body. In this weakened state the body is susceptible to diseases that usually occur only in older, debilitated people or in people whose immunity is otherwise altered, such as transplant recipients who are on immunosuppressive drugs.

AIDS, therefore, is a collapse of the body's immune defense system, resulting in death by rare forms of cancer, pneumonia, or other overwhelming infections. This collapse is due to a virus that actually destroys the body's immune system, making it vulnerable to a wide range of other diseases.

Once a person has become HIV positive, he or she is then almost always infectious to any sexual partner for the rest of his or her life. In addition, if HIV positive persons give blood or pass bodily secretions to another person, it is possible for that other person to get the HIV virus from them.

1004 Who in the United States is most likely to have AIDS?

Male, sexually active homosexuals and drug users still make up the bulk of patients who have been infected with the HIV virus, but this is gradually changing. The virus is being spread through heterosexual transmission—from male to female and from female to male.

In 1997 the CDC reported that 19 percent of those with HIV were women. The significance of this is that the HIV organism has escaped the homosexual and drug world into the heterosexual world of the person who is having sex with someone down the street, in the office, or at the university.

In the early days of AIDS, it was thought that a promiscuous homosexual lifestyle or contaminated blood transfusions were necessary for a person to acquire AIDS. Studies today, however, show that is not true.

AIDS is now, in part, merely another sexually transmitted disease. However, it is one that kills almost every teenager, every coed, every person that becomes infected. There have been 375,000 reported deaths from AIDS in the United States as of 1997, according to the Centers for Disease Control.

One of the saddest aspects of AIDS is that women can pass it to their babies, either during pregnancy or at delivery. About one-fourth of babies born to women with HIV infection will have congenital HIV, and most of these babies will be dead within two to three years after delivery. If a pregnant woman with HIV infection is treated with AZT, her baby has a better chance of not becoming infected. In addition, the 7,000 HIV-infected women who deliver babies each year will die. That means all their babies will be motherless. Many will be orphans because their fathers will also die of AIDS. And, many of the babies will die too.

Although science is producing some medical relief for people who have become infected with AIDS, it is still incurable. It is sad that many people are continuing to ignore the health warnings and guidelines that would keep them from getting AIDS.

The only HIV-infected people who could not have avoided it are those who received it by blood transfusion, those who had intercourse with a marriage partner who was unfaithful, health-care workers who got it from patients, patients who got it from health-care workers, and a very few other groups. If people in our society would not use drugs and would not have sex outside of marriage, AIDS would be a problem for very few people.

There are some unsettling problems on the horizon having to do with AIDS. An HIV-2 has been identified in several countries. This means, of course, that the AIDS virus is mutating. It is hoped that the same drugs that control HIV-1 will be effective against HIV-2 and, as it appears, HIV-3, etc.

In addition, HIV is already showing some resistance to AZT. Fortunately, new drugs are emerging. DDI (didanosine) has now been approved and DDC (zalcitabine) is being tried for the treatment of AIDS.

AZT, the medicine that slows the progress of the disease, will cost approximately $3,000 a year. When the virus progresses into AIDS, the cost of the additional medications necessary for good care becomes staggering. The emotional cost is even higher. And finally, a person who becomes HIV infected knows that he or she is living with a death sentence.

Because you can get HIV from any men you have sex with (if they are carriers of HIV), I urge you to decide now not to have sex until you get married. If you have already had sex, don't have it again until you are married. If you are currently in a sexual relationship, determine now that if you break up with this man, you will not have sex with another man till he marries you. If you are concerned that you (or your partner) might have become infected with HIV, be tested for it as soon as possible.

An article in *AMA News* (June 1, 1990) can be a good warning to you:

> More than one-third of a group of HIV positive women continued to engage in unsafe sexual practices, despite having received intensive, repeated, HIV related education. Education efforts aimed at stemming transmission will be ineffective in the face of such strong denial, irrespective of intelligence or education level. Patients who are clearly in denial regarding their HIV status reported continued regular unprotected sex with several (HIV) negative partners, including fully informed spouses.

Studies show that this type of activity is as true for men as it is for women. You would think that if someone cares for another person, he or she would be honest about the possibility of being infected with HIV (or at least use some protection). Studies show over and over again, however, many of those people infected with HIV do not protect those with whom they have sex.

You must protect yourself, and I encourage you to do so by making a decision now not to have sex again until you get married and when you are married never have sex outside of that marriage relationship.

An Afterword

Whether or not we accept the fact that God created our bodies or that he has anything to say about how we use them, it seems reasonable to learn how our bodies function best. One way to do this is by observing what happens to other people; then we can develop guidelines for our own activity.

Let's review a few things.

> AIDS is a frightening new disease. It has no cure and results in death. It exists only because of sexual promiscuity and intravenous drug use in our world, and it infects more heterosexual men and women every month.
> Precancerous and cancerous growths of the cervix are now epidemic in our society. They almost never occur in virgins or in married women when neither husband nor wife has ever had intercourse with anyone except each other. The virus that causes genital warts seems to cause precancerous and cancerous

changes of the cervix; spread of this virus (HPV) is primarily by sexual intercourse.

One of the most common causes of infertility in our society is PID (pelvic inflammatory disease), usually caused by gonorrhea or chlamydia. People who get these infections are permanently sterile 10 to 20 percent of the time after only one infection.

Syphilis, if untreated, can lead to multiple, severe health problems. Worse, if a woman's syphilis has not been treated, it can lead to severe congenital abnormalities in any baby she might deliver.

STD infections are often present without symptoms. One can have intercourse with a person who has not had intercourse with anyone else in years and still become infected with a sexually transmitted disease from that sexual partner.

If the pattern of sexual activity we engage in has the potential for cutting out from under us the basics of life itself—health, fertility, and longevity—it seems reasonable to reevaluate that pattern. Albert Camus said: "What is natural is the microbe. All the rest—health, integrity, purity . . . is a product of human will, of a vigilance that must never falter."

I hope the facts discussed in this chapter will help you to be more satisfied with your sexual lifestyle if you are engaging in sex only in marriage. I urge you to reevaluate and change your sexual activity if you are engaging in sex outside of marriage. I hope you do not have to experience an irreversible process in your body that can affect you for the rest of your life.

If you contract one of these diseases, you can survive. Perhaps you can live with the infertility that you might experience from an episode of PID, but the regret and frustration of such an experience can affect you for the rest of your life.

Do not expect to hear much about this problem from your physician. Most physicians are afraid of sounding moralistic to their patients. They are so reluctant to come across this way, in fact, that they do not treat sexually transmitted disease as they do other infectious processes. There are laws, for example, in most states that force a person to be quarantined if he or she has infectious tuberculosis.

Most doctors treat STD differently, however. They almost never recommend that an infected person stay away from others so that the disease spread can be stopped. The emphasis is usually on treatment of the disease rather than on prevention.

The one practice that will absolutely stop the spread of sexually transmitted disease is for men and women to have intercourse with no one until they are married, and then only with their husband or wife. Of course, remarriage increases a person's sexual contacts, but this would be minimal when compared to the sexual exposure many in our society have today.

Perhaps we need some motivation other than fear of damage to our bodies from sexually transmitted disease to accept the validity of reserving sex for marriage. Could it be that the motivation we need to help us treat our bodies right might come from the One who made our bodies in the first place? I think so.

I believe that God made me and therefore knows how I will function best and how I will be happiest. He has written an "Owner's Manual" for the human being: the Bible. Just as I look in my Ford's owner's manual when I want to know how my car will function best (because it was written by the people who made my Ford), so I look into the Bible to see how my psyche and my body will work most efficiently.

The Bible has some specific guidelines about sexual function:

Marriage should be honored by all, and the marriage bed kept pure, for God will judge the adulterer and all the sexually immoral (Heb. 13:4).

Therefore what God has joined together, let man not separate (Mark 10:9).

Husbands, love your wives, just as Christ loved the church and gave himself up for her ["died for her"] (Eph. 5:25).

You shall not commit adultery (Exod. 20:14).

The wife's body does not belong to her alone but also to her husband. In the same way, the husband's body does not belong to him alone but also to his wife (1 Cor. 7:4).

God gave them over in the sinful desires of their hearts to sexual impurity for the degrading of their bodies with one another (Rom. 1:24).

God knows what will provide us with the happiest, healthiest life. His guidelines concerning sex say that we will enjoy sex most if we reserve it for marriage. In spite of that, some of us will try to use sex in ways outside God's guidelines. If we do, not only will we eventually have greater emotional instability and problems than we might otherwise have had, but we may also contract disease.

God knows we have a need for intimacy—he created us with it. But we will not find that intimacy by engaging in sexual intercourse. As a matter of fact, Dr. J. Dudley Chapman of Ohio University College of Osteopathic Medicine recently pointed out that "the sexual revolution with its emphasis on performance has caused some people to shy away from intimacy." We can enjoy true sexual intimacy only by developing a loving relationship with a person of the opposite sex, by becoming committed to him or her, and then becoming intimate with him or her in marriage, the environment God planned for sexual intimacy.

This is what God meant when he said, "A man will leave his father and mother and be united to his wife, and they will become one flesh" (Gen. 2:24).

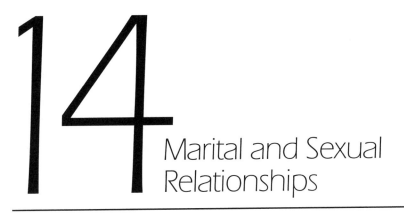

14

Marital and Sexual Relationships

Although this book is concerned primarily with the physical aspect of a woman's body, the sexual and relationship aspects of a woman's life are vitally important. Concerns about marital and sexual relationships: frustrations with husbands, a divorce, or grown children's marital problems dramatically affect our lives. You may be experiencing some soul-wracking emotions. If you are, you need to seek the cure for the spiritual and emotional "cancer," just as you would search diligently for treatment of a physical malignancy.

If you have a good marriage, do not blissfully assume that you will live happily ever after. If you are wise, you will do the things necessary to keep future problems from developing in your relationship with your husband. A good marriage takes a lot of work, sacrifice, and tender loving care. Such a marriage is worth the work, however, because the satisfying, harmonious, and secure relationship that characterizes it can help provide the environment for everyone in the family to develop to the maximum of their God-given potential.

Those who are trying to decide whether or not they want to get married and be committed to marriage may argue that since there are so few happy marriages in our society they would be better off not getting married. I feel that just as a woman should not get married only because society expects her to, so should she not avoid marriage because she fears the problems that society says exist in marriage. If she lives her life based on fear of what "might happen" she would never move away from home, drive a car, get married, or have children. For you who might fear marriage I am glad to report that statistics show the majority of happily married people consider their marriage partner to be their best friend, 75 percent of people entering their first marriage will remain married into old age, and married people have higher levels of sexual satisfaction than unmarried people.

It is important that if a woman does choose to get married, she not do it expecting her husband to fulfill all her needs completely. In her book *The Joy of Being a Woman*, Ingrid Trobisch says (p. xiii), "No man will ever be able to satisfy completely the innermost desires of a woman's heart for love, beauty, and shelteredness. I believe it is possible to live a full life, whether single or married, in spite of unfulfilled desires. We can only look to the One who says: 'My purpose is to give life in all its fullness' (John 10:10)."

Marriage can never be "perfect" since it reflects the imperfect natures of a man and woman. It can, however, provide the stage, direction, and raw materials for the emotional and spiritual growth of the couple.

Some Basic Marital Principles

1005 What can I do to help make sure I develop a good marriage or to improve the marriage I have?

The suggestions that follow are not all-inclusive, and you may not agree with all of them. They are, however, principles that many counselors who deal with marriage problems see couples frequently violating. I hope these suggestions can help you avoid some common problems in marriage. They may improve your marriage if you use them as a pattern to change things that need changing.

Never consider divorce as an option. Most problems that occur in life can be solved. Present-day technology has shown us that solutions can be found to seemingly impossible problems. This holds true for marriage, and yet we tend not to believe it. If we enter marriage considering divorce as an eventual option, when we encounter problems, which we definitely will, divorce will seem to be the only solution. Leaving even the possibility of divorce at the marriage altar will free our minds to find other solutions to the problems that inevitably will surface.

There may be times when you will want to bail out of your marriage. If you and your husband deny yourselves the option of ever considering divorce, you will spend your intellectual and emotional energy in working out your problems. This will greatly increase the chance that you and your husband will enjoy a long and happy life together.

Realize that no two people are perfect for each other. I am not saying that God has not chosen two people to be man and wife, but rather that those two people are neither perfect in themselves nor perfect for each other. Marion and I have often said that without our commitment to each other and to our God, we could have ended up in the divorce courts. Although our personalities are very different, with the help of God we have been able to work with our differences and find an exceedingly happy relationship.

Expect—but don't push—change. You should never enter marriage planning to make changes in your husband later. You should realize, however, that neither you nor he will stay the same person you were when you married. You will both change. It is important to accept this reality even though you do not know what changes the future may hold. If you have been married for a long time, you are probably quite aware that you are not the same person you were on your wedding day. Marriage is a constant process of adaptation to and acceptance of each other, and this flexibility is one of the things that adds spice and life to the marriage relationship.

Learn to love. Amazing to the Western mind is the fact that many marriages in the world are still arranged by the parents, often the two people not meeting more than a few weeks prior to their marriage. In many of these marriages the couples learn to live together and to love each other. Although most of us would probably deny it, we still have a Hollywood approach to love in our society, characterized by talk such as "falling in love" usually "across a crowded room." There will be times in your marriage when you do not feel love for your spouse. It is important that you know this beforehand, so that you will not think that all hope is gone. You can learn to love again, even when you feel that you have lost the spark that you had when you got married. In fact, it is only when you come to the point of losing the short-lived, emotional spark that you can start developing the deep, abiding, warm, and mature love that characterizes the sound marriage we all desire.

Sacrifice and compromise. Marriage is not a fifty-fifty proposition. It is a ninety-ten arrangement whereby the husband and wife both must give 90 percent and expect only 10 percent in return. I believe that this is one of the key elements in having a happy marriage. To be willing to give more than you get requires discipline, and both discipline and giving are completely opposite to the values society seems to be teaching us today. It is impossible for a person to be happy without giving, sacrificing, and compromising. If we try to find fulfillment by "getting," we will find that the more we receive, the more we want, and that there is no end to that cycle. Our only hope for happiness is in "giving," and our only hope for a good marriage is in being willing to sacrifice and give for our spouse. Amazingly, with that attitude, both partners usually end up receiving more than they expected!

Don't misuse pride. Pride is one of the most damaging forces in a marriage. Men in particular often find it difficult to say, "I'm wrong," or "I'm sorry." That attitude is caused by pride. Likewise, women are being told that if they "give in" to their husbands they are retreating from their rightful position as modern women. This too is a problem of overblown pride. Neither husbands nor wives can afford to tolerate unbending pride in themselves if they are to have a good marriage.

Never entertain the thought of being unfaithful. Most husbands or wives do not wake up suddenly one morning and say, "Today I am going to destroy my life, my marriage, and my children and have an affair." They are more likely to allow dissatisfaction to incubate, to grow, and then to produce the action that tears their homes apart. Once planted, the seed of lust or desire toward someone other than a mate can grow by leaps and bounds, nurtured by feelings of injustice, frustration, and self-pity. It soon becomes a full-grown plant, choking out any good fruits of the marriage and ultimately destroying the whole with its clutching, tearing tentacles. Just as the tallest mountains are moved one shovelful at a time, so adultery becomes reality one thought at a time. An improper thought rejected, however, will be quickly replaced by a better thought, and those of us who truly desire a good marriage ultimately learn that truth. We deliberately refuse the luxury of planting the seeds of self-indulgence, and choose instead to nurture the growth of our marriages. It is a matter of conscious choice.

Treat your mate as your best friend. Sadly, the people we love the most are often the people we treat the worst! We would never treat the people we work with or strangers on the street the way we all too often treat our families. Not only should the Golden Rule be in effect in our homes, but we should handle with the tenderest care the relationships that are of utmost importance to us.

Leave mother and father. A marriage in which either partner is still emotionally dependent on a parent is headed for trouble. A healthy marriage requires emotionally mature people. If a husband or wife is still dependent on his or her parents, that person is functionally immature and childish. Any person in a marriage who has this type of dependency should get counseling immediately if the problem cannot be solved.

Have a spiritual commitment together. A spiritual commitment creates a lasting foundation for the home. A mutual commitment to God gives the family security and a common purpose. God instituted marriage and the home, and on this foundation we can be assured of being in a God-ordained institution from which we can work out his will in our lives.

Realize the importance of sex. A marriage is not just a spiritual or emotional partnership. Marriage is also quite definitely a physical relationship. The Bible reveals how God integrated the physical aspect of marriage (including nakedness) into the sanctity of the home:

> A man shall leave his father and his mother, and shall cleave to his wife; and they shall become one flesh. And the man and his wife were both naked and were not ashamed.
>
> Genesis 2:24–25 NASB

And from the Song of Solomon 7:10–12 (NASB):

> I am my beloved's,
> And his desire is for me.
> Come, my beloved, let us go out into the country,
> Let us spend the night in the villages....
> There I will give you my love.

It is sometimes easy to focus on improving communication and solving problems and to forget about the importance of working on improvement of the sexual relationship in marriage.

Communicate. In his book, *Why Am I Afraid to Tell You Who I Am?* (Allen, Tex.: Argus, 1969), John Powell shares the following tremendous insight (pp. 43–44):

> Harry Stack Sullivan, one of the more eminent psychiatrists of interpersonal relationships in our times, has propounded the theory that all personal growth, all personal damage and regression, as well as all personal healing and growth, come through our relationship with others. There is a persistent, if uninformed, suspicion in most of us that we can solve our own problems and be the masters of our own ships of life, but the fact of the matter is that by ourselves we can only be consumed by our problems and suffer shipwreck. What I am, at any given moment in the process of my becoming a person, will be determined by my relationships with those who love me or refuse to

love me, with those whom I love or refuse to love.

> It is certain that a relationship will be only as good as its communication. If you and I can honestly tell each other who we are; that is, what we think, judge, feel, value, love, honor and esteem, hate, fear, desire, hope for, believe in and are committed to, then, and then only, can each of us grow.

These words eloquently emphasize the importance of communication in marriage. They also explain why destructive, unproductive, or nonexistent communication in a marriage can become intolerable and damaging. We would all agree that talking with a spouse is a higher priority than watching TV, but we sometimes find it hard to make the decision to turn off the TV to discuss a problem or just "visit" with each other. When we compare the ultimate value of TV with talking together as husband and wife, it is incredible that there is any difficulty in making the right decision.

Be willing to get help. From the day a couple is married, they need help. There are many sources of outside support; don't be afraid to learn from parents, trusted friends, or your pastor. If you and your husband develop some knotty problems you cannot untie, don't be afraid or ashamed to go to a psychologist, psychiatrist, counselor, or a member of the clergy for counsel. If your pastor, priest, or rabbi does not feel competent to counsel you, he or she will probably be able to suggest a professional counselor. It is important that you like your counselor and that you share a mutual value system. If a counselor suggests activities or solutions that offend your morality or values, you should find another source of counsel.

It is much better to go to a counselor for solutions to a problem when it starts rather than waiting until it has become ingrained.

Invest time and work. It is hard to overemphasize the importance of this particular aspect of marriage enrichment, yet it is one of the most neglected areas. Husbands and wives seem to feel that a good marriage should exist without working at it—but it will not. Men and women work at their jobs, in their homes, and at clubs or schools. It seems that we are willing to work at everything except our marriages and families. It is small wonder that in some cities there are more divorces than marriages.

Unfortunately, it is easier to pretend that a marriage is good than to spend time and effort fixing it. Yet couples must allow adequate time for the marriage relationship, even if it requires turning down a higher-paying job, or social and club activities. This "sacrifice," in the long run, will make for a happier life and marriage. Money cannot produce happiness in our later years, nor can fame. In fact, they seem merely to complicate life.

Envision the future. Each of us needs a vision of the years ahead and a willingness to invest whatever it takes to insure as happy and peaceful a future as possible. Much time, work, and dedication must be expended on a marriage today, to make it "profitable" in the future. It is nice to know, as the years go by, that our investment will pay rich dividends in a deep, close relationship with another human being who loves us and whom we love in return, who needs us and whom we need, and who is our best friend.

forms of communication between husband and wife. Physical intimacy should communicate the love, emotion, and commitment that each has for the other. Sexual intercourse is an almost unbelievable combination of emotional and physical communication between two people. Even more marvelous than this is the fact that such a union can produce a baby who is, in a true sense, the "one flesh" that two people become when they have intercourse.

It seems clear that from the beginning God created us as sexual persons with the ability to have intercourse as a way to express and experience the deepest form of personal relationship with each other. In addition, and just as important, is the ability to reproduce ourselves by that act. Because of this, it seems clear that no marriage can reach its highest potential for a loving, happy relationship between a husband and wife without a healthy, fulfilling sexual compatibility.

Preparing for Marriage

1006 When you say, "Realize the importance of sex," does that mean you believe that a couple's sexual relationship is a primary factor in marriage?

Yes. As a matter of fact, it is important enough to spend most of the rest of this chapter discussing.

Obviously one of the primary functions of a woman's body is sexual activity. This is evident not only by the way that the body is made, but also from statements in Scripture in which sexuality is discussed. Many sections of the Bible point out the importance of the physical/sexual aspect of married life.

There is no foolish naivete about a woman's body, about marriage, about sexuality, or about sexual intercourse in the Bible. God did not design one part of the body to be more important than another, nor did he create "good" parts and "bad" parts. Every part of a woman's body is important and was designed to be properly used.

Sexual intercourse is one of the most intimate

1007 What do I need to know about sex if I am about to get married?

Contrary to prevailing modern opinion, if you have not had intercourse before marriage, you have a head start in your marital sexual relationship over the woman who has already had intercourse. It is even better if neither you nor your husband has had intercourse before. You will be able to develop patterns of sexual activity together, unhindered by "comparisons" to former partners, sexual hang-ups carried over from past experience, guilt from former sexual activity, or physical problems (including infertility) that may have resulted from sexually transmitted disease or abortion.

I encourage you to read books about sexuality and sexual intercourse. One particularly good book is *The Joy of Being a Woman* by Ingrid Trobisch. In this book the author says, "The secret [to sexual fulfillment and happiness] lies in the self-acceptance of the woman as a woman and especially in saying Yes to her body with its special ways of experiencing life" (p. 7).

Trobisch's discussion of the wife's sexual involvement in marriage includes this statement: "This confidence in herself and complete trust in the sheltering love of her husband will enable her, figuratively speaking, to be able to jump off a cliff without any doubt in her heart that her husband will be there to catch her." It is important to develop that type of trust in your husband and acceptance of yourself as a woman that will enable you to have this abandonment of yourself to your husband in sexual intercourse. The end result is not self-deprecation in "giving yourself" to your husband, but rather the total fulfillment that comes with your emotional and physical immersion in a relationship with someone whom you love and trust implicitly.

If you have had sexual intercourse before marriage, it is best to try to put behind you any past experience and preconceived ideas about intercourse and enter marriage with an open mind. This will allow you and your husband to develop your own personal approach to your sexual interaction.

One of the most pleasant surprises about sex is that a husband and wife never achieve perfection. There is always an improvement or variation that can become a rewarding part of sexual relations, even when a couple has been married fifty or sixty years!

1008 Is it important to have a physical examination before marriage?

Yes. Consulting your doctor before marriage is a good idea for several reasons. If you are a virgin, a pelvic examination will reveal any abnormalities you may have: a hymen that might be too tight for intercourse (see Q. 12 and 600), a growth on an ovary or the uterus, or a major abnormality that might signal an infertility problem. If you have had sexual intercourse before, the physician can per-

form tests to see if you have any detectable sexually transmitted disease. The physician cannot tell just by the physical exam whether or not you have a sexually transmitted disease. If you think that there is any possibility that you might have a sexually transmitted disease, tell your physician so appropriate testing can be done. Even if you do not think it is likely, if you have had intercourse before, I suggest you ask the doctor to test your cervix for chlamydia and gonorrhea and to do blood tests for syphilis, hepatitis B, and HIV. If your fiancé has had sex before, he should also see a doctor and have the same tests.

A major reason women see a doctor before marriage is for counsel and advice concerning contraception. You might find it helpful to read chapter 12 before seeing your doctor for a premarital exam. Being knowledgeable and prepared for your appointment will allow you to utilize your time with the doctor much more effectively. If you have a good idea beforehand what kind of contraceptive you want to use, you can ask the doctor about it and he or she can give you a prescription if necessary.

In addition to performing the physical examination, most doctors will encourage you to discuss your attitudes concerning sexuality. If you are aware of having any hang-ups, say so. Your doctor can answer your questions and will refer you to a counselor if you need further information or advice about marital and sexual relations.

If you do have sexual problems or hang-ups, you should not feel guilty. Our perception of sex is a result of input from our families, our peers, what we read, movies we have seen, and so on. In one sense we are not really responsible for the way we feel, but we are responsible for allowing distorted views and misinformation to persist in our minds.

1009 Is premarital counseling really important?

Because there seem to be so many strikes against marriage today, expert premarital counseling is advisable. Marriage truly is wonderful but it is not the ethereal, live-happily-ever-after life that a couple might expect, and good counseling can prepare them for that reality. It will also underscore the truth that marriage takes hard work, sacrifice, and humility.

The human tragedy of divorce is everywhere around us, and each divorce represents an incredible amount of pain. The problems that lead to divorce can start at any time in a relationship between a man and a woman, even before they get married.

I encourage you to talk to your pastor, priest, or rabbi about premarital counseling. Take advantage of the opportunity to avoid some of the pitfalls of marriage. Learn more about your future mate before you marry him, so that you are not taken by surprise in the early, fragile days of your marriage. Such counseling can teach you how to have a oneness in marriage that truly is thrilling.

I also encourage you to read books and/or attend seminars. An excellent book by Michael J. McManus is *Marriage Savers* (Grand Rapids: Zondervan, 1995). Also check with your church about "Engaged Encounters," a weekend retreat that has been helpful to many engaged couples.

1010 Is a good knowledge of male and female sexual anatomy important to marriage?

It is vital that you know about your own and your husband's sex organs and their function. This information is important not only for the actual sex act but also for sex-related matters such as contraception, pregnancy, delivery, and so on.

In a wonderful little book, *Better Is Your Love than Wine*, by Jean Banyolak and Ingrid Trobisch (Downers Grove, Ill.: InterVarsity, 1979), this intuitive statement appears (p. 19): "The act of love is an intimate encounter of the whole masculine person with the whole feminine person. It is the total union of body, soul and spirit." If you are going to have this type of intimate contact with another person, you need to know what that person looks like naked and what he looks like sexually aroused.

It is each partner's responsibility to caress and stimulate the other in foreplay. You must, therefore, know what parts of your husband's body are sexually sensitive, where those parts are, and what they look like. (See chapters 1 and 10 for complete information on the female body and female organs.)

1011 What are the male sex organs and how do they function?

To help you understand the male genital organs, two illustrations are provided. Using these illustrations you can see where the sperm are produced and can follow their course from origin in the testicles (testes) through the internal and external male genitalia to the outside of the body.

The scrotum is the sack of skin that holds the man's two testicles. If a man has only one testicle, he generally still has more than enough sperm for fertility and more than enough testosterone production to be a totally normal male. Both testosterone and sperm are produced in the testicles. Testosterone, a male hormone, is secreted into the veins of the scrotum and distributed through the man's body by the blood-vessel system.

The man's seed (sperm) is produced continuously by the testicles, but the same amount of sperm is not produced each day. This is one reason a couple does not achieve pregnancy every time they have intercourse during the woman's fertile period.

The sperm produced by the testicles are passed into a collecting system called the epididymis. Each testicle has an epididymis contained entirely inside the scrotum.

The vas deferens is the tube that passes up from each epididymis, out of the scrotum, over the pubic bone, and back down into the pelvis to connect with a storage chamber for sperm, the ampulla, which is located just above the prostate gland. The ampulla penetrates through the prostate gland to connect to the urethra, the tube from the bladder that carries urine and sperm to the outside through the penis.

Just before the ampulla connects to the urethra, the seminal vesicles open into the ampulla. The seminal vesicles are glands that produce sem-

Adult Male Internal Sex Organs

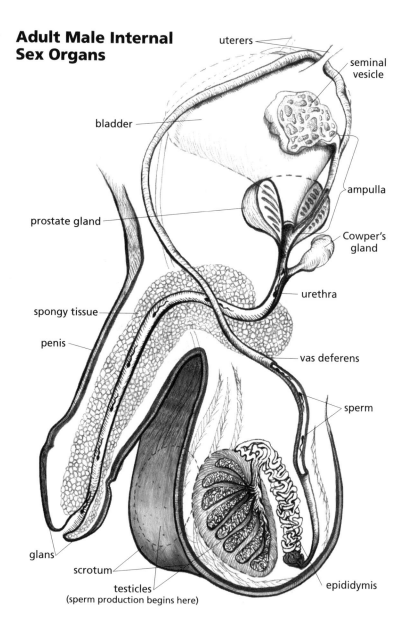

uterers

seminal vesicle

bladder

ampulla

prostate gland

Cowper's gland

urethra

spongy tissue

penis

vas deferens

sperm

glans

scrotum

testicles
(sperm production begins here)

epididymis

inal fluid that carries the sperm down the urethra and out of the penis. If all the sperm in a man's ejaculate were concentrated, there would be only a small mass of cells. Without the seminal fluid, they would not make up enough volume to leave the man's penis. Most of the material that comes out of a man's penis with ejaculation is, therefore, the mucus produced by the seminal vesicles and the prostate gland.

Attached to the upper urethra are two pea-size tubular glands, called Cowper's glands,

which discharge a mucous secretion into the urethra.

The urethra serves two functions: It is the tube through which urine is passed from the bladder and it is also the tube through which the seminal fluid is ejaculated. When ejaculation occurs, the semen is squirted forcefully and quickly through the urethra to the outside. Simultaneously, the base of the bladder clamps down, preventing the flow of semen back through the urethra into the bladder or of urine out of the bladder into the urethra at the time of ejaculation.

The penis is an ingenious organ, carefully created to perform three intricate functions: The first is the passage of urine from the bladder; the second is erection, which allows the penis to be inserted into the woman's vagina; and the third is the passage of semen from the ampulla.

The foreskin of the penis is merely loose skin that covers the head of the penis (the glans penis). When a man's penis is erect, the foreskin pulls back away from the glans. If a man has been circumcised the glans stays exposed all the time. If a man is not circumcised, he should retract the foreskin from the glans daily and wash under it.

A man's penis becomes erect when with sexual excitement blood flows into the spongy tissue of the penis. Valves in the veins that flow out of this spongy tissue keep the blood from flowing back out as fast as it flows in. It is interesting that a man's erection can become slightly flaccid and then rigidly erect again. Since an erection is emotionally controlled, a distraction can cause an erection to be lost or weakened.

An erect penis is important for pleasure and for conception. Intercourse would be impossible without it. Without a firm penis, the deposition of semen inside the woman's vagina against her cervix would be impossible. Incidentally, the force of the ejaculate does not push the semen up inside the woman's uterus, but merely deposits it high in the vagina, where the sperm have the best chance of swimming out of the semen into the cer-

Male Sex Organs

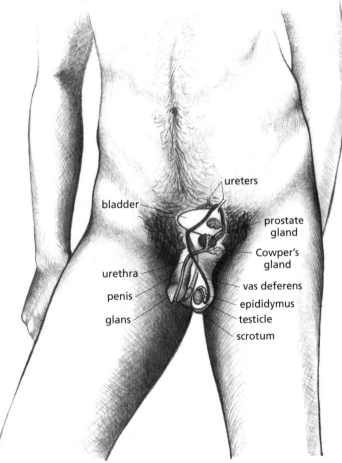

ureters

bladder

prostate gland

Cowper's gland

urethra

vas deferens

penis

epididymus

glans

testicle

scrotum

vical mucus. (See the complete discussion on conception in chapter 6.)

God ingeniously designed the female and male bodies to fit together perfectly. In doing this, he not only provided for procreation but for pleasure as well.

1012 Which areas of a man's body can be used to stimulate him sexually?

A sensitive partner can arouse her mate by touching him almost anywhere, but there are some areas that are more sexually sensitive than others. Most of these erogenous zones are in the genital area. A general rule for both men and women is that the closer the stimulation is to one of the openings of the body, the more arousing it is.

A man's nipples, like a woman's, are often sexually sensitive, and his scrotum can be gently touched to produce erotic stimulation. The closer to the urethral opening at the end of the penis a man is stimulated, the more likely he is to be sexually aroused. Often the area on the underside of the glans penis (where the glans attaches to the shaft of the penis) is one of the most sensitive areas of a man's body.

The area around the anus is often sexually sensitive, and the armpits and the inside of the thighs are areas that can often be used to arouse either a man or a woman.

In stimulating these areas, it is important to realize that the more sexually excitable an area is, the more likely it is to be delicate and sensitive. Stimulation should be gentle.

1013 Where are a woman's erogenous zones?

You will probably find that your areas of sexual sensitivity are much like those of the man. Stimulation of your mouth and ears and the areas around them will probably be pleasant to you, and sensitive stimulation of your breasts will probably be erotic. Just as a man's scrotum is sexually sensitive, so are both the labia minora and majora when

touched carefully and stimulated gently. Just as a man's penis is his most sensitive area sexually, so your clitoris is your most sexually responsive area. As a matter of fact, the clitoris is the only organ in either the male or the female body that is made only for sexual pleasure.

Maximizing Your Sexual Pleasure

1014 What is the best environment for sexual activity?

Both you and your husband will enjoy love play more when you know that you will not be interrupted. You need to be sure that the phone is covered with a pillow or disconnected. If there are other people in the house, make sure that the bedroom door is locked.

Personal hygiene for both of you is important. Just as you will not appreciate his body odor, he will not want your breath to smell of onions! Be sensitive to each other; learn what things are likely to make your total environment conducive to sexual arousal.

From the beginning it is important that you and your husband vary the place, atmosphere, and method of your sexual activity. Since sameness and routine become boring, it is important to occasionally change some aspect of the circumstance in which you make love.

Some couples have the mistaken romantic notion that sexual activity should take place only when there is complete unity of desire, intensity, and setting. This implies that each sexual experience is a perfect sexual experience and places unnecessary restraints and constrictions on your lovemaking. Sexual pleasure is elastic and as a couple spontaneously explores the range of sexual responsiveness, their enjoyment of each other intensifies. Don't wait to initiate sexual activity until you both are equally interested. If you do, you will cheat yourselves out of a broad range of interesting and exciting activity.

1015 What are the phases of sexual responsiveness?

Masters and Johnson, well-known researchers in human sexuality, describe a "sexual response pattern" in their book, *Human Sexual Response* (Boston: Little, Brown & Company, 1966). They identify four phases through which a couple normally passes during sexual excitement.

Excitement phase. It is during this phase that foreplay should occur. You should gently stimulate your husband, and he should gently stimulate your sensitive areas. As you become sexually aroused, your labia majora and minora will swell, and lubrication of your vaginal opening will occur. Your breasts and nipples will also become engorged and somewhat swollen. In addition, both your heart rate and your breathing rate will increase. As you stimulate your husband, his penis will become erect and hard. The skin around his testicles will become thickened, and the testicles themselves will be drawn up against his body more tightly.

The amount of time that you and your husband spend in foreplay is a completely personal matter. The key is that you allow enough time for each partner to become fully aroused. If you feel that your husband is rushing you, let him know. Likewise, if he feels that you are rushing him, he should tell you.

Plateau phase. Once you have stimulated each other into the "plateau phase," both will be ready for entry of the penis into your vagina. During this interval, the changes that occurred during the excitement phase will continue, but with greater intensity. This phase should last long enough to bring you both to orgasm, sometimes simultaneously. If your husband experiences premature ejaculation, he will lose his erection. In that case, the way for you to reach orgasm is for him to stimulate your clitoris with his fingers or, if mutually acceptable, with his tongue.

A husband can learn to hold back his orgasm for at least fifteen minutes of continual thrusting,

and he can also learn to keep his erect penis in your vagina for thirty minutes. Probably neither you nor he would want to have intercourse for this long every time, but it is possible. (See Q. 1018.)

Orgasm. Orgasm for a woman involves involuntary contractions of the muscles surrounding the outer portion of the vagina, which often includes a thrusting of the pelvis. Contractions of other muscles of the body may also occur. A woman may perspire and salivate, and her increased heart rate will peak. The feeling is one of intense pleasure and relief. It is unlike any other sensation a woman will ever experience. For a woman, orgasm is an all-encompassing event involving the whole body. A man's orgasm is much more localized; the majority of his intense feelings are directed toward his pelvis and penis.

A woman can have repeated orgasms. For some women this is a regular occurrence; for others it is rare. You may find that your husband will ejaculate after you have had one orgasm, but that he can continue to stimulate you and bring you to orgasm repeatedly. If you want him to do this, guide his hand to your clitoris or other erotically sensitive parts of your body and move his hand around in such a way that he brings you to climax again.

You may not always have an orgasm with intercourse and yet feel quite fulfilled with the lovemaking experience. It is important that you let your husband know that you can be satisfied with his lovemaking even without having an orgasm. Women occasionally tell me that they are not sure whether or not they have an orgasm, but most women definitely know when it occurs. If you feel satisfied and relaxed after intercourse, you have probably had a climax even though it may have been subdued.

A man's orgasm occurs only once during an episode of sexual excitement, but it involves multiple contractions of the prostate gland, the ejaculatory ducts, and the penis. These contractions usually occur five or six times and at tenth-of-a-second intervals. A man ejaculates about one teaspoon of seminal fluid, which contains an average of 100 million individual sperm.

Resolution phase. During this time, engorgement of a woman's pelvic structures and of her breasts gradually returns to normal. If she has had an orgasm this engorgement diminishes more quickly than if she has not been brought to climax. During this phase of resolution, a woman can sometimes be brought to orgasm again by stimulation.

Most of the time a man cannot immediately have another erection and orgasm. After intercourse a man will often relax and go to sleep more quickly than his wife. If your husband does this and it bothers you, ask him if he will stay awake with you a little while and hold and caress you until your resolution phase is complete. Some men can have an erection and ejaculation again in an hour or two. If your husband can do this, a little closeness can turn into more than that if you both want it to. However, many men must wait several hours or overnight to develop another erection, especially as they get past the age of fifty.

1016 How often is "normal" for couples to have intercourse?

The frequency of intercourse that satisfies you and your husband is the "normal" frequency for you. Some couples have intercourse only once a month; others have intercourse every day. Either one of these habits of intercourse—and anything in between or beyond—is normal if the couple is happy with it.

Most young to middle-aged couples, however, want to have intercourse about two or three times a week unless there is a medical or emotional problem. For the purpose of fertility, couples who have intercourse three to four times a week are the most likely to get pregnant during a one-year period.

One of the most down-to-earth directives to married couples concerning frequency of intercourse that I know of is in 1 Corinthians 7:3–5 where the apostle Paul states: "The husband should fulfill his marital duty to his wife, and likewise the wife to her husband. The wife's body does not belong to her alone but also to her husband. In the same way, the husband's body does not belong to him alone but also to his wife. Do not deprive each other except by mutual consent and for a time, so that you may devote yourselves to prayer."

If you (or your husband) are extremely dissat-

isfied with the frequency of your intercourse, don't pretend there is no problem. Get sexual counseling if you cannot work it out on your own. Too often a husband or wife will tolerate the frustration related to frequency of intercourse, suffering in silence until he or she is filled with anger and resentment, finally "bursting out" and saying and doing things that would never have been necessary if the dissatisfied partner had been more open earlier.

In most such cases the wife is satisfied with the frequency of intercourse, but the husband wants to have relations more often. He may need to adjust his demands to some extent, but the wife may also need to modify her willingness to satisfy his needs and desires. Compromise on both parts is the ideal, and communication is usually the key.

It is best to remember that you and your husband have promised yourselves to each other. You will want to enter into intercourse with your husband frequently enough to relieve the emotional tension that sexual need produces in him. He can become filled with resentment and anger if you habitually avoid having intercourse with him. He can feel trapped, caught between your resistance to his advances and moral values that deny him sexual release with anyone else. A situation like this can affect not only his happiness but your own as well.

1017 Is the desire for oral sex normal?

Oral sex, which refers to the stimulation of the sexual organs of either partner with the mouth or tongue of the other, is ultimately a matter of personal preference. The best discussion I have seen concerning oral sex is in the book, *The Gift of Sex: A Christian Guide to Sexual Fulfillment,* by Clifford and Joyce Penner (Waco: Word Books, 1981). I encourage you to get a copy and read this discussion.

The Penners point out that in the Bible's Song of Solomon, reference seems to be made to the lovers stimulating each other with their mouths. If this is so, it would seem to indicate that from God's perspective there is nothing wrong with the practice of oral sex (Song of Sol. 4:16–5:1). The authors do stipulate, however, that although there is nothing unnatural or wrong about oral sex, it would be wrong if it "violates" one of the partners. They state: "It does not violate anyone to *avoid* oral sex, but it certainly *may* violate someone to be pushed into it" (italics mine).

The Penners feel that there are three questions concerning this subject that should be answered.

Is it natural? A body part is still a body part, no matter where it is located. Oral stimulation of the genitals, therefore, can be accomplished as "naturally" as can oral stimulation of the breasts, the mouth, and the ears. What would make oral sex and other sexual variations "unnatural" would be in insisting that a partner participate against his or her wishes. Having intercourse should be an act of love, and it is unnatural to intentionally violate the one you love.

Is it right? Although the Penners use the Bible as their authority and refer to the passage in Song of Solomon, they point out that Scripture is not really clear on the matter of oral sex, and the Bible cannot be used to either support or incriminate it. They conclude: "The principle of what is loving and caring for the other person must be addressed; on the other hand, the teaching that our bodies are each other's to enjoy must also be incorporated."

Is it clean? There are three conditions that can exist in the bodily systems related to sexual relations: sterile, clean, or contaminated. The urinary system is normally "sterile" (it has no bacteria); the reproductive system, which includes the penis and the vagina, is "clean" (normally free of any disease-producing organisms); the rectal area and the mouth are "contaminated" (have disease-producing microorganisms). If the body is washed and clean and there are no infections present, the mouth would not be contaminated by the genitals nor the genitals by the mouth. If any contamination did take place it would be from the mouth to the genitals, but this is unlikely.

Just because something is not clearly wrong, dirty, or unnatural does not necessarily make it right, natural, or necessary for you. The factual data in this section is intended merely to clear up some myths and distortions concerning oral sex.

In conclusion the Penners make this statement: "To the one who desires oral activity but is inhibited by the hesitancy of your spouse, we offer encouragement. Many couples change over time, and what was uncomfortable for one becomes more natural as that one is cared for and loved without judgment and without demand."

1018 What can be done about the problem of premature ejaculation?

First, let me tell you that an occasional premature ejaculation is normal, and every man experiences it. When this happens, it is usually associated with anxiety, stress, extreme sexual excitement, or prolonged abstinence from sexual activity.

If premature ejaculation without apparent reason occurs frequently enough to be a problem to a couple, something should be done. Fortunately, premature ejaculation is almost always curable.

Premature ejaculation is defined as ejaculation that occurs too quickly for one sexual partner to achieve sexual satisfaction. Some sex therapists say that ejaculation is premature when intercourse lasts less than thirty seconds to a minute. Dr. Charles B. Williams, in *Medical Aspects of Human Sexuality* (May 1991), makes this statement: "A man should be able to ejaculate more or less when he chooses. If he has difficulty controlling ejaculation and finds that he regularly ejaculates before he wishes to, then ejaculation is premature." Dr. Williams continued by saying:

The famous sex researchers, Masters and Johnson, describe the start of orgasm, called the "stage of inevitability," as a point of no return. At this stage, semen starts collecting in the urethra where it passes through the prostate. Once you reach this stage of intense sexual excitement, ejaculation will always occur. Thus the keys to controlling ejaculation are:

1. Learning to recognize the feeling that comes just before the stage of inevitability, which is called the "plateau stage"; and

2. Learning to relax the right muscles so that the "plateau stage" goes no further until you want it to.

Dr. Williams encourages men to learn to recognize the "plateau stage" and to be able to stop the progress of their sexual excitement at that stage. He recommends that men practice this by masturbating. I would suggest that if a couple is uncomfortable about the husband masturbating, the wife can stimulate her husband using a good lubricant.

Dr. Williams suggests that the man masturbate (or be stimulated by his wife) until he feels that he is almost ready to ejaculate. Penile stimulation should stop at this point, and the man should relax all his muscles, breath out, and count to four before breathing in again. He can relax all the muscles around his penis and anus by bearing down as if he were blowing up a balloon. (Relaxing his abdomen and buttocks also helps.)

When the urgent feeling has subsided, penile stimulation can begin again. If the urgency returns immediately, the man is probably in the "late plateau stage," which Dr. Williams says is probably too close to the point of ejaculation to be reliably controlled. If he ejaculates after his penile stimulation has stopped, he has gone beyond the plateau stage to the stage of inevitability (which means he went too far with penile stimulation).

Dr. Williams recommends doing this exercise again the next day and continuing it daily until a man can relax his muscles well enough to continue masturbating (or continue penile stimulation) for fifteen minutes without ejaculating unless he chooses to.

Once a man has learned to identify the plateau stage and relax his muscles during penile stimulation without intercourse, he can use the same technique while having intercourse.

If you would like to have a reprint of the article by Dr. Williams, write to:

Editor
Medical Aspects of Human Sexuality
249 West 17th Street
New York, NY 10011

1019 Can drugs taken for a medical problem affect sexual responsiveness?

Yes. Drugs can definitely affect sexual responsiveness in both men and women. Unfortunately many people and many doctors do not associate drugs with sexual problems.

Men and women can lose their sexual desire because of certain drugs, and men may lose their ability to have an orgasm or their ability to ejaculate. Some drugs cause men to have persistent erections (called priapism), and others cause men and women to become sleepy and lose their energy, which can alter their desire for intercourse. Testosterone, occasionally used in ointments for postmenopausal women who have vulvar irritation, can cause vulvar and pelvic discomfort and distorted sexual interest.

Alcohol also can negatively affect sexual responsiveness. Although a small amount of alcohol can reduce tension from the day's activities or from anxiety about the sexual relationship, larger amounts of alcohol decrease libido and sexual interest in both men and women. For example, about 40 percent of alcoholic men are impotent and about 40 percent of alcoholic women have poor response to sexual stimulation. If either partner drinks excessively, the sexual relationship will suffer. Other drugs, such as marijuana and cocaine, may also affect sexual responsiveness.

Obviously this list does not include all the drugs that are dispensed in this country. It does show, however, that many drugs have a significant impact on sexual function. If you are having a problem with sexual function, you may want to consult your physician to see if the problem could be caused by a drug you are taking.

Problems That Hamper Sexual Enjoyment

1020 If we are having problems in our sexual relationship, what can we do?

Sexual problems occur frequently. In their book, *Human Sexual Inadequacy*, Masters and Johnson state that "a conservative estimate would indicate half of the marriages [in this country] are either presently sexually dysfunctional or imminently so in the future." These researchers are talking about problems such as so-called frigidity on the part of a woman, about women who find it difficult to be aroused, and about men with premature ejaculation and impotence.

In their research, Masters and Johnson found that they could help about 75 percent of people with such problems using a two-week therapy program. Since many of their patients had experienced difficulty for years, this is an astoundingly short treatment period to produce such success and is certainly worth the investment.

If you are experiencing a sexual problem in your relationship with your husband, don't tolerate it any longer. The longer the problem exists, the more difficult it will be for you to correct.

If your problem requires professional help, I would suggest that you see a counselor who employs the techniques espoused by Masters and Johnson. These counselors will not usually go into deep psychotherapy; they go directly to the problem and solve that problem, for most people, with short-term therapy.

Remember that the choice of a counselor is a very personal thing; if you find that the personality or morality of the one you have chosen bothers you, change. Do not, under any circumstances, cooperate with a "counselor" who suggests that sex with him will cure your problem, or that an affair with another man will help you. This is unsound and unethical counsel and can lead you into even more problems and guilt.

1021 What can I expect from sex counseling?

If a counselor recommends prolonged therapy for a sexual problem, be sure that your problem demands such a long period of therapy. Most problems of sexuality can be cured within a few short weeks. Compare the program your counselor recommends with the one outlined below. In *Understanding Human Sexual Inadequacy* by Fred Belliveau and Lin Richter (New York: Bantam, 1982), there is an excellent summary (pp. 87–110) of the Mas-

ters and Johnson treatment program. The program your sex counselors use will probably be similar to the following outline. (The days refer to days of counseling, not days of the week. The frequency of visits will be determined by the counselors.)

Day One: The couple and the co-therapists, usually a male and a female, meet together for the initial interview, then they separate. The male co-therapist goes with the husband and the female co-therapist goes with the wife for a history-taking session. These interviews involve thorough questioning about the specific sexual problem(s) and about each person's past life, including a social, sexual, and medical history. At the end of the session the couple is asked not to have any sexual activity until told to do so by the therapists.

Day Two: On this day the husband is interviewed by the female co-therapist and the wife by the male co-therapist. Masters and Johnson have found that a person being interviewed will often tell something to a therapist of the opposite sex that he or she would not tell to a therapist of the same sex. The second-day interview concentrates on the motivation of the patients for coming to therapy and includes a more relaxed discussion of the problem that brought the couple for therapy in the first place.

Day Three: Complete medical histories are taken, physical examinations are done, and diagnostic laboratory tests are performed. Following these procedures, a round-table discussion with the four people takes place. At this session the co-therapists share what they have found from the two history-taking interviews and the physical examinations. The patients are given the opportunity to discuss situations that the therapists seem not to understand thoroughly and to disagree with the therapists if they wish. Masters and Johnson say "the marital partners must continue while in therapy to represent positively their own social and sexual value systems and their preference in lifestyle."

At the round-table discussion the co-therapists give their ideas of what is probably causing the problem. At the end of this discussion the patients are given "physical direction." In essence this physical direction, or "sensate focus," relies on the principle that, for a couple to achieve fullest sexual expression, they must touch each other in a communicative way. Sensate focus is a concept devised by Masters and Johnson to help people learn to communicate by touching. They are told to choose two periods of time between the end of the round-table on Day Three and the therapy on Day Four, during which they will practice sensate focus.

Sensate-focus activity primarily involves pleasurable touching (except of the genitals) of the husband by the wife or the wife by the husband. The goal is for the person who is touching the other to discover what type of touching his or her partner finds the most pleasant. During this time the couple is not to have intercourse or touch each other's genitals or the woman's breasts.

Day Four: A therapy session is held to review the couple's experience with sensate focus. Further discussion is held, with instructions given for changing the sensate-focus technique slightly. On Day Three the one who received the touching was to be passive, doing nothing but keeping the other from doing anything that was unpleasant, distracting, or irritating. On Day Four the one who receives the touching is to participate actively by putting his or her hand on the hand of the one who is doing the touching to show the toucher which places to touch, how hard to touch, and in what direction to move his or her hand. In this session pleasurable stimulation is applied to all parts of the body, including the genitals and breasts, but without the demand of sexual response.

Day Five to End of Therapy: On this day in therapy the therapists start working with the patients on their specific problems, such as painful intercourse, premature ejaculation, and so on. This therapy continues to the end of the treatment program. During the entire treatment program, the couple may spend between twelve and thirty hours with the therapists in addition to the hours spent doing their "homework." Masters and Johnson have found that the results come quickly, and the patients themselves report rapid response to therapy.

For a more complete discussion of this mode of therapy I suggest that you get *Understanding Human Sexual Inadequacy*. (This book is basically a lay interpretation of Masters and Johnson's book *Human Sexual Inadequacy*, which was written for the medical profession.)

The reason that I emphasize that the counseling should resemble the procedures above is that I have had several patients tell me of horrible experiences with sex counselors. One patient said that a counselor recommended that she and her husband separate for a while and this almost ruined their marriage. One man was told that he had sexual problems with his wife because of a "hang-up" about his relationship with his grandmother. Generally, sex counseling does not require a psychotherapeutic approach. It can usually be short, straightforward, and simple and still be effective. It may require much more intensive counseling but usually does not. If your counselor gives you advice that does not seem right, get a second opinion.

There is no accrediting organization for sexual-dysfunction clinics in the United States, and the only list of these clinics that I know of is published annually by a magazine mailed to physicians, *Sexual Medicine Today*. The list is not all-inclusive, but it can give you the name of an organization in your area that could refer you to a local sexual dysfunction clinic or physician. For a copy of this list write to *Sexual Medicine Today*, 257 Park Avenue South, New York 10010. Carefully evaluate a counselor, even if the name is on this list.

1022 Is it normal for my husband and me to enjoy physical closeness without it culminating in sexual intercourse every time?

Not only is it normal, but it is good—and often necessary.

Most women like to be held and cuddled, and many times they need not only the comfort and security of their husband's arms but also the freedom that allows sex to be the furthest thing from their minds. Unfortunately, many women find that any attempt to have physical closeness with their husbands is interpreted as a "come-on" for sex. A husband should be sensitive to the needs of his wife in these cases, as should a wife be when her husband just "needs to be held." If either of you does not feel like having intercourse but does want to be physically close, this should be shared with the marriage partner.

There are times when one or the other of you cannot have intercourse—because of illness or pregnancy, for example—and there are times when one or the other of you will be too tired, disinterested, or distracted to have intercourse. A relationship that *must* always result in intercourse whenever there is private, physical intimacy is usually not a healthy relationship and can become confining. Usually one person or the other will begin to feel used, because closeness seems only to lead to the other's personal sexual gratification.

A husband and wife need to be able to express love and affection for each other without the feeling that it must always lead to intercourse. This can be a wonderful part of marriage. Such closeness can include massaging each other's backs, kissing, holding each other close, and going to sleep in each other's arms. The variety can be as endless as your love for each other.

This type of relationship assures your partner of your love for him (and you of his love for you) that is not dependent on intercourse each time there is any display of intimacy. Such a relationship is quite helpful if one of you develops a medical problem that makes intercourse impossible for a time, because you will know that you can still enjoy physical closeness.

Arousal, especially of the man, will occur occasionally when neither of you intends it to happen. This does not mean that your husband must have intercourse, or that you need to feel guilty if you do not want to have intercourse at that time. It will not hurt his body to let the arousal pass, any more than it hurts a person's body to feel hungry and let the hunger pass without eating for a while.

An Afterword

In conclusion I quote Ingrid Trobisch: "Marriage is not a destination, but a journey. As husband and wife make this journey together, growing and maturing and learning how to love, they will reach sexual harmony as a ripe fruit of their marriage" (*The Joy of Being a Woman and What a Man Can Do*, p. 30).

Glossary

abdomen   The portion of the body, below the chest, which contains the stomach, intestines, gallbladder, liver, spleen, pancreas, lymph glands, kidneys, bladder, and, in a woman, the female reproductive organs.

abortion   The loss of a pregnancy before the twentieth week of pregnancy. An abortion may be spontaneous or induced.

abscess   A collection of pus surrounded by an inflamed area.

acute illness, acute pain   "Acute" indicates a relatively sudden onset of pain or illness, with definite symptoms and limited duration, as opposed to "chronic" pain or illness, which is a recurring illness or pain of indefinite duration and less intensity.

adenoma   Noncancerous (benign) tumor composed of gland-like tissue.

adenomatous hyperplasia of the endometrium   Overgrowth of the uterine lining. Not malignant at this point.

adenomyosis   Endometriosis that is present in the muscular wall of the uterus. This condition exists when islands of tissue like the uterine lining are present in the muscular wall of the uterus.

adenosis   A condition in which areas of the vaginal lining (squamous epithelium) are replaced by tissue that is like the cervical lining (columnar epithelium). Often caused by exposure to DES (diethylstilbestrol) in the mother's womb.

adhesion   Scar tissue binding together structures of the body that are not ordinarily attached to each other. This may result from surgery, inflammation, or injury.

adolescence   The period of human life between puberty and adulthood.

adrenal glands   Part of the hormone system. These glands, one located on top of each kidney, produce hormones that control the body's defense mechanisms, regulate the body's water and salt, and help maintain correct blood pressure.

AIDS   Acquired immunodeficiency syndrome. A collapse of the body's immune defense system due to HIV, usually resulting in death by rare forms of cancer, pneumonia, and overwhelming infections.

albumin   A protein found in egg whites, in plants, and in animals. When found in the urine, it may indicate the presence of kidney disease.

allergy   A reaction to a substance (called an antigen) by a person sensitive to that substance. Symptoms may be so mild as to go unnoticed or may be severe enough to produce death.

amenorrhea   Absence of menstrual periods. Primary amenorrhea means that a woman has never had a period. Secondary amenorrhea means that a woman has had one or more periods and then stopped having them for a length of time.

amniocentesis   Removal of some of the fluid that surrounds the unborn baby during pregnancy, usually for testing purposes. This is done by insertion of a needle through the skin of the mother's abdomen into the pregnant uterus.

analgesic   A drug that reduces pain.

androgen   A male hormone that produces and controls the secondary male sex characteristics, such as the beard, muscles, and deep voice. Testosterone, the male sex hormone, is the primary male hormone (androgen). All normal women secrete androgens in small amounts from their ovaries and adrenal glands.

anemia   Low concentration of hemoglobin (oxygen-carrying material) in the red blood cells. A "blood count" tells if a woman is anemic.

anesthesia   The absence of pain sensation, with or without a loss of consciousness. *General anesthesia* involves loss of consciousness. *Regional anesthesia* produces loss of pain sensation in a particular area of the body by the use of epidural, spinal, or other nerve block. *Local anesthesia* is produced by injection of an anesthetic agent into localized tissue. *Topical anesthesia* is a lack of pain on a surface area from direct application of an anesthetic agent.

angioma   *See* vascular spider.

anorexia nervosa   A condition most often found in young women, characterized by loss of appetite, aversion to food, and marked weight loss. Death may result if the problem is not treated. Another related eating disorder is bulimia, a condition in which a person overeats and then induces vomiting. An aspect of this problem is that they often develop severe dental decay because of the effect of stomach acid on their teeth from the repeated vomiting. Bulimarexia is a condition that combines aspects of both diseases. Bulimia, bulimarexia, and anorexia nervosa are almost always emotional in origin.

antibiotics Drugs that kill or inhibit the growth of bacteria.

anticoagulant A drug that hinders clotting (coagulation) of the blood.

antihistamines Drugs that oppose the effects of histamine in the body. Used in allergic conditions, such as hay fever and serum sickness, and also for alleviation of cold symptoms.

anus The opening at the lower end of the bowel; the opening of the rectum through which bowel movements are eliminated from the body.

Apgar score A rating system used to document a newborn's condition after birth. Includes heart rate, muscle tone, respiration, color, and response to stimuli. It is normally used to evaluate the infant one minute and five minutes after birth.

appendicitis Inflammation of the appendix, a small organ (three to six inches long) that projects from the lower bowel in the lower right part of the abdomen. A potentially fatal condition, appendicitis must be treated with immediate surgery.

areola The ring of darkly pigmented skin around the nipple of the breast.

arteriosclerosis Hardening of the arteries, a condition in which the walls of the arteries become coated with deposits of a cholesterol-containing material. The resulting obstruction of these blood vessels can result in heart attacks, strokes, and gangrene of fingers and toes, arms and legs.

artificial insemination Instillation of sperm into the vagina or uterus by medical technique rather than by intercourse. Husband's sperm may be used (AIH), donor's sperm may be used (AID), or the insemination can involve putting washed sperm into the uterus (intrauterine insemination—IUI). Washed sperm may be from a woman's husband or from a donor. (See chapter 11 regarding this technique.)

aspiration A procedure in which fluid or material is drawn out of a cyst, growth, or body cavity with a needle or tube. Suction is usually applied with a syringe.

atypical endometrial hyperplasia A precancerous form of endometrial hyperplasia (overgrowth of the uterine lining). Not malignant, but 80 percent of women who have it will develop cancer if it is not treated.

augmentation mammoplasty An operation, performed by a plastic surgeon, in which an implant is put into the breast to make it larger or more shapely.

axilla The underarm or armpit.

bacterial vaginosis (BV) Vaginal infection. The most common infection of the vagina, not always transmitted sexually. This infection is characterized by a discharge that is watery, often heavy, with a fishy odor. This vaginal infection does not cause burning or itching of the vulva. Formerly called gardnerella (hemophilus) vaginitis.

Bartholin's glands Vulvar glands that secrete a clear, thin mucus to lubricate the vulva during intercourse. They increase their output of mucus during sexual excitement, adding to the lubrication for intercourse. The two glands are located on either side of the lower part of the vulva, with an opening just inside the labia minora.

basal body temperature Body temperature immediately on awakening in the morning, before any daily activity (including getting out of bed) has begun.

benign Not malignant, not cancerous.

bilateral salpingo-oophorectomy Surgical removal of both fallopian tubes and both ovaries.

biopsy Surgical removal of portions of the body's tissue for microscopic study and diagnosis.

birth-control pills ("the Pill") A pill containing synthetic estrogens and progesterones. Use of such pills produces an artificial menstrual cycle that prevents the release of the egg from the ovary each month.

bran Ground husks of cereal grains. A convenient source of fiber, useful for increasing the amount of bulk in a person's diet. *See also* fiber.

Braxton-Hicks contractions Sometimes called "false labor pains." The uterus contracts all the time, even when it is not pregnant, but the contractions are made more obvious by the enlarged uterus of pregnancy. Braxton-Hicks contractions do not prepare the uterus for labor, nor cause labor to start.

breast reconstruction Rebuilding the breast after surgical removal or deformity. Such plastic surgery can involve augmentation with implants and remodeling using other body tissue and skin.

breech birth A delivery in which a baby's bottom end (buttocks or feet) comes first, rather than its head.

BSE Breast self-examination.

bulimia or **bulimarexia** *See* anorexia nervosa.

carcinoma A technical word for certain types of cancer. It is important to remember that a growth can be a cancer (carcinoma) and, in its early stages, not be dangerous for an individual if proper treatment is obtained.

carpal tunnel syndrome Pain or numbness of the hands, produced by swelling in the wrists. This is often seen during pregnancy.

caruncle A condition in which the lining of the inside of the urethra seems to protrude from the urethral opening. This is not a malignant growth.

catheter Any of a variety of tubes for insertion into the body.

caudal anesthesia Often given in the past during childbirth (but not often used now), it numbs a woman from the waist down but usually allows her to move her body and to push, assisting in delivery. Injected in the lowest end of the spinal column, just above the tailbone, it differs from an epidural only by where the needle is inserted into the body. It is not the same as a spinal. *Compare* epidural and spinal anesthetic.

celibacy The state of remaining unmarried. The term most often used to define voluntary renunciation of sexual relations is abstinence.

centimeter A unit of measurement; .3937 inch; cc—cubic centimeter, there are about 30 cc in a fluid ounce.

cerclage operation An operation in which a "purse string" type of suture or band of material is put around the cervix to strengthen it so as to prevent miscarriages or premature deliveries.

cervical cap   A "miniature diaphragm" that fits over a woman's cervix and acts as a barrier between the sperm and the cervix.

cervical erosion   Properly termed *ectropion*. A reddish discoloration immediately around the opening of the cervix caused by the lining of the inside of the cervix extending from the cervical opening to cover a part of the external cervix. It is not an "erosion" of tissues. The term *erosion* was applied to this condition many years ago before careful study showed that it is a normal condition.

cervical intraepithelial neoplasia (CIN)   Precancerous cells of the cervix. Graded by physicians as to severity and extent:

CIN I—cells are mildly precancerous

CIN II—cells are moderately precancerous

CIN III—cells are severely precancerous

This is the terminology that most gynecologists are now using instead of "dysplasia."

cervical nabothian cyst   Small hard nodules on the cervix caused by clogged mucous glands. Not precancerous, dangerous, or painful. Does not usually need treatment.

cervix   The lower part of the uterus that includes the mouth of the uterus. It is about two inches long and one inch wide in an adult.

cesarean section   Surgical operation for delivering a baby through an incision in the abdomen when normal vaginal delivery is dangerous, impossible, or unwise.

chancre   A sore, usually painless, that is the entry site of syphilis into the body. *See also* syphilis.

chancroid   A sexually transmitted disease caused by *Hemophilus ducreyi* bacteria.

chemotherapy   The administration of medications for the treatment or prevention of a disease. Although this term usually refers to the treatment of cancer, technically it can apply to use of antibiotics and other drugs for any disease.

chlamydia   The most common bacterial sexually transmitted infection (STD) in the United States. A major cause of PID (pelvic inflammatory disease) and sterility. Caused by the bacterium *Chlamydia trachomatis.*

chloasma   "Mask of pregnancy." Various-sized brown patches that occasionally appear on the face of a pregnant woman as a result of hormonal effect on her skin. Birth-control pills may also cause these discolorations.

choriocarcinoma   *See* malignant molar pregnancy.

chorionic villi sampling   A procedure in which an instrument is inserted through the cervix into a pregnant uterus for the aspiration of some of the placenta. This placental tissue is then tested to determine whether or not the unborn baby has a genetic abnormality. This procedure can cause miscarriage.

chromosome   A microscopic piece of protein, several of which are present in the nucleus of every living cell. Each chromosome is made up of hundreds of smaller units called genes, which carry the genetic material that transmits human traits from generation to generation.

chronic   Long-continued or of long duration. A chronic disease is one that is prolonged, or one that progresses slowly, as opposed to "acute," which denotes a sudden onset and limited duration.

cilia   Small, hairlike structures. In this book the term refers to cilia that line the inside of the fallopian tubes and are also on the tubes' fimbriated ends. Cilia beat constantly, sweeping the egg (ovum) into and through the tubes.

circumcision   Surgical removal of the foreskin, the loose fold that covers the head of the penis.

climacteric   The period of life (usually beginning about age 40) when the ovaries begin having decreased estrogen production. Includes menopause and ends when all estrogen-sensitive tissues have thinned out and lost all the effect that estrogens have had on them (about age 65–70).

clinical pelvimetry   Physician's examination of a pregnant woman's pelvis. This is done to determine if her pelvic bones are normal and wide enough to allow the vaginal delivery of her infant. The physician does this through the vagina by feeling the woman's bone structures with his or her hand.

clitoris   A highly sensitive organ, consisting primarily of erectile tissue, which is located above the urethra on the vulva. It is one of a woman's external sex organs and corresponds to the male penis. Its purpose is solely for sexual pleasure.

coccyx   The vertebral bones at the lower end of the spine. The tailbone.

colitis   Inflammation of the colon.

colon   The part of the large intestine that extends from the cecum to the rectum.

colostomy   A surgically constructed opening of the large intestine to the outside, usually through the lower left side of the abdomen, which allows evacuation of stools through that opening. A colostomy is made necessary by surgical removal of a portion of the colon and may be temporary or permanent.

colostrum   A thin, bluish fluid produced by the mother's breasts after childbirth. Often precedes the true milk by two or three days. It can also be secreted by the breasts during pregnancy. Such production can start months before delivery and is totally normal.

colposcopy   An examination of the vulva, vagina, or cervix by magnification of these areas by a colposcope. This is done primarily to detect precancerous or cancerous growths.

colpotomy   An operation in which the abdomen is entered through an incision in the upper back part of the vagina. This procedure is not often used, having been replaced by another technique. *See also* laparoscopy.

conception   The union of sperm and ovum, the male and female sex cells, in the human body that leads to the development of a new life.

condom (female)   A contraceptive used by the female to prevent pregnancy and infection with sexually transmitted diseases. It is a soft, plastic tubelike device that a woman can insert into her vagina to collect sperm and secretions.

condom (male)   A contraceptive used by the male. A rubber sheath that covers the penis and prevents the sperm from being deposited in a woman's vagina.

condyloma acuminata   *See* genital warts.

congenital   Existing at birth.

conization An operation in which the doctor removes a cone-shaped piece of tissue from the portion of the cervix that can be seen through the vagina.

contraception A method, device, or substance used to prevent conception.

contraceptive foam A barrier-type contraceptive that coats the cervix and vagina with a sperm-killing agent. It contains the same chemical agent used in the contraceptive jelly and suppositories.

contraceptive shots Injections of 150 mg of Depo-Provera (a long-lasting progesterone) that prevent pregnancy for about three months. Not FDA-approved.

contraceptive vaginal suppository A suppository that contains a sperm-killing chemical and is inserted into the vagina prior to intercourse. It is a relatively unreliable method of contraception.

corpus luteum The structure left in the ovary after ovulation has occurred, formed from the follicle in which the egg developed. The corpus luteum is actually a short-lived gland. After ovulation, it begins producing progesterone and continues this for two weeks, unless pregnancy occurs. (It also produces estrogen.) If pregnancy does occur, the corpus luteum continues to produce progesterone for a few weeks longer.

couvade syndrome Symptoms of pregnancy experienced by the male. May mimic the symptoms of pregnancy a woman may have, including nausea, abdominal pain, and vomiting.

"crabs" (pubic lice) Small parasites that live in body hair. Treatment is with medicated shampoo. Pubic lice are a different parasite from the head lice that so often occur in children. Usually passed by sexual contact, pubic lice are found primarily in pubic hair.

CT (computerized tomography) scan A sophisticated technique for taking an X-ray across a portion of a person's body instead of in the usual manner. The typical X-ray view is much like a photograph. The CT scan is done as though a part of the body were cut through with a knife and a picture made of the severed end. A computer is used to put together several X-ray exposures to produce this type of X-ray.

curettage The scraping of a body cavity with an instrument to remove tissue and secretions. *See also* D&C.

cyst A sac containing fluid or semisolid material. Some cysts are present in the body as a normal part of its function (i.e., follicle cysts of the ovary that release an egg each month). Some cysts in the body are abnormal growths.

cystitis Inflammation of the bladder caused by infection or irritation.

cystoscopy An operation in which a physician looks into the bladder with a lighted telescope called a cystoscope.

D&C Dilatation and curettage. An operation performed on a woman's uterus through the vagina. Some type of anesthesia is usually required. The cervix is dilated with a series of increasingly larger round dilators. When the cervix is dilated enough, a scraping instrument is inserted into the uterus to scrape (curette) the lining of the uterus. Occasionally, a hollow scraping instrument, through which suction can be applied, is used for doing the curettement.

dermoid cyst Benign cystic teratoma, a tumor of the egg cells of the ovary. This tumor develops when an unfertilized egg begins growing. It is capable of containing any of the tissues that are in a human body. Typically, such tumors can contain hair, teeth, oil and sweat glands.

DES (diethylstilbestrol) A synthetic compound that produces the same effect in a woman's body as estrogen. Formerly prescribed to prevent miscarriage (but it did not), it can cause sexual organ abnormalities and cancer in the offspring of women who take this drug while pregnant.

diagnostic ultrasonography *See* ultrasound.

diaphragm A dome-shaped rubber cup with a flexible spring rim. When inserted in the vagina, this device holds contraceptive jelly against the cervix so that sperm are killed before they can enter the uterus and cause pregnancy.

dilatation and curettage *See* D&C.

diuretic Medication that causes the kidneys to withdraw more fluid from the bloodstream than they normally do, causing decrease in fluid retention (swelling) in the body and an increase in frequency of urination.

douche A method of cleansing or treating the vagina by irrigating it with water or a water-based preparation.

Down syndrome Often called mongolism. Caused by an abnormality in certain chromosomes resulting in mental retardation, a large tongue, cardiovascular abnormalities, and other physical abnormalities.

dry labor A nonmedical term that is often incorrectly used to describe the type of labor a woman will have if her "bag of waters" breaks several days or weeks before labor and delivery. Dry labor does not usually happen, however, because the amniotic fluid can be replaced completely by the body as often as every three hours. If all the fluid were lost and not replaced, the baby would die almost immediately.

dysmenorrhea Painful menstruation; menstrual cramps.

dyspareunia Painful intercourse.

dysplasia of the cervix *See* cervical intraepithelial neoplasia.

eclampsia A very serious disorder of late pregnancy. Preeclampsia becomes eclampsia when a woman develops convulsions. This abnormality can cause death of both the mother and the baby. It is characterized in a pregnant woman by protein in her urine, high blood pressure, generalized swelling, and convulsion. *See also* toxemia of pregnancy.

ectopic pregnancy A form of pregnancy in which the embryo begins developing outside the uterus. It is considered an ectopic pregnancy whether the pregnancy is in the fallopian tubes (tubal pregnancy), in the ovaries, or in the abdominal cavity.

ectropion *See* cervical erosion, for which ectropion is the correct medical term.

edema Increased amounts of fluid in body tissues.

effacement Shortening and thinning of the cervix, a process associated with pregnancy and labor. The cervix is usually about one inch long. Late in pregnancy or in early labor, the cervix can become shorter than one inch (partially effaced). Labor completes the effacement process as the contractions of labor cause the cervix to totally thin out (100 percent effacement).

ejaculation The ejection of seminal fluid through a man's urethra to the outside. *See also* semen. Women do not have a true ejaculation, although some women excrete fluid from their urethras at the apex of sexual excitement. Whether or not this is the equivalent of a male's ejaculation, no one knows for certain.

embryo An organism in the earliest stage of development. A human is considered to be an embryo from conception through the first six weeks of life. *See also* fetus.

endocrine glands Any of the ductless glands, such as the adrenals, the thyroid, the pituitary, the ovaries, the testes, whose secretions pass directly into the bloodstream. The secretions they produce are called hormones.

endolymphatic stromal myosis An overgrowth of the connective tissue of the uterus that causes uterine enlargement and bleeding. It may be a semimalignant growth.

endometrial biopsy A procedure in which a doctor inserts an instrument into the uterus and scrapes out a portion of the lining of the uterus (endometrium) for evaluation.

endometrial hyperplasia Nonmalignant overgrowth of the tissue of the lining of the uterus (endometrium).

endometrial polyp An overgrowth of the lining of the uterus (endometrium) that develops as a projection from the wall of the uterus.

endometrioma (chocolate cyst) Endometriosis (see below) that results in the collection of enough blood, scar, and tissue to form a cystic mass. When opened, an endometrioma will drain a chocolate-colored fluid that is a result of the monthly bleeding of endometriosis tissue. These accumulations are most often found in ovaries, but can be present wherever endometriosis is growing.

endometriosis The lining of the uterus is called the endometrium. When this tissue is present anywhere else in the body (except in the uterine muscular wall where it is called adenomyosis), it is called endometriosis. It can be found on a woman's intestines, in abdominal skin incisions, and in other parts of a woman's body. Surprisingly, it has even been found in men.

endometrium The membrane that lines the inner surface of the uterus.

endorphins The body's own natural, opiatelike hormones. These hormones are produced by the body to relieve its own pain.

epidermal inclusion cyst Small harmless vulvar bumps (much like pimples on facial skin) that may appear on the outer surface of the labia majora.

epididymis Sperm-collecting ducts that are present on each testicle.

epidural An anesthetic given through a needle in the lower back, sometimes used during labor and delivery. This anesthetic numbs a woman from the waist down but still allows her to move her legs and to bear down, assisting in the delivery of her infant. Although the needle is put into the back in the same place as the needle for a "spinal," it is not a spinal. For an epidural, the needle is not inserted as deeply as that for a spinal and does not actually penetrate the fluid sac that surrounds the spinal nerves. *Compare* spinal anesthetic.

episiotomy A surgical incision at the outer end and backside of the vagina that allows more room for delivery of the baby. This procedure is used to prevent tearing of the vagina during delivery.

epulis Swelling of a person's gums in such a way that the enlargement resembles a growth.

estrogen The primary female sex hormone. A woman's estrogen is principally produced in her ovaries. When the ovaries stop working at menopause, a woman's body will contain very little natural estrogen.

external cervical os The opening of the cervix into the vaginal canal.

fallopian tubes Structures attached to the upper corner of the uterus on either side. They are about the same shape and size as a large earthworm. The outer ends of the fallopian tubes are open, and it is through them that an egg passes from the ovary to the uterus. *See also* fimbriae.

fascia Sheets of fibrous tissue that hold muscles and various body organs in place.

fertile Able to conceive.

fertilization The union of the male sperm and the female egg (ovum).

fetoscope A stethoscope-like instrument that allows a listener to hear the heartbeat of a baby inside its mother's uterus.

fetus A term used for the unborn baby from the start of the seventh week of pregnancy until it is delivered. *See also* embryo.

fiber The part of food that is not digested. Fiber adds bulk to the stools and is an essential part of a healthy diet.

fiber-optic light This light technique has made it possible for physicians to brightly illuminate cavities of the body so they can be viewed with small "telescopes." The lightbulb is outside the body and is projected at one end of a bundle of flexible glass fibers. This special fiber bundle carries the light to the inside of the body for laparoscopy, hysteroscopy, and other procedures, such as arthroscopy, cystoscopy, and so on. The advantage of this procedure over the old technique of using a lightbulb at the end of the telescope is that the light can be much brighter, but without the telescope getting too hot. *See also* laparoscopy.

fibroadenoma A benign growth of the breast that comes from the lining of the gland tissue inside a woman's breasts.

fibrocystic breast change Used here as it applies to the breast. An overreaction of breast tissue to normal female hormones. Causes pain and lumpiness.

fibroid tumor A common benign growth of smooth muscle fibers of the uterus. Since fibroid tumors almost never become malignant, they are surgically removed for reasons other than the chance of malignancy.

fibromas Tumors composed of fibrous connective tissue that do not become malignant, but can get quite large.

fimbriae Small tentacles on the end of the fallopian tube that sweep over the surface of the ovary to capture the released egg.

fissure A slit, break, or crack in a part of the body. An example is a break in the nipple of a nursing mother.

fistula An abnormal, usually narrow passage from a body cavity to the outside skin or from one cavity to another. One of the more common fistulae of the female organs is an opening from the bladder into the vagina as a result of childbirth.

follicle-stimulating hormone (FSH) A hormone released from the pituitary that is responsible in the woman for the development of the egg-containing follicles of the ovaries.

follicular phase The part of a woman's monthly cycle during which her egg is developing. When the woman ovulates (releases the egg from the ovary), the follicular phase is ended and the luteal phase has begun. *See also* luteal phase.

forceps Instruments that fit around an infant's head and assist in its birth. Obstetrical forceps are designed so that they do not squeeze the baby's head. Pulling pressure is applied to the strongest part of the bones of the baby's head.

gardnerella (hemophilus) *See also* bacterial vaginosis (BV).

Gartner's duct cyst These cysts arise from tissues that lie in the walls of the vagina on either side. Gartner's duct cysts do not become malignant, are usually not painful, and do not need treating unless they become bothersome because of their size.

gastroenterologist Medical specialist who diagnoses and treats intestinal problems. Gastroenterologists do not perform surgery.

gene Part of a chromosome, a basic unit that determines hereditary traits.

general anesthesia An anesthetic that puts a person to sleep. General anesthesia is normally started with Pentothal or some similar drug in the veins and then continued with a gas administered with a mask or a tube into the lungs. General anesthesia given today has an outstanding safety record because of new developments in the field.

genital warts (condyloma acuminata) Virus-caused growths on the external genitalia, anus, urethra, vagina, or cervix. These may occur in both men and women and are not cancerous. Venereal warts can be spread by sexual contact, but that is not always the case. Special attention is required if they are present during pregnancy.

gestation *See* pregnancy.

gestational diabetes Diabetes that develops during pregnancy but was not present before the pregnancy started. It usually ends when the pregnancy is over. If it does not, the mother is then a true diabetic.

GIFT (gamete intrafallopian transfer) An adaptation of the IVF procedure in which eggs and semen are injected directly into the fallopian tubes by means of a thin tube threaded through an incision made during a laparoscopy or minilaparotomy.

glans penis or **glans clitoris** The head of the penis or head of the clitoris.

gonad Sex organ in which the reproductive cells develop and sex hormones are produced. Ovaries are female gonads; testes are male gonads.

gonadotrophin A hormone produced by the pituitary gland capable of promoting ovarian or testicular growth and function. *See also* follicle-stimulating hormone (FSH) and luteinizing hormone (LH). These are the two gonadotrophin hormones.

gonorrhea A contagious venereal disease, characterized by inflammation of the internal genitalia and caused by a microorganism known as the gonococcus.

graafian follicles The tiny sacs, each containing an egg, that are present in the ovaries of even newborn baby girls. Starting at puberty, one follicle generally matures and ovulates each month, making it possible for pregnancy to occur.

grade When applied to cancer, a technical term used to describe the aggressiveness of the cancer cells.

granulation tissue "Proud flesh." Red sensitive tissue that often forms in the vagina after a hysterectomy, which can cause bleeding, spotting, discharge, and pain with intercourse. This tissue may remain for months or years unless a doctor eliminates it by cauterizing it. This type of tissue can develop at the site of an injury of the skin, mouth, or vagina.

granuloma inguinale A venereal disease whose main symptom is ulceration of the external genital organs. It is rare in the United States.

granulosa-theca cell tumor Nonmalignant, ovarian tumor. Produces increased amounts of female hormones and, occasionally, male hormones.

gynecology The branch of medicine dealing with diseases of women, particularly those of the reproductive organs and the breasts.

hemangiomas Benign accumulation of blood vessels.

hematoma Mass of clotted blood present in a person's tissue. If it is present under the skin, it is seen as a bump, with bruising around and over the area. A hematoma that develops inside a person's body from a severe injury or from surgery can contain from a small amount of blood to several pints of blood, and can cause a person to become so anemic that transfusion is necessary.

hemophilus *See* bacterial vaginosis.

hemorrhage Excessive bleeding from the body. Hemorrhage can be internal or external. If not controlled, hemorrhage can lead to shock and even death.

hermaphrodite A person who has both testicular and ovarian tissue present in the body, with ambiguous genitalia.

hernia Protrusion or bulging of a body organ through the tissues that normally contain it.

herpes Virus-caused infection of two types. Herpes simplex virus type I produces fever blisters; herpes simplex virus type II is the sexually transmitted form of herpes. Both types of herpes are characterized by small blisters that break open, leaving small, shallow, sensitive ulcers.

hormone A substance, produced by specialized body tissue called endocrine glands, that is carried by the bloodstream to another part of the body. It has a specific effect on hormone-responsive cells, thereby exerting its effect on the body. Hormones can also be manufactured synthetically. *See also* endocrine glands.

human chorionic gonadotrophin (HCG) A hormone produced by the placenta in pregnancy that is necessary for the maintenance of pregnancy. Because HCG has an effect in the body similar to luteinizing hormone, it is often given by injection to make the ovary release its egg at the appropriate time in the monthly cycle.

hydatid cysts of Morgagni Small, grapelike structures usually found near the open end of fallopian tubes. About one-fourth to one-half inch in diameter, they are fairly common, nonmalignant, and do not need to be removed unless they seem to be distorting the open end of the tube because of their size or position. Occasionally a hydatid cyst will grow large enough that a doctor will be able to feel it during a pelvic exam. Surgery may be necessary to make sure that the growth is not a tumor on the ovary.

hydatidiform mole An abnormal pregnancy in which the placenta has developed as a mass of grapelike cysts. *See* molar pregnancy.

hymen The membrane at the opening of the vagina that partially blocks the entrance to the vagina. Laypeople have named this the "maidenhead." This is the membrane that is broken with a woman's first act of intercourse, following which she is no longer a virgin.

hyperthyroidism Overactivity of the thyroid gland, producing weakness, heat sensitivity, sweating, weight loss despite increased appetite, restlessness, heart palpitation, staring, tremor, and protrusion of the eyes.

hypoglycemia A condition of the body in which a person's pancreas does not control the level of sugar in the blood properly. Because of the resulting low blood sugar, a person will often feel ill, experiencing headaches, hunger, trembling, dizziness, and weakness.

hypothalamus A portion of the brain at its base, just above and attached to the pituitary gland. The hypothalamus is the "master control unit" for the female hormone cycle, but also controls the body's other glands and their hormone production.

hypothyroidism The underfunctioning of the thyroid gland. The condition may produce dry, cold skin, puffiness of the glands and face, slow speech, weight gain, mental apathy, constipation, hearing loss, and memory impairment.

hysterectomy Surgical removal of the uterus.

hysterosalpingogram An X-ray procedure in which dye is injected through the cervix into the uterus and out through the fallopian tubes. As the dye is injected, X-rays are taken to facilitate evaluation of a woman's uterus and fallopian tubes. The evaluation is very reliable for the uterus but not quite so reliable for the fallopian tubes.

imperforate hymen A hymen that has no opening. If this condition is not found before a girl starts her menstrual periods, it can cause problems with the female organs as blood backs up into them. The hymen is normally open enough to allow the menstrual flow to exit from the body through the vagina.

impotence A man is impotent when he cannot develop an erection adequate for penile entry into the vagina or when he cannot maintain an erection long enough after entry for ejaculation to occur there. A woman is not considered impotent unless she has a physical condition or emotional problem that prevents the entry of a man's penis into her vagina.

incompetent cervix A cervix that is too weak to hold a pregnancy.

incontinence Leakage of stool or urine. Women may leak urine with an occasional hard cough or vigorous laugh, and such occasional episodes of loss of urine or stool are not abnormal. If they occur often enough to be embarrassing or bothersome, however, treatment may be necessary. Any persistent leakage of stool is abnormal and should be evaluated.

infertility A condition in which a supposedly fertile couple does not achieve pregnancy after twelve to eighteen months of regular, normal intercourse. "Sterility" is a condition in which factors exist in either male or female that permanently prevent pregnancy from occurring.

intraductal papillomas Small, tumorlike growths of the ducts of the breast. May cause oozing of fluid (sometimes bloody) from the nipples.

intrauterine growth retardation (IUGR) A condition in which the fetus is not growing as rapidly as it should inside the mother's uterus. This problem may be due to many factors, and may or may not be a cause of abnormalities in the newborn.

invasive molar pregnancy (chorioadenoma destruens) Pregnancy in which abnormal placental tissue grows into (invades) the uterine wall. *See also* molar pregnancy and malignant molar pregnancy.

in vitro (test tube) fertilization (IVF) A technique whereby a woman's egg is taken from her body and placed in a culture dish to which sperm are added. After fertilization has occurred, the embryo is placed in the woman's uterus, where it develops as any normal pregnancy would.

IUD (intrauterine contraceptive device) A small device that is inserted into a woman's uterus to prevent conception. It normally remains in place until removed by the physician.

IUGR *See* intrauterine growth retardation.

Kegel's exercises Exercises of a woman's pelvic muscles to increase vaginal strength and thereby reduce vaginal looseness.

labial agglutination A condition seen in young girls in which the edges of the two labia majora stick together, making the vagina appear closed. This is usually due to minor inflammation and is not dangerous, since the labia do not actually grow together.

labia majora The large outer lips of the vulva. Normally covered with hair in adult females.

labia minora The small folds (lips) within the larger labia majora that surround the vaginal opening.

lactation Production and secretion of milk by the female breast following childbirth and during the months of nursing.

lactiferous sinus The widened part of the milk ducts in the breast, just under the nipple, that act as a reservoir for milk during the nursing process.

laparoscopy A procedure that allows the physician to view the female organs in the abdominal cavity with an optical telescope that is passed through a small incision in the abdominal wall (usually through the lower edge of the navel). Some procedures, such as sterilization, laser operations, and cutting apart adhesions can be done at laparoscopy.

laparotomy An operation on a person's abdomen in which the abdominal cavity is opened with an incision. For example, an appendectomy is a laparotomy done for removal of an appendix.

leukoplakia White patches on the "skin" of the vulva, the vagina, or the cervix. Not malignant, or premalignant, as was thought in the past.

leukorrhea A discharge from the vagina due to an infection or growth.

libido Sexual drive.

lichen sclerosus A condition in which the skin of the vulvar tissues becomes thin and somewhat shrunken. Vulvar itching often accompanies the condition.

linea nigra A dark line that appears on the abdomen (especially of pregnant women) from the navel to the pubic hair.

lipoma Painless, nonmalignant tumor made up of fatty cells. Since lipomas rarely become malignant, they generally do not need to be removed unless a doctor is unsure what they are, or if they are in some way bothersome.

local anesthetic An anesthetic administered by injecting an anesthetic agent directly into the tissues that need to be made painless.

lumpectomy A nonmedical term referring to breast surgery in which only the cancerous lump—not the entire breast—is removed.

lupus erythematosus Connective tissue disorder that occurs most often in young women. May be limited to the skin, producing a butterfly-shaped red rash on the nose and cheeks. In its more serious form, it may affect joints, lungs, or kidneys, producing fever and muscle/joint pain. The cause is unknown.

luteal phase The part of a woman's monthly cycle that lasts from the moment she ovulates (releases an egg) until her menstrual period starts (usually fourteen days). It is called the luteal phase because, as soon as ovulation occurs, the ovary is left with a small cystic structure, called the corpus luteum, which produces both estrogen and progesterone until menstruation starts. *See* follicular phase.

luteinizing hormone (LH) A hormone produced by the pituitary that stimulates the ovary to release its egg. LH is one of the two gonadotrophin hormones (the other is FSH).

lymphogranuloma venereum (LGV) A sexually transmitted disease (STD) that produces enlarged lymph nodes in the groin and a rectal infection with discharge of mucus and pus from the anus and from the open sores that develop.

magnetic resonance imaging *See* MRI.

malignant Cancerous.

malignant molar pregnancy (choriocarcinoma) A condition of the uterus containing highly invasive and malignant tissue developing from placental tissue. Choriocarcinoma can occur after a normal, a tubal, or a molar pregnancy.

mammography (Xerogram or film screen) A special X-ray of the breast for early detection of malignancy. It can help in the diagnosis of breast lumps.

mastectomy Surgical removal of the breast. *See* radical mastectomy, simple mastectomy, subcutaneous, lumpectomy, and resection.

mastitis The precise definition of mastitis is "breast infection," which occurs most commonly either immediately after the delivery of a baby or during the nursing of a baby. Mastitis is also used in reference to women who have tender, cystic breasts (cystic mastitis). *See also* fibrocystic breast change.

meconium Material that is passed from the bowels of an unborn baby into the fluid surrounding it. This can be a normal occurrence, but it is frequently an indication that the baby is under stress. This term also applies to the stools that normal newborn babies pass before they have had anything to eat. Such stools are dark green, very sticky, and without odor.

Meig's syndrome A condition in which an ovarian tumor, called a fibroma, is associated with fluid in the chest cavity (around the lungs) and excessive fluid in the abdominal cavity.

menarche The term used for the first menstrual period.

menometrorrhagia Bleeding from the uterus that is excessive and irregular.

menopause The term used for a woman's last menstrual period.

menstrual extraction A smoke-screen term used by some people to refer to a very early abortion. A small suction apparatus is used to remove the uterine lining and the embryo if it is present immediately after a woman has missed a period.

menstruation The periodic (monthly) flow of blood and debris from her uterus during a woman's reproductive years.

metrorrhagia Bleeding between menstrual periods.

miscarriage *See* abortion.

mittelschmerz "Mid pain." Abdominal discomfort at the time of ovulation.

molar pregnancy (hydatidiform mole) A pregnancy in which an abnormal placenta is produced. The abnormal placenta is characterized by the presence of multiple, grapelike cysts. *See* invasive molar pregnancy and malignant molar pregnancy.

molluscum contagiosum An infection caused by a virus which is mildly contagious. It is usually sexually transmitted. This infection is characterized by small, dome-shaped bumps that grow primarily on the inside of the upper thighs. It is not dangerous and can be cured by scraping away the small, pearly-appearing center of each bump.

mongolism *See* Down syndrome.

monilia vaginitis Also called fungus, candidal, or yeast infection, this is the most common vaginal infection. Characterized by itching, vulvar redness, and a cheesy, white discharge.

mons pubis, mons veneris The pubic mound, or fatty pad overlying the pubic bone and over which the pubic hair grows.

MRI (magnetic resonance imaging) A technique for taking pictures of the inside of the body, much like a CT scan but without ionizing radiation (X-ray). Formerly called NMR. This technique uses a large magnet rather than an X-ray machine. *See also* CT scan.

mucous cystadenomas Nonmalignant ovarian tumors that contain mucuslike material. If left alone, they can grow and rupture, or can become malignant.

müllerian duct cells The cells in a female embryo that develop into the fallopian tubes, the uterus, and the upper portion of the vagina.

myomectomy A surgical procedure in which fibroid tumors of the uterus are removed but the uterus itself is preserved.

natural family planning Sometimes called the "rhythm method." With this contraceptive technique, which involves no devices or medications, a couple will avoid intercourse around the time of ovulation, when there is an egg present for fertilization. The same principle may be used in reverse by a couple wishing to increase the chance of pregnancy, by scheduling intercourse around the probable ovulation time.

neural tube defect A congenital abnormality of a baby, characterized by abnormalities of the central nervous system. An example is *spina bifida*, a condition in which the spinal cord can be exposed because of a defect in the bones and skin overlying it.

nevus *See* vascular spider.

nipple The small protuberance on the breast from which, in females, the milk glands discharge milk. Contains erectile tissue and is surrounded by the areola, a darker-pigmented circle.

nodule A small, hard lump.

nonstress test (NST)   A diagnostic evaluation of an unborn baby, based on the heartbeat of the baby as recorded by a fetal monitor. When a healthy fetus moves, its heartbeat increases (just as yours does when you exercise). The nonstress test records the baby's heartbeat to see if it increases with movement as is normal.

obstetrics   The branch of medicine that deals with pregnancy and childbirth.

oophorectomy   Surgical removal of an ovary.

orgasm   The climax of sexual excitement.

osteoporosis   Weakened and brittle bones, most common in women after menopause. When osteoporosis is present, the bones can break easily. When postmenopausal women break a bone, it is usually because they have developed osteoporosis. The "dowager's hump" and loss of height that are sometimes seen in postmenopausal women are caused by recurrent fractures of the vertebrae.

ovaries   Two sex glands, located in the lower part of the abdomen on either side of the uterus. Their primary function occurs between menarche (first menstrual period) and menopause. During this time, they release an egg each month, making pregnancy possible if the egg is fertilized. The ovaries also produce the female hormones, estrogen and progesterone, responsible for changing a girl's body into that of a woman and preparing the body for the occurrence of pregnancy.

ovulation   The process in which the egg (ovum) is released from the ovary. In sexually mature females, ovulation usually occurs every twenty-eight days, halfway between the menstrual periods. Ovulation usually starts a fourteen-day chain of events that ends with a menstrual period if pregnancy does not occur. *See also* follicular phase and luteal phase.

ovum   Egg cell. When fertilized, it is capable of developing into a person similar to its parents in traits that are hereditary, or transmitted by the genes of the chromosomes.

oxytocin challenge test (OCT)   Also called "stress test." A diagnostic evaluation of an unborn baby's condition. This evaluation is different from a "nonstress test" in that Pitocin is given intravenously to cause the uterus to contract. Since an unhealthy baby cannot tolerate the normally decreased blood flow through the uterus that results from a contraction, its heartbeat will drop, indicating a problem.

papilloma   A small tumorlike growth that may or may not be malignant. Papillomas may be present in the breast or in other parts of the body.

Pap smear   In gynecology, the term *Pap smear* refers to a smear of scrapings from a woman's cervix or vagina that is transferred to a glass slide. After being stained, the cells in the scraping can be viewed by pathologists to determine whether or not malignancy exists. Such a smear may also show infection, though it is not widely used for that purpose. Pap smears can be taken from other parts of the body and are helpful in determining if there is cancer in the lungs, in the breasts, and other parts of the body.

paracervical block   An anesthetic technique in which an anesthetic drug is injected into the tissues on either side of the cervix at the top of the vagina. Paracervical block is very useful for procedures done on the cervix or uterus in a doctor's office. It is rarely used during labor because it often causes a baby's heartbeat to slow down.

PCOS   *See* polycystic ovarian syndrome.

pelvic congestion syndrome   A condition in which the pelvic tissues become swollen, boggy, and congested. Because of these changes in the tissue, women will often feel pelvic discomfort and pain.

penis   The male organ of intercourse. Also contains the urethra, which carries urine from the body.

perineum   The part of the perineum that a woman can see is the tissue between her vulva and her anus. The woman's perineum is actually a much more extensive structure than this, including the muscles and tissues of her lower pelvis, through which the vagina and rectum exit to the outside. It is the tissues of the perineum that hold the intestines and internal organs inside a woman's body.

peristalsis   Rhythmic contractions of tubular structures in the body that propel their contents. The intestines' peristalsis, for example, propels food through the intestines; and the fallopian tubes have rhythmic peristaltic contractions that propel the egg down the tube.

peritoneal fluid   The fluid that bathes the internal organs and is contained inside the peritoneal cavity (the space between all the organs inside the abdominal cavity).

peritoneum   The membrane that lines the internal abdominal wall and all the internal abdominal organs.

peritonitis   An infection or inflammation of the peritoneal cavity (the space between all the organs inside the abdomen). Such a condition causes a great deal of pain. Peritonitis may be caused by infections of the female organs, appendicitis, or a ruptured gallbladder. This condition must be accurately diagnosed and quickly treated, because death can result.

placenta   An organ through which the fetus is fed and provided oxygen while in the mother's uterus. The placenta also removes waste from the amniotic fluid. It filters out germs, keeping them from getting into the uterus from the cervix. It produces the hormones necessary for maintaining the pregnancy in a healthy condition. The placenta is a temporary organ that develops on fertilization of an ovum and is delivered soon after the baby is born. *See also* umbilical cord.

placenta previa   A term applied to a placenta that is located completely or partially in the lower part of the uterus. Because the cervix tends to stretch during the latter part of pregnancy, a placenta previa will often bleed. If the placenta previa is too low in the uterus, a woman must deliver her baby by cesarean section, since death from blood loss can result for both mother and baby if a vaginal delivery is attempted.

PMS (premenstrual syndrome)   A term applied to the symptoms a woman may experience prior to her menstrual period. They may begin at ovulation and last until the period begins, approximately fourteen days. The symptoms may include cramps, backache, tension, depression, irritability, mood swings, swelling, breast tenderness, and so on.

polycystic ovarian syndrome (PCOS, Stein-Leventhal syndrome, sclerocystic ovaries)   An abnormality of the ovaries that produces irregular periods and can result in infertility. The drug Clomiphene citrate (Clomid, Seraphene) usually causes such ovaries to release eggs.

polyp   A usually nonmalignant tumor that hangs by a pedicle, or stalk, from a body cavity. Polyps are often found hanging from the cervix. They may be present in the uterine cavity itself.

postmature syndrome A term used to describe the condition of a baby who is born more than two weeks past the due date and who has been affected by that situation. For example, weight loss may have resulted because adequate nutrition has not been able to pass through a placenta that has been gradually deteriorating because of the length of the pregnancy.

postpartum sterilization Sterilization procedure done immediately after delivery or during the next few days. *See also* sterilization.

precocious puberty Sexual development before the age of eight. If a girl has menstrual periods before the age of eight, she has precocious puberty. If she has significant breast or pubic hair development much before that age, she may have precocious puberty and should be evaluated by a physician.

preeclampsia *See* toxemia of pregnancy.

pregnancy The state of a woman from conception to delivery of a child, usually 280 days.

premature menopause (premature ovarian failure) Cessation of ovarian function before age forty.

premenstrual syndrome *See* PMS.

presacral neurectomy This procedure, often associated with infertility treatment, involves cutting the sympathetic and parasympathetic nerves that spread out inside the abdomen to the uterus and tubes. The theory is that such an operation relieves any uterine and tubal spasm that might be inhibiting fertility. This procedure does not affect sexual feeling at all. Most women are aware of having had this procedure only because they have less menstrual cramping and often will not feel any pain with labor. This operation is now often done to eliminate severe, debilitating menstrual cramps.

progesterone A female hormone produced by the ovaries after ovulation.

prolapsed uterus A condition in which the uterus loses its support and falls down into the lower vagina, or even out of the vagina. If the uterus protrudes from the vagina, it can cause a great deal of discomfort, but if it is only down into the lower vagina, it may cause no discomfort at all. If a woman has no discomfort with a prolapsed uterus, she need not have surgery done; if she does have discomfort, surgery will usually eliminate the discomfort.

puberty The period of life during which a person becomes capable of reproduction and manifests such secondary sex characteristics as growth of pubic and underarm hair, and development of breasts in the female.

pudendal block An anesthetic procedure in which the anesthetic agent is injected through the wall of the vagina, about halfway up on either side, producing anesthesia of the pudendal nerves and numbing the lower half of the vagina and the vulvar and anal areas.

pulmonary embolism A blood clot, or an embolus of amniotic fluid, etc., that is carried by the flow of blood to the lungs. It results in chest pain, a cough, and labored breathing. This is a critical problem that can result in death. Specialized medical care is required.

radical mastectomy Removal of the entire breast, the underlying chest muscles (pectorals), and the lymph nodes under the arm (axilla).

rectovaginal fistula A hole from the vagina into the rectum. A fistula of this type will usually allow stools to pass from the rectum into the vagina. This condition can almost always be successfully repaired surgically.

rectum The lowest segment of the digestive tract. Terminates in the anus, through which solid waste is evacuated from the body.

resection of breast tissue (segmental or quadrant) Surgical procedure involving excising as much as one quarter of the breast tissue and, usually, the lymph nodes in the axilla, or underarm.

Rh factor A hereditary factor in the blood that can cause complications if the mother is Rh negative and the fetus is Rh positive.

rhythm method *See* natural family planning.

round ligament pain Pain during pregnancy caused by stretching or pulling of the round ligaments of the uterus. These ligaments are located on each side of the uterus and help hold it in position. Such pain is not dangerous, but it can be as severe as that of appendicitis and it may last for several days.

salpingitis isthmica nodosa Nodular thickening along the course of the fallopian tubes. This condition usually results in infertility. It can occasionally be diagnosed by a hysterosalpingogram, but will often require a laparoscopy or laparotomy and direct visualization for diagnosis.

scabies Infection caused by mites (parasites that burrow under the skin).

scan A term often used by obstetricians and gynecologists to refer to an ultrasound study or a sonogram.

scrotum The sac of skin that holds the male's testicles.

semen The material that is expelled from a man's penis at ejaculation. The largest component of semen is mucus, the result of secretions from the prostate gland and seminal vesicles. In the mucus of the semen is contained the sperm, the most "important" element but the smallest in volume. If all the sperm from a semen specimen were gathered together, they would amount to only a small pellet of material, no more than one-eighth of an inch across.

septate uterus Incomplete fusion of the two halves of the uterus, resulting in an inner wall in the uterus.

serous cystadenomas Nonmalignant ovarian tumors that contain cystic areas of fluid. If left alone, they can grow and rupture or become malignant.

severe atypical endometrial hyperplasia The most extremely abnormal form of uterine hyperplasia (overgrowth of the uterine lining). Considered malignant (but completely curable by hysterectomy), it is confined to the surface of the uterine lining. Continued change will result in true invasive cancer.

sexually transmitted disease *See* STD.

simple mastectomy Removal of the entire breast, leaving the pectoral (chest) muscles.

Sims-Huhner Test (SHT) Also called postcoital test (PC test). A diagnostic procedure used to evaluate the receptivity of a woman's cervical mucus to her husband's sperm. It is normally done a day or two before ovulation and several hours after intercourse. It is painless and is much like a routine Pap smear.

skin tags   Small, skin-colored projections of skin, about the size of small ticks, that often proliferate during pregnancy. Such growths most often occur on a woman's neck and upper chest. They generally, but not always, disappear after pregnancy.

smegma   Secretions that may accumulate either where the labia minora overlie the clitoris or under the foreskin of the male penis.

sonogram, sonography   *See* ultrasound.

sperm   The male reproductive cell. *See also* semen.

spinal anesthetic   A technique in which the anesthetic agent is injected through the lower back into the spinal fluid. This produces complete numbness and paralysis of the muscles from the waist down, stopping both pain and movement. If a woman has a spinal for delivery, the baby must be low in the birth canal before the spinal is given because she cannot effectively push the baby out while so anesthetized. Using today's improved technique, a spinal is an extremely safe form of anesthesia, both for the baby and the mother. *See* epidural.

stage (of cancer)   Technical term used to define the extensiveness of cancer in the body, whether it is just in the organ where it started or has spread to other parts of the body.

STD (sexually transmitted disease)   The new and modern term for venereal disease. This type of disease is passed almost exclusively by sexual contact.

Stein-Leventhal syndrome   *See* polycystic ovarian syndrome.

sterility   Incapacity to produce children, in either the female or the male. *See* infertility.

sterilization   A procedure whereby permanent birth control is provided. Such a surgical operation may involve surgery to the fallopian tubes in the female (tubal ligation) or surgery on the vasa in a male (vasectomy). A sterilization may be reversible, except in the case of a hysterectomy, removal of ovaries, or removal of testicles.

stress test   *See* oxytocin challenge test.

striae gravidarum   "Stretch marks." Pinkish lines, resembling scars, that appear on the abdomen, breasts, and thighs of some pregnant women, and usually remain after pregnancy.

subcutaneous mastectomy   Removal of most of the breast tissue while leaving the surface skin and nipples intact.

supracervical hysterectomy   Removal of only the upper part of the uterus, leaving the cervix in place.

surgical menopause   Cessation of ovarian function due to removal of the ovaries by surgery.

syphilis   If untreated, a most dangerous STD. Caught only by sexual contact with a person who has it. Caused by the germ *Treponema pellidum*, syphilis is a horrible, destructive disease. *See also* chancre.

telangiectasia   *See* vascular spider.

teratomas (dermoids)   *See* dermoid cyst.

testicles, testes   The two male sex glands that hang outside the body in a sac called the scrotum. They produce sperm and testosterone, the male sex hormone.

testosterone   The primary male sex hormone.

thrombophlebitis   Blood clots with resulting inflammation in a person's vein or veins.

toxemia of pregnancy   "Poisoning" of pregnancy. A disorder of pregnancy (cause unknown) characterized by hypertension (high blood pressure), edema (swelling), and albuminuria (protein in the urine). Doctors use the term *preeclampsia* for toxemia without convulsions and *eclampsia* for toxemia with convulsions. *See also* eclampsia.

toxic shock   A condition caused by the *Staphylococcus aureus* bacterium. Affects both men and women, but sometimes associated with use of high-absorbency tampons. Symptoms may be mild or severe and include any or all of the following: fever, chills, vomiting, diarrhea, dizziness, fainting, sore throat, sunburnlike rash.

trichomoniasis   An infection of the vagina caused by a microscopic organism called *Trichomonas vaginalis*. This infection is usually characterized by a frothy, green discharge that causes significant itching. It can be transmitted sexually, and, if a woman is treated for it, her husband should also be treated.

trophoblastic cells   Cells that contribute to the formation of the placenta and make up much of the tissue of the placenta.

tubal ligation   Tubal sterilization. A procedure that blocks the fallopian tubes by cutting, clamping, cauterizing, or (occasionally) tying them, making it impossible for an egg to pass through.

tubal pregnancy   *See* ectopic pregnancy.

tuberculosis   Infectious disease characterized by tubercles (small, round nodules), that may appear on various parts of the body, especially the lungs. Symptoms include weight loss, appetite loss, persistent fever and cough (with expectoration), nausea, and spitting up of blood. This infection is caused by the tubercle bacillus *Mycobacterium tuberculosis*.

tumor   A growth. A mass of cells that may or may not be malignant.

twilight sleep   Childbirth anesthetic that alleviates pain and erases memory of the birth process. Rarely used today.

ultrasound (diagnostic ultrasonography, sonogram, sonography)   Diagnostic tool based on the use of high-frequency sound waves, radiated into the body by a handheld transmitter, "bounced back" to the transmitting device, and projected onto a screen for evaluation.

umbilical cord   The connecting tube for the fetus with the placenta through which blood flows back and forth between baby and mother. This blood, of course, carries the baby's oxygen and nutrition. *See also* placenta.

umbilicus (navel)   The depressed scar in the abdomen where the umbilical cord was attached to the baby while in the mother's uterus.

ureter   The tube through which urine moves from the kidney to the bladder.

urethra   The tube through which urine moves from the bladder to the exterior of the body.

urologist   Bladder and kidney specialist. These physicians treat kidney or bladder problems. They also often treat men for problems of male infertility.

uterus (womb)   Hollow, pear-shaped organ in the female pelvis that carries an unborn child for nine months. It is from the uterus that the menstrual flow originates. When the uterus is removed, there will be no more menstrual flow, even though a woman's ovaries may still be functioning normally and producing hormones and an egg each month.

uterus didelphus A congenital abnormality in which the two halves of the uterus failed to fuse together during intrauterine life. In this condition, a woman has two partial uteri. Such a uterus can usually carry a normal pregnancy and the condition does not usually cause infertility.

vagina Female genital passage that extends from the vulva to the uterus.

vaginal discharge A woman may have various types of secretions from her vagina. Mucous secretions that occur just before a period or at ovulation time are usually totally normal, even though they may at times be somewhat heavy. Secretions that smell or cause itching, or are discolored, are often a sign of infection. For such discharge, a woman should see a physician. *See also* bacterial vaginosis; monilia vaginitis; trichomoniasis.

vaginitis Inflammation of the vagina, usually characterized by discharge.

vaporization conization Laser treatment of the cervix involving vaporization of the tissue of the center portion of the cervix as seen by the doctor through the vagina. The portion of tissue that is evaporated by the laser is similar to the cone-shaped tissue that is removed at a conization done with a surgical knife. *See also* conization.

varicocele An accumulation of veins around the testicle that occasionally result in a man's sperm count or sperm quality being lower than normal, with resulting fertility problems. Such a condition can usually be cured with a minor operation.

varicose veins Veins that become so dilated that they can be seen and felt above the surface of the skin. They appear most frequently in the legs. Women often confuse small spiderlike veins or bluish discolorations of their legs with varicose veins. However, varicose veins are usually as large as a person's little finger lying under the skin. Smaller visible veins are not varicose veins and ordinarily do not have the potential for becoming varicose veins.

vascular spider (nevus, angioma, telangiectasia) Small red discolorations of the skin that may occur in pregnant women, in men, or nonpregnant women, appear most commonly on the face, neck, upper chest, and arms. Red lines extend outward from their center. They are not dangerous, and, after pregnancy, will often become much less numerous.

vas deferens or "vas" The narrow tube through which sperm travel from the testes of the male to the seminal vesicles.

vasectomy Sterilization surgery on the male accomplished by cutting the vas, the tube that carries the sperm from the testicles to the internal sex organs.

venereal disease (sexually transmitted disease) Any disease that is contracted through sexual intercourse or intimate contact. *See* STD.

vernix The white greasy film that covers an unborn child. Composed of secretions from oil glands of the body, hair that has fallen from the skin, and other secretions.

vesico-vaginal fistula A hole from the vagina into the bladder. Such an opening allows constant drainage of urine. This drainage of urine causes a woman's vulva to be constantly wet, irritated, odorous, and uncomfortable. This problem can result from vaginal surgery or hysterectomy. It can be surgically repaired. In pregnancies in which the child's head is too large for the mother's pelvis and in which labor lasts for several days, both vesico-vaginal and recto-vaginal fistulae can result from the baby's head eroding through the vaginal wall.

vulva External sex organs of the female.

vulvectomy Surgical removal of the labia majora and minora and, often, of the clitoris, to remove premalignant or malignant tissue of the vulva.

wedge resection (of ovary) Surgical removal of a segment of the ovary in an effort to establish regular menstrual periods and thus fertility. A woman should have this only if suggested and performed by a gynecologist or other specialist experienced in caring for women with infertility problems. Inexperienced physicians might recommend this procedure when it is unnecessary. It is rarely done today. If it is not done with careful technique and using fine suture, it can result in adhesions of the tubes and ovaries that can result in worse infertility.

wolffian duct cells Cells in the body of the male fetus that will become his vas deferens, epididymis, and seminal vesicles as development proceeds.

womb *See* uterus.

Xerogram, Xeroradiography *See* mammography.

Index

Numerals in *italics* refer to illustrations and charts.